# Developmental Care
# of Newborns & Infants
## A GUIDE FOR HEALTH PROFESSIONALS

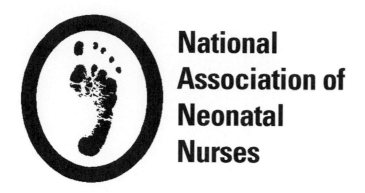

**National Association of Neonatal Nurses**

# Developmental Care of Newborns & Infants
## A GUIDE FOR HEALTH PROFESSIONALS

**Carole Kenner,** DNS, RNC, FAAN
Dean and Professor
University of Oklahoma College of Nursing
Oklahoma City, Oklahoma

**Jacqueline M. McGrath,** PhD, RN, NNP, CCNS
Assistant Professor
Coordinator, Neonatal Nursing Specialty Track
Arizona State University
Tempe, Arizona

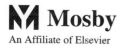
**Mosby**
An Affiliate of Elsevier

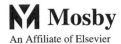
## Mosby

An Affiliate of Elsevier

11830 Westline Industrial Drive
St. Louis, MO 63123

DEVELOPMENTAL CARE OF NEWBORNS & INFANTS:      ISBN 0-323-02443-2
  A GUIDE FOR HEALTH PROFESSIONALS

---

### NOTICE

Nursing is an ever-changing field. Standard safety precautions must be followed, but as new research and clinical experience broaden our knowledge, changes in treatment and drug therapy may become necessary or appropriate. Readers are advised to check the most current product information provided by the manufacturer of each drug to be administered to verify the recommended dose, the method and duration of administration, and the contraindications. It is the responsibility of the treating licensed prescriber, relying on experience and knowledge of the patient, to determine dosages and the best treatment for the patient. Neither the publisher nor the author assumes any liability for any injury and/or damage to persons or property arising from this publication.

---

**Library of Congress Cataloging-in-Publication Data**
Developmental care of newborns & infants: a guide for health professionals/[edited by]
  Carole Kenner, Jacqueline McGrath.
      p.   ; cm.
  Includes bibliographical references and index.
  ISBN 0-323-02443-2
    1. Neonatal intensive care.   2. Infants (Newborn)—Development.   3. Infants
  (Newborn)—Nursing.   4. Infants (Newborn)—Care.   I. Title: Developmental care of
  newborns and infants.   II. Kenner, Carole.   III. McGrath, Jacqueline.
      [DNLM:   1. Intensive Care, Neonatal—methods.   2. Child Development.   3. Family.
  4. Intensive Care Units, Neonatal.   5. Neonatal Nursing—methods. WS 421 D489 2004]
  RJ253.5.D486 2004
  618.92′01—dc22                                                        2004040225

*Executive Editor:* Michael S. Ledbetter
*Developmental Editor:* Amanda Sunderman Politte
*Editorial Assistant:* Mary Parker
*Publishing Services Manager:* Catherine Albright Jackson
*Project Manager:* Clay S. Broeker
*Senior Designer:* Amy Buxton

Printed in the United States of America

Last digit is the print number:  9  8  7  6  5  4  3  2  1

# CONTRIBUTORS

**Heidelise Als, PhD**
Associate Professor of Psychiatry (Psychology)
Harvard Medical School
Director, Neurobehavioral Infant and Child Studies
Children's Hospital Boston
Boston, Massachusetts

**Kelly A. Amspacher, MSN, RN**
Independent Consultant
Neonatology/Perinatology
Havertown, Pennsylvania

**Diane D. Ballweg, MSN, RNC, CNS**
Newborn Developmental Specialist
Memorial Hermann Southwest Hospital
Houston, Texas

**Maryann Bozzette, PhD, RN**
Assistant Professor
University of Illinois at Chicago
College of Nursing
Chicago, Illinois

**Deborah Winders Davis, DNS, RNC**
Research Associate, Neonatal Follow-Up Program
Associate Professor, Department of Pediatrics
Research Associate, Cognitive Development Lab
Associate Clinical Professor, Department of
  Psychological and Brain Sciences
Adjunct Associate Professor, School of Nursing
University of Louisville
Louisville, Kentucky

**Bette Liberman Flushman, MA**
Infant Developmental Specialist
Intensive Care Nursery
Children's Hospital and Research Center
Oakland, California

**Gay Gale, MS, RNC**
Neonatal Development Nurse
Children's Hospital and Research Center Oakland
Oakland, California;
Staff Nurse III, NICU
Alta Bates Summit Medical Center
Berkeley, California

**Lois V. S. Gates, MS, RNC, CNA**
Case Coordinator, NICU
Penn State Children's Hospital
Milton S. Hershey Medical Center
Hershey, Pennsylvania

**Chrysty D. Graves, OTR/L**
Children's Medical Ventures, Respironics
Sales Account Manager
Norwell, Massachusetts

**Teresa Gutierrez, PT, MS, PCS**
Physical Therapy Supervisor
Mary Bridge Children's Health Center
Coordinator Instructor, NDTA
Tacoma, Washington

**Lynda Law Harrison, PhD, RN, FAAN**
Professor and Co-Deputy Director
World Health Organization
Collaborating Center on International Nursing
School of Nursing
University of Alabama
Birmingham, Alabama

**Mary Claire Heffron, PhD**
Early Childhood Mental Health Program
Division of Developmental and Behavioral
  Pediatrics
Children's Hospital and Research Center
Oakland, California

**Jan Hunter, MA, OTR**
Neonatal Clinical Specialist
Infant Special Care Unit
University of Texas Medical Branch
Galveston, Texas;
Assistant Professor
Occupational Therapy
School of Allied Health
Galveston, Texas

**Katherine M. Jorgensen, MSN, MBA, RNC, HonD**
Neonatal Nurse Consultant
KMJ Consulting, Inc.
Daniel Island, South Carolina

**Cheryl Ann King, MSN, CCRN**
Neonatal Clinical Nurse Specialist
Mother and Child Hospital
Presbyterian/St. Luke's Medical Center
Denver, Colorado

**Joyce L. King, PhD, RN, FNP, CNM**
Assistant Professor (Clinical)
Nell Hodgson Woodruff School
  of Nursing
Emory University
Atlanta, Georgia

**gretchen Lawhon, PhD, RN**
Vice President
NIDCAP® Federation International
Ohio

**Anjanette Lee, MS, CCC/SLP**
Speech-Language Pathologist
Developmental Unit Consultant
Memorial Hermann Hospital Southwest
Houston, Texas

**Terrie Lockridge, MS, RNC**
Neonatal Clinical Nurse Specialist
Northwest Regional Perinatal Program
Children's Hospital and Regional
  Medical Center
Seattle, Washington

**Marilyn J. Lotas, PhD, RN**
Associate Dean for Student Services
Director of the BSN Program
Frances Payne Bolton School of
  Nursing
Case Western Reserve University
Cleveland, Ohio

**Linda M. Lutes, BS, MEd**
Infant Development Specialist, Educator,
  and Consultant
Product Trainer and Senior Account
  Manager
Children's Medical Ventures/
  Respironics
Mustang, Oklahoma

**Rita H. Pickler, PhD, RN, CS, PNP**
Associate Professor
School of Nursing
Virginia Commonwealth University
Richmond, Virginia

**Shawn Pohlman, PhD, RN, NCCNS**
St. Louis, Missouri

**Jana L. Pressler, PhD, RN**
Associate Professor of Nursing
PhD Program Director
School of Nursing
University of Missouri—Kansas City
Kansas City, Missouri

**Lynn B. Rasmussen, PhD, RNC, NNP**
Assistant Professor
NNP Program Director
University of Missouri—Kansas City
Kansas City, Missouri

**Linda Rector, MS, CCLS**
Neonatal Child Life Specialist
Consultant
Houston, Texas

**Barbara A. Reyna, MS, RNC, NNP**
Neonatal Nurse Practitioner
VCU Health System
MCV Hospitals and Physicians
Richmond, Virginia

**Tanya Sudia-Robinson, PhD, RN**
Faculty Associate in Healthcare Ethics
Emory University
Center for Ethics
Atlanta, Georgia

**Jane K. Sweeney, PhD, PT, PCS**
Professor and Graduate Program
  Director
Doctor of Science Program in Pediatric Physical
  Therapy
Rocky Mountain University of Health Professions
Provo, Utah;
President
Pediatric Rehab Northwest, LLC
Gig Harbor, Washington

**Nancy Sweet, MA**
Director of Early Intervention
  Services
Division of Developmental and
  Behavioral Pediatrics
Children's Hospital and Research Center at
  Oakland
Oakland, California

**Lauren T. Taquino, MS, RN, CCRN**
Neonatal Clinical Nurse Specialist
Children's Hospital and Regional
  Medical Center
Seattle, Washington

**Carol Spruill Turnage-Carrier, MSN, RN, CNS**
Neonatal Clinical Nurse Specialist
Texas Children's Hospital
Newborn Center
Houston, Texas

**Kathleen A. VandenBerg, MA**
Center Director, West Coast NIDCAP®
  Training Center,
Co-Director, Special Start Training
  Program
Mills College, Department Education
Oakland, California

**Marlene Walden, PhD, RNC, NNP, CCNS**
Assistant Professor
Baylor College of Medicine;
Neonatal Nurse Practitioner
Texas Children's Hospital
Houston, Texas

**Charlotte Ward-Larson, PhD, RNC, CS**
Associate Professor
Union University School of
  Nursing
Germantown, Tennessee

# REVIEWERS & ORIGINAL CONTRIBUTORS

This project was created in several phases. We want to acknowledge the many people who worked on the beginning phases of this text.

**Janice Ancona**
St. Joseph Hospital
Milwaukee, Wisconsin

**Joy Voyles Brown, Ph.D., RN**
University of Colorado Health Sciences Center
Denver, Colorado

**Anita Catlin, MSN, FNP, RN**
Professor
Napa Valley College
Napa, California

**Karen D'Apolito, PhD, RN**
Vanderbilt University
Nashville, Tennessee

**Deana DeMars, PT**
The Children's Regional Hospital
Camden, New Jersey

**Linda Gilkerson, PhD**
Erikson Institute
Chicago, Illinois

**Terry Griffin, MS, RNC, NNP**
Rush Children's Hospital
Chicago, Illinois

**Julie Harrell**
Columbus Children's Hospital
Columbus, Ohio

**Dianne Hicks, RN, MA**
Doctors Medical Center
Modesto, California

**Sonia Imaizumi, MD**
The Children's Regional Hospital
Camden, New Jersey

**Beverly Johnson, PhD**
Institute for Family Centered Care
Bethesda, Maryland

**Barbara Kellam, MSN, RN**
Savannah, Georgia

**Kimberly LaMar, ND, RNC, CNNP**
College of Nursing
Arizona State University
Tempe, Arizona

**Margaret (Meg) McLincha, RN**
Buford, Georgia

**Laure Mouradina, ScD, OTR, BCP**
University of Oklahoma Health Sciences Center
Oklahoma City, Oklahoma

**Virginia A. Passero, Ph.D., RNC**
Madison, Connecticut

**Katherine Peters, PhD, RN**
University of Alberta
Alberta, Canada

**M. Kathleen Philbin, Ph.D., R.N.**
Philadelphia, Pennsylvania

**Laura Robison, MSN, RNC**
Sinai Samaritan Medical Center
Milwaukee, Wisconsin

**Elsa Sell, MD**
Taos, New Mexico

**Catherine Shaker, MS, CCC**
St. Joseph's Hospital
Milwaukee, Wisconsin

**Karen M. Smith, BSN, RNC, M.Ed.**
St. Luke's Regional Medical Center
Boise, Idaho

**Kathy Walburn**
University of Nebraska Medical Center
Omaha, Nebraska

**Maribeth White, RN, NNP**
Emory University
Atlanta, Georgia

**Robert White, MD**
Chair, NICU Design Standards
Memorial Hospital
South Bend, Indiana

## DEVELOPMENTAL CARE TASK FORCE LIST (1998–2000)

**Heidelise Als, PhD**
Children's Hospital
Boston, Massachusetts

**Maryann Bozzette, PhD, RN**
University of Illinois at Chicago
Chicago, Illinois

**Catherine Bush**
Children's Medical Ventures, Inc.
Norwell, Massachusetts

**Stanley Graven, MD**
University of South Florida
Tampa, Florida

**Jeanie Hallaron, MS, RN**
Past NANN BOD
Orlando, Florida

**Leslie Jackson, OT**
The American Occupational Therapy Association, Inc.
Bethesda, Maryland

**Pat Johnson, MSN, MPH, RN, NNP**
Past President of NANN
Phoenix, Arizona

**Katherine M. Jorgensen, MSN, MBA, RNC, HonD**
KMJ Consulting Inc.
Charleston, South Carolina

**Carole Kenner, DNS, RNC, FAAN**
Past President of NANN
Chicago, Illinois

**Lynn Lynam, MS, RNC, NNP**
Past President of NANN
Ohmeda Medical
Columbia, Maryland

**Read McCarty**
Children's Medical Ventures, Inc.
Norwell, Massachusetts

**Jacqueline M. McGrath, PhD, RN, NNP, CCNS**
Arizona State University
Phoenix, Arizona

**Lu-Ann Papile, MD**
University of New Mexico
Albuquerque, New Mexico

**Suzanne Staebler, MSN, RNC, NNP**
Past Co-Chair NANN Education and Practice
  Committee
Plano, Texas

**Sandra Swanson, BSN, RN, MSOD**
Past Co-Chair NANN Education and Practice
  Committee
Loyola Medical Center
Maywood, Illinois

**Jane K. Sweeney, PT, PCS, PhD**
Northwest Pediatric and Neurologic
  Rehabilitation
Gig Harbor, Washington

# PREFACE

Individualized, family-centered, developmental care (IFDC) is a framework for providing care that enhances the neurodevelopment of the infant through interventions that support both the infant and family unit. This foundation of caregiving requires collaboration among the health care team, and it views the family as an integral part of this team. Research has shown that developmental caregiving enhances the outcomes of high-risk infants who require neonatal intensive care, yet accurate and expedient implementation of evidence-based interventions has been difficult given the existing intensive care environment and the medical priorities established by the needs of the high-risk infant. Additionally, many interventions are still not well tested by research and require cautious implementation. The basis of developmental caregiving is acknowledgment of the individual needs of the infant and family, yet this cannot be done without standardized and essentially sound education and support of neonatal intensive care unit (NICU) professionals.

In response to these concerns, the National Association of Neonatal Nurses (NANN) formed an interdisciplinary task force to develop a "core curriculum" that has evolved into *NANN's Developmental Care of Newborns & Infants* to serve as a cornerstone for education of and clinical practice by NICU professionals. This text provides evidenced-based guidelines for implementation of developmentally supportive caregiving with infants and families served through the NICU and beyond. It reviews the impact of the prenatal and postnatal environment on development. It stresses the need for a family-centered, individualized approach to care. Families are partners in this process. This text represents an integrated, interdisciplinary approach.

The interdisciplinary task force developed the following philosophy statement:

Developmental care is a philosophy that embraces the concepts of dynamic interaction between the infant, family, and surrounding environment. Developmentally supportive care provides a framework in which the environment of care and the process of delivering care are modified and structured to support the individualized needs of the developing newborn and family. This concept of care represents a continuum that begins antenatally, through the intrapartal period, at birth, throughout hospitalization, discharge as the infant transitions home, and outcomes in infancy and later childhood. Links to care in the community are made prior to discharge.

What is developmental care? It is awareness, an intuitiveness to observe the infant and family and their interactions with the environment. It is a framework for providing care that supports the neurobehavioral development of the infant. It involves a broad prevention orientation targeted to improve developmental processes and competence for infants at risk. It is a philosophy that is predicated on human needs and cues and not on administrative facility tasks and schedules. It is a willingness to look holistically at the infant, family, and environment and provide interdisciplinary care accordingly. It is not a type of intervention for when the infant is stable; it is a method of care to promote stability and reduce the prevalence of signs and symptoms of identifiable disorders, thereby minimizing the ultimate effect upon normal functioning (i.e., how the care is provided). It is an approach to care that is, for the most part, infant driven. It requires collaboration among the health care team and views the family as an integral part of this team. To accomplish this integration of care, all health team members must be educated in the fundamental principles of developmental care.

Both the "macroenvironment" (the surrounding room lights and sounds of the unit or home environment) and the "microenvironment" (the immediate infant, including touch and positioning, as well as the family environment) are affected by alterations made in either milieu. Most often these alterations within the developmental context are done to better match the environment of the infant to the infant's maturation, as well as help simulate the once-protective intrauterine environment in the infant's extrauterine life. The process of care delivery is adjusted in response to communications from the infant, or behavioral cues. The aim is to decrease associated stress and increase the potential of the available skills possessed by the infant as he or she attempts to regulate and organize his or her responses.Within the continuum, it also involves early screening to detect and abbreviate the course of action and the extent of any behavioral disruptions before they develop into additional problems. This cue-based integration of caregiving depends on a multidisciplinary focus that is attuned to this type of care. Nurses; physicians; physical, occupational, and respiratory therapists; developmental specialists; and other ancillary personnel who touch or interact with the infant or family must be synchronized, familiar with, and practice the concepts of developmental care if it is to be accomplished. Developmental care requires that each member of the health care team, including the family, have a working knowledge of what developmental care is, how to "read" behavioral cues, and what significance these cues have on the baby's growth and development. Families are an integral part of the team because family-centered care concepts support partnerships between parents and healthcare providers that facilitate the parental role as primary care provider.

The clinical implications and future goals of the work represented in this text include holistic yet standardized implementation of evidence-based interventions with infants and families who are served by those in the NICU, as well as support for further testing through clinical research of these interventions. Lastly, it cannot be underscored enough that developmental caregiving is evolving; thus, gaps as well as evidence to support this care must be acknowledged and changes in suggested practice may be expected to continue. To build on this process, NICU staff orientation and basic and advanced professional education programs must incorporate IFDC into their routine curricula. It is essential content that needs to be viewed as such in order to move developmental care to the next level of full implementation in the NICU and beyond.

Gendron (1994) uses the analogy of a tapestry to describe the integration of new and different kinds of knowledge into caregiver activities. She describes warp and weft threads as woven together on a structure to create the tapestry. When applied to caregiving in the NICU, warp threads can be described as the sterile, highly technologic, and sometimes unwelcoming environment, including the rigorous schedule of assessments, procedures, and tests that must be followed; the unending medications to be given; and the tedious implementation of medical and nursing interventions. Weft threads can be described as the integration of individualized, family-centered, developmental interventions into routine practices. They are the blending of complimentary agendas and the synchrony of caregivers with infants. They are the fluid performance of medical and nursing tasks. They are the gentle and calming bathes to be given; the balancing of feeding with comforting; and the matching of awake periods to family visits and kangaroo care. They are the moments to be treasured, the lessons to be learned, and the joys to be shared. They are the art and excellence of neonatal care, and sometimes they are "an act of love" (Swanson, 1990).

## ACKNOWLEDGMENTS

This project has been a long time coming and has had support from many, many developmental care experts. First of all we would like to thank the National Association of Neonatal Nurses (NANN) for its foresight to bring together a team of interdisciplinary experts to write this "core" individualized, family-centered, developmental care text. NANN entrusted us with this most needed project, and we are grateful for having been a part of the process that will continue to make the concepts of IFDC grow in the environment of the NICU. We also wish to thank Catherine Bush, Vice President, Children's Medical Ventures, Norwell, MA for providing funding to get this project off the ground.

Dr. Stanley Graven gave the interdisciplinary planning team space to meet at his annual *"Physical Environment of the High-Risk Newborn and Family"* and guidance on how to bring an interdisciplinary focus to this text. Thank you so much for your continued support.

Finally we owe a big thanks to the team who worked behind the scenes to get this book to press.

Jan Zasada *(The In Bin)*, who spent hours getting materials ready to go to Elsevier; Amanda Politte, Developmental Editor at Elsevier, who made sure we were on target with our publication date and processed the manuscript; and Michael Ledbetter, Executive Editor at Elsevier, who gave us support when we needed it most.

**Carole Kenner, DNS, RNC, FAAN**
**Jacqueline McGrath, PhD, RN, NNP, CCNS**

Gendron, D. (1994). The tapestry of care. *Advances in Nursing Science, 17*(1), 25–30.
Swanson, K.M. (1990). Providing care in the NICU: Sometimes an act of love. *Advances in Nursing Science, 13*(1), 60–73.

# CONTENTS

# Developmental Care: An Overview

**Jana L. Pressler, Carol Spruill Turnage-Carrier, and Carole Kenner**

1

For caregivers to fully comprehend the paradigm shift in caregiving to newborn developmental caregiving, they must first have a background in the history of the evolution of hospital-based caregiving for neonates and young, sick infants. As emphasized in part in the past by Gottfried and Gaiter (1985) in the edited book, *Infant Stress Under Intensive Care: Environmental Neonatology*, and by Newborn Individualized Developmental Care and Assessment Program (NIDCAP®) (Boston, MA) trainers during their initial training session with trainees (James M. Helm, personal communication, March 3, 1994). This chapter begins with an overview of frontiers of neonatal caregiving in hospitals to provide a foundation and to embed developmental care into a relevant context. Then we will sequentially discuss hospital-based caregiving and the preterm infant, infant development and developmental care, the Frontier of Cost Savings, and what the future might hold.

## FRONTIER OF MOLECULAR BIOLOGY

### Historical Perspective of Caregiving in Nurseries

#### Care of Preterm Infants in Hospitals

The year 2000 marked a century of formalized hospital care for preterm infants. The first institutional care of preterm neonates can be traced to 1880 in France and the development of the earliest infant incubator, the Tarnier-Martin Couveuse (Gottfried & Gaiter, 1985) that was modeled after incubators that were being used for hatching chicken eggs (Figure 1-1). According to Gottfried and Gaiter, the first hospital nursery, housing preterm infants, was established 13 years later (in 1893) by one of Tanier's students, Dr. Pierre Budin. In 1900, seven years after the first preterm nursery was developed, the first textbook discussing the care of preterms, or weaklings, was published. In his initial lecture, Budin wrote (1900, as translated by W. J. Maloney in Budin &

Maloney, 1907): "We shall begin with the study of infants affected with congenital feebleness. They are classed as weaklings, and are, as a rule, the product of premature labor." Budin's philosophy of infants as weaklings is consistent with thinking at that time because for hundreds of years, newborns had been erroneously conceptualized and cared for as though their minds were a "blooming, buzzing confusion" (James, 1890) and, for the most part, "tabula rasas," or blank slates, on which adults created the individual features of newborns. Through the years, developmental psychology and (later) neonatology has made significant progress from viewing neonates strictly from the blank slate perspective characterized by these early times (Figures 1-2 and 1-3).

### Specifics Pertinent to a Historical Overview of the Frontiers of Neonatal Caregiving

***The First Frontier: Minimal Handling, Skill Mastery, Limited Access, and the Concept of Viewing.*** Budin (Budin & Maloney, 1907) focused on support of body temperature, feedings, and control of infection. Before the inception of his approach, the goals for caring for preterm infants were limited to the care of the digestive tube and prophylaxis of contagious diseases. Based on his principles, one of Budin's students, Dr. Martin Couney, exhibited preterm infants to the public for profit (Budin & Maloney, 1907). With infants housed in incubators, the mothering of Couney's preterms was replaced by nursing care. The goal of caregiving was minimal handling. To accomplish this goal, infection control procedures were rigorously maintained. The paradigm of neonatal treatment that evolved from Couney's exhibitions, or mainstays, were: minimal handling, emphasis on mastery and application of special nursing skills and procedures, and limited access to preterm infants. Because Couney's paradigm, or portions of it, continues to persist in preterm infant care, our attention is being refocused on what the goals of caregiving should be beyond Couney's theories (Figure 1-4).

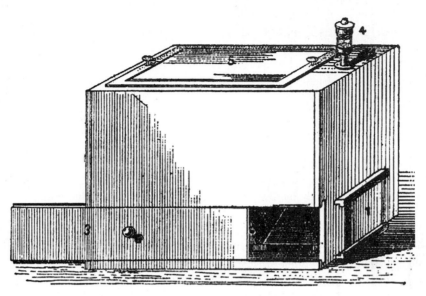

FIG. 3.—TARNIER'S INCUBATOR.

1. Air entry.   2. Hot-water bottles.   3. Sliding door.   4. Air exit.   5. Glass cover.

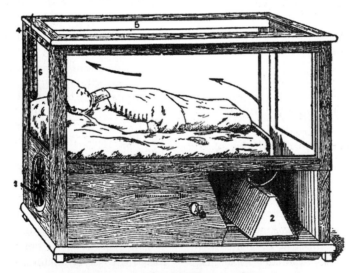

FIG. 5.—INCUBATOR OF WOOD AND GLASS.

1. Air entry.   2. Hot-water bottles.   3. Horizontal partition on which the infant rests.
4. Holes by which the air escapes.   5. Glass cover.   6. Thermometer.   The
arrows indicate the course taken by the air in the incubator.

Figure 1-1 Sketches of Tarnier's earliest incubator. (*From Auvard, A. [1883]. De la couveuse pour infants. Archives de Tocologie des Maladies des Femmes et des Enfants, 10[Oct.], 577-609.*)

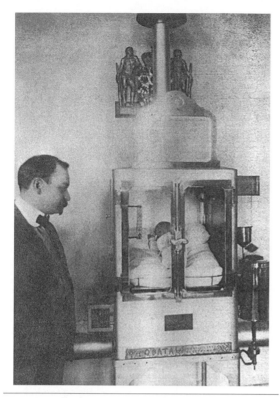

Figure 1-2 A very small preterm infant in an incubator. The unidentified onlooker might be Martin Couney.

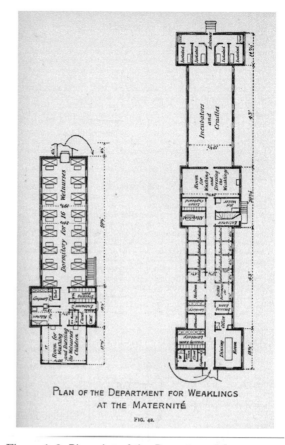

PLAN OF THE DEPARTMENT FOR WEAKLINGS
AT THE MATERNITÉ

FIG. 42.

Figure 1-3 Blueprint of the Department for Weaklings at the Maternité in Paris, France, showing the separate anteroom for staff hand washing, weakling dormitory, anteroom for washing and dressing weaklings, and incubator center.

***The Second Frontier: The Miniaturization of Technology, Infant Ventilators, and the Development of Neonatology into a Specialty.*** Between 1960 and 1970, neonatology developed into a specialty, with board specialization offered to physicians from the American Academy of Pediatrics (AAP). This change occurred as a result of technologic improvements in caring for infants, primarily in terms of thermoregulation and the development of radiant warmers, and the development of more finite scaling of ventilator settings to meet the lower inspiratory and expiratory pressures required by very small neonates. Neonatology further expanded with the development of total parenteral nutrition and intralipid therapies and the use of central lines for infusions. With support from the March of Dimes (MOD) in 1970, transport teams came into formal existence. These teams supported the regionalization of care by both ground and air transport so that more sophisticated care could be efficiently delivered to the largest number of infants and families.

***The Third Frontier: Sophisticated Respiratory Treatments, Family-Centered Care, and the Concept of Touring.*** Given that neonates could reach tertiary care centers, and neonatal growth and development was enabled through use of central lines, by 1980 the emphasis for care returned to the neonates' oxygenation status. Transcutaneous oxygen monitors were invented first, followed by pulse oximeters. These devices were used along with high-frequency ventilation, surfactant replacements,

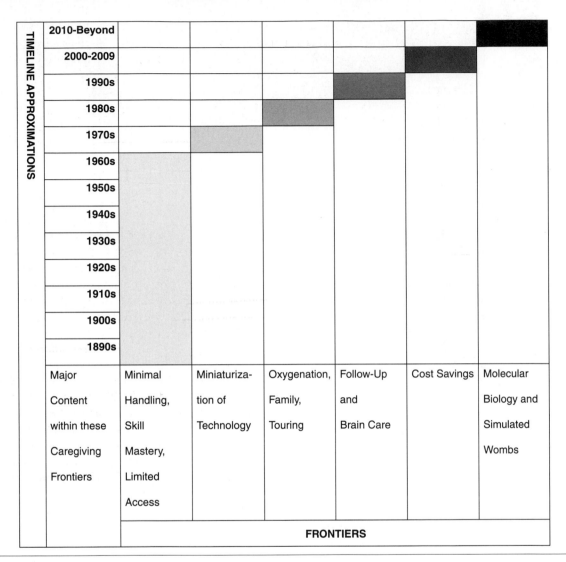

| TIMELINE APPROXIMATIONS | Major Content within these Caregiving Frontiers | Minimal Handling, Skill Mastery, Limited Access | Miniaturization of Technology | Oxygenation, Family, Touring | Follow-Up and Brain Care | Cost Savings | Molecular Biology and Simulated Wombs |
|---|---|---|---|---|---|---|---|
| 2010-Beyond | | | | | | | ■ |
| 2000-2009 | | | | | | ■ | |
| 1990s | | | | | ■ | | |
| 1980s | | | | ■ | | | |
| 1970s | | ■ | | | | | |
| 1960s | | | | | | | |
| 1950s | | | | | | | |
| 1940s | | | | | | | |
| 1930s | | | | | | | |
| 1920s | | | | | | | |
| 1910s | | | | | | | |
| 1900s | | | | | | | |
| 1890s | | | | | | | |
| | | | **FRONTIERS** | | | | |

Figure 1-4 Frontiers of caregiving.

extracorporeal membrane oxygenation, and nitric oxide therapy in addressing the neonates' oxygenation requirements.

With the 1986 implementation of the Education for All Handicapped Children Amendments, family-centered care emerged. To date, these amendments are the most important and far-reaching pieces of legislation ever enacted for developmentally vulnerable young infants. This statute requires "a statewide, comprehensive, coordinated, multidisciplinary, inter-

agency program of early intervention services for all handicapped infants and their families" (PL 99-457, Sec. 671). Although this bill did not mandate universal services for all children younger than 6 years of age, it did establish a discretionary program (Part H of the statute) that provides services for children from birth through 3 years. The law requires that early intervention services be made available for those experiencing developmental delay at the time of referral and assessment and for those having a condition diagnosed as having a high probability of resulting in subsequent developmental delay. Each state also has the option of including children who are "at risk of having substantial developmental delays if early intervention services are not provided" (PL 99-457, Sec. 672). For more information, see Chapter 23. Children falling within that discretionary category have typically been characterized as biologically at risk and/or environmentally at risk (Tjossem, 1976).

Family birthing centers and labor, delivery, recovery, and postpartum care units were created, and hospitals started competing for the patient care dollars that were attached to deliveries. Some institutions have decided to focus their time and efforts relatively exclusively on pursuits within this frontier. The AAP (Hauth & Merenstein, 1997) continues to emphasize that general neonatal respiratory care and family goals are included in this third frontier. However, some physicians are in the process or have already changed their caregiving emphasis toward a different set of goals. Family care is an area in which nursing has excelled for years. Emphasis on family-centered care and their needs is addressed in the guidelines put forth by White and the Committee to Establish Recommended Standards for Newborn ICU Design (2002). In its fifth report of the consensus conference, there are several standards that incorporate aspects of the family as an integral part of the newborn intensive care unit (NICU) and the care provided. These recommendations are used worldwide to influence the neonatal environment. Developmental care and inclusion of the family is a global issue.

### The Fourth Frontier: Brain Care and an Increased Focus on Infant Follow-Up.

Partly crossing over from its start in the third frontier, the fourth frontier consists of four distinct phases that are grounded in concerns related to infant development. Since the middle of the 1970s, when major research efforts were being solidified in molecular biology, neonatal research began centering more on the uniqueness of newborns as individuals, as well as on dynamic relationships between human genetics and the environment, with newborns viewed as contributors to the care given to them and, subsequently, to their environments. Infants are active participants in their own

development and can interact and react to the environment around them. The importance of providing a stimulating environment for infants has become increasingly recognized.

**The First Phase.** The first phase of the fourth frontier became evident around 1980, when infant follow-up clinics were formalized and physicians and developmental specialists became concerned about a number of negative infant outcomes they had observed in infant patients evaluated at these clinics. In response to the findings from infant follow-up clinics, infant stimulation programs emerged and became popular across the United States. Professionals from diverse disciplines pursued certificate programs in infant stimulation, with many of the programs supported by Area Health Education Centers (AHEC). Nursing care was becoming more specialized as neonatal nursing care was becoming a specialty, and the advanced practice role of the neonatal nurse practitioner or clinical nurse specialist was moving to graduate nursing education. For more information, see Chapter 25.

**The Second Phase.** The second phase of this frontier appeared when health care professionals became concerned about the noxiousness of iatrogenic stimuli and infant stimulation protocols, and took on advocacy positions to protect infants from sensory bombardment. This second phase is sometimes referred to as the age of *environmental neonatology*. The health professionals began to examine the macro- and microenvironments that surrounded the infant and the family and their interaction with both the infant and the family.

**The Third Phase.** Following closely behind Brazelton's (1973) development and refinement (Brazelton & Nugent, 1995) of the Neonatal Behavioral Assessment Scale, the third phase of this fourth frontier emerged. Neonatal care became less stereotypic, was individualized to meet the needs of particular neonates, and was based on individualized developmental assessments primarily spearheaded by Als (1979, 1981). The National Association of Neonatal Nurses (NANN) voiced their support of the developmental goals supported within this frontier with their creation of the Infant Developmental Care Guidelines (NANN, 1993), which were later revised in 2001. Also included in this frontier is the growing knowledge and understanding of the neonatal brain and its plasticity as related to neurologic insult and injury.

**The Fourth Phase.** The fourth phase of the fourth frontier evolved to an even higher level when developmental care subsequently became embedded within the context of the infant's family, so that care met the infants' needs in accordance with their assimilation as family members. It was recognized that the family was an important part of the neonatal care team, and family-centered guidelines for caregivers and institutions were outlined by the Institute for Family-Centered Care. Much of the hospital environment as a whole has been influenced by this movement; but, the NICU environment continues to be at the forefront of this movement. As indicated earlier, the inclusion of family and family-centered care principles into the recommended standards for NICU design (White, 2002) is helping to forge parent-partnerships in care within the confines of the NICU. Specialty groups such as the AAP; Association for the Care of Children's Health; Association of Women's Health, Obstetrics, and Neonatal Nurses (AWHONN); Institute for Family-Centered Care; International Society of Nurses in Genetics (ISONG); NANN; Parent Care; and Society of Pediatric Nursing, are just some of the many examples of organizations that have addressed the issue of the need for family-centered, individualized care for infants, and continue to do so.

**The Newest Frontier of Neonatal Caregiving: Cost Savings.** With infant outcomes at the forefront of care, developmental caregiving as an umbrella approach continues to evolve—but at whose and what expense? The frontier of neonatology within the information age of the new millennium focuses on balancing costs with benefits and deciding where and how much money should be spent, for what services and for whom. Health care has taken a 360-degree about-face in addressing the dollar savings of insurers. This turnaround stems from three historic events:

I. The creation of Health Maintenance Organizations (HMOs) and reliance on both team and primary nursing in the mid-1980s;

II. The articulation and implementation of case management and use of all licensed personnel by the late 1980s;

III. In the 1990s, a shift to managed care, a nursing shortage of critical proportion, a re-institution and use of nonlicensed caregivers, and widespread hospital mergers.

Cost-savings will continue to be a focus as we move into the 21st century.

***The Frontier Ahead: Molecular Biology and Simulated Wombs.*** The new advances that are currently being made by molecular biologists in gene identification, genomics, and biogenetics are going to create a context for health care never before seen or known capable in the 20th century. By 2010, it seems highly likely that innovative strategies will have been determined for dealing with massive amounts of multidimensional data collected throughout gestation. Also, although controversy persists, new types of simulated womblike environments for extremely young gestation neonates will likely have been developed and tested. Based on reviews of human and animal early stimulation research, Schaefer, Hatcher, and Barglow (1980) have claimed that the stimulation present in utero is optimal and would best facilitate development of preterm infants. However, Als, Lester, Tronick, and Brazelton (1980) have disagreed, arguing that an artificial re-creation of the intrauterine-environment would not appropriately meet the needs of preterm infants, because transitions occurring at birth automatically trigger independent functioning of the respiratory, cardiac, and digestive systems needed for extrauterine survival. This frontier will be filled with new and uncertain ethical dilemmas because the capacity to care for younger and sicker infants is imminent with high technologic advances, computerized decision making, and the untapped potential for revised and updated methods of patient assessment and treatment. It calls into question the age-old chat of the definition of viability in terms of use of technology and the very immature infant. What is the age of viability? It also begs the question: Just because we can, should we? Part of the dilemma arises from the lack of systematic studies that examine long-term developmental and physical problems of the extremely low-birthweight infant and the family. The developmental care movement is challenging us to look at these outcomes, to provide evidence to support our clinical decisions.

## DEVELOPMENTAL CARE AS A FOCAL POINT

Focus on infant development and the importance of developmental care requires untangling and sorting through the critical origins of knowledge concerning infant development. Developmental care is an outgrowth of explorations of the effects of institutionalized care on infants that dates back 55 years to the First Frontier of Neonatal Caregiving.

### Hospitalism and Infant Intelligence

Whereas the first theoretical basis for institutional effects on development came from Spitz's (1945, 1946) and Spitz and Wolf's (1946) work on hospitalism, based on an extensive review, Linn (1980) contended that the first theoretical basis of early environmental effects on infant development came from Hebb's (1949) classic writing on the foundations of intelligence. Spitz (1945, p. 53) was very concerned about the long lasting "evil effect of institutional care on infants," specifically the morbid conditions of infant foundling homes. However, Hebb was concerned more globally about the effects of early environments on infants' development of intelligence. According to Hebb, primary learning arose through perceptual experiences, and the foundational units of cognitive functioning were images of those experiences. Therefore, intelligence quotient (IQ) indices used without an understanding of an individual's early environment offered, at best, only part of the picture. According to Hebb (1949, p. 300):

We cannot, in any rigorous sense, measure a subject's innate endowment, for no two social backgrounds are identical and we do not know what the important environmental variables are in [the] development of intellectual functions.

### Emotional Problems, Environmental Retardation, and Essential Maternal Behavior

With caregiving and caregiving environments at the forefront, Escalona (1952) went on to identify and elaborate on significant emotional problems in infancy. Subsequently, Coleman and Provence

(1957) investigated environmental retardation of infants, whereas Rheingold (1956, 1960, 1963) and Stevenson, Hess, and Rheingold (1967) introduced empiric studies concerning the impact of essential mammalian maternal behavior on offspring. Not only were infant environments being studied, but also the role that human nurturing played as a natural constituent of those environments.

### Institutionalized Care, Maternal Deprivation, and Sensory Stimulation

Around the same time as infant environments were investigated, Provence and Lipton (1962) analyzed the longitudinal effects of institutionalized care on infants' behavior using sequences and detailed descriptions. In examining the important influences on infant development from a slightly different angle, Yarrow (1961) reviewed literature on maternal deprivation through 1960 in completing an extensive critique of empiric support for the role of environments in contributing to maternal deprivation. After finding only one study, conducted by Rheingold (1960), that made any attempt to objectively describe an institutional setting, Yarrow speculated that institutional environments might differ in the quantity and quality of sensory stimulation that they had available overall, as well as in specific stimuli, such as the consistency of personnel and predictability of caregiver responsivity.

### The Conceptualization of Early Experience in Terms of Socioeconomic Status

In both the 1960s and the 1970s, researchers moved from a gross categorization of early experience as being "deprived" or "not deprived" to classification of groups in terms of "socioeconomic status" (SES) (Tulkin, 1977). The use of SES as an independent variable demonstrated moderate and consistent correlations with psychological dependent measurements (Horowitz, Sullivan, & Linn, 1978). But relying on SES as an accurate summary variable was not supported by studies conducted within a single socioeconomic class completed during that same time period (Elardo, Bradley, & Caldwell, 1975; Lewis & Goldberg, 1969; Yarrow, Pedersen, & Rubinstein, 1977). Richards (1977) pointed out that researchers' use of SES as a grouping variable led to the inaccurate assumption of homogeneity within SES groups.

## Transitioning from the Organization of Behavior to Assimilation and Accommodation

Triggered by Hebb's (1949) focus on the organization of human behavior into patterns and Werner's (1957) orthogenetic principle explaining human behavior as both developmental levels and stages, Piaget's (1973) concepts of assimilation and accommodation revolutionized the prevailing view of an infant's interactions with the environment. Piaget's ideas took hold in the United States at some time between the examination of maternal deprivation and the examination of SES. Piaget's ideas serve as groundwork for current thoughts regarding developmental care in that his concepts of assimilation and accommodation of an infant's perceptual experiences helped to identify the importance of environmental stability and environmental variety.

Detailed assessments of neonatal development, such as the Neonatal Behavioral Assessment Scale (NBAS) (Brazelton, 1973), incorporated the idea of optimal behavior into the scales used for scoring behavior. Although the concept of optimality and optimal behavior had been described prior to the work of Piaget (Prechtl, 1968), it did not play as significant a role in infant assessments until Brazelton emphasized it in the NBAS. Play has resurfaced lately in relationship to infant sleep and the impact on achievement motor milestones (Salls, Silverman, & Gatty, 2002).

Following the development of the NBAS and recognition of the importance of environmental stability and variety, other researchers also suggested that a "match" between an infant's cognitive level and the experiences made available to an infant produced what they thought represented optimal developmental progress (Hunt, 1976; Wachs, 1976). The concept of developmental care, the concept of newborn competencies, and the benefits of individualized developmental care all emanated from the idea of optimal developmental progress (Figure 1-5).

Individualized developmental assessments are being used more sparingly by many NICUs, although this is not necessarily the best approach,

particularly because of the training needed and the cost to conduct and translate the examinations into practice applications. Instead of individualized examinations, many NICUs are applying developmental care now more generally to the preterm infant population (e.g., no examination before using a Snuggle-Up or offering a Wee Thumbie [Children's Medical Ventures, Norwell, MA] pacifier to a newborn). Others are introducing the staff and care providers to developmental care through the Wee Care® program (see Appendix C). Although optimal developmental progress was and continues to be the crucial link to the future evolution of neonatal developmental care, many caregivers have loosened their hold on the notion that assessments of individual infants' developmental progress are essential to provide appropriate developmental care.

## Major Assumptions Underlying Development

The progression from global descriptions of early infant environments, to an emphasis on environmental specificity, and ultimately to the organization of behavior into patterns, led to the generation of instruments designed to describe infant development and infant environments. These naturalistic measurement tools can be prefaced by a number of general assumptions concerning child development. Such assumptions provide a framework for both the development and organization of developmental care. It is important to recognize assumptions in preparing the stage for what will be needed in a *nursery setting* that establishes and provides intensive neonatal care. Seven important assumptions discussed by developmental experts (Gesell & Thompson, 1934; Horowitz, 1990, 1995; Illingworth, 1987; Werner, 1957) underlie infant development and appear applicable and relevant to developmental care (Box 1-1).

## The Birth of Individualized Developmental Caregiving

The most widely used and well-recognized naturalistic, noninvasive infant and environmental coding scheme NIDCAP®, developed more than 20 years ago (Als, 1979, 1981). The NIDCAP® is based on four assumptions and further grounded in synactive

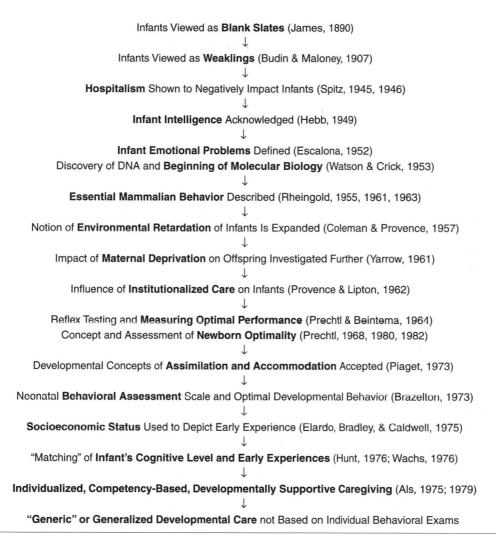

Infants Viewed as **Blank Slates** (James, 1890)
↓
Infants Viewed as **Weaklings** (Budin & Maloney, 1907)
↓
**Hospitalism** Shown to Negatively Impact Infants (Spitz, 1945, 1946)
↓
**Infant Intelligence** Acknowledged (Hebb, 1949)
↓
**Infant Emotional Problems** Defined (Escalona, 1952)
Discovery of DNA and **Beginning of Molecular Biology** (Watson & Crick, 1953)
↓
**Essential Mammalian Behavior** Described (Rheingold, 1955, 1961, 1963)
↓
Notion of **Environmental Retardation** of Infants Is Expanded (Coleman & Provence, 1957)
↓
Impact of **Maternal Deprivation** on Offspring Investigated Further (Yarrow, 1961)
↓
Influence of **Institutionalized Care** on Infants (Provence & Lipton, 1962)
↓
Reflex Testing and **Measuring Optimal Performance** (Prechtl & Beintema, 1964)
Concept and Assessment of **Newborn Optimality** (Prechtl, 1968, 1980, 1982)
↓
Developmental Concepts of **Assimilation and Accommodation** Accepted (Piaget, 1973)
↓
Neonatal **Behavioral Assessment** Scale and Optimal Developmental Behavior (Brazelton, 1973)
↓
**Socioeconomic Status** Used to Depict Early Experience (Elardo, Bradley, & Caldwell, 1975)
↓
"Matching" of **Infant's Cognitive Level and Early Experiences** (Hunt, 1976; Wachs, 1976)
↓
**Individualized, Competency-Based, Developmentally Supportive Caregiving** (Als, 1975; 1979)
↓
**"Generic" or Generalized Developmental Care** not Based on Individual Behavioral Exams

Figure **1-5** Conceptual trajectory of infant development leading to individualized caregiving.

theory (Als, 1979). Als' assumptions are extensions and refinements of those contained in the previous abbreviated set for general child development, with the exception of the third one, which essentially is a restated assumption from Werner (1957) mentioned earlier (Box 1-2).

The NIDCAP® is a means of recording observations of the behavior of a newborn, and using these observations to produce recommendations for caregiving that could meet the infant's goals as suggested by his/her behavior. Groups of specific autonomic, motor, and state behaviors are documented every 2 minutes for at least 20 minutes prior to a caregiving episode, during caregiving, and for at least 20 minutes following caregiving, or until an infant has settled. Notations concerning the infant's neonatal environment, including bed space, bed type, bedding, sound, light, room activity levels, the infant's medical history, and infant's current status are all considered.

## Box 1-1    Assumptions Underlying Development

1. It is believed that the most rapid time period of growth of all body systems, including the brain, are the first five years of postnatal life (Gesell & Thompson, 1934).
2. Development is orderly. The order of development is very similar for all infants (Gesell & Thompson, 1934).
3. Development occurs from gross to specific and proceeds in a cephalo-caudal sequence (Gesell & Thompson, 1934).
4. Development is directional and proceeds from an ordered series of levels of organization in which the constituent parts are less differentiated and less integrated to levels in which constituent parts are more differentiated and more integrated (Werner, 1957).
5. Development is a continuous process that is ongoing from conception to maturation (Illingworth, 1987).
6. Development takes place at distinct rates for each individual person (Horowitz, 1990; Illingworth, 1987).
7. Development occurs within a framework of interaction with care providers, including care by family members (Horowitz, 1995).

## Box 1-2    Assumptions Underlying Synactive Theory

1. The infant is in continuous interaction and transaction with the environment.
2. Behavior has meaning and is species-specific.
3. Development occurs from a global state to a state of increasing differentiation, articulation, and hierarchic integration (specific state).
4. The organism strives for smoothness of integration, with underlying tensions existing between approach and avoidance (Als, 1982).

Relying on the synactive theory and systematic NIDCAP® observations of an infant's behaviors, an individualized plan for caregiving can be developed by a trained and reliable NIDCAP® examiner (Als, 1984, 1991) (see *www.nidcap.com*, *www.nidcap.exe* or *www.nidcap.net* for up-to-date information regarding training). Based on the behaviors exhibited by each infant, the immediate environment and caregiving approach are customized to meet the particular infant's goals. The goals of these approaches are to facilitate the infant's self-regulatory behaviors while reducing stress to the infant (Cole, Begish-Duddy, Judas, & Jorgensen, 1990). This approach is highly individualized and specific to each infant's unique needs and behavioral competencies (Brazelton, 1979). Competencies are generally believed to result from deliberate efforts on the part of a person (White, 1959). A sense of competence becomes a source for fueling repetition, with an infant becoming increasingly more proficient and motivated as awareness and learning builds. The concept of competency, both those previously and newly established, provides an essential part of the core for the nursing care of neonates (Lawhon, 1997). As delineated earlier in the historical perspective, it has taken many decades for professionals and researchers to fully realize that newborns have the capabilities for being or demonstrating competencies.

Also based on synactive theory and many of Als' ideas, the Assessment of Preterm Infant Behavior (APIB) (Als, Lester, Tronick, & Brazelton, 1982; Als, Duffy, & McAnulty, 1988a, 1988b) is a more sophisticated assessment tool designed to document the competencies of the newborn for both research and clinical purposes. The APIB measures the degree of smoothness and modulation, regulation, and differentiation of five behavioral subsystems of functioning: (1) autonomic, (2) motor, (3) state regulation, (4) attentional/interactional, and (5) self-regulatory, in continuous interaction with each other and the environment at large. The APIB relies on techniques included in the NBAS (Brazelton & Nugent, 1995) in completing a sequence of incre-mentally demanding stimuli that extend from distal to proximal, from nontactile to tactile, and occur during sleep to wakefulness. According to Als, Duffy, and McAnulty (1988b), the APIB can provide stable groupings of infants by behavioral competencies regardless of gestational age. However, costs in terms of training and time allocation might be pro-hibitive for general use of the APIB in the NICU.

There are several for-profit companies and programs that are aimed at educating health professionals and parents in the philosophy of developmental care. Children's Medical Ventures (Norwell, MA), Contemporary Forums (Dublin, CA), Hill-Rom, Inc. (Batesville, IN), and Ohmeda Medical (Columbia, MD) are just a few of the many examples of developmental care programs.

More than a decade ago, Horowitz and Columbo (1990) reported that they believed that the field of infancy had yet to see much imaginative research because the field lacked necessary theoretical advances. They stated that without theoretical advances, the simple accrual of information, characteristic of a focus on specific concepts, would continue. Horowitz and Columbo believed that future researchers would benefit significantly from theoretical frameworks that involved information on infant competencies and developmental perspectives. Guided by the underpin-nings of the synactive theory, Als has attempted to contribute to the field of infancy in this way (Als, 1982, 1986). However, it appears that other researchers have not followed this path quite as closely.

## Other Individualized Neonatal Assessment Tools

Not derived from specific identifiable developmental theories, but also containing aspects of neonatal and infant development, at least four other tools have emerged since the creation of the APIB and NID-CAP®. Reflecting a mixture of somewhat different types of indices and not purely infant development, these tools include: the Neurobehavioral Assessment

of the Preterm Infant (NAPI) developed by Korner (1987) in the 1980s and later refined during collabo-rative investigations with colleagues in the early 1990s (Constantinou & Korner, 1993; Korner, Constantinou, Dimiceli, et al., 1991); the Test of Infant Motor Performance (TIMP) developed by Campbell et al. during the early 1990s (Campbell, 1999; Campbell, Osten, Kolobe, & Fisher, 1993; Murney & Campbell, 1998); Clinical High Risk Neonatal Pathways, developed by Gretebeck et al. during the mid- to late 1990s (Gretebeck, Shaffer, & Bishop-Kurylo, 1998); and the NICU Network Neurobehavioral Scale (NNNS), which was recently developed by Boukydis and Lester (1999). Use of these tools might perpetuate the earlier tradition of simply accumulating information by focusing on specific concepts, as might be deduced from the descriptions of the tools that follow.

### Neurobehavioral Assessment of the Preterm Infant

Korner, Constantinou, Dimiceli, et al., (1991) devel-oped the Neurobehavioral Assessment of the Preterm Infant (NAPI) in three phases: a pilot study, an exploratory study, and a validation study. In their exploratory study, behavioral clusters were system-atically subjected to statistical analyses to determine whether they also had high test-retest reliability and developmental validity. In their validation study, a shortened version of the NAPI was used with an independent cohort of 290 preterm infants on whom 533 examinations were completed. A step-wise methodologic process was used to test whether results from the exploratory study would generalize over cohorts, different versions of the test, different hospitals, and different examiners. This process yielded preterm neurobehavioral functions that generalized over both the exploratory and the vali-dation studies. The neurobehavioral functions included motor development and vigor, scarf sign, and vigor of crying. These functions were a revision of the eight dimensions that had been identified earlier by Korner (1987): (1) active tone/motor vigor, (2) alertness and orientation, (3) excitation proneness, (4) inhibition proneness, (5) scarf sign, (6) popliteal angle, (7) maturity of vestibular response, and (8) vigor of crying.

Constantinou and Korner (1993) assessed the effect of incorporating parents in the process of evaluating the behavior of preterm infants. Administration of NAPI in the presence of the parents was performed with 17 preterm infants, and the impact on the parents' perception of their infants was quantified. The extent to which parents validated their observations and increased their confidence in their infants' competence as a result of observing changes in their infant's behavior was evaluated. Parental presence during the administration of the NAPI was found to have educational benefits in offering reassurance and enhanced parental awareness.

## Test of Infant Motor Performance

The TIMP is a relatively new test of motor and postural control for infants younger than 4 months of age. Campbell, Osten, Kolobe, et al. (1993) developed this psychomotor instrument for completing clinical assessments of newborn movement that could be used to reflect motor responses to environmental stressors and to identify and predict infant motor problems and diagnoses.

Murney and Campbell (1998) have recently used the TIMP tool to examine the relationship between the environmental demands placed on infants in daily life and the demands placed on infants during administration of the TIMP Elicited Scale to 22 preterm and full-term infants and their caregivers. The infants were evenly divided into groups at low and at high medical risk for motor disability. The infants were videotaped while being handled by a parental caregiver during undressing, bathing, dressing, and playing in a naturalistic setting (hospital or home). Videotapes were analyzed for the environmental demands placed on the infants during caregiving. Demands were coded according to pre-established definitions, which represented descriptions for administering TIMP items. The researchers found that environmental demands that corresponded to 23 of the 25 TIMP items were present during caregiving activities. The number of environmental demands placed on the infants during caregiving that corresponded to the 25 TIMP Elicited Scale items corresponded to 23 of the 25 TIMP items observed during caregiving activities. They concluded that the demands placed on infants

during administration of the TIMP appeared representative of typical environmental demands.

In a psychometric investigation, Campbell (1999) explored the test-retest reliability of the TIMP over a 3-day period and compared the effect of using the same or different raters on two occasions on test-retest reliability of the TIMP. One hundred and sixteen test-retests of TIMP examinations were performed on 106 infants (white, black, and Latino). Infant participants, ranging in age from 32 weeks' postconceptional age to 16 weeks past term, were categorized by medical risk for motor disability (high, medium, or low). Ten raters (physical therapists and occupational therapists with documented TIMP reliability) were used in the study. Multiple regression analyses were completed to assess the relationship between pairs of test scores and to evaluate the effect of same versus different raters on the similarity between scores on the 2 days. Test scores on the 2 days were correlated significantly. The score on the first testing session explained most of the variance in the score on the second testing. There was no significant difference between pairs of scores based on rater. About 54% of the scores differed by fewer than eight points of a possible 170 points. Campbell's findings supported the conclusion that the TIMP has sufficient test-retest reliability for use in clinical practice to assess infant motor performance across the infant age range of younger than 4 months for which the test was designed.

## Clinical High Risk Neonatal Pathways

A research team headed up by Gretebeck (Gretebeck, Shaffer, & Bishop-Kurylo, 1998) from southwestern Pennsylvania studied a practical and more logistic approach for introducing developmental care principles into an intensive care nursery. This neonatal research team consolidated developmental interventions into five topical areas: (1) environmental organization, (2) structuring of nursing care, (3) feeding, (4) family involvement, and (5) family education, then threaded them into three acuity-based clinical pathways for caregiving. Each pathway incorporated developmental principles applicable to a different care acuity; the level III pathway was designed for acutely ill or very premature infants, the level II pathway was designed for infants recovering from acute illness or older premature infants, and the level I pathway was designed for full-term infants. Based on both cost and hospital stay analyses, the introduction of the developmental care pathways was thought to have had a positive impact on infants cared for in the intensive care nursery at Allegheny General Hospital in Pittsburgh. For examples of clinical pathways, please see Appendix A.

### NICU Network Neurobehavioral Scale

Boukydis and Lester (1999) have been working diligently on devising a shorter and more expeditious evaluation tool for assessing the behavior of preterm infants primarily for research purposes. They now have developed a comprehensive tool that: is comparable to that represented by the APIB; produces behavioral dimensions similar to the NBAS; is able to extract subtle neurobehavioral indicators of high risk preterms while requiring less training time and examination time. Boukydis and Lester (1999) claim that their NNNS examination not only provides these impressive research measurement advantages but also has been extended to routine use in clinical hospital practice. More research with this tool needs to be done by other scientists to increase evidence and support of the developer's claim.

## CONTEMPORARY INTENSIVE CARE AND ITS RELATIONSHIP TO INFANT OUTCOMES

Contemporary institutional neonatal care began about 30 years ago with the use of mechanical ventilation for managing respiratory problems stemming from hyaline membrane disease (Gottfried, 1985). During the first 10 of those years, the primary emphasis of health care was resuscitation and stabilization of ill, 29-week and older gestation infants, chiefly because younger infants' hyaline membrane status was severe enough that they rarely survived. With the advent of exogenous surfactant administration, the neonatal survival rate of younger neonates improved dramatically with morbidities, with increasing concern about how to prevent and treat them. Due to the higher incidence of surviving infants cared for in incubators for many weeks, these younger surviving infants were exposed to an

excessive amount of sensory stimuli from the environment and caregivers. Therefore, concerns about the effects of such stimuli on infant outcomes and functioning, as well as what was needed in terms of early interventions were warranted.

Developmental outcomes associated with the NICU environment and NICU care have been emphasized as critical in the follow-up of all low-birthweight (LBW) infants hospitalized in NICUs. During 15 years of follow-up of very low birthweight (VLBW) infants, it has been found that most infants are "grossly normal" neurologically. Between 1970 and 1980, the incidence of cerebral palsy, major sensory deficits, and mental retardation for VLBW infants born at less than 36 weeks' gestation was 5% to 10% (Eilers, Desai, Wilson, et al., 1986; Vohr & Garcia-Coll, 1985). But for those VLBW infants of 23 to 26 weeks' gestation, the risk of these handicaps was more than three times that of LBWs, or 35%. Because there has been little reduction in the number of VLBW infants born, improvements in the incidence of handicaps associated with VLBW are crucial (Graven, Bowen, Brooten, et al., 1992a). This need to focus on handicaps of VLBW infants is noted further in that bronchopulmonary dysplasia (BPD) has been associated with significant developmental delays (Koops, Abman, & Accurso, 1984), cognitive deficits (Hack & Fanaroff, 1999; Markestad & Fitzhardinge, 1981; Lindeke, Stanely, Else, et al., 2002), and strokes (Scher, Klesh, Murphy, et al., 1986).

Trying to decrease specific handicaps and their associated developmental sequelae using predictions based on assessments of infants during the first 6 months has not proven effective (Aylward, Verhulst, & Bell, 1989). Poor prediction from the first 6 months postnatally could be due to the infants' still developing nervous system, family psychosocial issues, environmental factors, psychometric issues relative to measurement or testing, or a combination of such reasons. One important point is that the influence of environmental and psychosocial risk factors on infant outcomes is often not weighed heavily in follow-up studies; however, these might be critical in attempts made to decrease handicaps and their associated sequelae. In fact, Aylward and Pfeiffer (1989) found that environmental and psychosocial variables were taken into account less than 2% of the time in a meta-analysis of 10 years of infant follow-up studies completed between 1979 and 1989.

## WHAT IS CURRENTLY KNOWN ABOUT THE OUTCOMES OF HOSPITALIZED PRETERM NEONATES

In general terms, what is currently known about the sequelae and risks associated with the NICU per se for VLBW (i.e., <1500 g) and very preterm (i.e., <30 weeks) gestation neonates is that it is not uncommon for these infants to have insecure attachment relationships during infancy and toddlerhood (Wille, 1991), and information processing deficits and attention deficit hyperactivity disorders (ADHD) during the preschool (Klein, Hack, Gallagher, & Fanaroff, 1985) and school-age years (McCormick, 1989, 1997; Hack, Breslau, Weissman, et al., 1991; Hack & Fanaroff, 1999; Lindeke, Stanely, Else, et al., 2002). It is possible that these problems might reflect these infants' earlier inability to cope with and attend to stresses and/or care received while hospitalized in the NICU. Although these areas of developmental difference might not seem grave to caregivers, they can be overwhelming to a family. Even though it is still less common for these children to have more severe developmental deficits, the impact for these children and their families cannot be ignored. Developmental issues are more common for preterm and younger infants than for those who are older and spend less time in the NICU. Maturation and environment at the time of early birth go hand-in-hand in affecting long-term development.

To date, studies of ways in which the NICU could be changed to optimize the growth and development of lowered birth weight (i.e., <2500 g) and preterm (i.e., <36 weeks) infants can be grouped according to: (1) providing supplemental stimulation to correct for deficits in the environment (Lester & Tronick, 1990); (2) providing contingent care based on infant cues (Barnard & Bee, 1983); (3) reducing stimulation (Lawson, Daum, & Turkewitz, 1977); and (4) eliminating inappropriate or overstimulating sensory variables or other experiences (Glass, Avery, Subramania, et al., 1985; Long, Lucey, & Philip, 1980).

### Supplemental Stimulation

The structure of intervention programs for preterm infants has been influenced by whether or not the preterm was considered to be an extrauterine fetus (also referred to as a fetal infant), and by assumptions concerning the preterm's development. If the preterm was considered to be an extrauterine fetus, intervention programs were designed to simulate the womb, thereby curbing the infant's exposure to exogenous stimuli. For example, tactile, kinesthetic/vestibular, circadian, and auditory stimulation have been provided to compensate for the absence of: (1) total cutaneous somasthetic input from the amniotic fluid; (2) kinesthetic input from a contingently reactive amniotic sac; (3) maternal diurnal rhythms; and (4) muted sensory stimuli to vision and audition (Als, 1982). If the preterm was considered to be developing differently from the fetus, programs were designed to stimulate the maturation of the senses. Such maturational programs might include tactile (e.g., gentle touch, massage), kinesthetic (e.g., blanket nests), vestibular (e.g., rocking and rocker-beds), visual (e.g., presenting human faces and a variety of visual patterns), and auditory (e.g., audiotapes of soothing classical music) stimulation (Graven, Bowen, Brooten, et al., 1992b). Because randomized clinical trials have not been completed comparing the advantages and disadvantages of the two different approaches to exogenous stimulation with preterm infants, the effectiveness of each, based on the degree of appropriateness for differing gestational ages, is unknown. Research is ongoing in this area, but, to date, the reports have not been consistent in their inclusion of the same outcome variables nor in their study populations (Symington & Pinelli, 2001).

The fact that neither the full extent of appropriateness nor the full extent of effectiveness of supplemental stimulation programs for preterm infant development is known reflects a continuing knowledge gap in terms of the preterm infant's extrauterine adaptation. Although researchers are investigating potential regulatory mechanisms within infants in terms of their coping with extrauterine life, for example, the roles of primitive newborn reflexes (Allen & Capute, 1990), the autonomic nervous system (Als, 1982; Hatch, Klatt, Porges, et al., 1986; Porges, 1991, 1992; Porges & Byrne, 1992; Porges, Matthews, & Pauls, 1992) and self-stimulating behaviors (Guess & Carr, 1991), such investigations are either system-specific, completed over short time spans, or have failed to adequately account for the interactive complexity of infants' dynamic functioning.

An exciting area of self-stimulation that has received support—some research and expert opinion—is nonnutritive sucking (NNS) (Aucott, Donohue, Atkins, et al., 2002; Pinelli & Symington, 2000). Used for decades as a method of calming an infant, especially if the child was NPO (nothing by mouth) or uncomfortable, it has come into fashion as a nonpharmacologic pain management technique, included in end-of-life and palliative care protocols, and as part of developmental care (Gibbins, Stevens, Hodnett, et al., 2002). This reminds us that we have to consider whether or not this is really a benign intervention or a legitimate therapy. Proponents champion the cause of decreased length of stay and increased comfort on infants when NNS is used. Pinelli, Symington, and Ciliska, (2002) suggest that in a review of published studies and literature, no short- or long-term negative effects have been found but that the therapy has not been systematically studied.

Despite the problems with gaining clear evidence to support our practice interventions, as an outgrowth of precision-based (compared with approximation-based) research methods, work on some elements of neonatal nursing and health care has shown encouraging results. Interventions that are believed to support successful coping of preterms of varying, but not specific, gestational ages include: cue-based care rather than pre-established time regimens (Als, 1982; Als, Lawhon, Brown, et al., 1986; Horns, 1998); using oscillating waterbed floatation and individually programmed breathing teddy bears for regulating respirations (Thoman, Ingersoll, & Acebo, 1991); containing infants in flexed postures (Als, 1982; Als, Lawhon, Brown, et al., 1986); limiting bright light exposure

and dimming light intensities (Glass, 1990); curbing inappropriate and excessively loud noise levels (Thomas, 1989); clustering care activities (Shields & Tenorio, 1988); nonnutritive sucking to modulate behavioral state (Gill, Behnke, Conlon, et al., 1992; Gill, Behnke, Conlon, et al., 1988); assisting mothers with breastfeeding their preterms (Meier & Pugh, 1985); encouraging early Kangaroo care to stimulate parental involvement, proximity, and bonding (Anderson, 1991); gentle touch (Harrison, Leeper, & Yoon, 1990) and massage; (Field, 1990; Scafidi, Field, Schanberg, et al., 1991; White-Traut & Nelson, 1988; White-Traut & Pate, 1987). However, how and why such interventions become developmentally therapeutic, are processed by infants in useful ways in coping with NICU stressors, or are differentially effective in supporting maturation across gestational ages is unclear.

On the other hand, if VLBW and/or very preterm infants were best treated as fetal infants, one solution would be to create bed spaces in intensive care nurseries that are more like womb surrogates. Although it is difficult to speculate and visualize exactly how a psychophysiologic intrauterine surrogate would be designed and used, this might prove fundamental in terms of providing for the best growth and developmental outcomes and for future care related to use of perfluorocarbon liquid ventilation. With increasing technologic developments using extracorporeal membrane oxygenation (ECMO) via the umbilical cord combined with an aqueous, physiologic-surrogate uterine sac (maintaining fetal circulation within an aqueous synthetic womb until extrauterine life is advised as safe) will undoubtedly be forthcoming within the next decade.

The theoretical premise underlying the preceding and subsequent description of caregiving is that of treating the VLBW and/or very preterm infant more like a fetus than like a neonate until the infant demonstrates sufficient developmental readiness for increasing his/her extrauterine transition. Birth and the loss of the umbilical lifeline can place excessive demands on preterm infants, some of which potentially could be ameliorated. Until knowledge gaps concerning the normal characteristics of VLBW and/or very preterm extrauterine adaptation are addressed, appropriate intervention cannot be guaranteed with any degree of certainty.

## Providing Contingent Care Based on Infant Cues

Supporting much of her life's work in the assessment, intervention, and evaluation of infant outcomes, the significance of providing care based on infants' cues has been identified, emphasized, and re-emphasized by Barnard (Barnard, 1978, 1999a, 1999b; Barnard, Booth, Mitchell, & Telzrow, 1983; Barnard, Hammond, Booth, et al., 1989), one of the most well-respected nurse researchers of newborns and infants. Barnard (1990, 1999a) defines cues as nonverbal forms of communication and as special forms of communication that newborns and young infants use widely to express their needs and wants. Typically classified as being of two types, engaging or disengaging, and of two distinct levels, subtle and potent, Barnard (1999a) has pointed out that no one cue has singular value and that it is of critical importance to search for an infant's predominant cues in order to determine whether he/she is primarily engaging or disengaging.

Although not validated in intensive care settings per se, Barnard's notion of the importance of providing contingent, cue-based care is conceptually strengthened by research completed by Sander (1962); Watson (1967); Bell and Ainsworth (1972); Ainsworth, Bell, and Stayton (1974); Brazelton, Koslowski, and Main (1974); Stern (1974); Tjossem (1976); and numerous others, who have investigated the microorganization of infant and interactional behavior; infant memory and learning; infant crying and caregiver responsiveness; attachment and social development; early experiences and reciprocity; facial, vocal, and gaze behaviors of infants with their mothers; and early intervention with infants, respectively.

The obvious significance of the cue-based caregiving approach is that it is dynamic, grounded in real time, and relevant to here-and-now. This approach is in contrast with intermittent infant developmental assessments that are used to produce reports of observed infant competencies and serve as the basis for planning future caregiving. Advantages of the cue-based approach is that it is never outdated; it can be closely linked with ongoing interactions covering a variety of caregiving situations and crossing over a number of different caregivers; and it is a vital piece of developmentally appropriate care (Holditch-Davis, Blackburn, & VandenBerg, 2003; Horns, 1998). One distinct disadvantage of the approach is that it requires caregivers to be informed and educated about recognizing infant cues, as well as the importance of, and how, to provide contingent and sensitive caregiving. By strictly basing caregiving on previous developmental assessments of infants' competencies, there might be more consistency in caregiving approaches that are used, and greater planning for periods of infant rest and sleep, although at times they might be not as up-to-date or appropriate with what is going on with the infant and new abilities that previously were not evident.

In her model of caregiver and infant behavior, Barnard (1978) points out areas for caregiver focus. These include: clarity and sensitivity to an infant's cues, alleviation of an infant's distress, providing social-emotional and cognitive growth-fostering situations, and the responsiveness of an infant to a caregiver's behavior. These areas of focus help to direct caregivers to a better understanding about their specific responsibilities during interactions with infants. Furthermore, sensitive caregivers time their stimulation with infants so that their stimulation is contingent and appropriate to an infant's behavioral cues. Because newborns are believed to have memories that last approximately 5 seconds (Lewis & Goldberg, 1969; Watson, 1967), newborns who are responded to within this short period of time learn that their behaviors are important and that they, as newborns, affect people in their environments.

Although this work emanated from the late 1960s and 1970s, the principles hold true today. Incorporation of infants' cues is part of the NIDCAP® educational program and most developmental care models for health professionals and families. The extension of the work is the foundation of today's developmental care that espouses a philosophy of individualized infant and family care. It is based on recognition of infant behavioral responses to stimuli (Byers, 2003). Full-term and premature infants appear to benefit from our ability to base care on cues. The first step in this process is education of staff and caregivers (Loo, Espinosa, Tyler, et al., 2003; White, Simon, & Bryan, 2002).

Verklan (2002), in her work on physiologic variability during the transition to extrauterine life, has found that some of our assumptions about normal physiologic transition do not hold when physiologic paramenters are measured over time. Her research has found that physiologic variability is a function of the interaction of the sympathetic and parasympathetic nervous systems. However, our primary knowledge of physiologic transition was based on time periods and not patterns of interaction among variables of time (after birth), gestational age, heart and respiratory rates, oxygen saturation, and other linear and nonlinear measures. What does this research have to do with developmental, cue-based, relationship-based care? Again, the basis of developmental care is our awareness of an infant's and family's response to stimulation and to plan our care accordingly. This care should be based on cues, responses, and behaviors, not how many hours old the infant is.

## Reduced Stimulation

Infants who are hospitalized for prolonged periods of time and/or infants suffering from maternal deprivation can exhibit classic signs of institutionalized infants, such as difficulties with expressive language, insecure attachment relationships to primary caregivers, indiscriminate friendliness, and difficulty in making transitions (Carlson & Earls, 1997; Frank, Klass, Earls, & Eisenberg, 1996; Gardner, 1982; Gardner & Goldson, 2002; Spitz, 1945). Modifying the hospital environment so that it is more appropriate, or "normalizing" it, might be one way of preventing these classic institutionalized infant signs as well as improving long-term infant outcomes (Als, Duffy, & McAnulty, 1996; Mouradian & Als, 1994; Resnick, Armstrong, & Carter, 1988). Normalizing the environment begins with an evaluation of the stimuli to which the infant is exposed, with classic signs of institutionalization, or hospitalism, including flat affect, apathy, and generalized fearfulness, observed through an infant's behavior (Brown, Pearl, & Carrasco, 1991; Buehler, Als, Duffy, et al., 1995; Provence & Lipton, 1962). Infants' behavior patterns can be used as one means by which to gauge change, with environmental

and caregiving changes made to promote more desirable infant behaviors.

## Decreasing or Eliminating Inappropriate or Overstimulating NICU Experiences

Graven, Bowen, Brooten, et al. (1992a) claimed that there were three distinct areas within the NICU that needed to be studied specifically in relation to infant outcomes. These include:

1. NICU environmental and caregiving factors contribute to physiologic instability of infants and might inhibit recovery, growth, and development;
2. Parents' involvement in NICU caregiving and parents' bonding to their infants are essential to infants' long-term development, but parents' involvement and bonding are adversely affected by the NICU environment;
3. Considerably more sophisticated methods are required to examine questions related to NICU environmental factors and infants' adverse neurologic outcomes.

## NICU Environmental and Caregiving Factors

To isolate some clinical examples that highlight the first area identified by Graven, Bowen, Brooten, et al. (1992a), one could examine the sensory environmental inputs included within NICU sounds, lighting, and tactile handling. The NICU has been shown to have sound levels that can be excessively high and potentially hazardous enough to be classified as pollutants (Cornell & Gottfried, 1976; Gottfried, Wallace-Lande, Sherman-Brown, et al., 1981). Researchers have documented NICU sound levels ranging from 50 to 120 decibels (dB) (Long, Lucey, & Philip, 1980; Thomas, 1989). Ninety decibels is the highest sound level that does not produce measurable damage, irrespective of duration (Lotas, 1992). As pointed out by Thomas (1989), loud sounds or prolonged exposure to sounds up to 120 dB are not uncommon in NICUs, which can permanently damage the cochlea. In fact, in VLBW infants, who typically require prolonged intensive care to survive, the incidence of sensorineural hearing loss is three and a half times higher than in LBW infants who are between 1501 and 2500 g in birthweight and require shorter stays in NICUs (Thiringer,

Kankkunen, Liden, & Niklasson, 1984). Exposure to bright light intensities is not uncommon for all infants cared for in NICUs. The range of ambient light levels has been reported to range from 35 to 190 foot-candles (ftc); however, most preterm infants cared for in NICUs are exposed to additional light sources, owing to natural light exposure from outside windows, their need for frequent diagnostic procedures, and frequent routine nursing procedures (Glass, Avery, Subramania, et al., 1985). Illumination levels recommended for business offices are 40 to 50 ftc (Lotas, 1992). The AAP contends that the maximum light needed for most procedures is a maximum of 60 ftc (Hauth & Merenstein, 1997). The *Recommended Standards for Newborn ICU Design* (White, 2002) recommends that ambient lighting be held between 1 to 60 ftc. When procedural lighting is needed, it should be adjustable, directed, and afford protection to any infants adjacent. Research has shown significantly higher incidences of retinopathy of prematurity (ROP) in preterms exposed to higher levels of ambient illumination (Glass, Avery, Subramania, et al., 1985). But in the past decade, STOP ROP studies and other research projects continue to probe the association of light exposure and ROP or other eye damage (Fielder & Moseley, 2000; Fielder & Reynolds, 2001; Phelps & Watts, 2001; Reynolds, Dobson, Quinn, et al., 2002; Winslow & Jacobson, 1999). Light exposure is also being examined for its role in stimulating positive growth and development (Brandon, Holditch-Davis, & Belyea, 2002). The premise is that cycled lighting promotes infant growth. So the aspect of light can be both positive and negative but is an important part of developmental care.

Handling or disturbing an infant, whether she is asleep or awake, every 20 to 30 minutes has been characteristic and documented within NICU caregiving environments (Korones, 1976). This handling frequency might be associated with high patient acuities, given that nurses are typically assigned to care for a two–NICU infant patient assignment. Frequent touching and/or disturbing infants enough to rouse them to obtain a blood sample, administering or regulating intravenous therapies of one type or another, and performing chest auscultation, physiotherapy, or endotracheal suctioning has resulted in a state of disorganization (High &

Gorski, 1985), sleep deprivation (Gottfried, 1985), and hypoxemia (Long, Philip, & Lucey, 1980). In contrast to these high degrees of auditory, visual, tactile, and handling stimulation associated with NICU environments, according to Gottfried (1985) and Blackburn and Barnard (1985), NICU infants receive infrequent social and soothing experiences. These findings might be explained by the severity of illness of these infants, the absence of oral feedings, the NICU culture, and the current knowledge base available pertaining to preterm infants' needs for these experiences.

Current research is focusing on the impact of stress mediated by individualized care on length of stay, complications, hormonal and chemical values, such as cortisol, growth hormone, and other factors associated with a physiologic stress response, and long-term outcomes. Byers (2003), in a summary article, reviews the evidence that we have acquired over the past few decades to support the need for developmental care related to infant and family responses. The difficulty with this area of research is due to lack of randomized clinical trials and the compounding variables of prenatal exposure to factors that resulted in a premature or sick infant's birth. Perlman (2002) acknowledges this difficulty in the report on cognitive and behavioral deficits in graduates of the NICU. The other area that has grown from the foundation of the need for soothing stimuli to enhance outcomes is in the area of pain. There is mounting evidence to support a rewiring of the infant's brain when exposed to painful treatments without proper intervention (Grunau, 2002). Another difficulty in this area is the actual measurement of pain (Gallo, 2003). Thanks to many devoted researchers and clinicians from several disciplines, we are making tremendous progress in this area.

## Parents' Involvement in NICU Caregiving and Parents' Bonding to Their Infants

To present some examples that address the second area circumscribed by Graven, Bowen, Brooten, et al. (1992a), one could look at the physical set-up of the NICU environment in terms of encouraging parental involvement and facilitating bonding. The experience of being cared for in an NICU might itself predispose infants of all gestations to disturbances in emotional well-being. The average length of stay in NICUs is somewhere between 15 to 20 days, with infants weighing less than 1.5 kg averaging a minimum of 40 days. Although family members are encouraged to visit their infants while they are being cared for in NICU settings, normal patterns of family member interactions have not been documented as being established easily with NICU infants who are preterm (Brown, Gennaro, York, et al., 1991; Minde, Whitelaw, Brown, et al., 1983). Parental visitation can be discouraged by inadequate social and emotional support for parents by neonatal nurses (Gottfried, 1985), the infants' confining bed space of 80 to 100 sq ft, lack of family privacy, and infants' daily caregiving activities being completed primarily by NICU nurses instead of by the infants' parents (Casteel, 1990). Parents' needs might go unmet in that: (1) they might not be helped to feel comfortable with the surrounding technology (McGrath, 2000); (2) they feel unwanted at their infant's bedside; (3) they are given inadequate information regarding activities that they could be doing while at the bedside; (4) they are not given recommendations concerning which sections of parent NICU information books, such as *Neonatal Intensive Care: What Every Parent Needs to Know* (Zaichkin, 2002) they could be reading to supplement their growing knowledge. In addition, a mother's concerns are representative of her needs at any given time and likely impact on her infant. It has been shown that unless a mother's own needs are met, a mother might be unable to meet the needs of her infant (Bull, 1981). Therefore, if a mother's needs preclude her infant's needs and are one precondition to her meeting her infant's needs and, therefore, her needs, addressing maternal concerns become an integral part of an infant's needs and subsequent developmental progress.

The importance of family involvement has been long associated with teaching mothers and female caregivers while in the NICU and during immediate follow-up. But more recently, fathers have received attention. Researchers such as Boechler, Harrison, and Magill-Evans (2003) and Shawn Pohlman (see Chapter 19 for more information on her research) are adding to our knowledge of the important role fathers have in individualized developmental care.

## Considerably More Sophisticated Methods Are Required

The third area delineated by Graven, Bowen, Brooten, et al. (1992a) can be illustrated by examining the methods of assessing NICU environmental factors in relation to infants' adverse neurologic outcomes. Neurologic outcomes can be evaluated using measures such as neurologic reflexes, head ultrasounds, intracranial pressure readings, measures of cerebral blood flow, and nuclear magnetic resonance images (Volpe, 2001). Using head ultrasounds to screen 85% of 1765 VLBW infants delivered at seven NICUs between 1987 and 1988, Hack, Breslau, Weissman, et al. (1991) found that 45% had experienced either a periventricular or parenchymal hemorrhage, of which 18% were severe. However, how environmental variables related to these intracranial hemorrhages was not specified because Hack, Breslau, Weissman, et al. did not evaluate environmental variables. Similarly, in other studies reporting the incidence of major neurologic sequelae, such as hydrocephalus, intracranial hemorrhage, hypoxic or ischemic encephalopathy, periventricular leukomalacia, cerebral palsy, neurosensory hearing loss, retinopathy of prematurity, and mental retardation (Fitzhardinge, Pape, Arstikaitis, et al., 1976; Grogaard, Lindstrom, Parker, et al., 1990; Hirata, Epcar, Walsh, et al., 1983), the influence of NICU environmental variables were not measured or discussed. As noted by Linn, Horowitz, Buddin, et al. (1985), studying the NICU environment is a difficult, tedious, and cumbersome task. Moreover, neurologic sequelae, such as those mentioned previously, have been associated most strongly with young gestational ages (Bowen, 1992; Boyce, Smith, & Castro, 1999). Researchers have demonstrated that the lower the gestational age, the more likely the infant was to have had a prolonged NICU stay and to have experienced a larger "dose" of the NICU environment.

The problem of dealing with the complexity of infants' neurologic functioning is potentiated by the fact that infant assessment itself is a very complex process. Completing infant assessments facilitates understanding of infants' change over time. Thus, caregivers can diagnose health problems and meet infants' short-term goals, establish significant positive and negative baseline parameters essential for identifying infants' needs, and meet infants' long-term goals of general well-being and health.

## ENVIRONMENTAL NEONATOLOGY AS A DISCIPLINE IN ITS OWN RIGHT

Environmental Neonatology was introduced first by Gottfried and Gaiter (1985) in the title of a book on infant stress in intensive care. Defined as the study of the effects of newborn intensive care facilities and microenvironments on the growth, development, behavior, and health conditions of infants, it has been thought to constitute an applied discipline in its own right (Wolke, 1987a). Prior to use of this new disciplinary category, there were both informal and formal concerns that the implementation of technologic and medical advances had outpaced considerations made regarding the psychosocial, emotional, and behavioral development of sick infants in hospitals (Korones, 1976; Lawson, Daum, & Turkewitz, 1977; Lucey, 1977), although little was being done to formally address these concerns.

Environmental Neonatology is an outgrowth of diverse neonatal research investigations, including neonatal environmental studies (Barnard & Bee, 1983; Korner, Guilleminault, Van den Hoed, & Baldwin, 1978; Tuck, Monin, Duvivier, et al., 1982), basic research of sensorimotor responses of full-term and preterm newborns (Field, 1977; Leijon, 1982; Palmer, Dubowitz, Bercholte, et al., 1982), iatrogenic sequelae resulting from medical treatments (Greenough, Dixon, & Robertson, 1984; Keating, 1976; Nelson, 1976), and the architectural design of NICUs (Korones, 1985). Today, however, much of the field of inquiry comprising Environmental Neonatology has been integrated with developmental caregiving (Wolke, 1987b), such that Environmental Neonatology is not considered in isolation, but instead as both a valid backdrop for and part of whatever caregiving activities are being completed or planned. For example, Als's (1981, 1984, 1991) NIDCAP® write-ups include recommendations for the nursery environment at large, bed space and bedding, and direct caregiver interactions based on each infants' current developmental competencies and goals.

Additionally, Environmental Neonatology can be subdivided further into those elements comprising early experiences of infants within the NICU. These include: the physical nursery structure, functional organization, levels of care, caregiving procedures and events, caregiver behavior, diurnal periodicity, heat transfer, thermoregulation, humidification, air velocity, illumination, phototherapy, sound levels and types, social contacts, medical-nursing contacts, handling, touch, vestibular-kinesthetic stimulation, family participation, infant behaviors, infant states, infant state modulation, gases, disinfectants, parenteral solutions, and pharmaceuticals.

### "Generic" Developmental Care Practices

To some extent, Environmental Neonatology has been translated and reduced to that provided by broad-spectrum, or generic, care practices. "Generic" developmental care tends to be equated with setting up environmental conditions that can be generalized across infants, irrespective of their developmental status. Examples of these types of practices are keeping an infant housed within an isolette or incubator routinely instead of in a radiant warmer bed, using blankets to create a nest for the infant, talking softly, keeping the lights in the room dimmed, covering the isolette or incubator to shield the infant from light, positioning an infant using blanket rolls, clustering caregiving activities to promote longer time blocks of uninterrupted rest, and only minimally handling the infant (McGrath & Conliffe-Torres, 1996; McGrath & Valenzuela, 1994; Young, 1996). These practices cut corners for practicing nurses, in that they do not require a developmental assessment of the infant to be implemented, but still appear to be developmentally appropriate in addressing issues involving the caregiving environment at large, bed space and bedding, and general issues relevant to direct caregiving. Because these generic practices are not specific to the behavioral cues or competencies of infants on an individual basis, they may or may not be precisely or sufficiently addressing most of their needs and developmental goals. However, given some of the recent success with Wee Care® products (Children's Medical Ventures, Norwell, MA) (Jorgensen, 2002), it might not matter. Generic developmental care might be an adequate treatment to meet most infants' goals without becoming more specific. The appropriateness of generic developmental care will not be known and cannot be ascertained without additional randomized clinical trials that will be difficult to systematically implement given the widespread use of many of these interventions. But our evidence is growing (Byers, 2003).

## Infant and Environmental Assessments

As suggested by the world-renowned mathematician Zadeh (1990), more than a decade ago in his construct of fuzzy logic, because complexity and fuzziness are positively correlated, approximations, rather than precise assessments, might be what are really needed to understand the complex and uncertain situations surrounding the care of VLBW and very preterm infants in NICUs. Such approximations might be achieved using time series and spectral analyses of longitudinal infant and environmental data. For example, when one considers some of the more subtle types of developmental disabilities experienced by VLBW and very preterm infants, it seems possible that if one tracked the development of disabilities across time, that some might be explained by asynchronous rhythmic functioning in response to environmental stimuli. Specifically, in dyslexia, the way that children use their eyes in combination with their ears is such that when they attempt to read, they do not visually lock in and hear what is being read but instead lump words in ways that the words do not make sense. For example, this asynchronous rhythmic functioning might have developed earlier in infancy as a response to overly stressful or incomprehensible stimuli that were part of being cared for in an intensive care nursery.

Use of chaos theory (Lorenz, 1963, 1993; Williams, 1997) and its accompanying nonlinear, dynamic mathematical solutions might be another complex avenue called upon as part of developing the sophisticated methods recommended by Graven, Bowen, Brooten, et al. (1992a) in exploring NICU environmental factors and infants' adverse neurologic outcomes over time. Chaos is no longer a new field, a fad, or a dead end. It is based on the rock-solid foundation of physics, Newton's laws, and nonlinear, nonintegral equations, the solution of which requires an appreciation of unstable behavior, new mathematical tools, and the advent of computer visualization. Williams (1997) and a list of other mathematicians

too long to mention believe that chaos methods can be extended to understanding complex social and environmental systems as well as neural networks. This might be another piece of the frontier awaiting NICU caregivers in the coming years.

## Sensitivity and Specificity

The complexity of infant assessments brings up the added issues of sensitivity and specificity. The sensitivity of an assessment is the ability to correctly identify all persons with the condition, problem, or disease. If developmental assessments are insensitive, there will be false negatives, leading to an under-referral for developmental problems. Likewise, if assessments are hypersensitive, there will be false positives, leading to over-referral. The issues of economics and cost-effectiveness of the assessments themselves enters into both situations.

The specificity of an assessment is its ability to identify all persons without the condition, problem, or disease in a stated population, the true positives and the true negatives, so that patients are not "over" treated. This concept is particularly important for case finding and for controlling the cost of case finding. To provide for economic balance in relation to possible expenditures for health care as a whole, case finding needs to be a continuing process and not a "once-and-for-all" endeavor.

All of the preceding concerns about assessing infant outcomes along with the environmental concerns discussed by Graven, Bowen, Brooten, et al. (1992a)—the physiologic instability of the infant; restricted parental involvement/disrupted parental bonding; and the need for more sophisticated methods—might be studied using approaches that combine ecology and technology. What is clear from prior infant outcome studies is that the present methods have had shortcomings that must be dealt with to prevent inaccurate assessments and unwise decision-making with respect to interventions for individual infants cared for in NICUs. It is also clear that there is a complexity inherent in describing the behavioral patterns of VLBW and very preterm infants that has not been adequately addressed. The use of a combined ecologic and technologic approach to studying preterm infants might be one valid way of addressing both infants' biobehavioral complexities and dynamic functioning. This approach might lead to

ghts into the initial manifestations and differ-
ong infants' outcomes, be invaluable in terms
of the prevention of subsequent developmental disorders, as well as be consistent with at least five items on
the prevention agenda of the nation established as
*Healthy People 2010* (U.S. Department of Health and
Human Services, 2000):

11.2 Reduce the prevalence of serious mental
retardation among school-aged children to no
more than 2 per 1000 children.

14.1 Reduce the infant mortality rate to no more
than seven per 1000 live births.

14.9 Increase to at least 75% the proportion of
mothers who breastfeed their babies in the early
postpartum period and to at least 50% the proportion who continue breastfeeding until their babies
are 5 to 6 months old.

22.1 Develop a set of health status indicators
appropriate for federal, state, and local health agencies and establish use of the set in at least 40 states.

22.4.1 Develop and implement a national process to
identify significant gaps in the Nation's disease prevention and health promotion data, including data
for racial and ethnic minorities, people with low
incomes, and people with disabilities, and establish
mechanisms to meet these needs.

In general, developmental care implemented based
on use of the NIDCAP® and APIB have shown
improved subsequent infant functioning in terms of
shorter lengths of hospital stay, fewer days of high
acuity intensive care, and reduced hospital costs (Als,
et al., 1986, 1994, 1996; Buehler, Als, Duffy, et al, 1995;
Fleisher, VandenBerg, Constantinou, et al, 1995;
Mouradian & Als, 1994). The major disadvantages
have been that, due to the start up costs of implementing and evaluating developmental care on an ongoing
basis, samples have been small, sites have been few, and
neither samples nor sites have been randomly selected.
Of six studies based on Als' developmental tools, only
5 NICUs in the United States have been involved in
clinical trials out of more than 130 existing tertiary
level NICUs (U.S. Department of Statistics, 1998). The
respective samples in these studies have included: 8
control and 8 treatment, 21 control and 24 treatment,
18 randomly assigned control and 20 randomly
assigned treatment, 13 randomly assigned control and
12 randomly assigned treatment participants. Samples
have been evaluated to generalize concerning populations at large. However, to be sure that samples are
truly representative of the population to which one
desires to generalize, samples must be selected randomly (Campbell & Stanley, 1963).

Improvements, developmental and otherwise,
that have been detected include:

1. Better autonomic functioning, present and future
2. Better motor functioning, present and future
3. Better state functioning, present and future
4. Improvement in brain functioning as seen using
   brain electrical activity mapping (BEAM)
5. Faster weight gain
6. Required fewer days of total parenteral nutrition
   (TPN)
7. Began enteral feedings earlier
8. Required fewer days of oxygen therapy
9. Improved lung functioning
10. Was younger in age than those previously upon
    discharge from the hospital
11. Required fewer days of ICU care
12. Duration of hospital stay was shorter
13. Improved mental performance on Bayley
    Mental Development Index (MDI) at 9 months
14. Improved psychomotor performance on Bayley
    Physical Development Index (PDI) at 9 months
15. Lower patient hospital costs

Other dynamic considerations that address consumer issues involving empowerment and family
satisfaction could greatly enhance the need for developmental care. Additional advantages to families and
the infants that are highly likely but have not been
evaluated involve:

I. Parental participation in routine baby care
II. Parental participation in more specialized care-
giving
III. Privacy issues viewed as important relative to
baby
IV. Parental communication with caregivers
V. Caregiver communication with and about baby
VI. Special caregiver attentiveness
VII. Parental social interactions with baby

The reason for these measurement oversights is a
direct reflection of the degree of difficulty with measurement, as identified earlier by Graven, Bowen,
Brooten, et al. (1992a) as an area needing further
study. Because dollar figures cannot be directly

attributed to any of these factors, and the fact that evaluation and documentation would require additional observations and tool development, these important areas have yet to be explored.

## FAMILY-CENTERED CARE

The movement today is to forge partnerships with parents/caregivers to provide continuing care, ease the transition to home from the NICU, and to improve long-term outcomes for both infant and family. Developmental, individualized care is a philosophy that embraces the family as a partner, not a visitor or an appendage of the infant, but an integral part of the healthcare plan. Chapters in this text are devoted to family issues and inclusion of the family including the father (see Chapters 18 and 19).

Ashpaugh and Leick-Rude (1999) conducted a survey of NICUs in the United States to determine how many used the developmental care approach for care. They found that 64% of all the NICUs practiced developmental care with another 24% indicating they were planning its incorporation in the future. Despite the high numbers, Griffin (2003) acknowledges that many of our institutional policies put a distance between the infant and their families. Moore, Coker, DuBuisson, et al. (2003) conducted a multisite study to examine use of family-centered care in the NICU. Four areas were examined. They were: the unit's vision and philosophy, unit culture, family participation in care, and the consideration of families as advisors. They found that although units espoused support of visitation policies, lack of ties to personnel education and performance indicators, and the unit's culture regarding family participation still acted as barriers to the implementation of family-centered care. Therefore, it appears that much work is needed in this area to move from a philosophy of care on the "books" and one that is truly implemented.

## ECONOMICS OF HEALTH CARE
### Business Factors
### Budgeting for Start-Up and Maintenance of Developmental Care

Few NICUs would say, if asked, that they do not incorporate some aspect of developmental care into their daily practice. However, to move toward a fully integrated developmental care approach or adopt an approach, such as that of NIDCAP®, or onsite training, such as that offered by Children's Medical Ventures or Ohmeda Medical, a substantial amount of money would be needed to train staff and change the environment. This initial start up cost is high, and the maintenance can be as well if there is a high turnover in staff. Developmental care teams are used in some units. In those cases, these positions become line item budget costs that must be part of an overall developmental care operating cost. These are recurring costs that in most institutions must be justified to continue. The justification is normally through cost savings and increased consumer satisfaction. However, ongoing educational and support costs must be considered in addition to salaries and fringe benefits. A difficulty with justifying these positions according to some administrators has been the lack of clarity of the roles that various team members play—no standardized job descriptions tend to exist nor do fully developed standards of care to guide such a team (Ashpaugh, Leick-Rude, & Kilbride, 1999). Much remains to be considered if developmental care is to be implemented.

Developmental care can be done on various levels, as indicated in other sections of this chapter at the macro level—unit structural design or micro level—at the infant's bedside and the immediate environment. In either case, to make an informed decision about how and to what degree to implement developmental care, an economic model should be applied.

To determine if developmental care makes a difference in costs, preimplementation data should be collected regarding outcomes. The typical benchmarks for outcomes of care include: laboratory and diagnostic tests; procedures; complications—short-term such as infection rates and long-term such as learning problems; hearing deficits; musculoskeletal problems; length of stay; days to full feedings; ventilator days; growth parameters; and parent satisfaction (Ohmeda Medical, 2003). Each of these benchmarks has a cost attached to it and has the potential of a cost savings after introduction of a new therapy such as developmental care. For example, in 1994, Als, Lawhon, Duffy, et al. reported a comparison study of traditional versus developmental care. The sample was very small but the findings suggested the length of stay was almost cut in half and almost $90,000 in savings were realized, when developmental care according to the NIDCAP® approach was introduced. The premise behind NIDCAP® is that relationship-based, developmentally supportive care will result in more positive, cost-effective outcomes for infants and their families (Als & Gilkerson, 1997; Als, 1998). However, the criticism of all developmental care programs has been that they have failed to help NICUs examine the cost-effectiveness of these models in relationship to short- and long-term outcomes.

Another consideration of the economics of developmental care is the need to cost out the survey development, distribution, and analyzation of data that must occur if benchmarking and outcomes measurement are to be part of the organizational culture. For example, there is more emphasis today in health care on consumer satisfaction. Although neonatal and pediatric health professionals have prided themselves on their involvement of parents/families in care, the measurement of their satisfaction has usually been part of an overall continuous quality improvement program and not aimed at looking at any particular aspect of care. Pink, Murray, and McKillop (2003) examined hospital efficiency and patient satisfaction. This study was an example of a hospital-wide effort at measuring satisfaction and not aimed at any one aspect. Yet their findings suggested that efficiency of an environment and satisfaction were not linked. What does this have to do with infants, families, and developmental care? The same principle holds true in most NICUs—the emphasis or survey done by a hospital to measure patient/family satisfaction does not necessarily get at the unit level of factors that contribute to the variable satisfaction. Family satisfaction as part of the consumer involvement in health care is very important, when developmental care with family as a central feature is considered.

a. Family empowerment has been an important aspect of developmental care. Treating parents as partners and not visitors in the NICUs has been espoused in the literature for the past decade. But what does it mean? That depends on the family and their cultural values and beliefs. Participation in care for one family might be of tantamount importance but to another just being at the bedside and not "responsible" for the care might be enough to empower them to voice concerns. Aspects that should be considered include family participation in routine care, such as bathing, feeding, and diaper changes. Some families might want to learn specific aspects of care, such as suctioning, nasogastric feedings, and dressing changes. The level of family participation should be determined by the family and health professional—working together, on an individualized plan of care. The privacy of the family must also be considered. Some might want to participate in group-parent support group activities whereas others want to remain by themselves not sharing all aspects of the infant's problems with others. These needs must be respected. In turn, communication with the family should be done in a private place or area where conversations, questions, and concerns cannot be overheard by others in the unit. If the parent/family cannot be present, there are video connections with some units now where families can view their infants in the privacy of their own home or get updated information via a private website. Few units have these capabilities, but these aspects of keeping the family informed are other areas that must be costed out in terms of infant and family outcomes as well as the comparison to start-up costs for such technology.

b. Observations of the family interacting with their infants or the questions that they pose to the healthcare professionals are other aspects of outcomes of care in need of study. Sometimes these observations lead to a better understanding of how well the family is coping with their infant's illness or their understanding of care—even to the point of knowing what follow-up care is necessary for them after discharge.

c. The key to the "economics" of developmental care is tied to the need for research to determine what is effective—physiologically, psychologically, and fiscally sound interventions. Systematic, controlled trials would be the ideal, but because of the nature of neonatal care and the fact that in many instances it would be unethical to withhold or try an unproven treatment, most neonatal studies represent convenience, small samples of infants and families, leaving the findings suspect. Worse yet, the approach or successful intervention in one setting might not work in another NICU. Mirmiran, Baldwin, and Ariagno (2003) found that environmental lighting had no effect on infant circadian rhythms. This finding is the opposite of other experts' theories. Does this mean we ignore these findings or the previous ones? No. It means we need more replicated studies to determine the factors that influence circadian rhythm. That is a given of our modern NICU. Some of the examples of studies that have been done that need to be re-examined include: Als, Lawhon, Duffy, et al. (1994); Bray, Shields, Wolcott, et al. (1969); Caine (1991); Coleman, Practt, Stoddar, et al., (1998); Hack, Breslau, Weissman, et al. (1991); Peters, 1999; Petryshen, Stevens, Hawkins, et al. (1997); Schwartz, Ritchie, Sacks, et al. (1997); and Walsh-Sukys, Reitenbach, Hudson-Barr, et al. (2001). This situation should not discourage us from trying to replicate studies, do randomized controlled trials when possible, and gain more evidence to support our care. We must apply standards to our care, use practice guidelines that are evidence based, and then test their efficacy in our settings. We can no longer afford to take an approach to care just because it "feels right." We need evidence and the economic principles to support our change in practice. It is another challenge of modern health care that those involved in developmental care must face.

## SCOPE OF PRACTICE— DEVELOPMENTAL CARE

Developmental care application is far-reaching in scope. Implications for direct and indirect caregivers in the NICU have to be addressed regarding impact on infants, the environment, and the competency in the delivery of developmental care. Changing the model of care from the traditional clinically focused model to individual family and neonatal supportive care requires that NICUs evaluate and reorganize every aspect of care delivery. Moving from procedure-guided care to process-guided care necessitates a complete change in thinking and caregiving practices that affects every aspect of the NICU environment, from development of protocols and purchasing of equipment to staffing and interaction among caregivers and families. With such enormous scope of practice, developmental care is not accomplished quickly or without great introspection, education, analysis, planning, preparation, and implementation. From policy to individual staff competency, the commitment to Developmental Care must be evident. As the survey previously cited by Ashpaugh and Leick-Rude (1999) implies, ties to performance evaluations, unit culture, and education of staff and caregivers are essential if developmental care is to be fully implemented into the NICU.

Several organizations, including NANN (1993, 2001), have published guidelines for the delivery of developmental care, which include the family-centered care component.

Standards that are consistently emerging include:
1. Individualized, flexible, hands-on care
2. Recognition and responsiveness to each infant's competencies, vulnerabilities, and thresholds
3. Developmentally supportive infant environment
4. Support of the parent-infant relationship
5. Recognizing parents' rights and ownership of their infant
6. Collaborative interdisciplinary practice by all caregivers

A coordinated plan of discharge care must be developed and implemented by health professionals and the family, if the impact on outcomes is to be optimal (Robinson, Pirak, & Morrell, 2000). Thigpen (2002) suggests that developmental care principles need to be applied to develop resuscitation standards for the delivery room and NICU. In her article, Thigpen offers guidelines for consideration of physiologic and developmental care needs during resuscitation efforts. Another study reports the need for awareness of physiologic stability in relationship to oxygen saturation using an individualized approach versus standard guidelines (Harrison, Berbaum, Stem, et al. (2001). What does this have to do with "standards" and scope of practice of developmental care? This study and the other articles presented earlier indicate the need for NICUs to adopt guidelines of developmental care and standards of care that are formulated at a unit, institution, state, or national level that are embedded in individualized, family-centered, developmental care (IFDC).

Standards and guidelines for IFDC must include accountability of the caregiver, consistency of the caregiver, awareness and inclusion of sensitivity to infant and family cues in relationship to behavioral responses, and use of interventions based on individualized needs, not arbitrary schedules for treatments or broad physiologic parameters that do not consider individualized differences.

## INTENSIVE CARE NURSERY DESIGN STANDARDS AND DEVELOPMENTAL CARE

Since the time of Florence Nightingale, who recognized the importance of the environment, we have included factors of light, sound, smell, and touch into care. But, have we? If you are a supporter of individualized, family-centered, developmental care, the answer is "yes." However, often the NICU environment, or, rather, its design, is not conducive to positive growth and development of the infant and family. Several national healthcare groups recognized the need for standards and guidelines to assist in better patient outcomes. From the 1970s and the leadership of March of Dimes to create healthier perinatal/neonatal outcomes in their publication *Towards Improving the Outcome of Pregnancy* (White Plains, NY), to the American Academy of Pediatrics and American College of Obstetricians and Gynecologists (AAP/ACOG) *Guidelines for Perinatal Care* (Elk Grove Village, IL), the momentum started to look at the patient, family, and environment together when planning/implementing care.

Dr. Stanley Graven, an eminent neonatologist, also recognized years ago that the physical environment of the high-risk infant and family was critical to neonatal care and outcomes. He and the University of South Florida at Tampa, Florida, sponsor a conference each year devoted to this topic.

With his help, and national funding from Ross Planning Associates/Ross Products Division/Abbott Laboratories, a task force grew that now has international prominence. This group is the Committee to Establish Recommended Standards for Newborn ICU Design under the leadership of Robert White, neonatologist. This interdisciplinary group, including architects, infection control specialists, infant developmental specialists, family advocates, nurses, and physicians, reviews the recommendations and updates every 2 to 3 years. This group is part of the Graven conference each year to gain visibility for the need to consider the design of the NICU to foster positive developmental outcomes and to look at the effects the environment has on the caregiver. These recommendations can be found at *www.nd.edu/kkolberg/~DesignStandards.htm*. The standards addressed by this group are:

1. Unit configuration
2. NICU location within the hospital
3. Minimum area, clearances, and privacy
4. Electric and gas supplies, and mechanical needs
5. Isolation rooms
6. Family entry and reception area
7. Scrub areas
8. General support space
9. Staff support space
10. Parent-infant rooms
11. Family support
12. Ancillary needs
13. Administrative space
14. Ambient lighting in infant care areas
15. Procedural lighting in infant care areas
16. Illumination of support areas
17. Daylighting
18. Floor surfaces
19. Wall surfaces
20. Countertops, casework, and cabinetry
21. Ceiling finishes
22. Ambient temperature and ventilation
23. Noise abatement
24. Safety/infant security

These standards are all related to the NICU environment and, ultimately, its impact on infant and family health outcomes. This listing is intended to serve as a framework for the rest of this book, which develops central tenets of these standards as they relate to individualized family-centered developmental care.

## THE FUTURE OF DEVELOPMENTAL CARE

Obviously, this text is an example of the view that individualized, family-centered developmental care is not a fad or a trend that will pass, but a philosophy of care that can impact positively on the infant and family. The support of a national organization such as NANN to gather interdisciplinary experts, including families to present the "core knowledge" necessary to embrace this philosophy, presents a strong case for the belief that this form of care is the "right thing to do." It embraces the physiologic principles, psychosocial measures, and holistic principles of the mind-body connection. Its research base still needs work. Harrigan, Ratliffe, Patrinos, et al. (2002) acknowledge the methodologic problems of studying medically fragile infants and present a thorough review of the literature available on the topic. They and others do not suggest that we should not continue to try to gain the evidence we need to support or refute aspects of developmental care.

The areas of developmental care that have received the most attention and research are identified by Byers (2003) as follows: management of the environment, clustering of care, nonnutritive sucking, co-bedding of multiples, kangaroo care, swaddling of infants, and family-centered care. These areas form the pillars of developmental care and are covered in detail in the remainder of this text. As acknowledged by many who embrace developmental care, this is a journey in the frontiers of neonatal, infant, and family care. We must continue this journey.

## CONCLUSION

This chapter has set the stage for the rest of this text. It provides an overview of individualized, family-centered, developmental care and the various aspects that must be considered.

## REFERENCES

Ainsworth, M.D., Bell, S.M., & Stayton, D. (1974). Infant-mother attachment and social development: Socialization as a product of reciprocal responsiveness to signals. In M. Richards (Ed.), *The integration of the child into a social world* (pp. 99-135). Cambridge, England: Cambridge University Press.

Allen, M.C., & Capute, A.J. (1990). Tone and reflex development before term. *Pediatrics, 85*(3)(Pt 2), 393-399.

Als, H. (1979). Social interaction: Dynamic matrix for developing behavioral organization. *New Directions for Child Development, 4,* 21-39.

Als, H. (1981). *A manual for the naturalistic observation of the newborn (preterm and full-term).* Cambridge, MA: Harvard Medical School.

Als, H. (1982). Toward a synactive theory of development: Promise for the assessment of infant individuality. *Infant Mental Health Journal, 3,* 229-243.

Als, H. (1984). *A manual for the naturalistic observation of the newborn (preterm and full-term).* Cambridge, MA: Harvard Medical School.

Als, H. (1986). A synactive model of neonatal behavioral organization: Framework for the assessment of neurobehavioral development in the premature infant and for the support of infants and parents in the neonatal intensive care environment. *Physical & Occupational Therapy in Pediatrics, 6,* 3-53.

Als, H. (1991). *A manual for the naturalistic observation of the newborn (preterm and full-term).* Cambridge, MA: Harvard Medical School.

Als, H. (1998). Developmental care in the newborn intensive care unit. *Current Opinion in Pediatrics, 10,* 138-142.

Als, H., Duffy, F.H., & McAnulty, G.B. (1988a). Behavioral differences between preterm and full-term newborns as measured with the APIB system scores: I. *Infant Behavior & Development, 11,* 305-318.

Als, H., Duffy, F.H., & McAnulty, G.B. (1988b). The APIB, an assessment of functional competence in preterm and full-term newborns regardless of gestational age at birth: II. *Infant Behavior & Development, 11,* 319-331.

Als, H., Duffy, F.H., & McAnulty, G.B. (1996). Effectiveness of individualized neurodevelopmental care in the newborn intensive care unit (NICU). *Acta Paediatrica, 416*(Suppl), 21-30.

Als, H., & Gilkerson, L. (1997). The role of relationship-based developmentally supportive newborn intensive care in strengthening outcome of preterm infants. *Seminars in Perinatology, 21*(3), 178-189.

Als, H., Lawhon, G., Brown, E., et al. (1986). Individualized behavioral and environmental care for the very low birth weight preterm infant at high risk for bronchopulmonary dysplasia: neonatal intensive care unit and developmental outcome. *Pediatrics, 78,* 1123-1132.

Als, H., Lawhon, G., Duffy, F.H., et al. (1994). Individualized developmental care for the very low-birth-weight preterm infant. Medical and neurofunctional effects. *Journal of the American Medical Association (JAMA), 272*(2), 853-858.

Als, H., Lester, B.M., Tronick, E.C., & Brazelton, T.B. (1980). Towards a research instrument for the assessment of preterm infant's behavior (A.P.I.B.). In H.E. Fitzgerald, B.M. Lester, & M.W. Yogman (Eds.), *Theory and research in behavioral pediatrics* (Vol. I, pp. 35-63). New York: Plenum Press.

Als, H., Lester, B.M., Tronick, E., & Brazelton, T.B. (1982). Manual for the assessment of preterm infant's behavior (APIB). *Theory and Research in Behavioral Pediatrics, 1,* 65-132.

Anderson, G.C. (1991). Current knowledge about skin-to-skin (kangaroo) care for preterm infants. *Journal of Perinatology, 11*(3), 216-226.

Ashpaugh, A., & Leick-Rude, M.K. (1999). Developmental care teams in the neonatal intensive care unit: Survey on current status. *Journal of Perinatology, 19*(1), 48-52.

Ashpaugh, J.B., Leick-Rude, M.K., & Kilbride, H.W. (1999). Developmental care teams in the neonatal intensive care unit: Survey on current status. *Journal of Perinatology, 19*(1), 48-52.

Aucott, S., Donohue, P.K., Atkins, E., et al. (2002). Neurodevelopmental care in the NICU. *Mental Retardation & Developmental Disabilities Research Reviews, 8*(4), 298-308.

Aylward, G.P., & Pfeiffer, S.L. (1989). Follow-up and outcome of low birthweight infants: Conceptual issues and a methodology review. *Australian Paediatric Journal, 25*(1), 3-5.

Aylward, G.P., Verhulst, S.J., & Bell, S. (1989). Correlation of asphyxia and other risk factors with outcome: A contemporary view. *Developmental Medicine & Child Neurology, 31*(3), 329-340.

Barnard, K.E. (1978). *Nursing child assessment training instructor's learning manual.* Unpublished manuscript available from the University of Washington, School of Nursing, Seattle, WA.

Barnard, K.E. (1990). *Keys to caregiving study guide.* Seattle: NCAST Programs, University of Washington.

Barnard, K.E. (1999a). *Keys to caregiving study guide* (rev. ed.). Seattle: NCAST Programs, University of Washington.

Barnard, K.E. (1999b). *Beginning rhythms: The emerging process of sleep wake behavior and self-regulation.* Seattle: NCAST, University of Washington.

Barnard, K.E., & Bee, H.L. (1983). The impact of temporally-patterned stimulation on the development of preterm infants. *Child Development, 54,* 1156-1167.

Barnard, K.E., Booth, C.L., Mitchell, S.K., & Telzrow, R.W. (1983). *Newborn nursing models.* Final report of a three year grant (R01 NU-00719). Division of Nursing, Bureau of Health Manpower, HRA, DDHS, Washington, DC.

Barnard, K.E., Hammond, M.A., Booth, C.L., et al. (1989). Measurement and meaning of parent-infant interaction. In F. Morrison, C. Lord, & D. Keating (Eds.), *Applied developmental psychology* (Vol. III, pp. 39-80). New York: Academic Press.

Bell, S.M., & Ainsworth, M.D. (1972). Infant crying and maternal responsiveness. *Child Development, 43,* 1171-1190.

Blackburn, S. (1998). Environmental impact of the NICU on developmental outcomes. *Journal of Pediatric Nursing: Nursing Care of Children & Families, 13,* 279-289.

Blackburn, S.T., & Barnard, K.E. (1985). Analysis of caregiving events relating to preterm infants in the special care unit. In A.W. Gottfried, & J.L. Gaiter (Eds.), *Infant stress under intensive care: Environmental neonatology* (pp. 113-129). Baltimore: University Park Press.

Boechler, V., Harrison, M.J., & Magill-Evans, J. (2003). Father-child teaching interactions: The relationship to father involvement in caregiving. *Journal of Pediatric Nursing, 18*(1), 46-51.

Boukydis, C.F., & Lester, B.M. (1999). The NICU Network Neurobehavioral Scale. Clinical use with drug exposed infants and their mothers. *Clinics in Perinatology, 26,* 213-230.

Bowen, F. (1992). Neurologic evaluation of the preterm infant. *NAACOG's Clinical Issues in Perinatal & Women's Health Nursing, 3*(1), 75-95.

Boyce, G.C., Smith, T.B., & Casro, G. (1999). Health and educational outcomes of children who experienced severe neonatal medical complications. *Journal of Genetics and Psychology, 160*(3), 261-269.

Brandon, D.H., Holditch-Davis, D, & Belyea, M. (2002). Preterm infants born at less than 31 weeks' gestation have improved growth in cycled light compared with continuous near darkness. *Journal of Pediatrics, 140*(2), 192-199.

Bray, P.F., Shields, W.D., Wolcott, G.J., et al. (1969). Occipitofrontal head circumference—An accurate measure of intracranial volume. *The Journal of Pediatrics, 75*(20), 303-305.

Brazelton, T.B. (1973). *Neonatal behavioral assessment scale.* London: Spastics International Medical Publications.

Brazelton, T.B. (1979). Behavioral competence of the neonate. *Seminars in Perinatology, 3,* 35-44.

Brazelton, T.B., Koslowski, B., & Main, M. (1974). The origins of reciprocity: The early mother-infant interaction. In M. Lewis, & L.A. Rosenblum (Eds.), *The effect of the infant on its caregiver* (pp. 49-76). New York: John Wiley & Sons.

Brazelton, T.B., & Nugent, J.K. (1995). *The Brazelton neonatal behavioral assessment scale* (3rd ed.). London: Spastics International Medical Publications.

Brown, L.P., Gennaro, S., York, R., et al. (1991). VLBW infants: Association between visiting and telephoning and maternal and infant outcome measures. *Journal of Perinatal & Neonatal Nursing, 4*(4), 39-45.

Brown, W., Pearl, L.F., & Carrasco, N. (1991). Evolving models of family-centered services in neonatal intensive care. *Children's Health Care, 20,* 50-55.

Budin, P., & Maloney, W.J. (1907). (translated). *The nurseling: The feeding and hygiene of premature and full-term infants.* London, England: Caxton Publishing.

Buehler, D.M., Als, H., Duffy, F.H., et al. (1995). Effectiveness of individualized developmental care for low-risk preterm infants: Behavioral and electrophysiologic evidence. *Pediatrics, 96*(5)(Pt 1), 923-932.

Bull, M.J. (1981). Change in concerns of first-time mothers after one week at home. *Journal of Obstetric, Gynecologic, and Neonatal Nursing, (JOGNN), 10*(5), 391-394.

Byers, J.F. (2003). Components of developmental care and the evidence for their use in the NICU. *MCN: American Journal of Maternal/Child Nursing, 28*(3), 174-181.

Caine, J. (1991). The effects of music on the selected stress behaviors, weight, caloric and formula intake, and length of hospital stay of premature and low birth weight neonates in a newborn intensive care unit. *Journal of Music Therapy, 18,* 88-100.

Campbell, D.T., & Stanley, J.C. (1963). *Experimental and quasi-experimental designs for research.* Boston: Houghton Mifflin.

Campbell, S.K. (1999). Test-retest reliability of the Test of Infant Motor Performance. *Pediatric Physical Therapy, 11,* 60-66.

Campbell, S.K., Osten, E.T., Kolobe, T.H.A., et al. (1993). Development of the Test of Infant Motor Performance. *Physical Medicine & Rehabilitation Clinics of North America, 4,* 541-550.

Carlson, M., & Earls, F. (1997). Psychological and neuroendocrinological sequelae of early social deprivation in institutionalized children in Romania. *Annals of the New York Academy of Sciences, 807,* 419-428.

Casteel, J.K. (1990). Affects and cognition of mothers and fathers of preterm infants. *Maternal Child Nursing Journal, 19*(3), 211-220.

Cole, J.G., Begish-Duddy, A., Judas, M.L., & Jorgensen, K.M. (1990). Changing the NICU environment: The Boston City Hospital model. *Neonatal Network, 9*(2), 15-23.

Coleman, J.M., Practt, R.R., Stoddar, R.A., et al. (1998). The effects of male and female singing and speaking voices on selected physiological and behavioral measures of premature infants in the neonatal care unit. *International Journal of Arts Medicine, 5*(8), 4-11.

Coleman, R.W., & Provence, S. (1957). Environmental retardation (hospitalism) in infants living in families. *Pediatrics, 19*(2), 285-292.

Constantinou, J.C., & Korner, A.F. (1993). Neurobehavioral assessment of the preterm infant as an instrument to enhance parental awareness. *Children's Health Care, 22,* 39-46.

Cornell, E.H., & Gottfried, A.W. (1976). Intervention with premature human infants. *Child Development, 47*(1), 32-39.

Eilers, B.L., Desai, N.S., Wilson, M.A., et al. (1986). Classroom performance and social factors of children with birth weights of 1250 grams or less: Follow-up at 5 to 8 years of age. *Pediatrics, 77*(2), 23-208.

Elardo, R., Bradley, R., & Caldwell, B.M. (1975). The relationship of infants' home environments to mental test performance from six to 36 months: A longitudinal analysis. *Child Development, 46,* 71-76.

Escalona, S.K. (1952). Emotional development in the first year of life. In M.J.E. Senn (Ed.), *Problems of infancy and childhood* (6th ed., pp. 11-91). New York: Josiah Macy, Jr. Foundation. Federal Register. (1986). *The Education for All Handicapped Children Act Amendments* (P.L. 99-457, Secs. 671-672).

Field, T. (1990). Alleviating stress in newborn infants in the intensive care unit. *Clinics in Perinatology, 17*(1), 1-9.

Field, T.M. (1977). Effects of early separation, interactive deficits, and experimental manipulation on infant-mother face-to-face interaction. *Child Development, 48,* 763-771.

Fielder, A.R., & Moseley, M.J. (2000). Environmental light and the preterm infant. *Seminars in Perinatology, 24*(4), 291-298.

Fielder, A.R., & Reynolds, J.D. (2001). Retinopathy of prematurity: Clinical aspects. *Seminars in Neonatology, 6*(6), 451-475.

Fitzhardinge, P.N., Pape, P., Arstikaitis, M., et al. (1976). Mechanical ventilation of infants less than 1,501 gram birth weight: Health, growth, and neurologic sequelae. *Journal of Pediatrics, 88*(4)(Pt 1), 531-541.

Fleisher, B.E., VandenBerg, K., Constantinou, J., et al. (1995). Individualized developmental care for very-low-birth-weight premature infants. *Clinical Pediatrics, 34,* 523-529.

Frank, D.A., Klass, P.E., Earls, F., & Eisenberg, L. (1996). Infants and young children in orphanages: One view from pediatrics and child psychology. *Pediatrics, 97,* 569-578.

Gallo, A.M. (2003). The fifth vital sign: Implementation of the Neonatal Infant Pain Scale. *Journal of Obstetric, Gynecologic, and Neonatal Nursing, 32*(2), 199-206.

Gardner, L.I. (1982). Deprivation dwarfism. *Scientific American, 227,* 76-78.

Gardner, S.L., & Goldson, E. (2002). The neonate and the environment: Impact on development. In G.B. Merenstein, & S.L. Gardner (Eds.), *Handbook of neonatal intensive care* (5th ed., pp. 219-282.). St. Louis: Mosby.

Gesell, A., & Thompson, H. (1934). *Infant behavior: Its genesis and growth.* New York: McGraw-Hill.

Gibbins, S., Stevens, B., Hodnett, E., et al. (2002). Efficacy and safety of sucrose for procedural pain relief in preterm and term neonates. *Nursing Research, 51*(6), 375-382.

Gill, N.E., Behnke, M., Conlon, M., et al. (1992). Nonnutritive sucking modulates behavioral state for preterm infants before feeding. *Scandinavian Journal of Caring Sciences, 6*(1), 3-7.

Gill, N.E., Behnke, M., Conlon, M., et al. (1988). Effect of nonnutritive sucking on behavioral state in preterm infants before feeding. *Nursing Research, 37*(6), 347-350.

Glass, P. (1990). Light and the developing retina. *Documents of Ophthalmology, 74*(3), 195-203.

Glass, P., Avery, G.B., Subramania, K.N., et al. (1985). Effect of bright light in the hospital nursery on the incidence of retinopathy of prematurity. *New England Journal of Medicine, 3133*(7), 401-404.

Gottfried, A.W. (1985). Environmental neonatology: Implications for intervention. In A.W. Gottfried, & J.L. Gaiter (Eds.), *Infant stress under intensive care: Environmental neonatology* (pp. 251-263). Baltimore: University Park Press.

Gottfried, A.W., & Gaiter, J.L. (eds). (1985). *Infant stress under intensive care: Environmental neonatology.* Baltimore: University Park Press.

Gottfried, A.W., Wallace-Lande, P., Sherman-Brown, S., et al. (1981). Physical and social environment of newborn infants in special care units. *Science, 214*(4521), 673-675.

Graven, S.N. (1997). Clinical research data illuminating the relationship between the physical environment & patient medical outcomes. *Journal of Healthcare Decisions, 9*, 15-19, 21-24.

Graven, S.N., Bowen, F.W., Jr., Brooten, D., et al. (1992a). The high-risk infant environment. Part 1. The role of the neonatal intensive care unit in the outcomes of high-risk infants. *Journal of Perinatology, 12*, 164-172.

Graven, S.N., Bowen, F.W., Jr., Brooten, D., et al. (1992b). The high-risk infant environment. Part 2. The role of caregiving and the social environment. *Journal of Perinatology, 12*, 267-275.

Greenough, A., Dixon, A.K., & Robertson, N.R.C. (1984). Pulmonary interstitial emphysema. *Archives of Disease in Childhood, 59*, 1046-1051.

Gretebeck, R.J., Shaffer, D., & Bishop-Kurylo, D. (1998). Clinical pathways for family-oriented developmental care in the intensive care nursery. *Journal of Perinatal & Neonatal Nursing, 12*(1), 70-80.

Griffin, T. (2003). Facing challenges to family-centered care. I: Conflicts over visitation. *Pediatric Nursing, 29*(2), 135-137.

Grogaard, J.B., Lindstrom, D.P., Parker, R.A., et al. (1990). Increased survival rate in very low birth weight infants (1500 grams or less): No association with increased incidence of handicaps. *Journal of Pediatrics, 117*(1 Pt 1), 139-146.

Grunau, R. (2002). Early pain in preterm infants: A model of long-term effects. *Clinics in Perinatology, 29*(3), 373-394.

Guess, D., & Carr, E. (1991). Emergence and maintenance of stereotypy and self-injury. *American Journal of Mental Retardation, 96*(3), 299-319, 321-344.

Hack, M., Breslau, N., Weissman, B., et al. (1991). Effect of very low birth weight and subnormal head size on cognitive abilities at school age. *The New England Journal of Medicine, 325*(4), 231-237.

Hack, M., & Fanaroff, A. (1999). Outcomes of children of extremely low birthweight and gestational age in the 1990s. *Early Human Development*, 53, 193-218.

Harrigan, R.C., Ratliffe, C., Patrinos, M.E., et al. (2002). Medically fragile children: An integrative review of the literature and recommendations for future research. *Issues in Comprehensive Pediatric Nursing, 25*(1), 1-20.

Harrison, L., Berbaum, M.L., Stem, J.T., et al. (2001). Use of individualized versus standard criteria to identify abnormal levels of heart rate or oxygen saturation in preterm infants. *Journal of Nursing Measurement, 9*(2), 181-200.

Harrison, L.L., Leeper, J.D., & Yoon, M. (1990). Effects of early parent touch on preterm infants' heart rates and arterial oxygen saturation levels. *Journal of Advanced Nursing, 15*(8), 877-885.

Hatch, J.P., Klatt, K., Porges, S.W., et al. (1986). The relation between rhythmic cardiovascular variability and reactivity to orthostatic, cognitive, and cold pressor stress. *Psychophysiology, 23*(1), 48-56.

Hauth, J.C., & Merenstein, G.B. (1997). *Guidelines for perinatal care* (4th ed.). Elk Grove, IL: American Academy of Pediatrics and the American College of Obstetricians and Gynecologists.

Hebb, D.O. (1949). *The organization of behavior.* New York: Wiley.

Helm, J.M. (personal communication, March 3, 1994). *Introduction to the NIDCAP®.* Lecture presented at Wake Medical Center, Raleigh, NC.

High, P.C., & Gorski, P.A. (1985). Recording environmental influences on infant development in the intensive care nursery: Womb for improvement. In A.W. Gottfried, & J.L. Gaiter (Eds), *Infant stress under intensive care: Environmental neonatal* (pp. 131-155). Baltimore: University Park Press.

Hirata, T., Epcar, J.T., Walsh, A., et al. (1983). Survival and outcome of infants 501 to 750 gm: A six-year experience. *Journal of Pediatrics, 102*(5), 741-748.

Holditch-Davis, D., Blackburn, S.T., & VandenBerg, K.A. (2003). Newborn and infant neurobehavioral development. In C. Kenner, J.W. Lott, & A.A. Flandermeyer (Eds.), *Comprehensive neonatal nursing: A physiologic perspective* (3rd ed., pp. 236-283). St Louis: W.B. Saunders.

Horns, K.M. (1998). Being In-Tune Caregiving. *Journal of Perinatal and Neonatal Nursing, 12*(3), 38-49.

Horowitz, F.D. (1990). Developmental models of individual differences. In J. Colombo, & J.W. Fagen (Eds.), *Individual differences in infancy: Reliability, stability, prediction* (pp. 3-18). Hillsdale, NJ: Lawrence Erlbaum Associates, Inc.

Horowitz, F.D. (1995). The nature-nurture controversy in social and historical perspective. In F. Kessel (Ed.), *Psychology, science, and human affairs: Essays in honor of William Bevan* (pp. 89-99). Boulder, CO: Westview Press.

Horowitz, F.D., & Columbo, J. (1990). Future agendas and directions in infancy research. *Merrill-Palmer Quarterly, 36*, 173-178.

Horowitz, F.D., Sullivan, J.W., & Linn, P. (1978). Stability and instability in the newborn infant: The quest for elusive threads. In A.J. Sameroff (Ed.), Organization and stability of newborn behavior: A commentary on the Brazelton Neonatal Behavioral Assessment Scale. *Monographs of the Society for Research in Child Development, 43*(5-6, Serial No. 177), 29-45.

Hunt, J.McV. (1976). Environmental programming to foster competence and prevent mental retardation in infancy. In R.N. Walsh, & W.T. Greenough (Eds.), *Environments as therapy for brain dysfunction* (pp. 201-255). New York: Plenum.

Illingworth, R.S. (1987). Normal development. In *The development of the infant and young child: Normal and abnormal* (9th ed., pp. 83-128). New York: Churchill Livingstone.

James, W. (1890). *Principles of psychology 2.* New York: Publisher unknown.

Jorgensen, K. (2002). Moving forward with developmental care: Education and beyond. *Newborn and Infant Nursing Reviews, 2*(1), 5-8.

Keating, J.B. (1976). Therapeutic misadventures: Total parenteral alimentation. In T.D. Moore (Ed.), *Iatrogenic problems in neonatal intensive care. Report of the 69th Ross Conference on Pediatric Research* (pp. 35-42). Columbus, OH: Ross Laboratories.

Klein, N., Hack, M., Gallagher, J., & Fanaroff, A.A. (1985). Preschool performance of children with normal intelligence who were very low birth weight infants. *Pediatrics, 75*, 531-537.

Koops, B.L., Abman, S.H., & Accurso, F.J. (1984). Outpatient management and follow-up of broncopulmonary dysplasia. *Clinical Perinatology, 11*(1), 101 122.

Korner, A.F. (1987). Preventive intervention with high-risk newborns: Theoretical, conceptual, and methodological perspectives. In J.D. Osofsky (Ed.), *Handbook of infant development* (2nd ed., pp. 1006-1036). New York: John Wiley & Sons.

Korner, A.F., Constantinou, J., Dimiceli, S., et al. (1991). Establishing the reliability and developmental validity of a neurobehavioral assessment for preterm infants: A methodological process. *Child Development, 62,* 1200-1208.

Korner, A.F., Guilleminault, C., Van den Hoed, J., & Baldwin, R.B. (1978). Reduction of sleep apnea and bradycardia in preterm infants on oscillating waterbeds: A controlled polygraphic study. *Pediatrics, 61,* 528-533.

Korones, S.B. (1976). Disturbance and infants' rest. In T.D. Moore (Ed.), *Iatrogenic problems in neonatal intensive care. Report of the 69th Ross Conference on Pediatric Research* (pp. 94-97). Columbus, OH: Ross Laboratories.

Korones, S.B. (1985). Physical structure and functional organization of neonatal intensive care units. In A.W. Gottfried, & J.L. Gaiter (Eds.), *Infant stress under intensive care: Environmental neonatology* (pp. 7-22). Baltimore: University Park Press.

Lawhon, G. (1997). Providing developmentally supportive care in the newborn intensive care unit: An evolving challenge. *Journal of Perinatal and Neonatal Nursing, 10*(4), 48-61.

Lawson, K., Daum, C., & Turkewitz, G. (1977). Environmental characteristics of a neonatal intensive care unit. *Child Development, 48*, 1633-1639.

Leijon, I. (1982). Assessment of behavior on the Brazelton Scale in healthy preterm infants from 32 conceptional weeks until full-term age. *Early Human Development, 7,* 109-118.

Lester, B.M., & Tronick, E.Z. (1990). Guidelines for stimulation with preterm infants. *Clinical Perinatology, 17*(1), xv-xvii.

Lewis, M., & Goldberg, S. (1969). Perceptual-cognitive development in infancy: A generalized expectancy model as a function of the mother-infant interaction. *Merrill-Palmer Quarterly, 15,* 81-100.

Lindeke, L.L., Stanely, J.R., Else, B.S., et al. (2002). Neonatal predictors of school-based services used by NICU graduates at school age. *MCN: American Journal of Maternal Child Nursing, 27*(1), 41-46.

Linn, P.L. (1980). Newborn environments and mother-infant interactions. *Dissertation Abstracts International, 41*(1-B), 378-379.

Linn, P. L., Horowitz, F.D., Buddin, B.J., et al. (1985). An ecological description of a neonatal intensive care unit. In A.W. Gottfried, & J.L. Gaiter (Eds.), *Infant stress under intensive care: Environmental neonatology* (pp. 83-111). Baltimore: University Park Press.

Long, J.G., Lucey, J.F., & Philip, A.G. (1980). Noise and hypoxemia in the intensive care nursery. *Pediatrics, 65*(1), 143 145.

Long, J.G., Philip, A.G., & Lucey, J.F. (1980). Excessive handling as a cause of hypoxemia. *Pediatrics, 65*(2), 203-207.

Loo, K.K., Espinosa, M., Tyler, R., et al. (2003). Using knowledge to cope with stress in the NICU: How parents integrate learning to read the physiologic and behavioral cues of the infant. *Neonatal Network, 22*(1), 31-37.

Lorenz, E.N. (1963). Deterministic nonperiodic flow. *Journal of the Atmospheric Sciences, 20*, 130-141.

Lorenz, E.N. (1993). *The essence of chaos.* Seattle: University of Washington Press.

Lotas, M.J. (1992). Effects of light and sound in the neonatal intensive care unit environment on the low-birth-weight infant. *NAACOG's Clinical Issues in Perinatal & Women's Health Nursing, 3*(1), 34-44.

Lucey, J.F. (1977). Is intensive care becoming too intensive? *Pediatrics, 59*(Suppl.), 1064-1065.

Markestad, T., & Fitzhardinge, P.M. (1981). Growth and development in children recovering from bronchopulmonary dysplasia. *Journal of Pediatrics, 98*(4), 587-602.

McCormick, M. (1989). Long term follow-up of infants discharged from neonatal intensive care units. *Journal of the American Medical Association (JAMA), 261,* 1767-1772.

McCormick, M.C. (1997). The outcomes of very low birth weight infants: Are we asking the right questions? *Pediatrics, 99*(6), 869-876.

McGrath, J.M. (2000). Developmentally supportive caregiving and technology: Isolation or merger of intervention strategies? *Journal of Perinatal and Neonatal Nursing, 14*(3), 78-91.

McGrath, J.M., & Conliffe-Torres, S. (1996). Integrating family-centered developmental assessment and intervention into routine care in the neonatal intensive care unit. *Nursing Clinics of North America, 31*, 367-386.

McGrath, J.M., & Valenzuela, G. (1994). Integrating developmentally supportive caregiving into practice through education. *Journal of Perinatal & Neonatal Nursing, 8*(3), 46-57.

Meier, P., & Pugh, E.J. (1985). Breast-feeding behavior of small preterm infants. *MCN: American Journal of Maternal Child Nursing, 10*(6), 396-401.

Minde, K., Whitelaw, A., Brown, J., et al. (1983). Effect of neonatal complications in premature infants on early parent-infant interactions. *Developmental Medicine & Child Neurology, 25*(6), 763-777.

Mirmiran, M., Baldwin, R.B., & Ariagno, R.L. (2003). Circadian and sleep development in preterm infants occurs independently from the influences of environmental lighting. *Pediatric Research, 53*(6), 933-938.

Moore, K.A., Coker, K., DuBuisson, A.B., et al. (2003). Implementing potentially better practices for improving family-centered care in neonatal intensive care units: Successes and challenges. *Pediatrics, 111*(4 Pt 2), e450-e460.

Mouradian, L.E., & Als, H. (1994). The influence of neonatal intensive care unit caregiving practices on motor functioning of preterm infants. *American Journal of Occupational Therapy, 48*, 527-533.

Murney, M.E., & Campbell, S.K. (1998). The ecological relevance of the Test of Infant Motor Performance Elicited Scale items. *Physical Therapy, 78*, 479-489.

NANN. (1993). *Infant and family-centered developmental care guidelines*. Petaluma, CA: NANN.

NANN. (2001). *Infant and family-centered developmental care guidelines*. Glenview, IL: NANN.

Nelson, N.M. (1976). Therapeutic misadventures: Oxygen. In T.D. Moore (Ed.), *Iatrogenic problems in neonatal intensive care. Report of the 69th Ross conference on Pediatric Research* (pp. 17-22). Columbus, OH: Ross Laboratories.

Ohmeda Medical. (2003). *Economics of prematurity and developmental care: Clinical Series*. Columbia, MD. Available online at *http://www.ohmedamedical.com/index2.cfm?act = file&file = /clinical_services/Economics%20of%20Prematurity%20and%20Developmental%20Care_Web%20Sample.pdf*.

Palmer, P.G., Dubowitz, L.M.S., Bercholte, N., et al. (1982). Neurological and neurobehavioral differences between preterm infants at term and full-term newborn infants. *Neuropediatrics, 13*, 183-189.

Perlman, J.M. (2002). Cognitive and behavioral deficits in premature graduates of intensive care. *Clinics in Perinatology, 29*(4), 779-797.

Peters, K.L. (1999, January). Physiological and behavioral responses of ill premature neonates to various types of touch in a routine procedure (abstract). In S.N. Graven (Ed.), *Proceedings of the Sixth conference on The Physical and Developmental Environment of the High Risk Infant*, Clearwater Beach, FL.

Petryshen, P., Stevens, B., Hawkins, J., et al. (1997). Comparing nursing costs for preterm infants receiving conventional vs. developmental care. *Nursing Economics, 15*(3), 138-150.

Phelps, D.L., & Watts, J.L. (2001). Early light reduction for preventing retinopathy of prematurity in very low birth weight infants. *Cochrane Database Systematic Review*, CD0000122.

Piaget, J. (1973). *The child and reality: Problems of genetic psychology*. New York: Grossman Publishers.

Pinelli, J., & Symington, A. (2000). How rewarding can a pacifier be? A systematic review of nonnutritive sucking in preterm infants. *Neonatal Network, 19*(8), 41-48.

Pinelli, J., Symington, A., & Ciliska, D. (2002). Nonnutritive sucking in high-risk infants: Benign intervention or legitimate therapy? *Journal of Obstetric, Gynecologic, and Neonatal Nursing (JOGNN), 31*(5), 582-591.

Pink, G.H., Murray, M.A., & McKillop, L. (2003). Hospital efficiency and patient satisfaction. *Health Services Management Research, 16*(1), 24-38.

Porges, S.W. (1992). Vagal tone: A physiologic marker of stress vulnerability. *Pediatrics, 90*(3 Pt 2), 498-504.

Porges, S.W. (1991). Vagal mediation of respiratory sinus arrhythmia: Implications for drug delivery. *Annals of New York Academy of Science, 618*, 57-66.

Porges, S., & Byrne, E.A. (1992). Research methods for measurement of heart rate and respiration. *Biology and Psychology, 34*(2-3), 93-130.

Porges, S.W., Matthews, K.A., & Pauls, D.L. (1992). The biobehavioral interface in behavioral pediatrics. *Pediatrics 90*(5 Pt 2), 789-797.

Prechtl, H.F.R. (1968). Neurological findings in newborn infants after pre- and perinatal complications. In J.H.P. Jonxis, H.K.A. Visser, & J.A. Troelstra (Eds.), *Aspects of prematurity and dysmaturity* (pp. 52-77). Springfield, IL: C.C. Thomas.

Prechtl, H.F.R. (1980). The optimality concept. *Early Human Development, 4*, 201-205.

Provence, S.A., & Lipton, R.C. (1962). *Infants in institutions: A comparison of their development with family-reared infants during the first year of life*. New York: International Universities Press.

Resnick, M.B., Armstrong, S., & Carter, R.L. (1988). Developmental intervention program for high-risk premature infants: Effects on development and parent-infant interactions. *Journal of Developmental & Behavioral Pediatrics, 9*, 73-78.

Reynolds, J.D., Dobson, V., Quinn, G.E., et al. (2002). Evidence-based screening criteria for retinopathy of prematurity: Natural history data from the CRYO-ROP and LIGHT-ROP studies. *Archives of Ophthalmology, 120*(11), 1470-1476.

Rheingold, H.L. (1956). The modification of social responsiveness in institutional babies. *Dissertation Abstracts International,* AATT-02957.

Rheingold, H.L. (1960). The measurement of maternal care. *Child Development, 31,* 565-575.

Rheingold, H.L. (Ed.). (1963). *Maternal behavior in mammals.* New York: Wiley.

Richards, M.P.M. (1977). An ecological study of infant development in an urban setting in Britain. In P.H. Leiderman, S.R. Tulkin, & A. Rosenfeld (Eds.), *Culture in infancy: Variations in the human experience* (pp. 469-493). New York: Academic Press.

Robinson, M., Pirak, C., & Morrell, C. (2000). Multidisciplinary discharge assessment of the medically and socially high-risk infant. *Journal of Perinatal & Neonatal Nursing, 13*(4), 67-86.

Salls, J.S., Sliverman, L.N., & Gatty, C.M. (2002). The relationship of infant sleep and play positioning to motor milestone achievement. *American Journal of Occupational Therapy, 56*(5), 577-580.

Sander, L.W. (1962). Issues in early mother child interaction. *Journal of the American Academy of Child Psychiatry, 1*(1), 141-166.

Scafidi, F.A., Field, T.M., Schanberg, S.M., et al. (1991). Massage stimulates growth in pre term infants: A replication. *Infant Behavioral Development, 13,* 167-188.

Schaefer, M., Hatcher, R.P., & Barglow, P.D. (1980). Prematurity and infant stimulation: A review of research. *Child Psychiatry and Human Development, 10,* 199-212.

Scher, M.S., Klesh, K.W., Murphy, T.F., et al. (1986). Seizures and infarction in neonates with persistent pulmonary hypertension. *Pediatric Neurology, 2*(6), 332-339.

Schwartz, F.J., Ritchie, R., Sacks, L., et al. (1997). Perinatal stress reduction, music and medical cost savings. *Journal of Prenatal and Perinatal Psychology and Health, 12*(1), 19-29.

Shields, P.J., & Tenorio, K.E. (1988). Cluster care nursing: Maricela's story. *Pediatric Nursing, 14*(2), 125-127.

Spitz, R. (1945). Hospitalism: An inquiry into the genesis of psychiatric conditions in early childhood. In O. Fenichel, P. Greenacrre, H. Hartmann, E.B. Jackson, E. Kris, L.S. Kubie, B.D. Lewin, M.C. Putnam, R.A. Spitz, A. Freud, W. Hoffer, & E. Glover (Eds.), *The psychoanalytic study of the child,* (Vol. 1, pp. 53-74). New York: International Universities Press.

Spitz, R. (1946). Hospitalism: A follow-up report. In A. Freud, H. Hartmann, & E. Kris (Eds.), *The psychoanalytic study of the child,* (Vol. 2, pp. 113-117). New York: International Universities Press.

Spitz, R., & Wolf, K.M. (1946). Analitic depression: An inquiry into the genesis of psychiatric conditions in early childhood. In A. Freud, H. Hartmann, & E. Kris (Eds.),

*The psychoanalytic study of the child,* (Vol. 2, pp. 313-342). New York: International Universities Press.

Stern, D.N. (1974). Mother and infant at play: The dyadic interaction involving facial, vocal, and gaze behaviors. In M. Lewis, & L.A. Rosenblum (Eds.), *The effect of the infant on its caregiver* (pp. 187-213). New York: John Wiley & Sons.

Stevenson, H.W., Hess, E.H., & Rheingold, H.L. (Eds.). (1967). *Early behavior: Comparative and developmental approaches.* New York: Wiley.

Symington, A., & Pinelli, J. (2001). Developmental care for promoting development and preventing morbidity in preterm infants. *Cochrane Database Systemic Review, 4,* CD00001814.

Thigpen, J. (2002). Developmental considerations for resuscitation of the VLBW infant. *Neonatal Network, 21*(4), 21-26.

Thiringer, K, Kankkunen, A. Liden, G., & Niklasson, A. (1984). Perinatal risk factors in the aetiology of hearing loss in preschool children. *Developmental Medicine & Child Neurology, 26*(6), 799-907.

Thoman, E.B. (1990). Temporal patterns of caregiving for preterm infants indicate individualized developmental care. *Journal of Perinatology, 23*(1), 29-36.

Thoman, E.B., Ingersoll, E.W., & Acebo, C. (1991). Premature infants seek rhythmic stimulation, and the experience facilitates neurobehavioral development. *Journal of Developmental and Behavior Pediatrics, 12*(1), 11-18.

Thomas, K. (1989). How the NICU environment sounds to a preterm infant. *MCN American Journal of Maternal Child Nursing, 14*(4), 249-251.

Tjossem, T. (1976). Early intervention: Issues and approaches. In T. Tjossem (Ed.), *Intervention strategies for high risk infants and young children* (pp. 3-33). Baltimore: University Park Press.

Tuck, S.J., Monin, P., Duvivier, C., et al. (1982). Effect of a rocking bed on apnea of prematurity. *Archives of Disease in Childhood, 57,* 475-477.

Tulkin, S.R. (1977). Social class differences in maternal and infant behavior. In P.H. Leiderman, S.R. Tulkin, & A. Rosenfeld (Eds.), *Culture in infancy: Variations in the human experience* (pp. 495-537). New York: Academic Press.

U.S. Department of Health and Human Services. (2000, November). *Healthy People 2010: Understanding and improving health* (2nd ed.). Washington, DC: U.S. Government Printing Office.

Verklan, M.T. (2002). Physiologic variability during transition to extrauterine life. *Critical Care Nursing Quarterly, 24*(4), 41-56.

Vohr, B.R., & Garcia-Coll, C.T. (1985). Neurodevelopmental and school performance of very low-birth-weight infants: A seven-year longitudinal study. *Pediatrics, 76*(3), 345-350.

Volpe, J.J. (2001). *Neurology of the newborn* (4th ed.). Philadelphia: W.B. Saunders.

Wachs, T.D. (1976). Utilization of a Piagetian approach in the investigation of early experience effects: A research strategy and some illustrative data. *Merrill-Palmer Quarterly, 22,* 11-30.

Walsh-Sukys, M., Reitenbach, A., Hudson-Barr, D., & De Pompei, P. (2001). Reducing light and sound in the neonatal intensive care unit: An evaluation of patient safety, staff satisfaction, and costs. *Journal of Perinatology, 21*(8), 230-235.

Watson, J.S. (1967). Memory and "contingency analysis" in infant learning. *Merrill-Palmer Quarterly, 13,* 55-76.

Werner, H. (1957). The concept of development from a comparative and organismic point of view. In D.B. Harris (Ed.), *The concept of development: An issue in the study of human behavior* (pp. 125-148). Minneapolis: University of Minnesota Press.

White, C., Simon, M., & Bryan, A. (2002). Using evidence to educate birthing center nursing staff about infant states, cues, and behaviors. *MCN: American Journal of Maternal/Child Nursing, 27,* 294-298.

White, R. (Committee to Establish Recommended Standards for Newborn ICU Design). (2002). *Recommended standards for newborn ICU design: Report of the fifth consensus conference on newborn ICU Design.* Clearwater Beach, FL. Available online at *www.nd.edu/~kkolberg/DesignStandards.htm.*

White, R.W. (1959). Motivation reconsidered: The concept of competence. *Psychological Review, 66,* 297-333.

White-Traut, R.C., & Nelson, M.N. (1988). Maternally administered tactile, auditory, visual, and vestibular stimulation: relationship to later interactions between mothers and premature infants. *Research in Nursing & Health, 11,* 31-39.

White-Traut, R.C., & Pate, C.M.H. (1987). Modulating infant state in premature infants. *Journal of Pediatric Nursing, 2,* 96-101.

Wille, D.E. (1991). Relation of preterm birth with quality of infant-mother attachment at one year. *Infant Behavior & Development, 14,* 227-240.

Williams, G.P. (1997). *Chaos theory tamed.* Washington, DC: Joseph Henry Press.

Winslow, E.H., & Jacobson, A.F. (1999). Does light reduction prevent retinopathy of prematurity? *American Journal of Nursing, 99,* 14.

Wolke, D. (1987a). Environmental neonatology. *Archives of Disease in Childhood, 62,* 987-988.

Wolke, D. (1987b). Environmental and developmental neonatology. *Journal of Reproductive and Infant Psychology, 5,* 17-42.

Yarrow, L.J. (1961). Maternal deprivation: Toward an empirical and conceptual reevaluation. *Psychological Bulletin, 58,* 459-490.

Yarrow, L.J., Pedersen, F.A., & Rubenstein, J. (1977). Mother-infant interaction and development in infancy. In P.H. Leiderman, S.R. Tulkin, & A. Rosenfeld (Eds.), *Culture in infancy: Variations in the human experience* (pp. 539-564). New York: Academic Press.

Young, J. (1996). *Developmental care of the premature baby.* London: Bailliere Tindall.

Zadeh, L.A. (1990, April). *Fuzzy logic: Approximate reasoning in solving complex problems.* Unpublished manuscript presented at Vanderbilt University School of Nursing, Nashville, TN, April 20, 1990.

Zaichkin, J. (Ed.). (2002). *Newborn intensive care: What every parent needs to know* (2nd ed). Santa Rosa, CA: NICU Ink.

# 2 Individualized Care: Actions for the Individualized Staff Member

**Diane D. Ballweg**

Developmental care implementation requires comprehensive changes in newborn intensive care unit (NICU) system processes as well as in individual staff knowledge and practice. The complexity of this change process makes the transition from traditional, task-directed care to holistic, relationship-based care challenging for NICUs as a whole and for personnel members as individuals.

Practicing developmental care means providing ongoing, individualized, developmentally supportive experiences for maturing newborns and their families, to promote their optimal development (Als, 2002; Lawhon, 1997). Developmentally supportive caregivers realize that "the infant brain is designed to be molded by the environment it encounters" (Schore, 2002), including the social and emotional as well as the physical environment (Figure 2-1). Working within a developmental framework, caregivers view human development as an ongoing process, that is, layers building upon those previously developed and supporting those yet to come. Thus, newborn developmental care begins at birth, continues throughout the infant's hospitalization, and supports the transition to home and to the community (Als, 1992).

Historically NICU healthcare team members have not appreciated the impact of their individual and collective contributions to overall high-risk infant development. Therefore, their practice and systems processes typically do not reflect this caregiving model. As such, implementation of the necessary comprehensive changes to provide developmentally supportive care is typically lengthy and involves a high level of difficulty, as it frequently requires alterations in not only staff knowledge and attitude, but also individual and group behavior (Hersey & Blanchard, 1977). Staff and administration often feel overwhelmed and frustrated by the number and magnitude of changes involved in implementation. The complex process requires expert guidance in program development and maintenance, content, systems and individual change, and multidisciplinary collaboration. Hospital and unit administrators are increasingly aware of the data to support this change and of the growing consumer expectations for this model of caregiving (Als, Lawhon, Brown, et al., 1986; Als, Lawhon, Duffy, et al., 1994; Ashbaugh, Leick-Rude, & Kilbride, 1999; Becker, Grunwald, Moorman, & Stuhr, 1991; Brink, 2002; Browne & Paul, 1999; Buehler, Als, Duffy, et al., 1995; Fleisher, VandenBerg, Constantinou, et al., 1995; Hanson, Johnson, Jeppson, et al., 1994; Harrison, 1993; Heller, Constantinou, VandenBerg, et al., 1997; Johnson, 1995; Kleberg, Westrup, & Stjernqvist, 2000; Kleberg, Westrup, Stjernqvist, & Lagercrantz, 2002; Leyden, 1998; Owens, 2001; Parker, Zahr, Cole, & Brecht, 1992; Peters, 2001; Petryshen, Stevens, Hawkins, & Stewart, 1997; Philbin, Ballweg, Tsakiri, et al., 1998; Shannon & Gorski, 1994; Shonkoff, Phillips, & Committee on Integrating the Science of Early Childhood Development, 2000; Westrup, Kleberg, von Eichwald, et al., 2000). They might, however, hesitate to use personnel and monetary resources to begin the process. If support is initiated, they might become unwilling to continue when dramatically improved outcomes are not quickly realized (Lawhon, 1997). Alternatively, if progress is realized, they might then believe the unit provides sufficient developmental care and reduce or even discontinue support because of a lack of appreciation of the current maintenance needs of this care model.

Staff members convinced of the value of the developmental approach might feel any attempt at implementation is futile without complete support

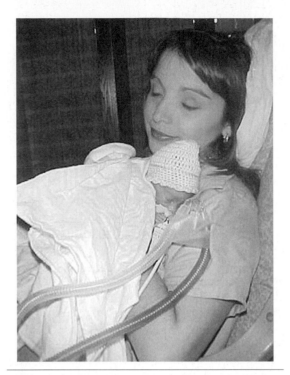

Figure **2-1** Provide nurturing experiences for maturing newborns and their families. (*Courtesy of the Hill family, Houson, TX.*)

for global changes such as unit renovation and facility-wide, comprehensive, family-centered care. Contrary to these beliefs, staff members can integrate supportive care knowledge and skills into their individual practice despite the lack of systemwide changes. The extent to which they are able to individually implement developmental care principles will differ from unit to unit. Consequently, the resulting impact on unit function and patient outcomes will also vary.

This chapter outlines some actions for the individual staff member when unit-wide changes are not supported, or are in process, but not yet fully implemented. Challenges that might be encountered when individual staff members begin providing components of developmentally supportive care are also presented. Specific information regarding supportive interactive and physical environments and the various roles and respective qualifications needed to support individual and system-wide implementation is reviewed in subsequent chapters of this text.

## INDIVIDUAL ACTIONS TO PROMOTE DEVELOPMENTALLY SUPPORTIVE CARE IN THE NICU

### Commitment and Self-Education

Commitment to the process and self-education are the first steps to implementing developmental care. Any individual or group change process begins with an awareness of the need and the subsequent motivation to alter practice (Hersey & Blanchard, 1977; VandenBerg, 1997). Educational content should include both informational and practical components, owing to the comprehensive nature of developmental care. The caregiver should seek information that includes, but is not limited to, basic human neurobehavioral development and organization, synactive theory, subsystem interaction (autonomic, motoric, state), sensory development and support, infant communication, and infant-family relationships. VandenBerg (1997) identified four basic principles of developmental care that are necessary for the caregiver to understand to employ a developmentally sensitive approach to caregiving. These include learning that developmental care:

• Is family-centered
• Is relationship-based
• Involves skillfully observing infant behaviors
• Is based on individualized care

Caregivers should also cultivate skills such as supportive handling, holding, positioning, relationship building, providing support surrounding and during necessary care procedures, timing and prioritization of care, support of sensory development, supportive feeding and bathing, promoting sleep-wake state regulation, and reflective communication (Als & McAnulty, 1998; VandenBerg, 1997). Educational resources include the multidisciplinary literature, unit-based, local, and national education and/or consultation programs and professional networking (Als, 1996, 2002; Ballweg & Lee, 2004), discussed elsewhere in this text.

### Relationship Building

Relationship building is key to implementation because humans are innately social and require positive, supportive relationships for growth (Als, 1992; Brazelton & Cramer, 1990; Gilkerson & Als, 1995). This is true for NICU employees as well as for infants and their families. The support of nurturing, compassionate relatedness, and, subsequently, humane care are basic tenets of the nursing profession and should be a goal for all NICU staff (Als, 1998; Kennell, 1999; Levin, 1999; Watson, 1992). Two of the recurring components of contemporary nursing identified by Watson (1992, p. 84) as being consistent with Nightingale's view of the nursing profession are "honor of the wisdom of connected oneness, wholeness, the interrelationship between and among person-nature-environment/caring-health-healing" and "recognition of the interrelationship between and among the personal, the political, the social, and the scientific."

Providing developmental care is more than just being nice to families and infants. It is "a process of give and take" (VandenBerg, 1997). That is, it involves forming relationships with genuine, respectful, two-way interaction, even with newborns. According to Als (1999a), developmental care emphasizes the following four key concepts:

- The personhood, humanity, value and integrity of each infant
- The importance of parents and family
- The affective connectedness and mutual relatedness of all persons
- The responsibility and opportunity entailed on the social nature of all humans

The relationship, that is, the appropriateness of interaction with the infant, is the foundation for all caregiving. Thus, how the caregiver feels about the baby as a human being will influence the manner and timing of all care practices.

## Relationship to the Infant

The caregiver needs to empathize with the infant's experience to establish a supportive relationship. Staff who can appreciate what the infant is experiencing in the intensive care setting provide more supportive care than those who do not (Lawhon, 1997). "As NICUs begin to define themselves not only as physical care settings but also as settings that support emotional well-being, the infants and families in that care will benefit" (Als, 1996, p. 68).

The caregiver should strive to respect and understand the meaning of infant behavior, including the identification of the infant's current goals and

thresholds for disorganization, and learn how to adjust care accordingly. Additionally, appreciation that the infant is learning from and responding to the caregiver as well is vital (Als, 1999b; Brazelton & Greenspan, 2000). VandenBerg (1997) reminds caregivers "We have an impact that affects the infant's responses, and we must recognize that our hands, our voice, our touch, and our own body rhythms are affecting the way the infant is reacting to our care" (p. 69).

A basic principle of developmental care is the need to respect the individuality of each infant. Care should be based on the individual infant's neurobehavioral and physiologic goals instead of on categoric criteria such as gestational age or weight, protocols, or strict pathways (Lawhon, 1997). Flexibility and focus are necessary to continually assess infants and adapt care to their ever-changing needs (Als, 1998).

## Support of the Infant-Family Relationship

The caregiver needs to acknowledge the short- and long-term value of supporting the developing family-infant relationship. "Relationship-based caregiving implies that the nurse makes a human connection with the infant and, consequently, is invested in furthering the beginning parent-infant relationship" (Lawhon, 1997, p. 55). Caregiving that includes positive, respectful interactions with families, supports families to be with and care for their infant whenever they choose, and respects their privacy with their infant, demonstrates that the caregiver truly values the family-infant relationship (Klaus, Kennell, & Klaus, 1995; Lawhon, 2002).

A developmentally sensitive caregiver respects the strengths and individuality of the family. Many families today consist of a diversity of relationships, not necessarily the traditional core of mother, father, and infant. Caregivers guide families to identify their own strengths, empower them to make informed choices for their infants, and then respect those choices (Browne & Smith-Sharpe, 1995; Hurst, 2001; Johnson, 1995; McGrath, 2001). This empowerment includes supporting families to share equally in making decisions regarding the timing and process of daily care activities, such as bathing or feeding the infant, as well as those decisions associated with life-threatening situations.

Recognition of the family as the primary care-givers and "most important life-long nurturers" of the infant is necessary (Als & McAnulty, 1998, p. 2). This recognition of family can be accomplished despite barriers presented by the physical design of the unit (Figure 2-2). "When family members are truly acknowledged and respected as primary collaborators in their infants' care, they will feel comfortable being with their son or daughter, regardless of the available space or furniture" (Lawhon, 1997, p. 56). This kind of caregiving includes acknowledging that parents and families are partners in caregiving and not "visitors to the NICU environment."

### Relationship to the Staff

Staff should strive to respect the strengths and individuality of each fellow staff member as well as those of the infant and family. This is important and yet can be the most challenging when others do not share the same views (Gilkerson & Als, 1995). This topic is discussed later in this and subsequent chapters.

Caregivers who are functioning as advocates for the infants and their families' need to practice using reflective process when interacting with other staff. Reflection involves the individual being fully aware of the behaviors observed, the emotions experienced, and their own responses as an interaction is occurring. A flexible mind and willingness to practice and learn is necessary to become proficient in this process (Gilkerson & Als, 1995).

### Supportive Care Practices

Many supportive care practices can be implemented by the individual staff member despite the status of unit-wide integration of developmental care. Just how many depends on organizational issues of the particular unit such as staffing ratios, the time

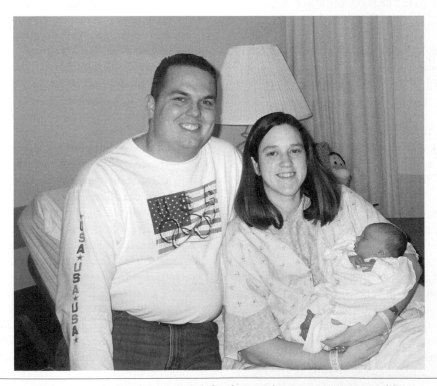

Figure 2-2 Support families in their roles as their infant's most important nurturers. (*Courtesy of the Rosson family, St. Louis, Mo.*)

required for nondirect care duties, and general attitudes regarding developmentally supportive care. A major premise of these changes should be to nurture and guide the family in supporting their infant. Thus, the infant's family should be assisted to become confident in their role as the primary caregivers for the infant.

### Direct Caregiving

The essence of developmental care is supporting the infant to experience life in the NICU in the most nurturing way possible, building the foundation for continued development. Every interaction between the caregiver and the infant is a part of their relationship and needs to be appropriate for that individual infant. The goal is to support infants so that they can reach out and engage their world rather than simply tolerate or always be defending themselves from the world (Figure 2-3). To do this and support optimal development, caregiving

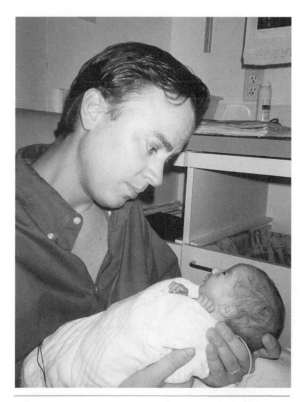

Figure **2-3** Preterm infant engaging her father (*Courtesy of the Geen family, St. Louis, Mo.*)

needs to be appropriate in type, timing, and amount of interaction or interventions for the individual infant (Lickliter, 2000). The following examples summarize some specific interventions for the caregiver (Als, 1999b; Als & McAnulty, 1998; VandenBerg, 1997).

1. *Approach* the infant gently by speaking softly and resting a hand on the baby before moving them or beginning any care activity. Keep the baby's face in view during caregiving so that subtle signs of discomfort or relaxation are recognizable.

2. *Position* the infant, whether lying in bed, being held or moved, or experiencing a procedure or other caregiving, to support flexion and midline orientation based on the infant's individual needs for support. Moving should be done slowly and smoothly, taking care to help the baby gradually adjust.

3. Ensure *feeding* is a pleasurable, nurturing experience for the infant. Strive to arrange calm surroundings and focus full attention on the baby's behavior to guide the pace of the feeding. Support the baby to gently fall asleep after the feeding.

4. When the baby indicates the need for *burping,* support relaxation by holding him or her upright against the shoulder. Again, move the baby gradually when repositioning to resume feeding.

5. Gather all supplies needed for *diaper changing* and *skin care* before approaching the baby. Support the infant to maintain a tucked position and to remain comfortable.

6. Ensure *bathing* is a relaxing, soothing experience for the infant. When intravenous and arterial lines are no longer needed, provide swaddled immersion bathing. Immerse the baby in warm water using hands, a blanket, or a towel to keep the baby's arms and legs tucked and the baby comfortable.

7. Coordinate *timing and sequencing of caregiving interactions* with the family's schedule, to support the infant's developing sleep-wake cycles, and to conserve the infant's energy for feeding and alert periods. Strive to coordinate examinations by specialists, ultrasonographers, and

others to also support the infant's growth and development. Work with the care team to eliminate unnecessary interventions.

8. Prepare the baby for *procedures*, including common ones, such as suctioning and IV insertions by planning ahead to provide comfort measures, such as swaddling, pacifier, and arranging for a second supportive person. Support the infant's position and comfort during procedures. Continue support afterwards to help settle the infant.

9. *Comfort* the baby quickly and consistently when he or she is upset or uncomfortable during or between caregiving. Responding quickly decreases the detrimental physiologic effects of crying, including changes in cerebral blood volume and oxygenation (Brazy, 1988), and begins building trust in the caregiver. If crying is not responded to within 90 seconds, the infant will likely be more difficult to console (Johnson & Johnson Pediatric Institute, Ltd., 1998).

10. *Support developing alertness* by speaking softly and being carefully attuned to the baby's behaviors that indicate enjoyment or distress related to the interaction. Respond to signs of enjoyment by continuing the interaction. If the baby shows even subtle signs of distress or exhaustion, discontinue the interaction and hold the baby quietly.

### The Immediate Sensory Environment

The nurse can arrange appropriate bedding and control the environment immediately surrounding the infant (Als, 1999b; Als & McAnulty, 1998; VandenBerg, 1997). However, the general physical environment and design of the NICU will affect the extent of control that can be achieved.

1. Arrange the infant's *bedspace* so it appears welcoming to the family with available chairs and as much privacy as possible. Encourage the family to decorate the space. This can be achieved even in crowded units.

2. Protect the infant from bright, direct *lighting* to facilitate sleep and also alertness when appropriate for the infant. Adjust the lighting to provide diurnal cycling as appropriate for the infant's developmental level. Lighting perceived by the infant can be dimmed by shielding the visual field with blankets or other coverings while still allowing visibility of the infant for safe caregiving and permitting the infant to see the environment.

3. Lower *sound* levels by speaking and moving softly, answering alarms quickly, and closing drawers and doors quietly. Remember that entering the NICU means entering the room of an intensive care patient.

4. Strive to keep the *activity level* calm despite the intensive nature of the care provided. Even emergency situations can be handled expertly in a nonfrantic, controlled manner.

5. Carefully arrange objects in the infant's *visual field* according to the infant's ability to handle inanimate visual stimulation without distress. Provide new objects only when the baby is calm and alert. Remove them if the infant becomes distressed. Babies often prefer the responsive faces of their parents or caregivers to inanimate objects.

6. Minimize *noxious and unfamiliar odors*, such as hair spray, perfume, and alcohol swabs in the infant's environment. Open packages of necessary products with strong odors away from the baby's face to lessen the initial impact of the smell. Skin-to-skin holding increases the infant's comfort and their familiarity with their parents' bodies and scents.

7. Use supportive *bedding and clothing* according to the baby's individual needs and comfort. Encourage parents to hold their baby skin-to-skin, as they are the best beds for their premature baby (Figure 2-4).

8. Provide *regulatory supports* whenever needed to help the infant become increasingly proficient in self-comforting. These include buntings, their own fingers and hands for sucking, pacifiers, soft rolls for grasping, hand and blanket containment, holding, and skin-to-skin contact with family members (Figure 2-5).

9. Ensure *medical equipment and attachments* are as comfortable as possible for the

infant. Adjust tubes, wires, and tapes so they do not pull on the infant's skin. Size IV boards to maximize range of motion and comfort while still adequately supporting the IV site.

## Reflection While Providing Individualized Care and a Supportive Environment

Use of reflective process is necessary for establishing developmentally supportive relationships with infants as well as with staff members, as mentioned previously

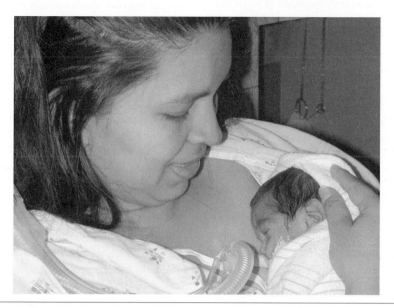

Figure **2-4** Kangaroo care.

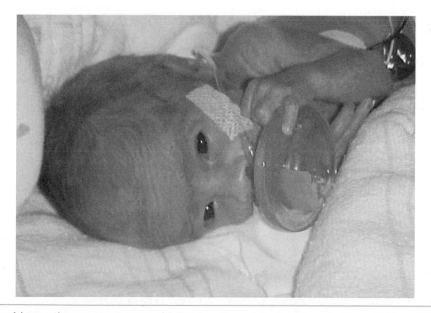

Figure **2-5** Provide regulatory supports to aid the development of self-comforting abilities. (*Courtesy of the Hill family, Houston, TX.*)

(Als & Gilkerson, 1997; Als & McAnulty, 1998; Gilkerson & Als, 1995; Lawhon, 1997). Reflection requires the individual to focus fully on the present interaction while providing the necessary healthcare interventions; to appreciate the goals and needs for support that the infant is communicating; to be fully aware of the individual's own behaviors and their effect on the infant's behavior; and to simultaneously adjust caregiving based on the content and appropriateness of the interaction for the infant.

## WORKING THROUGH COMMON CHALLENGES

The individual staff member works within the nursery system. As such, individual practice is affected by and, in turn, affects the larger system of the NICU. Attempting to incorporate developmental care into practice is often challenging on many levels. The effort, however, might lead to unit awareness, the first of six common stages of unit-wide implementation (Browne & Smith-Sharpe, 1995). Additionally, staff members who attempt early integration of principles into their individual practice are frequently later identified as developmental care resources for the NICU (Smith, 1999).

### Process Challenges

The staff needs to appreciate the time and difficulty involved in complex change, such as that of moving from task-directed to relationship-based care. This involves changes at four levels: knowledge, attitude, individual behavior, and group behavior. Each level must change before the next one can do so; however, aspects of these changes can be somewhat overlapping (Hersey & Blanchard, 1977). Patience with oneself and with coworkers is necessary as new information and skills are learned and integrated into practice. Persistent, active pursuit of this change, however, should also be an expectation. Fragile, preterm infants are experiencing the NICU 24 hours a day, 7 days a week as they continuously mature, laying the foundation for the future. The infants and families who must traverse the NICU are depending on the individual caregiver and the staff to create a NICU experience that supports optimal development.

### Personal Challenges

A staff member might become frustrated with the slow process of change. Furthermore, once skilled at understanding the meaning of infant behavior and the impact of the interaction with the environment and caregivers, she/he might experience emotional anguish when an infant or family is observed to be struggling to deal with a less than optimal situation. If this struggling occurs under the care of another staff member who is less proficient in providing neurobehavioural and family support, he or she might feel torn between preserving the harmony between staff members and interjecting to support the family and infant. It is important for the caregivers to seek out someone who shares their understanding to provide an outlet for exploration of feelings, support, and problem solving.

### Challenges for Families

As individual staff members begin to implement components of developmentally supportive care, families might find themselves "caught in the middle" between staff members that practice very differently. A particular staff member cannot be there for the infant and family all the time. For example, the evening shift caregiver might feel quite comfortable encouraging the family to provide care including skin-to-skin holding, whereas the day shift caregiver might not. One caregiver might cover the incubator and discuss the benefits of this with the family only to have the next shift caregiver remove the cover and refute its value. Staff members should prepare the family for what they might encounter, explaining the differences in practice and the evolving nature of newborn care.

### Challenges for Staff

Staff members should be aware that although the changes involved in developmental care are satisfying to some, they might be threatening to other staff members who view the changes as a loss instead of a benefit. This is especially true for staff members who pride themselves on providing highly technical care. Often polarization occurs between those who support developmental care and those who do not (Als & Gilkerson, 1997). Both covert and overt sabotage of implementation efforts can occur. A change this large brings out a variety of uncomfortable feelings among the staff, including guilt over the effects of past caregiving, a sense of loss of socialization opportunities in a quieter unit, and the loss of previously held roles, such as that of the expert neonatal caregiver.

Resistance, although negative, is energy that needs to be understood and directed. Caregivers need to strive to "acknowledge and value each person, regardless of their beliefs" (Gilkerson & Als, 1995, p. 22) and "have empathy for what motivates others, believe that people have good reasons for their behavior, and stay connected in a way that is useful" (p. 26). Remember that all caregivers share the same goal of wanting to do what they believe is best for the baby. It is the disagreement of the definition of "best care" that is the challenge. This disagreement results from different levels of knowledge, experience, and attitude.

## System Support Challenges

System issues, such as staff-to-infant ratios, the time required for nondirect care tasks, the acceptance of flexibility in and deviation from scheduled, task-oriented care, and the commitment to providing care that supports human development, will impact the ability of staff members to implement developmentally supportive care (Browne & Smith-Sharpe, 1995). The individual staff member should consider forming or joining unit practice or process teams to stimulate change in the NICU (Als, 1999b; Ballweg, 2001). Collaboration between the various members of the healthcare team, including the family, is necessary to structure the infant's 24-hour NICU experience, to support optimal development. Ultimately, systems changes, not just individual changes, are required to move the unit forward. The need for new and/or redefined roles will become apparent. Outside consultation or evaluation of progress might also be needed (Ballweg & Lee, 2004).

## Challenges for Infants

When some staff members provide care from a developmentally supportive framework and others do not, infants, like families, will find themselves "caught in the middle" between staff members that practice very differently. This lack of consistency of the quality of collaborative interaction is a mismatch analogous to learning how to waltz with ever-changing partners. Each partner has a different rhythm, a different touch, a different style of leading, following, and adjusting to the changing dance steps (Walburn, 1992). This unpredictability of experience can be especially costly to fragile preterm infants (Als, 1997; Als & McAnulty, 1998). Despite this, staff should not believe it is too "confusing" for the infant to receive supportive care only some of the time and, therefore, abandon efforts to collaborate with the infant when providing care. They should continue to strive to provide developmentally nurturing, reciprocal caregiving as consistently and with as few different caregivers as possible (Als & McAnulty, 1998; Brazelton & Greenspan, 2000; Stern, 1977).

## CONCLUSION

Developmental care is a philosophy of, a framework for, and a culture of providing relationship-based care that guides the quality, quantity, and timing of all interactions, including the social, environmental, and physical impacting infants and their families and, thus, providing individualized, developmentally supportive experiences that encourage optimal development. Developmental care is a system-wide intervention that crosses all disciplines and work shifts. Achieving optimal medical and behavioral outcomes requires unit-wide implementation. It is important, however, for individual staff members to integrate developmentally supportive knowledge and skills into their practice to the extent they are able. The appropriateness of the interaction between infant and caregiver and the caregiver's support of the developing infant-family relationship are the essence of developmental care. Additionally, each individual staff member creates the NICU culture and environment. Therefore, the journey toward full implementation begins with the first small step of the individual and continues with the persistent pursuit of change. The extent to which the individual caregiver can successfully integrate developmentally supportive practices will vary from unit to unit and depend on the particular challenges faced. The knowledge and skills of each staff member influence the experience of the infant and family in the NICU.

Every individual matters.

Every individual has a role to play.

Every individual makes a difference.

   Jane Goodall (Goodall & Berman, 1999)

## REFERENCES

Als, H. (1992). Individualized, family-focused developmental care for the very low-birthweight preterm infant in the NICU. In S.L. Friedman & M.D. Sigman (Eds.), *The psychological development of low birthweight children* (pp. 341-388). Norwood, NJ: Ablex Publishing.

Als, H. (1996). Earliest intervention for preterm infants in the newborn intensive care unit. In M.J. Guralnick (Ed.), *The effectiveness of early intervention* (pp. 47-76). Baltimore: Brookes Publishing.

Als, H. (1997). Neurobehavioral development of the preterm infant. In A.A. Fanaroff & R.J. Martin (Eds.), *Neonatal-perinatal medicine: Diseases of the fetus and infant* (6th ed., Vol. 2). St. Louis: Mosby.

Als, H. (1998). Developmental care in the newborn intensive care unit. *Current Opinion in Pediatrics, 10,* 138-142.

Als, H. (1999a, October). *Tenth anniversary address: As NIDCAP® marks its first decade, challenge and opportunity lie ahead.* Symposium conducted at the 10th Annual NIDCAP® Trainers' Meeting, Stowe, VT.

Als, H. (1999b). Reading the premature infant. In E. Goldson (Ed.), *Developmental interventions in the neonatal intensive care nursery* (pp. 18-85). New York: Oxford University Press.

Als, H. (2002). *Program guide: Newborn individualized developmental care and assessment program (NIDCAP®).* (rev. ed.). Boston: Children's Medical Center Corporation.

Als, H., & Gilkerson, L. (1997). The role of relationship-based developmentally supportive newborn intensive care in strengthening outcome of preterm infants. *Seminars in Perinatology, 21*(3), 178-189.

Als, H., Lawhon, G., Brown, E., et al. (1986). Individualized behavioral and environmental care for the VLBW preterm infant at high risk for bronchopulmonary dysplasia: NICU and developmental outcome. *Pediatrics, 78*(6), 1123-1132.

Als, H., Lawhon, G., Duffy, F.H., et al. (1994). Individualized developmental care for the very-low-birth-weight preterm infant: Medical and neurofunctional effects. *Journal of the American Medical Association (JAMA), 272*(11), 853-858.

Als, H., & McAnulty, G. (1998). *Developmental care guidelines for use in the newborn intensive care unit (NICU).* Boston: Children's Medical Center Corporation.

Ashbaugh, J.B., Leick-Rude, M.K., & Kilbride, H.W. (1999). Developmental care teams in the neonatal intensive care unit: Survey on current status. *Journal of Perinatology, 191,* 48-52.

Ballweg, D.D. (2001). Implementing developmentally supportive family-centered care in the newborn intensive care unit as a quality improvement initiative. *Journal of Perinatal Neonatal Nursing, 15*(3), 58-73.

Ballweg, D.D., & Lee, L.A. (2004). New roles for developmental care. In C. Kenner & J. McGrath (Eds.), *Developmental care of newborns and infants: A guide for health professionals.* St. Louis: Mosby.

Becker, P.T., Grunwald, P.C., Moorman, J., & Stuhr, S. (1991). Outcomes of developmentally supportive nursing care for very low birth weight infants. *Nursing Research, 40*(3), 150-155.

Brazelton, T.B. & Cramer, B.G. (1990). *The earliest relationship: Parents, infants, and the drama of early attachment.* New York: Addison-Wesley.

Brazelton, T.B., & Greenspan, S.I. (2000). *The irreducible needs of children: What every child must have to grow, learn, and flourish.* Cambridge, MA: Perseus Publishing.

Brazy, J.E. (1988). Effects of crying on cerebral blood volume and cytochrome $aa_3$. *Journal of Pediatrics, 112,* 457-461.

Brink, S. (2002, May 27). Little patients. *U. S. News and World Report,* 52-53.

Browne, J.V., & Paul, D.J. (1999). Developmentally supportive care in the NICU: A nurturing approach for premature and sick multiples. *Twins,* March/April, 24-25.

Browne, J.V., & Smith-Sharpe, S. (1995). The Colorado consortium of intensive care nurseries: Spinning a web of support for Colorado infants and families. *Zero to Three, 15*(6), 18-23.

Buehler, D.M., Als, H., Duffy, F.H., et al. (1995). Effectiveness of individualized developmental care for low risk preterm infants: Behavioral and electrophysiological evidence. *Pediatrics, 96*(5), 923-932.

Fleisher, B.E., VandenBerg, K., Constantinou, J., et al. (1995). Individualized developmental care for very low birth weight premature infants. *Clinical Pediatrics, 34,* 523-529.

Gilkerson, L., & Als, H. (1995). Role of reflective process in the implementation of developmentally supportive care in the newborn intensive care nursery. *Infants & Young Children, 7*(4), 20-28.

Goodall, J., & Berman, P. (1999). *Reason for hope.* (pp. 281). New York: Warner Books.

Hanson, J.L., Johnson, B.H., Jeppson, E.S., Thomas, J., & Hall, J.H. (1994). *Hospitals moving forward with family-centered care.* Bethesda, MD: Institute for Family-Centered Care.

Harrison, H. (1993). The principles for family-centered care. *Pediatrics, 92*(5), 643-650.

Heller, C., Constantinou, J., VandenBerg, K., et al. (1997). Sedation administered to very low birth weight premature infants. *Journal of Perinatology, 17,* 107-112.

Hersey, P., & Blanchard, K.H. (1977). *Management of organizational behavior: Utilizing human resources.* 3rd edition. Englewoood Cliffs, New Jersey: Prentice-Hall.

Hurst, I. (2001). Vigilant watching over: Mothers' actions to safeguard their premature babies in the newborn intensive care nursery. *Journal of Perinatal Neonatal Nursing, 15*(3), 39-57.

Johnson, B.H. (1995). Newborn intensive care units pioneer family-centered change in hospitals across the country. *Zero To Three, 15*(6), 11-17.

Johnson & Johnson Pediatric Institute, Ltd. (1998). *Amazing talents of the newborn. Emerging perspectives in perinatal care: A reference guide for the healthcare professional.* Skillman, NJ: Johnson & Johnson Pediatric Institute, Ltd.

Kennell, J.H. (1999). The humane neonatal care initiative. *Acta Paediatrica, 88*, 367-370.

Klaus, M.H., Kennell, J.H., & Klaus, P.H. (1995). *Bonding: Building the foundations of secure attachment and independence.* New York: Addison-Wesley.

Kleberg, A., Westrup, B., & Stjernqvist, K. (2000). Developmental outcome, child behavior and mother-child interaction at 3 years of age following Newborn Individualized Developmental Care and Intervention Program (NIDCAP®) intervention. *Early Human Development, 60*, 123-135.

Kleberg, A., Westrup, B., Stjernqvist, K., & Lagercrantz, H. (2002). Indications of improved cognitive development at one year of age among infants born very prematurely who received care based on the Newborn Individualized Developmental Care and Assessment Program (NIDCAP®). *Early Human Development, 68*, 83-91.

Lawhon, G. (1997). Providing developmentally supportive care in the newborn intensive care unit: An evolving challenge. *Journal of Perinatal Neonatal Nursing, 10*(4), 48-60.

Lawhon, G. (2002). Facilitation of parenting the premature infant within the newborn intensive care unit. *Journal of Perinatal Neonatal Nursing, 16*(1), 71-82.

Levin, A. (1999). Humane neonatal care initiative. *Acta Paediatrica, 88*, 353-355.

Leyden, C.G. (1998). Consumer bill of rights: Family-centered care. *Pediatric Nursing, 24*(1), 72-73.

Lickliter, R. (2000). The role of sensory stimulation in perinatal development: Insights from comparative research for care of the high-risk infant. *Developmental and Behavioral Pediatrics, 21*(6), 437-447.

McGrath, J.M. (2001). Building relationships with families in the NICU: Exploring the guarded alliance. *Journal of Perinatal Neonatal Nursing, 15*(3), 74-83.

Owens, K. (2001). The NICU experience: A parent's perspective. *Neonatal Network, 20*(4), 67-69.

Parker, S., Zahr, L., Cole, J.G., & Brecht, M. (1992). Outcome after developmental intervention in the neonatal intensive care unit for mothers of preterm infants with low socioeconomic status. *Journal of Pediatrics, 120*(5), 780-785.

Peters, K.L. (2001). Association between autonomic and motor systems in the preterm infant. *Clinical Nursing Research, 101*, 82-90.

Petryshen, P., Stevens, B., Hawkins, J., & Stewart, M. (1997). Comparing nursing costs for preterm infants receiving conventional vs. developmental care. *Nursing Economics, 15*, 138-145, 150.

Philbin, M.K., Ballweg, D.D., Tsakiri, S., et al. (1998). Hospital cost savings and physiologic benefit of developmentally supportive care for very low birth weight newborns. *Pediatric Research, 43*, 40A.

Schore, A.N. (2002, October). *Interactive regulation: An organizing principle of prenatal and postnatal development.* Symposium conducted at the Developmental Interventions in Neonatal Care, San Francisco, CA.

Shannon, J.D., & Gorski P.A. (1994). Health-care professionals' attitudes toward the current level and need for developmental services in neonatal intensive care units. *Journal of Perinatology, 14*(6), 467-472.

Shonkoff, J.P., Phillips, D.A., & Committee on Integrating the Science of Early Childhood Development. (2000). *From neurons to neighborhoods: The science of early childhood development.* Washington, DC: National Research Council Institute of Medicine, National Academy Press.

Smith, K.M. (1999). The journey of a staff nurse. *American Journal of Maternal/Child Nursing, 24*(1), 46-47.

Stern, D. (1977). *The first relationship: Infant and mother.* Cambridge, MA: Harvard University Press.

VandenBerg, K.A. (1997). Basic principles of developmental caregiving. *Neonatal Network, 16*(7), 69-71.

Walburn, K. (1992, November). *Developmental priorities for the "chronic" infant in the neonatal ICU.* Symposium conducted at the Developmental Interventions in Neonatal Care, Chicago, IL.

Watson, J. (1992). Notes on nursing: Guidelines for caring then and now. In D.P. Carroll (Ed.), *Notes on nursing: What it is and what it is not,* Commemorative Edition (pp. 80-85). Philadelphia: J.B. Lippincott.

Westrup, B., Kleberg, A., von Eichwald, K., et al. (2000). A randomized, controlled trial to evaluate the effects of the newborn individualized developmental care and assessment program in a Swedish setting. *Pediatrics, 105*(1), 66-72.

# 3 Theoretic Perspective for Developmentally Supportive Care

Heidelise Als and gretchen Lawhon

Advances in neonatal care have led to significant changes in the survival rates of preterm infants. In nearly 4 million live births annually in the United States, 12% of all newborns each year are born prematurely, and 18% of African-American newborns are preterm (U.S. Department of Health and Human Services Center for Disease Control, 2002). Approximately 1.3% are born weighing less than 1500 g (Guyer, Strobino, Ventura, et al., 1996). Survival rates for those very low birthweight infants (<1500 g) have been stable during the past few years, and are estimated at 80% to 90%, if the infant is admitted to a newborn intensive care unit (NICU) (Hack, Horbar, Malloy, et al., 1991; Herdman, Behney, & Wagner, 1987). Beyond the newborn period preterm infants experience a disproportionate amount of morbidity and need for medical services (Collin, Halsy, & Anderson, 1991; McCormick, Bernbaum, Eisenberg, et al., 1991). Even for those infants who escape major medical complications, very low birthweight infants represent a larger proportion of children with learning problems and developmental limitations, especially in visual-perceptual-motor skills (El-Metwally, Vohr, & Tucker, 2000; Ment, Vohr, Allan, et al., 2003; Peterson, Vohr, Staib, et al., 2000; Vohr & Msall, 1997; Vohr, Wright, Busick, et al., 2000). There is a growing concern and effort to reduce the inherent stress of the newborn intensive care environment while encouraging and facilitating the emerging competence of the infant.

The purpose of this chapter is to provide the theoretic perspective for developmentally supportive care for the newborn. Appreciation of the evolution of newborn development within a neurobiologic social context leads to an understanding of the newborn's behavior that guides the professional caregiver's approach. Because infants' behavior is their main channel of communication, it is para-mount that the professional caregiver appreciates the importance in understanding the meaning of behavior. This requires both sensitivity and vigilance on the part of the caregiver in recognizing and appreciating the subtle nuances of the infant while simultaneously performing the necessary interventions in a therapeutic manner (Franck & Lawhon, 2000). Through trust in the meaningfulness of the infant's behavior, the traditional task-oriented care model is transformed into a collaborative model, with the infant guiding the caregiver as an active participant. Supportive research findings that test this theoretic perspective in the clinical arena are reviewed. Finally, a review of the Newborn Individualized Developmental Care and Assessment Program (NIDCAP®) (Boston, MA) guidelines for provision of individualized developmentally supportive family-centered care is summarized.

## BRAIN DEVELOPMENT

In the full-term child, axonal and dendritic proliferation, and the massive increase in outer-layer cortical cell growth and differentiation leading to the enormous gyri and sulci formation of the human brain (Cowan, 1979), occurs in an environment of mother-mediated protection from environmental perturbations. There is a steady supply of nutrients, temperature control, and the numerous regulating systems, including those of chronobiologic rhythms afforded by the intrauterine environment (Reppert & Rivkees, 1989). In contrast, for the preterm infant, these are absent and are replaced by stimuli from a very differently organized NICU environment. There is increasing evidence that the NICU environment involves sensory overload and stands in stark sensory mismatch to the developing nervous system's growth requirements (Freud, 1991; Gottfried & Gaiter, 1985; Wolke, 1987). It has been shown that prolonged, diffuse sleep states; unattended crying (Hansen & Okken, 1979; Martin, Okken, & Rubin, 1979); supine positioning (Martin, Herrell, Rubin, & Fanaroff, 1979); routine and excessive handling (Danford, Miske, Headley, & Nelson, 1983; Long, Philip, & Lucey, 1980; Murdoch & Darlow, 1984; Norris, Campbell, & Brenkert, 1982); ambient sound (Long, Lucey, & Philip, 1980); lack of opportunity for sucking (Anderson, Burroughs, & Measel, 1983; Burroughs, Asonye, Anderson-Shanklin, & Vidyasagar, 1978; Field, Ignatoff, Stringer, et al., 1982); and poorly timed social and caregiving intera_____ ____ Hale, Leonard, & Martin, 1983) hav_____ ____ tal effects. How does one estir_____ on the infant's nervous syst_____ the relative equilibrium of _____ environment to the extraut_____ ment of the NICU (Albert_____ does one identify and fos_____ strengths in doing so? H_____ infant's current vulnerab_____ engender in the face of t_____ expectation and the input ____ _____ _____ These questions will be considered in this chapter and within other chapters in this text.

## DEVELOPMENTAL THEORY

The principle of phylogenetic and ontogenetic adaptation concerns the individual organism as an evolving member of a species. The ethologist's construct of adaptation (Babson, 1970; Jones, 1972, 1974, 1976) suggests that each organism at any stage of development is evolved to implement not only a species-appropriate but also a species-parsimonious level of adaptedness to its particular niche. Because the process of selection takes place at the level of behavior over generations, many essentials of a species' repertoire can become hardwired, as experimental animal and human studies have documented (Lettvin, Maturana, McCulloch, & Pitts, 1959). In the course of a species' evolution, a surprisingly specific and effective organism-environment fit is ensured at the level of the organism's central nervous system (CNS). The more primitive and simple the organism's nervous system, the more behavioral configurations, or sequences, are likely to be hardwired on a simpler level. The more complex the organism

and the more complex and flexible the behavioral interconnections necessary to ensure species survival, the larger is the association cortex in comparison with the primary sensory cortex. The more likely also is there to be softwiring, which allows flexibility and complexity of response backed up by a system of multiple checks and balances. The more complex and flexible the organism, the larger also is the buffering plasticity and organismic Spielraum, the idling or play space (Als, 1982b, 1992, 1999; Als & Brazelton, 1981; Als, Lester, Tronick, & Brazelton, 1982b).

Ethologic studies of the interaction between newborn and caregiver have identified, from the prenatal period on, the importance, complexity, and subtlety of parent-infant interactions. Although the human newborn shares in the ventroventral primate Tragling (being carried) configuration (Hassenstein, 1973), the human newborn depends on the parents' active physical support to hold on to make being carried successful.

Positive elicitors, which emotionally fuel the caregiver, are not only available but, it appears, are required early on to keep parents socially and affectively close to human infants, who are motorically ineffectual in ensuring the closeness to the parent that is necessary for their survival. Immediately after birth the connections between the newborn's eye opening and visual attention and the parent's affectionate behavior demonstrate a complex homeostatic regulation (Als, 1975, 1977; Grossman, 1978; Minde, Morton, Manning, & Hines, 1980; Robson, 1967). These behaviors appear to function as mutual releasers launching both partners on their path of complex affective and cognitive interchange, fueling mutual competence well beyond discomfort removal, caretaking, and feeding. The ethologist's principle of adaptedness thus sharpens one's observations in taking seriously all of the organism's behavior at each stage of species adaptation. It further identifies the human newborn as a socially competent and active partner in a feedback system with the caregiver, eliciting and seeking that physiologic, motor, state, and attention interactive organization from the environment that the newborn requires to ensure self-actualization.

The evolutionary importance of this earliest extrauterine social-affective connection is underscored by the simultaneous evolutionary differentiation of facial musculature, highlighting the species-specific facial repertoire of the human that supports subtle, complex, and flexible facial expression from birth on. This repertoire of behaviors stands in relationship to the highly differentiated, complex, and flexible social nature and structure of humans, which is the postulated species adaptation ensuring species survival (Als, 1982a). This relationship suggests that from birth on, human newborns are structured to actively elicit the emotional and affective/cognitive support and input that launches and fuels their own increasing behavioral differentiation and organization (Als, 1977). Human newborns are active shapers of their own development, and a high value appears to be placed on their interactive attention capacity in keeping with their species-specific humanness.

The application of the principles of organism-environment transaction to the study of the human newborn (Sander, 1962, 1964, 1970, 1976, 1980) has led to the identification of the interplay of various subsystems of functioning within the organism. These systems influence the infant's physiologic functioning, motor activity, and state organization as they interact with the caregiving environment. The adaptive tasks for the infant are to achieve phase synchrony between periodicities that characterize these different systems, as well as synchronization between internal events and the environment (Sander, 1975, 1980; Sander, Stechler, Burns, & Lee, 1979). Stimuli that are poorly timed are seen to penetrate and disrupt all subsystems, whereas appropriately timed stimuli appear to maintain and enhance functional integration and support growth. The task of support lies in the identification of synchronous and cohesive functioning and of the thresholds to disruption.

According to Denny-Brown (Denny-Brown, 1962, 1966), a motor system physiologist, underlying the organism's evolving toward smoothness of integration is the tension between two basic antagonists of behavior, as seen in movement disorders such as athetosis. There are two basic physiologic types of responses—namely, the exploratory and the avoiding response; the 'toward' and the 'away'; the approaching or reaching out; and the withdrawing or defending response. The two responses at times are released together and are in conflict with one another. If a threshold of organization- is passed, one can abruptly ow basic these two poles of ated by the existence of sin- nsory cortex programmed toward movements upon r single cells produce total nts (Duffy & Burchfiel, rinciple has been shown to the gradual specialization ses leading to functionally stance, in altricial animals, e-grasping, huddling, and others (Als, 1982a, 1999; Als, Lester, & Brazelton, 1979; Rosenblatt, 1976; Schneirla, 1959, 1965; Schneirla & Rosenblatt, 1961, 1963).

The principles outlined are thought to be relevant to fetal infants who find themselves in the extrauterine environment too early. The principle of dual antagonist integration is helpful in understanding the behavioral patterns of preterm infants to assess thresholds from integration to disorganization. In the integrated performance, the 'toward' and 'away' antagonists modulate each other in bringing about an adaptive response. If an input is compelling to the infant and stimulates the infant's interest and internal readiness, the infant will approach the input, react and interact with it, seek it out, and become sensitized to it. If the input exceeds the infant's capacity to respond, the infant will actively avoid the input, and withdraw from it. Both responses mutually modulate each other. For example, a full-term newborn is drawn to the animated face of the interacting caregiver. As the attention intensifies, the infant's eyes widen, eyebrows rise, and mouth shapes toward the interactor (Als, 1975, 1977). If the dampening mechanisms of this intensity are not established, as in the immature or preterm infant, the whole head might move forward, arms and legs might thrust toward the interactor, and fingers and toes will extend toward the stimulus. The response, early on, involves the entire body in an undifferentiated way and gradually will become largely confined to the face (Als, 1979). The differentiation process appears to be regulated through such homeostatic infant behaviors as averting the eyes, yawning, sneezing, or hiccoughing, or it might be regulated by the caregiver through kissing, nuzzling, or moving the infant closer, thus resetting the cycle (Als, 1975, 1977). If neither of these regulation mechanisms is brought into play, or if the initial input is too strong, the infant might turn away, grimace, extend his arms to the side, arch his trunk, splay his fingers and toes, cry, hiccough, spit up, stop breathing, or defecate. In short, the infant will engage in avoidance behaviors at various levels of functioning. Therefore, it appears that very early behavioral functioning might be conceptualized as the continual negotiation of the fetal infant's developmental agenda (Als, 1978, 1979, 1982b, 1982c, 1983; Brazelton & Als, 1979).

The initial overriding issue with which the prematurely born human newborn appears to be grappling is the stabilization and integration of physiologic functions, such as respiration, heart rate (HR), temperature control, digestive function, and elimination, for which the preterm infant typically requires medical technologic support, such as a respirator, an incubator, or intravenous feeding. The prematurely born infant's motor system is the competent motor system at the corresponding fetal stage that is capable of initiating and maintaining flexion, rotation, bringing the hand-to-mouth, sucking, grasping, and so on.

State organization and other periodicities, no longer supported by the maternal sleep-wake, and rest-activity cycles, nor by the maternal hormonal and nutritional cycles, are now influenced by the rhythm of the NICU environment. Therefore, a model of subsystem differentiation emerges, called "synactive" (Als, 1982b), which highlights the simultaneity of all subsystems in their interaction with one another and with the environment. The process of development appears to be that of stabilization and integration of subsystems, which allow the differentiation and emergence of next capacities that, in turn, contribute toward a newly integrated system. In this model, the entire system continually reopens and progresses to a new level of more differentiated integration, from which, in turn, the next emerging subsystem differentiation occurs, progressing to more sophisticated and integrated levels of physiologic and behavioral organization throughout the lifespan (Als, 1979, 1982b, 1982c, 1983; Als, Lester, Tronick, & Brazelton, 1982a; Als, Lester, Tronick, and Brazelton, et al., 1982b). To paraphrase Erikson (Erikson, 1962), self-actualization is participation with the world and interaction with another with

a "minimum of defensive maneuvers and a maximum of activation, a minimum of idiosyncratic distortion and a maximum of joint validation."

## UNDERSTANDING NEWBORN BEHAVIOR

Taking into consideration the anatomic and functional development of the brain, it is hypothesized that it is feasible in this model to estimate the expectation of the fetal brain for input and the developmental goals of the infant for co-regulatory support by observing the infant's behavior. This approach postulates that the infant's own behavior provides the best information base from which to estimate the infant's current capabilities, and to infer what the infant attempts to accomplish and what processes are involved to achieve each level of differentiation. On the basis of this information, one should be in a position to estimate what supports might currently be useful in furthering the infant's competencies and supporting overall neurobehavioral organization, even in the face of necessary medical and nursing procedures. Because the infant is seen as continuously and actively self-constructing (Fischer & Rose, 1994), the task of care becomes that of collaborating with the infant. The formulation of observation and design of subsequent support for a prematurely born infant, therefore, is conceptually based in a combination of knowledge of the fetal brain and of behavioral developmental progression. The developmental functioning of the full-term infant provides a biologic blueprint, but is one that, for the preterm infant, is modified by the altered environment-fetus transaction, and by each infant's individual characteristics and needs. By accurately interpreting the infant's behavior, it should become possible to construct an appropriate caregiving environment (Als, 1982b).

It has been shown that even the earliest born and most fragile of infants displays reliably observable behaviors. These take the form of autonomic and visceral responses, such as respiration patterns, color fluctuations, spitting, gagging, hiccoughing, and straining. Other behaviors include movement patterns, postures, truncal tone, and the tone of extremities and face, reflected as finger splaying, arching, and grimacing, among others. Other parameters to consider are levels of awareness, referred to as "states," such as sleeping, wakefulness, and aroused upset, and their respective characteristics (Als, 1983, 1984; Als, Lester, Tronick, et al., 1982b).

The infant's behavioral repertoire thus far has been identified along the lines of three main subsystems: the autonomic system, the motor system, and the state system. The reasoning in support of this approach is that the infant's communication with the environment along these subsystem lines is readily accessible for observation, even without instrumentation, and will indicate whether what is currently going on around or within the infant is supportive of the infant's functioning or is taxing and demanding and potentially stressful for the infant (Als, 1982b; Als, Lawhon, Gibes, et al., 1986). The infant's behavior can be understood as involving these basic subsystems. The autonomic system's functioning is observable in the infant's breathing patterns, color fluctuation, and visceral stability or instability. Examples of the autonomic systems responses include respiratory regularities or irregularities, color changes, such as cyanosis or pallor, and visceral stability reflected in, for instance, hiccoughing, gagging, or spitting up. Observing the infant's body tone, postural repertoire, and movement patterns assesses the effects of the infant's motor-system integrity and functioning. Examples of these are reflected in facial and trunk tone; tone of the extremities, as well as in the extensor and flexor postures and movements of face, trunk, and limbs. The infant's state organization is observable in the infant's range of available states, the robustness and modulation of the states, and the patterns of transition from state to state. Some infants show the full continuum of states from deep sleep, to light sleep, to drowsy, to quiet alert, to active awake and aroused, to upset and crying (Brazelton, 1973). Alternately, some infants during interactions move from sleep to aroused states and immediately back down to sleep again, skipping the alert state. In a word, state stability and the smooth transition from state to state reflect intact state organization and CNS control, whereas the opposite would reflect CNS disorganization.

## NIDCAP®

NIDCAP® has created a clinically usable paper-and-pen methodology for recording detailed observations of the infant's naturally occurring behaviors in the NICU, and, thus, to document an infant's communication. The observer does not interact directly with the infant, but stands close by and watches the infant. To understand the infant's current functioning and thresholds of stability of the autonomic, motor, and state organizational systems, it has been found useful to observe the infant for at least 60 to 90 minutes. This includes approximately 10 minutes of observation before a caregiving interaction with the infant, the duration of the caregiving interaction, for instance, vital sign taking, suctioning, diaper changing, and feeding, and approximately 10 minutes following the caregiving interaction. Such an observation, especially if repeated on at least a weekly basis, yields specific information regarding an infant's robustness and development (Als, 1981; Als, et al., 1986; Als, Lawhon, Duffy, et al., 1994). The observations can then form the basis for caregiving suggestions and modifications in environmental structuring.

In integrating the observed behavioral communications into a descriptive narrative, the infant's environment is first described in terms of light, sound, and activity. The behavioral picture derived from the observation period preceding the caregiving interaction is then described, in its relationship to HR, respiratory rate (RR), and blood oxygen levels. Then, the caregiving interaction and its effect on the infant are documented, with specific behaviors being observed again in relation to HR, RR, and oxygen levels. The infant's efforts to integrate the effects of the interaction, and also the caregiver's efforts to aid the infant, are described. As pointed out, the infant has strategies and mechanisms available to move away from and avoid environmental demands or configurations that are inappropriate in complexity, intensity, and/or timing of the infant. The infant furthermore has strategies and mechanisms available to seek out and move toward inputs that are at the level of the infant's current intake capacities. Avoidance behaviors are thought of as reflecting stress. Approach and self-regulation behaviors might shift and become stress behaviors, and similarly, stress behaviors, when successful in reducing stress, might become self-regulatory strategies. In this model, extension behaviors largely are thought to reflect stress, and flexion behaviors are thought to reflect self-regulatory competence. Diffuse behaviors are thought to be reflective of stress, and well-defined robust behaviors reflective of self-regulatory balance. Self-regulatory balance, thus, is reflected in regular, smooth respirations, which are neither too fast nor too slow and are not interspersed with pauses. Other evidence of this balance is the presence of pink color; the absence of tremors, startles, and twitches; the absence of visceral signs; the absence of flaccidity; the presence of smooth, but not overly flexed active tone and arm, leg, and trunk position; smooth movements of arms, legs, and trunk; and efforts and successes at tucking trunk and limbs together. Suck-searching and sucking, hand and foot clasping, hand-to-mouth efforts, grasping and holding on, the presence of robust states, raising of eyebrows (face opening), frowning, forward shaping of the mouth (ooh face), looking, cooing, and speech movements, HR between 120 and 160; RR between 40 and 60, and oxygen saturation, using a pulse oximetry, between 92% and 98%, are typically interpreted as effective self-regulation. Stress and a low threshold to react, reflecting greater sensitivity, would be reflected by irregular respirations, overly slow or fast respirations, and respiratory pauses; and color other than pink—that is, pale, mottled, red, dusky, or blue. Other evidence for stress is the presence of tremors, startles, and twitches and visceral signs, such as spitting up, gags, hiccoughs, grunting, and bowel movement straining, sounds, gasps, and sighs. Motor signs of stress include flaccidity of the face, arms, legs, and trunk; frequent extensor movements of the arms and legs; stretching and drowning-like behavior; frequent squirming; arching; frequent tongue extensions; grimacing; specific finger, arm and leg extensions (splaying, airplaning, saluting, and sitting on air); frequent fisting, fussing, yawning, sneezing; floating eye movements; and visual averting. A HR less than 120 or greater than 160; RR of less than 40 or greater than 60; and blood oxygenation of less than 92% or higher than 98% are also considered potential signs of stress. A picture emerges from such a description as to the level of support or relative vigor of sensory input at which the infant moves from self-regulatory balance to stress. The behavioral record is written

with descriptions in a language understandable to parents as well as professionals. The record's purpose is to educate and support the caregivers in understanding the infant's behavioral functioning and seeing the infant as an active structurer and participant in his or her own development (Als, 1999).

## SUPPORTIVE RESEARCH

To test the efficacy of the NIDCAP® approach to caregiving in supporting CNS development in the lesion-free brain, a sample of healthy, low-risk, preterm infants, free of known focal and suspected lesions, was studied (Buehler, Als, Duffy, et al., 1995). Twenty-four consecutively inborn preterm singleton infants cared for in a 16-bed, level II, special care nursery (SCN) were randomly assigned to an experimental and a control group. They were younger than 34 weeks' gestational age at birth, of appropriate weight for gestational age, with uneventful labor and delivery histories; did not require mechanical ventilation for more than 24 hours; were genetically and neurologically intact; and had healthy mothers. The experimental group infants were formally observed within the first 24 hours after birth and every seventh day thereafter. A developmental psychologist in collaboration provided the group with ongoing individualized developmental care with a developmentally trained nurse clinician. Control-group infants received the standard of care practiced throughout the SCN. A group of 12 healthy, full-term infants was studied as a comparison group. Although the preterm experimental group infants showed no differences in terms of medical outcome compared with the preterm control group or the fullterm group, significant differences among the three groups were found on two behavioral outcome measures, the Assessment of Preterm Infant Behavior (APIB) (Als, Lester, Tronick, et al., 1982a) and the Prechtl Neurological Evaluation (Prechtl, 1977).

Four of the six APIB subsystem scores showed significant group differences. As the post hoc pairwise comparisons indicate, the preterm control group displayed the least well-organized behavioral performance, whereas the preterm experimental and full-term groups were behaviorally comparable. The preterm control group was significantly less well organized than the preterm experimental group on autonomic, motor, and attention parameters. The preterm control group also differed significantly from the full-term comparison group on measures of autonomic, motor, and regulatory organization. The preterm control group was the least well modulated, the preterm experimental group the second best modulated, and the full-term group the most well modulated.

Measures of electrophysiologic function also showed significant improvement for the intervention preterm group compared with the control preterm group. Thirteen of these significant correlations were found between the frontal lobe features and APIB variables measuring attention control and state organization. An additional nine features representing the temporal, parietal, and central regions also correlated significantly with APIB measures of attention. The remaining six correlations indicated significant relationships with measures of autonomic and motor organization. Thus, the medically healthy preterm infants who received individualized developmental care were better adjusted autonomically and motorically and, especially, in terms of state regulation and attention functioning than the preterm infants who received standard care. Furthermore, they were comparable to the healthy full-term infants with respect to these functions. These neurophysiologic differences were seen in spite of the fact that there were no medical differences between the groups at the time of the quantified electroencelogram (qEEG) study. The frontal region demonstrated significant correlation with behavioral indices of attention control and state organization, and appeared to show differential vulnerability in the preterm control group. This is not surprising given that, as pointed out earlier, neuronal organization of this region occurs relatively late in the developmental sequence (Huttenlocher, 1984; Schade & van Groenigen, 1961; Yakovlev & Lecours, 1967). Previous studies of prematurity have indicated the frontal region's differential vulnerability (Duffy, Als, & McAnulty, 1990). It appears that the intervention supports a more full-term–like differentiation of brain function for these healthy preterm infants, and might especially protect frontal-lobe functioning. A second study of medically low-risk, preterm infants born at 28 to 33 weeks' gestational age and appropriate in growth for age (AGA) found similarly encouraging behavioral and electrophysiologic results, and furthermore identified for the first time brain structural effects of NIDCAP® care. Total cerebral tissue volume of subcortical gray matter, as measured by three-dimensional magnetic resonance imaging (MRI) tissue segmentation techniques, was significantly increased, as was fiber development in frontal and internal capsule white matter, as measured by MR-diffusion tensor imaging (DTI) (Als, Duffy, McAnulty, et al., 2002).

The NIDCAP® approach to environmental support and care based on reading the preterm infant's behavioral cues as described is increasingly advocated also for the preterm infants at highest risk for later disability (Becker, Grunwald, Moorman, & Stuhr, 1993; Grunwald & Becker, 1990; Lawhon, 1986; Lawhon & Melzar, 1991; VandenBerg, 1990a, 1990b; VandenBerg & Franck, 1990; Wolke, 1987). In the past 20 years this approach has been tested in several studies. Als and Berger (1986) found improved medical outcome of very low birthweight (VLBW) ventilated preterm infants as evidenced by shorter stays on the respirator, and a decrease in the need for supplemental oxygen and gavage feedings. Improved behavioral outcome at 2 weeks' corrected age, as assessed with the APIB (Als, 1982a, 1982b), and at 9 months using the Bayley Scales of Infant Development Scores, were again found. Furthermore, there was improved behavioral regulation as assessed by using a videotaped play paradigm (Kangaroo-Box Paradigm) (Als & Berger, 1986; Als, Duffy, & McAnulty, in press). Becker, Grunwald, Moorman, et al. (Becker, Grunwald, Moorman, & Stuhr, 1991; Becker, Grunwald, Moorman, & Stuhr, 1993; Grunwald & Becker, 1990) found significantly lower scores of morbidity in the first 4 weeks of hospitalization, as measured with the Minde Daily Morbidity Scale (Minde, Whitelaw, Brown, & Fitzhardinge, 1983). There was significantly earlier onset of oral feedings, better average daily weight gain, shorter hospital stays, as well as, improved overall behavioral functioning at discharge, as measured with the NBAS (Brazelton, 1984). Long-term outcomes assessed for the Als study (Als, Lawhon, Gibes, et al., 1986) at 18 months and 3 years continue to show a consistent developmental advantage of the experimental group over the control group (Als, Duffy, & McAnulty, in preparation). The preliminary results from the longitudinal data available from this study show much improved performance of the experimental group at 7 years on several neuropsychologic measures (Als, in press).

Another study (Als, Lawhon, Duffy, et al., 1994) used random assignment of infants, weighing less than 1251g, born before 30 weeks gestational age, intubated within the first 3 hours after delivery, and requiring mechanical ventilation for at least 24 of the first 48 hours. Eighteen control and 20 experimental group infants met these criteria. For this study, a group of nurses were specially educated and trained in the behaviorally based approach of individualized caregiving. Staffing was structured in such a way that for the experimental group infants, during at least one shift in every 24-hour cycle, a nurse specially educated in the behavioral approach cared for the infant and family. Formal behavioral observations were conducted by a psychologist in collaboration with a developmental clinical nurse specialist, started within the first 24 hours, and were repeated every 10th day until discharge from the nursery. Again, these observations provided the basis for support to the primary teams for individualization of care for the experimental group infants and their families. Control group infants were identified to the NICU staff within 2 weeks before discharge so that staffing and care would not be influenced or biased in any way. The control and experimental groups were comparable on all background variables, including birthweight; gestational age at birth; Apgar scores at 1 and 5 minutes; mean and maximum fractions of inspired oxygen ($FiO_2$) in the first 48 hours and the first 10 days; the incidence of patent ductus arteriosus, maternal age, social class, Obstetric Complication Scale Scores (Littman & Parmelee, 1974), gender, ethnicity, birth order; and the use of prenatal corticosteroids. The experimental group infants showed a significant reduction in the length of hospitalization, were younger at discharge, had reduced hospital charges, and improved weight gain to 2 weeks after their due date. They had a reduced rate of intraventricular hemorrhage (IVH), and of the severity of chronic lung disease. They also showed improved developmental outcome at 2 weeks corrected age, as measured

with the APIB (Als, Lester, Tronick, & Brazelton, 1982b), with much better functioning in terms of autonomic regulation, motor system performance, and self-regulation. Systematic electrophysiologic group differences by qEEG with topographic mapping (Duffy, Burchfiel, & Lombroso, 1979) were also found at 2 weeks postterm, suggesting that there were differences in function in a large, central region of the brain as well as in a large portion of the right occipital hemisphere, in two left parietal, a right parietal, and an additional right occipital region.

By 9 months after the expected date of confinement (EDC), two infants in the control group were unavailable for study. On assessment with the Bayley Scales of Infant Development, the experimental group, compared with the control group, showed a significantly higher Mental Developmental Index (118.30 ± 17.35 vs 94.38 ± 23.31; F = 12.47; $df$ = 1, 34; $P \le 0.001$) and Psychomotor Developmental Index (100.60 ± 20.19 vs 83.56 ± 17.97; F = 6.97; $df$ = 1,34; $P \le 0.01$).

Furthermore, of 20 infant variables measured in the 6-minute Kangaroo Box Paradigm Play Episode, 16 showed differences favoring the experimental group. They ranged in significance level from less than 0.03 to less than 0.0001. The largest differences were found in gross and fine motor modulation, overflow postures and associated movements, complexity and modulation of combining object and social play, ability to stay engaged in the task, and degree of facilitation necessary to accomplish the task. In the 6-minute Still-Face Episode, 12 of 19 infant parameters showed significant group differences ($P < 0.04$ to $< 0.0001$), again favoring the experimental group infants. None of the 14 parent variables assessed showed a significant group difference, yet all three interaction variables (turn-taking, overall synchrony of the interaction, and overall quality of the interaction variables ($P < 0.0004$) favored the experimental group. Therefore, the infants in the experimental group appeared significantly better organized, better differentiated, and better modulated than the control group infants. Canonical correlation between the factors derived from the APIB variables and the factors derived from the Kangaroo-Box variables was statistically significant. This indicates a strong relationship between overall behavioral regulation at 2 weeks, as measured with the APIB, and overall regulation at 9 months, as measured with the Kangaroo Box Paradigm.

Neither IVH nor bronchopulmonay dysplasia (BPD) had significant indirect effects on any of the medical outcome variables. In terms of electrophysiologic outcome, IVH had a significant indirect effect on only one variable. However, even for this variable, the direct intervention effect was stronger. The presence of BPD had no indirect effect on any of the electrophysiologic findings. Neither IVH nor BPD had any significant indirect effects on any of the APIB or Bayley outcome measures. Furthermore, only two of the 32 Kangaroo Box measures showed significant indirect IVH effects, namely symmetry of motor performance in the play and in the still-face episode. None showed indirect BPD effects. Therefore, the direct effects of the intervention on outcome appear to go beyond the indirect contribution from reduction in IVH and BPD.

Two studies from other centers (Fleisher, VandenBerg, Constantinou, et al., 1995) focused on the same high-risk populations and were conducted since the introduction of surfactant in the NICUs. The studies found significant positive medical results and, in the one study testing behavioral outcome, also positive APIB results, although the NIDCAP® intervention in both studies involved only in-service orientations to the nursing staff, and relied in each of the two NICUs on an experienced NIDCAP® trained professional and leader to provide daily support to those caring for the experimental group infants. The study conducted in Sweden (Westrup, Kleberg, von Eichwald, et al., 2000) has also reported long-term, significantly improved neurodevelopmental outcome for the experimental group children at 1, 3, and 5 years of age (Kleberg, Westrup, & Stjernqvist, 2000; Kleberg, Westrup, Stjernqvist, & Lagercrantz, 2002; Westrup, Böhm, Lagercrantz, & Stjernqvist, 2003).

In another study (Als, Duffy, & McAnulty, in preparation) the integration of this individualized approach into the NICU was tested by assignment of experimental group high-risk infants to specially trained care teams supported on an ongoing basis by two developmental specialists, who, however, did not conduct serial behavioral observations. Preliminary analysis of outcome again showed reduction in

number of days on the ventilator and in need of gavage tube feedings, decreased length of hospitalization, and improved weight gain, as well as improved developmental outcome at 2 weeks and 9 months after the EDC. There was no decrease in incidence of IVH or severity of chronic lung disease. IVH effects might depend on developmental support in the acute first few hours of admission, when systematic feedback might be differentially productive.

A recent, multicenter study tested the NIDCAP® approach simultaneously in three different NICUs. Again, the design was that of a randomized clinical (multicenter) trial that focused on ventilator-dependent, very high-risk preterm infants born at 28 weeks' gestation or younger. The study involved an inborn as well as two transport NICUs, and NICUs that used primary care nursing and conventionally scheduled nursing. Results validated the effectiveness of the developmental care model in terms of significant improvement, especially in terms of weight gain and growth parameters, and in reduction of length of hospital stay and hospital cost. Developmental outcome, as measured with the APIB, also showed significant improvement. Furthermore, analysis of the assessment of family functioning showed that the experimental group parents were significantly more effective in understanding their infants as individuals and themselves as parents (Als, Gilkerson, Duffy, et al., in press). Furthermore, the consistency of NIDCAP® care implementation for the experimental groups was measured and found to be significantly higher than for the control group infants in all those parameters, which involved care aspects under the direction of the individual caregiver at the bedside (Als, Buehler, Kerr, et al., 1990, 1995, rev. 1997). The three NICU-wide parameters of light, sound, and activity level were not found to be different between the control and experimental group infants. This was interpreted to mean that NIDCAP® care involves more than light, sound, and activity control, and seems to include the quality of the individually sensitive caregiving interaction with the infant that relies on each infant's cues to guide the timing, intensity, and duration of all action sequences and subcomponents.

Results of the studies reviewed, which assessed the effectiveness of developmental care in the NIDCAP®

model for healthy preterm infants and for very early born, very low birthweight, and very high risk preterm infants, suggest that differences in experience during the last 16 weeks of gestation differentially influence infants' neurodevelopmental functioning. These differences are measurable at 2 weeks' and 9 months postterm and appear to foreshadow the developmental differences documented for preterm children at preschool and school ages.

## NIDCAP® GUIDELINES FOR COLLABORATIVE CARE

The clinical framework of developmental care, derived from the conceptual and empiric work previously outlined and referred to as NIDCAP®, offers training for professionals in the family-centered individualized approach to care described. To effectively integrate developmentally supportive, family-centered care into NICUs in the NIDCAP® framework, the following guidelines for the individualized structuring of the infant's 24-hour day, enhancement of the physical environment, and caregiving team collaboration are provided (Holmes, Sheldon, & Als, 1995; Vento & Feinberg, in press; Als & Gilkerson, 1995, 1997; Als & McAnulty, 1998; Gilkerson & Als, 1995). These guidelines have been derived from the experiences of the NIDCAP® research teams and should always be individualized to the needs of the infant and family.

## STRUCTURING OF THE INFANT'S 24-HOUR DAY

The primary care team coordinates all interventions across several 24-hour time epochs into individually appropriate clusters timed in accordance with the individual infant's sleep-wake cycles, state of alertness, medical needs, and feeding competence. All interventions are evaluated regarding their necessity and appropriateness for a particular infant. The goal is to provide restfulness and to support growth. Infants' caregiving schedules are coordinated with family schedules to support the integration of the infant into the family and the family into the NICU, and to foster the family's involvement and competence in the child's nurturance and care. During delivery of care, caregivers approach the infant and family in a calm, attentive manner, explaining to the

family the goal and approximate sequence of the care components considered.

Caregivers are encouraged to observe the infant first to understand the infant's current means of communication. They then introduce themselves to the infant using a soft voice and gentle touch, providing periods of rest and recovery between manipulations, containing the infant in a gentle embrace with their hands and/or encouraging the parent to do so. Hands-on containment, sucking on a pacifier or the finger, hand holding, and hand-to-mouth exploration are ways to support the dialogue between infant and caregiver and to foster the infant's and the parent's overall competence. During transition periods between caregiving components, caregivers should direct careful attention to the infant's behavior. Typically, increased support is needed as the infant awakens spontaneously, makes efforts to come to alertness, and return to sleep. This is especially the case for very prematurely born infants and those with dysmature or impaired nervous systems, such as infants who experienced birth asphyxia, intrauterine growth restriction, and narcotic or cocaine exposure. Such infants might demonstrate lower thresholds to disorganization. During alert periods caregivers attempt to balance sensory input from the caregiver and from the environment with the infant's current level of alertness and competence. Caregiver interactions are guided by the behavioral cues of the infant toward support of robust wakefulness, increasingly well-focused alertness, and well-modulated social interaction. Furthermore, caregivers should support softly flexed, comfortably aligned positions during sleep, routine care, feeding, bathing, and special procedures. Aids, such as blanket rolls, nesting, gentle swaddling, special buntings, and hands-on containment, might be helpful. Clothing the infant in soft cotton garments appropriately small in size and covering the infant with a soft cotton or silk blanket have been found to facilitate restfulness and comfort. The use of support is gauged to the infant's competence. Support is increased or decreased depending on the infant's autonomous maintenance of tone and well-adjusted positions and movements.

Feeding method and frequency is also individualized and is based on the infant's competence. The goal is to progress toward infant initiated and controlled feeding. To facilitate feeding competence, caregivers decrease environmental stimulation and securely cradle the infant in the caregiver's arms in semi-upright soft flexion, with hands in midline, free to grasp and hold on, and with legs and feet contained. Feeding success is not only judged by the infant's intake but also by the infant's overall energy levels, and autonomic, motor, and state functioning. Feeding is conceptualized as a pleasurable and nurturing experience.

Suctioning and providing pulmonary care is performed only when clinically indicated, never on a preset schedule and is always performed by a two-person team. Routine suctioning of the premature infant as well as chest physical therapy have been shown to lead to abrupt changes in blood flow velocity, associated with intraventricular hemorrhage and cerebral infarction and should, therefore, be avoided. When indicated and executed gently, support by the second caregiver (who, whenever possible, should be the parent) helps contain and stabilize the infant throughout the procedure, thereby lessening potential risks, and increasing support to the infant.

Opportunities for skin-to-skin holding and nesting are to be available at all times and to all families of NICU infants, including ventilated infants. Reclining chaise lounges with foot and head rests and large enough to accommodate two parents should be available at each bedside. Staff is specially trained in the care and comfort of postpartum parents and of infants for the provision of skin-to-skin nurturing. The parent's body has been found to provide warmth and maintain the infant's stable body temperature. The infant has been found to experience increased respiratory stability with decreased incidence of apnea and bradycardia. Such physical contact appears to result in more restful sleep in the infant and a sense of calm and fulfillment in the parent. Mothers who hold their infant skin-to-skin experience increased milk production as well as success and enjoyment in breastfeeding (see Chapter 15).

All infants with intact skin should be bathed by full immersion to the shoulder and neck level in suitably sized tubs filled with warm water. The infant can be supported placed in a deep warm water bath while loosely swaddled. Providing hands-on containment will further support the infant's relaxation and temperature stability. As soon and as frequently as possible, parents are the caregivers of choice to bathe their infant. Infants are weighed, softly swaddled in a blanket or bunting, with gentle movement from bed to scale and back, unless the bed simultaneously provides a scale. All special examination and assessment procedures, including physical examinations, ultrasound examinations of the head, chest radiographs, EEGs, eye examinations, neurologic examinations, and such, are performed collaboratively by the respective, specialist assisted by the infant's nurse, and facilitated by the parent, when possible, to support the infant's comfort and well-being in the course of required position changes, palpations, auscultations, and the like. The infant's face is shielded whenever possible from intense illumination. At all times the size and quality of equipment, materials, and devices required are apportioned to the size and strength of the infant's limbs and skin to ensure maximal comfort and physiologically appropriate alignment and movement of limbs, joints, and so on. Intravenous boards, whenever possible, support elbow flexion and finger grasp. Tape used is expected to be skin friendly. When bilirubin blankets are not sufficient and bilirubin lights and eye patches are necessary, rest periods from eye covers are provided with each caregiving interaction.

### Enhancement of the Physical Environment in Support of Infants and Families

Lighting is adjusted to support each individual infant's and family's best sleep and awake organization and deliver care without impinging on the development, comfort, and care of other infants. Individualized bedside-controlled lighting with dimmer capacity should be available. It is suggested that the general nursery lighting be indirect and readily adjusted in terms of brightness. Furthermore, nurseries should be quiet, soothing places. Suggestions for sound containment include creating a space within the NICU for admissions and special procedures; educating staff about preterm infant responses to various sound levels as part of the staff's training; moving daily rounds, discussions and conversations away from infant and family bed spaces; dampening sounds from equipment, such as telephones, waste receptacles, monitor alarms, sinks, doors, and movable equipment; eliminating radios, overhead pagers, and all other unnecessary sound; transferring infants from warming tables to incubators with quiet motors as soon after admission as possible; covering incubators with thick blankets fitted with special sound shielding material; choosing wall covering with sound-absorbent materials and structuring walls architecturally for maximal sound absorption, and carpeting all care areas.

Caregivers should avoid the use of perfumes, colognes, and scented hair sprays, as infants are very sensitive to these odors. The odor of tobacco on caregiver bodies and clothes as well as the odors of dry cleaning chemicals should also be avoided. Alcohol or sulfa-based chemicals should only be used when infants are removed from the care area. Care is taken to allow the cleaning fluids to dry and the vapors to evaporate before bedding the infant back in the incubator. While parents are holding the infant skin-to-skin, a soft cloth placed across the infant and their own breasts or chests or a mother's breast pads will enhance and extend the infant's comfort in the recognition of the parent's odor when the infant is returned to the incubator, tucked in with the parents' cloth or pad.

NICU environments are structured so that infants can be cared for in conjunction with their families. Specific aids such as soft bedding, buntings, water mattresses, and pacifiers are used to lessen the impact of necessary medical procedures and equipment. Homelike, individualized spaces or family coves for infant and family within the NICU; secure attractive cabinets to store belongings; communal space equipped with kitchen facilities; a library with written and audio-visual materials; washer and dryer facilities; rooms for sleeping; and bathroom and shower facilities for family members should be available. Twin and other multiple infants should be cared for in one family area and in one bed or incubator as possible. Parents are encouraged to consider their infants' care spaces as their space. They are encouraged to arrange the space to their aesthetic liking. Bedside telephones for family members are of great importance for all families. It is suggested that the NICU be structured for the 24-hour comfort not only of the parents, but also of the siblings and other family members in mind. Family participation is facilitated by readily available, trained child-care provision for siblings. Siblings who pass a screen for exposure to varicella and the presence of respiratory or other communicable illnesses present no increased risk to the infant. Because the infant's medical and nursing record (chart) are their parents' property, parents should be guided and encouraged to read the chart regularly and encouraged to enter their own observations and comments on a regular basis. This facilitates communication, builds mutual trust, and enhances the success of collaborative care.

## Collaboration of Care Providers

Implementation of developmental care in the NICU requires a multidisciplinary, collaborative approach. An analysis of the availability of resources and the unit's organizational functioning is an essential requirement prior to implementation of developmental care. Each infant has a primary team, which includes the family and specific representatives from nursing, medicine, respiratory therapy, and social work, identified within the first 24 hours of the infant's admission to the NICU. The primary team works collaboratively to develop an individualized plan of care. The care plan is reviewed daily during rounds; this includes the parents whenever possible. Regular team meetings are scheduled at the convenience of the family to ensure their continued observations and input into their infant's plan of care.

Specially trained developmental professionals should be full-time as an integral part of the staff in each NICU as developmental clinicians. These professionals are expected to have knowledge of high-risk newborn and family development, as well as infant, parent, and professional mental health, and support the primary teams in developmental care planning and implementation. They serve as resources and catalysts in developmental care collaboration. Institutions currently without developmental specialists should develop or acquire such persons and support the development of their role. A multidisciplinary developmental care committee should support the unit-wide implementation of developmental care. This committee focuses on coordinating unit-based developmental rounds, initiating a quality improvement project focusing on appropriate sound and light environments, organizing case presentations, developing a parent support group, and supporting developmental leadership in each of the NICU disciplines. A formal parent council with multicultural representation is also suggested.

As the nursery moves to becoming a family-integrated living environment, the needs of nursery staff for private space need to be considered very carefully. Resources and opportunities for personal and professional growth, such as regular meetings with a psychiatric clinical nurse specialist, psychiatrist, licensed clinical social worker, psychologist, or other mental health professional for the supportive discussion and reflection of family-staff and staff-staff issues needs to be provided. Ongoing collaboration with families in support of their appreciation of and pride in their infants' strengths and individuality will prepare families for their infants' discharge home from the NICU. Formal behavioral observation, using the NIDCAP® approach in conjunction with formal assessment with the APIB, prior to the infant's discharge from the NICU or transfer to a community hospital, is recommended in support of parents' and staff's understanding of the infant's current behavioral functioning and to guide referrals to community services and early intervention programs.

## CONCLUSION

For the purposes of this chapter, NIDCAP®'s approach has been used as the exemplar to illustrate the theoretic underpinnings of developmental care. The ultimate goal of any developmental care approach is to first adopt developmental care as the philosophic approach to care and then to make sure that all healthcare professionals and families work as a team to optimize neonatal/infant and family outcomes (Beyers, 2003).

## ACKNOWLEDGMENTS

This work was in part supported by a National Institutes of Health (NIH) grant RO1HD3826; U.S. Department of Education grants HO24S90003, HO23C970032, R305T990294; a grant from the Harris Foundation to H. Als; and grant P30HD18655 to J.J. Volpe.

## REFERENCES

Alberts, J.R., & Cramer, C.P. (1988). Ecology and experience: Sources of means and meaning of developmental change. In E.M. Blass (Ed.), *Handbook of Behavioral Neurobiology: Developmental Psychobiology and Behavioral Ecology* (Vol. 9, pp. 1-40). New York: Plenum Press.

Als, H. (1975). The human newborn and his mother: An ethological study of their interaction. (Doctoral dissertation, University of Pennsylvania, 1975). *Dissert Abs Int, 36,* 5.

Als, H. (1977). The newborn communicates. *J Commun, 27,* 66-73.

Als, H. (1978). Assessing an assessment: Conceptual considerations, methodological issues, and a perspective on the future of the Neonatal Behavioral Assessment Scale. *MSCDA, 43,* 14-28.

Als, H. (1979). Social interaction: Dynamic matrix for developing behavioral organization. In I.C. Uzgiris (Ed.), *Social Interaction and Communication in Infancy: New Directions for Child Development* (pp. 21-41). San Francisco: Jossey-Bass.

Als, H. (1981). *Manual for the naturalistic observation of the newborn (preterm and fullterm).* Boston, MA: Children's Hospital.

Als, H. (1982a). The behavior of the fetal newborn: Theoretical considerations and practical suggestions for the use of the APIB. In C.E. Seashore, D. Lewis, & D.L. Saetveit (Eds.), *Issues in neonatal care, WESTAR* (pp. 19-60). New York.

Als, H. (1982b). Toward a synactive theory of development: Promise for the assessment of infant individuality. *Infant Mental Health Journal, 3,* 229-243.

Als, H. (1982c). The unfolding of behavioral organization in the face of a biological violation. In E. Tronick (Ed.), *Human communication and the joint regulation of behavior* (pp. 125-160). Baltimore, MD: University Park Press.

Als, H. (1983). Infant individuality: Assessing patterns of very early development. In J. Call, E. Galenson, & R.L. Tyson (Eds.), *Frontiers of infant psychiatry* (pp. 363-378). New York: Basic Books.

Als, H. (1984). *Manual for the naturalistic observation of the newborn (preterm and fullterm)* (rev. Vol.). Boston: Children's Hospital.

Als, H. (1992). Individualized developmental care in the NICU: Estimating expectation for co-regulation. *IBD, 15,* 13.

Als, H. (1999). Reading the premature infant. In E. Goldson (Ed.), *Developmental Interventions in the Neonatal Intensive Care Nursery* (pp. 18-85). New York: Oxford University Press.

Als, H. (In press). Identification of behavioral disorganization in the newborn period: Opportunities for early intervention and outcome at school age. *Schweiz Z Psychol Anwend.*

Als, H., & Berger, A. (1986). *Manual and scoring system for the assessment of infants' behavior: Kangaroo-Box paradigm* (Unpublished manual). Boston, MA: Children's Hospital.

Als, H., & Brazelton, T.B. (1981). A new model of assessing the behavioral organization in preterm and fullterm infants: Two case studies. *Journal of the American Academy of Child Psychiatry, 20*, 239-263.

Als, H., Buehler, D., Kerr, D., et al. (1990, 1995, rev. 1997). *Profile of the nursery environment and of care components. Template Manual, Part I.* (Photocopy). Boston, MA: Children's Hospital.

Als, H., Duffy, F.H., & McAnulty, G.B. (In preparation). Long-term effects of very early individualized developmental care in the NICU to 3 and 7 years postterm.

Als, H., Duffy, F.H., & McAnulty, G.B. (In press). Neurobehavioral competence in healthy preterm and full-term infants: Newborn period to 9 months. *Developmental Psychology.*

Als, H., Duffy, F.H., McAnulty, G.B., et al. (2002). Earliest brain development and experience: Behavior, qEEG, and MRI. *Abstract Proceedings, Thirteenth Annual NIDCAP® Trainers Meeting, NIDCAP® Federation International, Williamsburg, VA, October 5-8.*

Als, H., & Gilkerson, L. (1995). Developmentally supportive care in the neonatal intensive care unit. *Zero to Three, 15*, 1-10.

Als, H., & Gilkerson, L. (1997). The role of relationship-based developmentally supportive newborn intensive care in strengthening outcome of preterm infants. *Seminars in Perinatology, 21*(3), 178-189.

Als, H., Gilkerson, L., Duffy, F.H., et al. (In press). A three-center randomized controlled trial of individualized developmental care for very low-birth-weight preterm infants: Medical, neurodevelopmental, parent and caregiving effects. *Journal of Developmental Behavior in Pediatrics.*

Als, H., Lawhon, G., Brown, E., et al. (1986). Individualized behavioral and environmental care for the very low birth weight preterm infant at high risk for bronchopulmonary dysplasia: Neonatal intensive care unit and developmental outcome. *Pediatrics, 78*, 1123-1132.

Als, H., Lawhon, G., Duffy, F.H., et al. (1994). Individualized developmental care for the very low birthweight preterm infant: Medical and neurofunctional effects. *Journal of the American Medical Association (JAMA), 272*, 853-858.

Als, H., Lawhon, G., Gibes, R., et al. (1986). *Individualized behavioral and environmental care for the VLBW preterm infant at high risk for bronchopulmonary dysplasia: I. NICU outcome.* Paper presented at the New England Perinatal Society, Woodstock, VT.

Als, H., Lawhon, G., Melzar, A., et al. (In preparation). Individualized behavioral and developmental care for the VLBW preterm infant at high risk for bronchopulmonary dysplasia and intraventricular hemorrhage: Study III: A clinical model.

Als, H., Lester, B.M., & Brazelton, T.B. (1979). Dynamics of the behavioral organization of the premature infant: A theoretical perspective. In T.M. Field, A.M. Sostek, S. Goldberg, & H.H. Shuman (Eds.), *Infants born at risk* (pp. 173-193). New York: Spectrum Publications.

Als, H., Lester, B.M., Tronick, E.Z., & Brazelton, T.B. (1982a). Manual for the assessment of preterm infants' behavior (APIB). In H.E. Fitzgerald, B.M. Lester, & M.W. Yogman (Eds.), *Theory and research in behavioral pediatrics* (Vol. 1, pp. 65-132). New York: Plenum Press.

Als, H., Lester, B.M., Tronick, E.Z., & Brazelton, T.B. (1982b). Towards a research instrument for the assessment of preterm infants' behavior. In H.E. Fitzgerald, B.M. Lester, & M.W. Yogman (Eds.), *Theory and research in behavioral pediatrics* (Vol. 1, pp. 35-63). New York: Plenum Press.

Als, H., & McAnulty, G. (1998). *Developmental care guidelines for use in the newborn intensive care unit (NICU)* (Unpublished manuscript). Boston, MA: Children's Hospital.

Anderson, G.C., Burroughs, A.K., & Measel, C.P. (1983). Non-nutritive sucking opportunities: A safe and effective treatment for preterm neonates. In T. Field & A. Sostek (Eds.), *Infants born at risk* (pp. 129-147). New York: Grune and Stratton.

Babson, S.G. (1970). Growth of low birthweight infants. *Journal of Pediatrics, 77*, 11-18.

Becker, P.T., Grunwald, P.C., Moorman, J., & Stuhr, S. (1991). Outcomes of developmentally supportive nursing care for very low birthweight infants. *Nursing Research, 40*, 150-155.

Becker, P.T., Grunwald, P.C., Moorman, J., & Stuhr, S. (1993). Effects of developmental care on behavioral organization in very-low-birth-weight infants. *Nursing Research, 42*, 214-220.

Brazelton, T.B. (1973). *Neonatal behavioral assessment scale.* London: Heinemann.

Brazelton, T.B. (1984). *Neonatal behavioral assessment scale* ( 2nd ed.). Philadelphia: J.B. Lippincott.

Brazelton, T.B., & Als, H. (1979). Four early stages in the development of mother-infant interaction. *The Psychoanalytic Study of the Child, 34*, 349-369.

Buehler, D.M., Als, H., Duffy, F.H., et al. (1995). Effectiveness of individualized developmental care for low-risk preterm infants: Behavioral and electrophysiological evidence. *Pediatrics, 96*, 923-932.

Burroughs, A.K., Asonye, U.O., Anderson-Shanklin, G.C., & Vidyasagar, D. (1978). The effect of non-nutritive sucking on transcutaneous oxygen tension in non-crying preterm neonates. *Research in Nursing Health, 1*, 69-75.

Butler, S.C., Als, H., McAnulty, G.B., et al. (2003). *Effectiveness of individualized developmental care for preterm infants: Neurobehavioral and neurostructural evidence.* Abstract proceedings, Biennial Meeting for the

Society for Research in Child Development, Tampa, FL, April 24-27, 2003.

Byers, J.F. (2003). Components of developmental care and the evidence for their use in the NICU. *MCN: American Journal of Maternal-Child Nursing, 28*(3), 175-182.

Collin, M., Halsy, C., & Anderson, C. (1991). Emerging developmental sequelae in the 'normal' extremely low birthweight infant. *Pediatrics, 88*(1), 115-120.

Cowan, W.M. (1979). The development of the brain. In *The brain: A scientific American book* (pp. 56-67). San Francisco: W.H. Freeman and Company.

Danford, D.A., Miske, S., Headley, J., & Nelson, R.M. (1983). Effects of routine care procedures on transcutaneous oxygen in neonates: A quantitative approach. *Archives of Disease in Childhood, 58*, 20-23.

Denny-Brown, D. (1962). *The basal ganglia and their relation to disorders of movement.* Oxford: Oxford University Press.

Denny-Brown, D. (1966). *The cerebral control of movement.* Springfield, IL: Charles C. Thomas.

Duffy, F.H., Als, H., & McAnulty, G.B. (1990). Behavioral and electrophysiological evidence for gestational age effects in healthy preterm and fullterm infants studied 2 weeks after expected due date. *Child Development, 61*, 1271-1286.

Duffy, F.H., & Burchfiel, J.L. (1971). Somato-sensory systems: Organizational hierarchy from single units in monkey area 5. *Science, 172*, 273-275.

Duffy, F.H., Burchfiel, J.L., & Lombroso, C.T. (1979). Brain electrical activity mapping (BEAM): A method for extending the clinical utility of EEG and evoked potential data. *Annals of Neurology, 5*, 309-321.

El-Metwally, D., Vohr, B., & Tucker, R. (2000). Survival and neonatal morbidity at the limits of viability in the mid-1990s: 22 to 25 weeks. *Journal of Pediatrics, 137*(5), 616-622.

Erikson, E.H. (1962). Reality and actualization. *Journal of the American Psychoanalysis Association, 10*, 451-475.

Field, T.M., Ignatoff, E., Stringer, S., et al. (1982). Nonnutritive sucking during tube feedings: Effects on preterm neonates in an intensive care unit. *Pediatrics, 70*(3), 381-384.

Fischer, K.W., & Rose, S.P. (1994). Dynamic development of coordination of components in brain and behavior: A framework for theory and research. In G. Dawson & K.W. Fischer (Eds.), *Human behavior and the developing brain* (pp. 3-66). New York: The Guilford Press.

Fleisher, B.F., VandenBerg, K.A., Constantinou, et al. (1995). Individualized developmental care for very-low-birth-weight premature infants. *Clinical Pediatrics, 34*, 523-529.

Franck, L.S., & Lawhon, G. (2000). Environmental and behavioral strategies to prevent and manage neonatal pain. In K.J.S. Anand, B.J. Stevens, & P.J. McGrath (Eds.), *Pain research and clinical management* (2nd revised and enlarged ed., Vol. 10, pp. 203-216): Amsterdam: Elsevier Science BV.

Freud, W.E. (1991). Das "Whose Baby" Syndrom. Ein Beitrag zum psychodynamischen Verständnis der Perinatologie. In M. Stauger, F. Conrad, & G. Haselbacher (Eds.), *Psychosomatische Gynäkologie und Geburtshilfe* (pp. 123-137). Berlin: Springer-Verlag.

Gilkerson, L., & Als, H. (1995). Role of reflective process in the implementation of developmentally supportive care in the newborn intensive care unit. *Infants and Young Children, 7*, 20-28.

Gorski, P.A., Hole, W.T., Leonard, C.H., & Martin, J.A. (1983). Direct computer recording of premature infants and nursery care: Distress following two interventions. *Pediatrics, 72*, 198-202.

Gottfried, A.W., & Gaiter, J.L. (1985). *Infant stress under intensive care.* Baltimore: University Park Press.

Grossman, K. (1978). Die Wirkung des Augenoffnens von Neugeborenen auf das Verhalten ihrer Mutter. *Geburtshilfe und Frauenheilkunde, 38*, 629-635.

Grunwald, P.C., & Becker, P.T. (1990). Developmental enhancement: Implementing a program for the NICU. *Neonatal Network, 9*(6), 29-45.

Guyer, B., Strobino, D.M., Ventura, S.J., et al. (1996). Annual summary of vital statistics—1995. *Pediatrics, 98*(6), 1007-1019.

Hack, M., Horbar, J.D., Malloy, M.H., et al. (1991). Very low birth weight outcomes of the National Institute of Child Health and Human Development Neonatal Network. *Pediatrics, 87*(5), 587-592.

Hansen, N., & Okken, A. (1979). Continuous TcPO2 monitoring in healthy and sick newborn infants during and after feeding. *Birth Defects, 4*, 503-508.

Hassenstein, B. (1973). *Verhaltungsbiologie des Kindes.* Muenchen: Piper Verlag.

Herdman, R.C., Behney, C.J., & Wagner, J.L. (1987). Neonatal intensive care for low birthweight infants: costs and effectiveness. *Health Technology Case Study 38, Publication OTA-HCA-38.*

Holmes, M., Sheldon, R., & Als, H. (1995). *Developmentally supportive and family centered care: Newborn Intensive Care Unit participation standards* (Unpublished manuscript). Oklahoma City: University of Oklahoma Health Sciences Center.

Huttenlocher, P.R. (1984). Synapse elimination and plasticity in developing human cerebral cortex. *American Journal of Mental Deficiency, 88*, 488-496.

Jones, N.B. (1972). Characteristics of ethological studies of human behavior. In N.B. Jones (Ed.), *Ethological studies of child behavior* (pp. 3-37). Cambridge: Cambridge University Press.

Jones, N.B. (1974). Ethology and early socialization. In M.P.M. Richards (Ed.), *The Integration of a Child into a Social World* (pp. 263-295). Cambridge: Cambridge University.

Jones, N.B. (1976). Growing points in human ethology: Another link between ethology and the social sciences. In P.P.G. Bateson & R.A. Hinde (Eds.), *Growing points in ethology* (pp. 427-451). Cambridge: Cambridge University.

Kleberg, A., Westrup, B., & Stjernqvist, K. (2000). Developmental outcome, child behavior and mother-child interaction at 3 years of age following Newborn Individualized Developmental Care and Intervention Program (NIDCAP®) intervention. *Early Human Development, 60,* 123-135.

Kleberg, A., Westrup, B., Stjernqvist, K., & Lagercrantz, H. (2002). Indication of improved cognitive development at one year of age among infants born very prematurely who received care based on the Newborn Individualized Developmental Care and Assessment Program (NID-CAP®). *Early Human Development, 68,* 83-91.

Lawhon, G. (1986). Management of stress in premature infants. In D.J. Angelini, C.M.W. Knapp, & R.M. Gibes (Eds.), *Perinatal neonatal nursing: A clinical handbook* (pp. 319-328). Boston: Blackwell Scientific.

Lawhon, G., & Melzar, A. (1991). Developmentally supportive interventions. In J.P. Cloherty & A.R. Stark (Eds.), *Manual of Neonatal Care* (3rd ed., pp. 581-584). Boston: Little, Brown, & Co.

Lettvin, J.Y., Maturana, H., McCulloch, W., & Pitts, W. (1959). What the frog's eye tells the frog's brain. *Proc. I. Radio Engineers, 47,* 1940-1951.

Littman, B., & Parmelee, A.H. (1974). *Manual for obstetric complications* (Unpublished manual). Infant Studies Project, Department of Pediatrics, School of Medicine, University of California, Los Angeles, CA.

Long, J.G., Lucey, J.F., & Philip, A.G.S. (1980). Noise and hypoxemia in the intensive care nursery. *Pediatrics, 65,* 143-145.

Long, J.G., Philip, A.G.S., & Lucey, J.F. (1980). Excessive handling as a cause of hypoxemia. *Pediatrics, 65*(2), 203-207.

Martin, R.J., Herrell, N., Rubin, D., & Fanaroff, A. (1979). Effect of supine and prone positions on arterial oxygen tension in the preterm infant. *Pediatrics, 63,* 528-531.

Martin, R.J., Okken, A., & Rubin, D. (1979). Arterial oxygen tension during active and quiet sleep in the normal neonate. *Journal of Pediatrics, 94,* 271-274.

McCormick, M., Bernbaum, J., Eisenberg, J., et al. (1991). Costs incurred by parents of very low birthweight infants after the initial neonatal hospitalization. *Pediatrics, 88*(3), 533-541.

Ment, L.R., Vohr, B., Allan, W., et al. (2003). Change in cognitive function over time in very low-birth-weight infants. *Journal of the American Medical Association, 289*(6), 705-711.

Minde, K., Whitelaw, A., Brown, J., & Fitzhardinge, P. (1983). Effect of neonatal complications in premature infants on early parent-child interactions. *Developmental Medicine and Child Neurology, 25,* 763-777.

Minde, K.K., Morton, P., Manning, D., & Hines, B. (1980). Some determinants of mother-infant interaction in the premature nursery. *Journal of the American Academy of Child Psychology, 19,* 1-21.

Murdoch, D.R., & Darlow, B.A. (1984). Handling during neonatal intensive care. *Archives of the Diseases of Childhood, 29,* 957-961.

Norris, S., Campbell, L., & Brenkert, S. (1982). Nursing procedures and alterations in transcutaneous oxygen tension in premature infants. *Nursing Research, 31,* 330-336.

Peterson, B.S., Vohr, B., Staib, L.H., et al. (2000). Regional brain volume abnormalities and long-term cognitive outcome in preterm infants. *Journal of the American Medical Association (JAMA), 284,* 1939-1947.

Prechtl, H.F.R. (1977). *The neurological examination of the full-term infant: A manual for clinical use* (2nd ed.). Philadelphia: J.B. Lippincott.

Reppert, S.M., & Rivkees, S.A. (1989). Development of human circadian rhythms: Implications for health and disease. In S.M. Reppert (Ed.), *Development of circadian rhythmicity and photoperiodism in mammals* (Vol. IX, Research in Perinatal Medicine, pp. 245-259). Ithaca, NY: Perinatology Press.

Robson, K. (1967). The role of eye-to-eye contact in maternal-infant attachment. *Journal of Child Psychology and Psychiatry, 8,* 13-25.

Rosenblatt, J.S. (1976). Stages in the early behavioral development of altricial young of selected species of non-primate mammals. In P.P.G. Bateson & R.A. Hinde (Eds.), *Growing points in ethology.* Cambridge: Cambridge University Press.

Sander, L.W. (1962). Issues in early mother-child interaction. *Journal of the American Academy of Child Psychiatry, 1,* 141-166.

Sander, L.W. (1964). Adaptive relationships in early mother-child interaction. *Journal of the American Academy of Child Psychiatry, 3,* 231-264.

Sander, L.W. (1970). Regulation and organization in the early infant-caretaker system. In R. Robinson (Ed.), *Brain and early behavior* (pp. 311-333). London: Academic Press.

Sander, L.W. (1975). Infant and caretaking environment: Investigation and conceptualization of adaptive behavior in a system of increasing complexity. In E.J. Anthony (Ed.), *Explorations in child psychiatry.* New York: Plenum Press.

Sander, L.W. (1976). Primary prevention and some aspects of temporal organization in early infant-caretaker interaction. In E. Rexford, L.W. Sander, & T. Shapiro (Eds.), *Infant psychiatry: A new synthesis* (pp. 187-204). New Haven: Yale.

Sander, L.W. (1980). Investigation of the infant and its environment as a biological system. In S.I. Greenberg & G.H. Pollock (Eds.), *The course of life: psychoanalytic contribution toward understanding personality development* (pp. 177-201). Washington, DC: National Institute of Mental Health.

Sander, L.W., Stechler, G., Burns, P., & Lee, A. (1979). Change in infant and caregiver variables over the first two months of life: Integration of action in early development. In E.B. Thomas (Ed.), *Origins of the infant's social responsiveness.* Hillsdale, NJ: Lawrence Erlbaum.

Schade, J.P., & van Groenigen, D.B. (1961). Structural organization of the human cerebral cortex. I. Maturation of the middle frontal gyrus. *Acta Anatomie, 41,* 47-111.

Schneirla, T.C. (1959). An evolutionary and developmental theory of biphasic processes underlying approach and withdrawal. In M.R. Jones (Ed.), *Nebraska Symposium on Motivation* (pp. 1-42). Lincoln: University of Nebraska Press.

Schneirla, T.C. (1965). Aspects of stimulation and organization in approach and withdrawal processes underlying vertebrate development. *Adv. Study of Behav., 1,* 1-74.

Schneirla, T.C., & Rosenblatt, J.S. (1961). Behavioral organization and genesis of the social bond in insects and mammals. *American Journal of Orthopsychiatry, 31,* 223-253.

Schneirla, T.C., & Rosenblatt, J.S. (1963). "Critical periods" in the development of behavior. *Science, 139,* 1110-1115.

U.S. Department of Health and Human Services Center for Disease Control. (2002). *National Vital Statistics Reports: Births: Final Data for 2001 (2).* Washington, DC.

VandenBerg, K.A. (1990a). Nippling management of the sick neonate in the NICU: The disorganized feeder. *Neonatal Network, 9*(1), 9-16.

VandenBerg, K.A. (1990b). Behaviorally supportive care for the extremely premature infant. In L.P. Gunderson & C. Kenner (Eds.), *Care of the 24-25 week gestational age infant (small baby protocol)* (pp. 129-157). Petaluma, CA: Neonatal Network.

VandenBerg, K.A., & Franck, L.S. (1990). Behavioral issues for infants with BPD. In C. Lund (Ed.), *BPD: Strategies for total patient care* (pp. 113-152). Petaluma, CA: Neonatal Network.

Vento, T., & Feinberg, E. (In press). Developmentally supportive care. In J. Cloherty & A. Stark (Eds.), *Developmentally supportive care* (4th ed.). Boston: Little, Brown.

Vohr, B.R., & Msall, M.E. (1997). Neuropsychological and functional outcomes of very low birth weight infants. *Seminars in Perinatology, 21,* 202-220.

Vohr, B.R., Wright, L.L., Dusick, A.M., et al. (2000). Neurodevelopmental and functional outcomes of extremely low birth weight infants in the national institute of child health and human development neonatal research network, 1993-1994. *Pediatrics, 105*(6), 1216-1226.

Westrup, B., Böhm, B., Lagercrantz, H., & Stjernqvist, K. (2003). Preschool outcome in children born very prematurely and cared for according to the Newborn Individualized Development Care and Assessment Program (NIDCAP®), *Developmentally supportive neonatal care: A study of the Newborn Individualized Developmental Care and Assessment Program (NIDCAP®) in Swedish settings.* Stockholm: Repro Print AB.

Westrup, B., Kleberg, A., von Eichwald, K., et al. (2000). A randomized controlled trial to evaluate the effects of the Newborn Individualized Developmental Care and Assessment Program in a Swedish setting. *Pediatrics, 105*(1), 66-72.

Wolke, D. (1987). Environmental and developmental neonatology. *Journal of Reproductive and Infant Psychology, 5,* 17-42.

Yakovlev, P.I., & Lecours, A.R. (1967). The myelogenic cycles of regional maturation of the brain. In A. Minkowsky (Ed.), *Regional development of the brain in early life* (pp. 3-70). Oxford: Blackwell.

# 4 Infant Mental Health: A New Dimension to Care

Gay Gale, Bette Liberman Flushman, Mary Claire Heffron, and Nancy Sweet

All infants require positive social relationships with their parents or primary caregivers to achieve healthy social and emotional development. The development of this relationship depends upon the interactional capabilities of both the parent and the infant. When communication between parent and infant goes smoothly, parents feel competent to care for and protect their infant, and the infant develops trust, the ability to regulate emotion, and a healthy sense of self (Sroufe, 1996). When this relationship does not go smoothly, as is often the case when the infant requires extended hospitalization, the future development of the child and the well-being of the family is placed at risk (Minde, 2000).

Infant family mental health is a broad, multidisciplinary field that provides a continuum of services to support the central role of these primary relationships between infants and their parents. Within this field, preventive interventions focus on the parents and children, whose relationships might be at risk due to developmental, environmental, or social risk factors (Knitzer, 2000). In this chapter, we describe how the principles of infant mental health can be integrated and made central to the work of the developmental care specialist in the neonatal intensive care unit (NICU). Special challenges that might occur because of parents' needs or preexisting concerns related to their own history of relationships are discussed. The chapter concludes with suggestions for strengthening parent-child relationships within the NICU and hospital environment through a mental health focus. We believe that developmental care will be enriched and strengthened if principles from the field of infant mental health are

identified and incorporated into the care of infants and their families.

## INFANT MENTAL HEALTH SERVICES
### Background

Although the term "mental health" has historical associations with the concept of mental illness, the term "infant mental health" refers to interventions and services aimed at wellness and problem prevention or reduction of risk (Heffron, 2000). Infant mental health programs are associated with broadly defined, early intervention programs that include preventive intervention and treatment services for the zero-to-three population and their families. These programs are designed to improve the social and emotional well-being of infants and families by strengthening relationships with caregivers and promoting age-appropriate social and emotional skills (Knitzer, 2000).

Medical or developmental factors, such as prematurity, birth trauma, congenital anomalies, and other chronic medical conditions, that place the child at risk for developmental delay contribute significantly to the family's need for infant mental health services (Minde, 2000). Programs in the community have many forms and are aimed at many specific populations, including parents with preexisting mental health problems or histories of problematic primary relationships, children in foster care, and families with such risk factors as poverty, father absence, minority status, teen parent status, low parental education, substance abuse, and recent immigration. Research indicates that as these risks accumulate, so do the deleterious

Box 4-1   WHAT IS INFANT MENTAL HEALTH CARE IN THE NICU?

Preventive strategies for infant mental health care in the NICU derive from those used in early childhood mental health.

1. Promote the emotional and behavioral well-being of infants, particularly those whose emotional development is compromised by environmental or biologic risks.
2. Help families of infants address whatever barriers they face to ensure their infant's emotional development is not compromised.
3. Expand the competencies of nonfamilial caregivers (in the NICU, this might include professional caregivers) to promote the emotional well-being of infants and their families.
4. Ensure that families with ineffective coping strategies have access to needed services and supports.

Adapted from Knitzer, J. (2000). Early childhood mental health services. In J.P. Shonkoff, & S.J. Meisels (Eds.), *Handbook of early childhood intervention* (2nd ed., pp. 416-417). Cambridge, UK: Cambridge Press.

*NICU*, Neonatal intensive care unit.

effects on the child's development (Garabino & Ganzel, 2000).

Preventive infant mental health interventions are geared toward providing support and understanding that nurture the mother or primary caregiver's ability to nurture the infant (Heffron, 2000). These interventions can and should be provided by a range of infant developmental specialists (IDSs). These specialists might include physical, occupational, and speech therapists; early childhood special education teachers; social workers; nurses; and others trained in facilitating positive social emotional relationships as well as other knowledge and skills related to an infant or family's well-being. IDSs working with this population assist mothers in their interpretation of their baby's cues, and foster skill development and development of mutual enjoyment that fosters attachment. Additionally, the IDSs assist the mother to identify needs, find resources, and facilitate connections with other families of children with similar challenges. Studies indicate that the quality and responsiveness of maternal care predicts security of attachment, and security of attachment has been shown to have long-term sequelae on developmental and social outcomes for children (Isabella, 1993; Isabella & Belsky, 1991; Sroufe, 1996). The caring, concern, and acceptance of the IDSs for the parent as well as for the baby can also provide a corrective emotional

experience for the parent, which supports the formation of a positive parent-infant bond.

## Infant Mental Health and Developmental Care in the NICU

Historically, the term "infant mental health program" has not included developmental care programs for at-risk infants hospitalized in the NICU. The approaches used by developmental care programs for hospitalized preterm babies do, however, frequently incorporate principles that overlap with the preventive roles of infant mental health programs in the community (Minde, 2000). Programs in the NICU that support healthy parent-infant attachment, such as family-centered care, are providing elements of preventive infant mental health care (Boxes 4-1 and 4-2).

Although in some cases a referral to a mental health professional might be indicated for parents, this chapter is focused on the work of strengthening parent-child relationships in the NICU through the IDS and collaborative caregiving of the caregiving team. As with the IDS in the community setting, the professional background of the developmental care specialist in the NICU might derive from different fields; the most common fields are early childhood education, psychology, nursing, physical therapy (PT), occupational therapy (OT), and speech pathology (see Chapter 26).

Box **4-2**   WHAT IS FAMILY-CENTERED CARE IN THE NICU?

1. Acknowledge that parents are the most important people in the infant's life and critical to the infant's well-being, especially when infants need life-saving technology and skilled professional staff to survive.
2. Recognize that over time, the family has the greatest influence on an infant's health and well-being.
3. Acknowledge that emotional, social, and developmental support comprise integral components of health care.
4. Promote practices that nurture strong bonds between infants and their families, and support those experiences throughout the intensive care experience.
5. Build on family strengths.

From Johnson, B.H. (1995). Newborn intensive care units pioneer family-centered change in hospitals across the country. *Zero to Three*, *15*(6), 11-17.

*NICU*, Neonatal intensive care unit.

## INTERVENTIONS THAT PROMOTE INFANT MENTAL HEALTH IN THE NICU

### Support Relationship-Based Developmentally Supportive Care

Als introduced the term "relationship-based developmentally supportive care" into the NICU in the mid-1990s (Als & Gilkerson, 1995; Gilkerson & Als, 1995). As envisioned by Als, this relationship-based care supports the parents' engrossment with their infant and the infant's expectation of nurturance from the family (Als & Gilkerson, 1997). In Als' model, the infant's care is guided by the infant's cues and the communication between the infant, parent, and caregiver. This collaboration recognizes the primacy of the infant's relationship with his or her parents in the infant's long-term development. The developmental care specialist works within an interdisciplinary team to facilitate the parent's understanding of the infant and to foster a mutual responsiveness between them (Als & Gilkerson, 1997). Interdisciplinary team members might represent the fields of neonatology, social work, psychiatry, nursing leadership, physical therapy/occupational therapy, nutrition, and lactation support.

An important goal of relationship-based care is assisting the baby in his or her efforts to maintain an organized and self-regulated state. Optimally, the routine care is offered according to the infant's readiness rather than a timed task-oriented schedule (Als, 1997). Relationship-based care supports physiologic stability, natural sleep-wake state cycling, neurosensory development, and social reciprocity primarily with the family. Ideally the developmental care specialist encourages all nursery staff to incorporate this perspective into their interactions with parents and infants (Als & Gilkerson, 1997).

Als has proposed that relationship-based care should become part of bedside caregiving (Als & Gilkerson 1997). Developmentally supportive, relationship-based bedside care acknowledges the relationship between the caregiver (nurse) and the infant and takes into account the infant's state and behavioral readiness for handling and interaction. Within this concept, no medical or nursing care is withheld, rather it is provided in the least disruptive way (Als & Gilkerson, 1997). Some examples of relationship-based care are the postponement of a physical examination or assessment until the sleeping infant has transitioned into a more active state, or placing an infant demonstrating rooting behavior at the mother's breast, although it is not the scheduled time for feeding.

### Promote Positive Interactions

Like the IDS working in the community setting, the developmental care specialist in the NICU provides preventive infant mental health care by promoting positive interactions within the parent-infant relationship. This approach focuses on building the parents' sense of confidence by increasing their feelings of competence with their infant. Preterm and sick infants are frequently unable to communicate their needs clearly, and these compromised abilities are a risk factor for the development of healthy infant-parent relationships. These infants can be difficult to soothe and feed. They might respond to their parents' attempts to interact with them by disengaging or with signs of discomfort. Many premature babies make sudden state shifts that can be confusing and even alarming. Parents frequently feel sad, guilty, confused, and worried by these types of responses. Having a baby in the NICU is a physically and emotionally exhausting experience. These and other factors, such as the parents' own attachment histories and lack of social support, can interfere with the development of a satisfying relationship and might lead the parents to perceive the infant as vulnerable or difficult (Miles & Holditch-Davis, 1997; Minde, 2000).

Because developmental care specialists are highly trained to observe and work with babies, they are ideal supports for parents or staff who are struggling to form relationships with infants whose immature nervous systems compromise their abilities to signal and respond. By identifying and responding appropriately to their infant's signals and cues, parents receive satisfaction in successfully meeting their infant's needs, and they can begin to appreciate the role they play in their infant's life. The developmental care specialist can promote this sense of competence through attuned coaching of the parent, acknowledgement of parental concerns, and voiced observations that provide praise and comment on successful attempts at interaction and caregiving.

## Promote Attachment

Attachment is defined as the unique relationship between two people that is specific and endures through time (Klaus & Kennel, 1982). The developmental care specialist promotes attachment and parental self-esteem by supporting the parents' ability to communicate reciprocally with their nonverbal infant. Reciprocity in the parent-infant relationship is an essential element of the attachment process (Klaus & Kennell, 1982). Klaus and Kennell (1976, 1982) were among the first experts to voice concern about how the inability of the sick or preterm infant to respond reciprocally to parents' attempts to interact (for example, mutual eye contact) puts the parent-infant attachment process at risk. They and

other experts noted that newborns hospitalized in the NICU were at greater risk for parental abuse and neglect and for failure to thrive following discharge than are infants who are not hospitalized (Hunter, Kilstrom, Kraybill, et al., 1978; Jeffcoate, Humphrey, & Lloyd, 1979; Klaus & Kennell, 1976; Leventhal, Garber, & Brady, 1989). These findings have led to the liberalization of NICU visiting hours to provide more opportunities for parents to engage with their infant and participate in their infant's care. Staff education has also led to greater sensitization of NICU staff about the needs of parents and the importance of supporting parent child attachments.

Among the many interventions suggested in the current literature to promote parent-child attachment in the NICU (Gale & Franck, 1998), one of the most effective is early holding. Early holding is defined as parental holding of the infant as soon as the infant is medically stable enough to tolerate holding. Although holding is essential to the development of the bond parents form with their infants early in life (Klaus & Kennell, 1976, 1982), holding policies vary widely in NICUs (Franck, Bernal, & Gale, 2002). For families at higher risk of attachment disorders due to chemical dependency issues or other family history factors, early holding and skin-to-skin (Kangaroo) holding can promote parental focus on the relationship with the child (Gale, Franck, & Lund, 1993). Furthermore, recent studies indicate that skin-to-skin holding in the NICU can have benefits for the infant's development and relationship with the parent that extend well into the first year of life (Feldman 2002; Feldman, Eidelman, Sireta, et al., 2002; Ohgi, Fukuda, Moriuchi, et al., 2002).

The developmental care specialist can play a pivotal role in facilitating early holding through negotiations with bedside caregivers about the infant's readiness for holding. Furthermore, by staying with the parent during the early holding experience, the developmental care specialist can facilitate the comfort of both the parent and the bedside nurse by observing the signals and cues of the medically stabile but behaviorally fragile infant. Infants are often moved in and out of their radiant warmer or incubator for routine procedures (e.g., weighing, bathing), and these activities can often be negotiated as times for parents to hold their fragile or less stable infant without disrupting routine care or unduly exposing the infant to the stress of the environment. During this special time, the developmental care specialist can facilitate the parent's sharing of long-term hopes for the child and the meaning of this early experience.

## Recognize and Acknowledge Parental Stress

Despite consistent improvements in NICU care, the needs of parents in the NICU can still be overlooked or treated as secondary, due to a focus on the acute needs of the baby (Affonso, Hurst, Mayberry, et al., 1992; Gale & Franck, 1998; Griffin, 1990). It is imperative that the parents' needs be assessed because the parents' psychologic well-being might be threatened by the deeply disturbing experiences they have been through with the birth and hospitalization of their infant (Affleck & Tennen, 1991). Miles and Holditch-Davis research studies have identified six major sources of stress for parents of prematurely born infants: (1) preexisting and concurrent personal and family factors; (2) prenatal and perinatal experiences; (3) infant illness, treatments, and perinatal experiences; (4) concerns about the infant's outcomes; (5) loss of the parental role; and (6) healthcare providers (Holditch-Davis & Miles, 2000; Miles & Holditch-Davis, 1997). Moreover, the stress experienced by parents during their infant's NICU stay continues to affect the parent-child relationship for years after discharge (Affleck, Tennen, & Rowe, 1991; Holditch-Davis & Miles, 2000; Miles, Funk, & Kasper, 1992; Miles & Holditch-Davis, 1997; Wereszczak, Miles, & Holditch-Davis, 1997). Additional factors, such as poor family functioning, lower levels of social support, and lower perceived control, might also increase parents' difficulties in adjusting to the NICU experience (Doering, Moser, & Dracup, 2000).

Parents need ongoing support to manage the stress they experience in the NICU (Holditch-Davis & Miles, 2000; Miles, Funk, & Kasper, 1992). Although bedside nurses are in an ideal role to provide this support, their time available to listen to families' worries might be limited by the attention that must be paid to the infant's medical needs. Mothers especially can be frustrated by feelings of loss of control and competition with nurses to protect and support their baby (Bass, 1991; Fenwick, Barclay, & Schmied, 2001; Griffin, 1990; Griffin, Wishba, & Kavanaugh, 1998;

Hurst, 2001a, 2001b; Kenner, 1990; Klaus & Kennell, 2001; Miles, Funk, & Carlson, 1993).

Therefore, one important mental health function of the developmental care specialist is supporting parents as they grieve for the loss of their hoped-for, perfect child (Shellabarger & Thompson, 1993). Many parents of NICU infants experience shock, anxiety, or depression related to this loss (Hummel & Eastman, 1991; Miles, Funk & Kasper, 1992). By listening to parental questions and concerns, the developmental care specialist can reduce the anxiety and fear that might interfere with the development of close feelings with their baby. The developmental care specialist encourages parents to talk about their feelings without minimizing these responses or attempting to cheer them up. The developmental care specialist can provide one-on-one counseling, a chance to discuss medical information that might be confusing and parent group meetings to move towards acceptance and understanding of this difficult period in their lives. The trust that builds from this nurturing connection creates a process that promotes parental investment in the relationship with the baby (Als & Gilkerson, 1995).

When a parent continues to have difficulty coping or is having prolonged difficulties interacting with the baby, the developmental care specialist is in an ideal position to discuss treatment with a mental health specialist. Using preventive infant mental health, the specialist helps the parents find their role despite barriers to the attachment process posed by a premature birth, the atmosphere of the NICU, persistent anxiety, and worries about the baby's survival. In spending time with the parent and the baby supporting responsive care, bonding, and attachment, the developmental care specialist can ascertain serious issues the parent is facing or might note problems in coping. In these cases, the specialist can assist the parent in locating other social work, mental health, or legal services when needs for support go beyond the scope of the work of developmental care.

## Provide Infants with Opportunities for Positive Social Interactions with Volunteers

Infants who "grow up" in the NICU without the opportunity for reciprocal interaction from a parent or consistent caregiver are at risk for alterations in growth and development. In describing her work as psychiatric consultant to the NICU, Goodfriend (1993) found that the lack of reciprocally positive contact from a consistent, caring adult contributed to irritability and failure to thrive in hospitalized premature infants who remained in the NICU for many months. She diagnosed these infants with reactive disorder of infancy and suggested that volunteers be assigned to provide the consistent positive human contact necessary for the development of normal mental health (Goodfriend, 1992). In many NICUs, the developmental care specialist trains and supports volunteers (often referred to as "cuddlers"), who offer touching, holding, and other positive sensory input when no parents or family are consistently available. For infants going into foster care, every attempt is made to work with the foster parent to provide this care as early as possible.

## THE ROLE OF THE BEDSIDE NURSE IN PROMOTING INFANT MENTAL HEALTH

Most NICUs do not have a developmental care specialist available to facilitate relationship-based care to all infants and their primary caregivers. Frequently, the person designated to provide developmental care also has other roles in the NICU or elsewhere in the hospital (see Chapter 26). Furthermore, this person might or might not be trained to provide relationship-based care to families or consultation and education to staff (Heffron, 2000). The bedside nurse can promote infant mental health and developmental care by integrating the following concepts into care.

### Promote Feelings of Parental Competence

Nurses in these environments have a crucial role in the immediate care of both the infant and the parent, and also in helping parents prepare for their ongoing care after discharge. Parents can best be supported when nurses hold both the baby and the parent in mind and shape interactions in a way that promotes feelings of competence and well-being, delivering the message that the parent is the most important person to this baby. A basic understanding of how a parent's own history with relationships can shape responses to the baby is important.

### Recognize and Acknowledge the Impact of Parents' Histories

It is important for bedside caregivers to recognize that the impact of premature birth will vary and will have specific meanings based on parents' own history of relationships, cultural context, family and spiritual support, and the particular meaning of the baby. The types of relational experiences that the parent has with nurses, the developmental care specialist, and medical staff can provide a corrective emotional experience for the parent or can have a long-term negative impact on feelings of competence and confidence.

### Recognize and Acknowledge Personal Feelings

Nurses who provide care to premature infants over time often develop protective feelings and can become irritated or angry with parents who are not visiting frequently, are hesitant to care for their babies, or who have questioned or criticized nursing care. Training and consultation should be available to nurses to help them understand parental reactions and their own responses (Griffin, 1990). This support can enable nurses working with challenging family situations to manage their own feelings and involve parents more and more inclusively in the care of their infants.

## SPECIFIC RECOMMENDATIONS FOR BEDSIDE CAREGIVERS

The importance of nurses' participation in facilitating the parent-infant relationship has been amply documented in the neonatal nursing literature (Gennaro, 1991; Griffin, Wishba, & Kavanaugh, 1998; Higley & Miller, 1996; Holditch-Davis & Miles, 2000; Miles, Carlson, & Funk, 1996; Saunders, 1994; Shellabarger & Thompson, 1993).

The following recommendations for bedside support of parenting are adapted from Gale and Franck (1998):

1. Provide maximal privacy for parents at the infant's bedside (e.g., curtains and screens) and private consultation rooms close to the NICU where staff can discuss the infant's care with the family in private.
2. Facilitate parents' participation in daily medical rounds by providing information about when

rounds occur and encouraging parents to ask questions they might have.

3. Welcome sibling visitation and participation in family activities at the bedside by talking with the sibling about the baby. An extra family member should be available in the event the sibling wants to leave the care area before the parent is ready.

4. Recruit primary nurses to provide consistency in caring for baby and the family.

5. Affirm the parents' role as the ultimate decision-makers about their infant's care, and make this part of staff discussions.

6. Encourage early holding, kangaroo care, and participation in the infant's routine care.

7. Invite parents to participate in their infant's pain care. Many parents want to be involved in providing comfort to their infant during or after a painful procedure (Franck, Scurr, & Couture, 2001).

8. Personalize the environment for each infant and the infant's parents by encouraging parents to individualize the infant's bedside with a quilt, photos, personal clothing, when appropriate, and always use the infant's and family members' names.

9. Promote breastfeeding through lactation consultation, a private space for breast-feeding, and provisions for lactation supplies, equipment, and storage of breast milk.

10. Provide praise, and support caregiving successes and efforts.

11. Reach out to hesitant or absent parents to encourage interaction.

The next section will include an example of the application of these principles to a case study.

## CASE STUDY

A young, first time mother precipitously delivered twins at 26 weeks' gestation. She saw her twins fleetingly after an emergency cesarean section as they were being transported to the NICU. After her discharge from the community hospital where the twins were delivered, she came directly to the NICU to see her babies. As she approached Monica, her baby girl, the nurse stopped her to inform her that Monica had just settled down following several procedures, and it would be best if the mother left her alone for now. The mother then went to Albert, her baby boy, where his bedside nurse also discouraged her from handling or touching him. The developmental care specialist was making rounds and introduced herself as she saw this young mother sitting stiffly at the bedside looking at all the technologic equipment. She acknowledged with empathy the mother's discomfort and her desire to touch and hold her babies. The mother described feeling unsure of whether her touch would be helpful or harmful to them. As they spoke, the mother was encouraged to put her hand inside the incubator firmly cupping Albert's small head with one hand and his feet with another. It was suggested that this was all he could handle at this time and her voice would be too much stimulation for now. She could, however, bring her face close to him and watch him. This mother was relieved and happy to be able to have this physical contact and closeness. Although it was uncomfortable for her, she held this position for 25 minutes. While the mother was engaged in this contact with Albert, the developmental care specialist talked to Monica's nurse. She pointed out how the mother was interacting with her baby and spoke of the benefits for this mother and her twins. Acknowledging the nurse's concern for the stressed twin girl, they decided that this mother could offer a similar approach for Monica. Here was a situation in which a young, new mother, who felt lost during her initial contact, was helped to assume a proactive role as the parent of very premature twins.

As time went on, the infants' individual tolerance levels for contact became more distinct, and the parents were guided in recognizing their differences. Albert had more effective self-regulation skills and an ability to maintain a calm state. Monica was more sensitive to handling and to the stimulation within the room. Their mother was able to respond appropriately to the needs of each baby. For example, Albert usually calmed when he heard her voice, whereas Monica often became active. Their mother would offer quiet touch to Monica without any voice until she was calmly settled.

The babies' beds were in the same room, but were spatially separated by several bed spaces. The mother developed a strong need to be in contact with both babies at the same time. Prior to attending to one of the twins, she would lift the corner of the incubator cover of the other twin so that she could see that baby while holding the other. This arrangement was interrupted one day when one infant became ill and, because of staffing needs, was moved across the room. The situation was extremely distressing to the mother because she could no longer see one twin while at the bedside of the other. The developmental care specialist listened to the mother's concerns and advocated for her needs with the staff. The babies were soon moved back into proximity where the mother could monitor them together. The mother's relief was apparent to all who came by the bedside.

From the beginning, this family had a great deal of support from extended family with several visitors taking turns visiting at both bedsides. The staff expressed concern to the developmental care specialist about the overstimulation to these babies through interactions with the several visitors'. The specialist worked with the staff to increase family members' awareness of and sensitivity to the babies' stress signals. It was decided by the parents to limit the visitors, thereby reserving the babies' energies for the parents' visits until their babies were ready for more interaction.

As with many babies who are hospitalized in the ICN for many weeks, the twins underwent numerous painful procedures. The developmental care specialist consulted with the parents about whether they wanted to be involved in supporting their infants during these times. The mother was interested, whereas the father initially decided he did not want this kind of involvement. The specialist met with the bedside nurses to work out ways the mother could offer support and comfort to Albert during a venipuncture that was to happen in the next hour. The nurse showed the mother how to offer a pacifier and hand swaddling during the procedure. The mother calmly provided the containment, the pacifier, and her soft voice. Following the procedure, Albert's mother held him for 45 minutes. She spoke of her satisfaction in going through this with him rather than going into the waiting room as she had previously been doing. She felt she came to know him even better as she participated in these procedures. When Monica needed similar care, her mother learned what subtle, but different, methods

worked for her. Through the support of the developmental care specialist and the staff, these parents gained confidence in their ability to contribute to the babies' care. The staff had worked together to ensure the building of a mutually satisfying relationship between these parents and their twins.

Additionally, the specialist provided reading materials about premature babies, contact with other families, and an introduction to the lactation consultant. She also introduced the parents to the follow-up case manager who would provide in-home care after discharge. This meeting took place in the NICU and helped the parents prepare for the transition to home. Once home, the parents commented that the doctors and nurses had saved the babies' lives, and the developmental care specialist had given them the confidence to be parents during this difficult time.

## CONCLUSION

The language of infant mental health is new to the NICU, but many of the underlying concepts, such as sensitivity to signals and cues, the importance of touch, and facilitating state regulation, have been practiced through the developmental care specialist role for many years. In the NICU, the goals of developmental care and infant mental health are the same: facilitate infant self-regulation and support the parent-infant attachment process to optimize long-term developmental outcomes for the infant and minimize the deleterious effects on the parent-infant experience. The use of a developmental care specialist and the role of infant mental health are rich areas for further research in the long-term outcomes of these infants. To conduct this research, nurses and developmental care specialists need a stronger focus on important aspects of infant mental health work. Key areas for learning include communication strategies that support parent competence and an understanding of transference, counter-transference, and this use of self. Additional areas of knowledge include issues related to parental history of relationships, an understanding of adult attachment and how babies and parents develop attachment over time, and specific techniques that support parent-child relationships in the NICU.

Development of parent-child attachment is a process that takes place over many months. However, the developmental care specialist is in an ideal position to mitigate the impact of a premature birth on the budding attachment. Indeed, we believe that application of the tenets proposed in this chapter in many cases can set the stage for the development of a more mature attachment in the subsequent months and years of an infant's life. Because there is ample evidence that secure relationships are central to positive developmental outcomes, we believe the effort and costs are warranted.

As developmental care specialists and nurses expand their roles to encourage secure parent-child attachment, training and consultation in the strategies of preventive infant mental health is essential. This is a growing area of developmental care that caregivers can advocate for in their own units.

## REFERENCES

Affleck, G., & Tennen, H. (1991). The effect of newborn intensive care on parents' psychological well-being. *Child Health Care, 20*(1), 6-14.

Affleck, G., Tennen, H., & Rowe, J. (1991). Mothers' remembrances of newborn intensive care. In G. Affleck, H. Tennen, & J. Rowe (Eds.), *Infants in crisis: How parents cope with newborn intensive care and its aftermath* (pp. 99-115). New York: Springer-Verlag.

Affonso, D.D., Hurst, I., Mayberry, L.J., et al. (1992). Stressors reported by mothers of hospitalized premature infants. *Neonatal Network, 11*(6), 63-70.

Als, H. (1997). Earliest intervention for preterm infants in the newborn intensive care unit. In M.J. Guralnick (Eds.), *The effectiveness of early intervention* (pp. 47-76). Baltimore: Paul H. Brookes Publishing.

Als, H., & Gilkerson, L. (1997). Relationship-based developmental NICU care. *Seminars in Perinatolgy, 21*(3), 178-189.

Als, H., & Gilkerson, L. (1995). Developmentally supportive care in the neonatal intensive care unit. *Zero to Three, 15*(6), 2-10.

Bass, L.S. (1991). What do the parents need when their infant is a patient in the NICU? *Neonatal Network, 10*(4), 25-33.

Doering, L.V., Moser, D.K., & Dracup, K. (2000). Correlates of anxiety, hostility, depression and psychosocial adjustment in parents of NICU infants. *Neonatal Network, 19*(5), 13-23.

Feldman, R. (2002). Intervention programs for premature infants: Considering potential mechanisms for change. *The Signal: Newsletter of the World Association for Infant Mental Health, 10*(3-4), 1-11.

Feldman, R., Eidelman, A.I., Sireta, L., et al. (2002). Comparison of skin-to-skin (kangaroo) and traditional care: Parenting outcome and preterm infant development. *Pediatrics, 110*(1),16-26.

Fenwick, J., Barclay, L., & Schmied, V. (2001). Struggling to mother: A consequence of inhibitive nursing interactions in the neonatal nursery. *Journal of Perinatal and Neonatal Nursing, 15*(2), 49-64.

Franck, L.S., Bernal, H., & Gale, G. (2002). Infant holding policies and practices Nursing in neonatal units. *Neonatal Network, 21*(2), 13-20.

Franck, L.S., Scurr, K., & Couture, S. (2001). Parent views of infant pain and pain management in the neonatal intensive care unit. *Newborn and Infant Nursing Reviews, 1*(2), 106-113.

Gale, G., & Franck, L.S. (1998). Toward a standard of care for parents in the neonatal intensive care unit. *Critical Care Nurse, 18*(5), 62-74.

Gale, G., Franck, L., & Lund, C. (1993). Skin-to-skin holding (kangaroo) holding of the intubated premature infant. *Neonatal Network, 12*(6), 49-57.

Garabino, J, & Ganzel, B. (2000). The human ecology of early risk. In J.P. Sholkoff & S.J. Meisels (Eds.), *Handbook of early childhood intervention* (2nd ed., pp. 76-93). Cambridge, UK: Cambridge Press.

Gennaro, S. (1991). Facilitating parenting of the neonatal intensive care unit graduate. *Journal of Perinatal and Neonatal Nursing, 4*(4), 55-61.

Gilkerson, L., & Als, H. (1995). Role of reflective process in the implementation of developmentally supportive care in the newborn intensive care nursery. *Infants and Young Children, 7*(4), 20-28.

Goodfriend, M.S. (1993). Treatment of attachment disorder of infancy in a neonatal intensive care unit. *Pediatrics, 91*(1), 139-142.

Griffin, T. (1990). Nurse barriers to parenting in the special care nursery. *Journal of Perinatal and Neonatal Nursing, 4*(2), 56-67.

Griffin, T., Wishba, C., & Kavanaugh, K. (1998). Nursing interventions to reduce stress in parents of hospitalized preterm infants. *Journal of Pediatric Nursing, 13*(5), 290-295.

Heffron, M.C. (2000). Clarifying concepts of infant mental health—Promotion, relationship-based preventative intervention, and treatment. *Infants and Young Children, 12*(4), 14-21.

Higley, A.M., & Miller, M.A. (1996). The development of parenting: Nursing resources. *Journal of Obstetric, Gynecologic, and Neonatal Nursing (JOGNN), 25*(9), 707-713.

Holditch-Davis, D., & Miles, M.S. (2000). Mothers' stories about their experiences in the neonatal intensive care unit. *Neonatal Network, 19*(3), 3-21.

Hummel, P.A., & Eastman, D.L. (1991). Do parents of preterm infants suffer chronic sorrow? *Neonatal Network, 10*(4), 59-65.

Hunter, R., Kilstrom, N., Kraybill, E., et al. (1978). Antecedents of child abuse and neglect in premature infants: A prospective study in a newborn intensive care unit. *Pediatrics, 61,* 629-635.

Hurst, I. (2001a). Vigilant watching over: Mothers' actions to safeguard their premature babies in the newborn intensive care nursery. *Journal of Perinatal and Neonatal Nursing, 15*(3), 39-57.

Hurst, I. (2001b). Mothers' strategies to meet their needs in the newborn intensive care nursery. *Journal of Perinatal and Neonatal Nursing, 15*(2),65-82.

Isabella, R.A. (1993). Origins of attachment: Maternal interactive behavior across the first year. *Child Development, 64,* 605-621.

Isabella, R.A., & Belsky, J. (1991). Interactional synchrony and the origins of infant-mother attachment: A replication study. *Child Development, 62,* 373-384.

Jeffcoate, J.A., Humphrey, M.E., & Lloyd, J.K. (1979). Disturbance in the parent-child relationship following preterm delivery. *Developmental Medicine and Child Neurology, 21,* 344-352.

Johnson, B.H. (1995). Newborn intensive care units pioneer family-centered care change in hospital across country. *Zero to Three, 15*(6), 11-17.

Kenner, C. (1990) Caring for the NICU parent. *Journal of Perinatal and Neonatal Nursing, 4*(3), 78-87.

Klaus, M.H., & Kennell, J.H. (2001). Care of mother, father, and infant. In A.A. Fanaroff & R.J. Martin (Eds.), *Neonatal-perinatal medicine* (5th ed., pp. 199-222). St. Louis: Mosby.

Klaus, M.H., & Kennell, J.H. (1982). Caring for the parents of premature or sick infants. In M.H. Klaus & J.H. Kennell (Eds.), *Parent-infant bonding* (pp. 151-226). St. Louis: Mosby.

Klaus, M.H., & Kennell, J.H. (1976). Caring for the parents of premature or sick infants. In M.H. Klaus & J.H. Kennell (Eds.), *Maternal-infant bonding* (pp. 99-166). St. Louis: Mosby.

Knitzer, J. (2000). Early childhood mental health services: A policy and systems development perspective. In J.P. Sholkoff & S.J. Meisels (Eds.), *Handbook of early childhood intervention* (2nd ed., pp. 416-438). Cambridge, UK: Cambridge Press.

Leventhal, J., Garber, R., & Brady, C. (1989). Identification during the postpartum period of infants who are at high risk of child maltreatment. *Journal of Pediatrics, 114,* 481-487.

Miles, M., & Holditch-Davis, D. (1997). Parenting the prematurely born child: Pathways of influence. *Seminars in Perinatology, 21*(3), 254-266.

Miles, M.S., Carlson, J., & Funk, S.G. (1996). Sources of support reported by mothers and fathers in a Neonatal intensive care unit. *Neonatal Network, 15*(3), 45-52.

Miles, M.S., Funk, S.G., & Carlson, J. (1993). Parent stressor scale: Neonatal intensive care unit. *Nursing Research, 42*(3), 148-152.

Miles, M.S., Funk, S.G., & Kasper, M.A. (1992). The stress response of mothers and fathers of preterm infants. *Research in Nursing and Health, 15,* 261-269.

Minde, K. (2000). Prematurity and serious medical conditions in infancy: Implications for development, behavior, and intervention. In C.H. Zeanah (Ed.), *Handbook of infant mental health* (2nd ed., pp. 176-194). New York: Guilford Press.

Ohgi, M., Fukuda, M., Moriuchi, H., et al. (2002). Comparison of kangaroo care and standard care: Behavioral organization, development, and temperament in healthy low-birth-weight infants through 1 year. *Journal of Perinatology, 22,* 374-379.

Saunders, A.N. (1994). Changing nurses' attitudes toward parenting in the NICU. *Pediatric Nursing, 20*(4), 392-394.

Shellabarger, S.G., & Thompson, T.L. (1993). The critical times: Meeting parental communication needs throughout the NICU experience. *Neonatal Network, 12*(2), 39-44.

Sroufe, L.A. (1996). *Emotional development: The organization of emotional life in the early years.* New York: Cambridge University Press.

Wereszczak, J., Miles, M., & Holditch-Davis, D. (1997). Maternal recall of the neonatal intensive care unit. *Neonatal Network, 16*(4), 33-40.

# The Neonatal Intensive Care Unit Environment

## Maryann Bozzette and Carole Kenner

In the 1960s, the neonatal intensive care unit (NICU) was established to provide care specifically for critically ill newborn infants. Since that time, the NICU has evolved into a state of the art technological center providing a myriad of health care facilities. Medical progress has been remarkable, with approximately a 90% survival rate of all premature infants. Some centers even report more than 80% of even the 500- to 800-g infants are surviving today (D'Agostino & Clifford, 1998; Harper, Rehman, Sia, et al., 2002). However, from a long-term developmental standpoint, these achievements have come at a great expense. The rapid progress in medical and technical innovations have been accompanied by continuing concern for developmental trajectories of infants receiving neonatal intensive care, particularly for very low birthweight (VLBW) infants.

The normal environment for the developing fetus at 23 to 40 weeks', gestation is the maternal womb. The intrauterine environment provides some protection from outside stimulation while surrounding the developing fetus with a dark, fluid environment for weightless movement, and intermittent filtered sounds. The uterine walls furnish boundaries that provide security for the developing human. Maternal activity and hormonal cycles provide rhythmic and cyclic stimulation. The fetus is gently rocked and moved as the mother moves. The placenta provides necessary nutrients that continuously meet all the metabolic needs of the growing fetus (Blackburn, 2003a, 2003b; Blackburn, 1998). The maternal-fetal system is an astonishing, self-sufficient unit for optimal development.

In contrast, the extrauterine environment of the NICU exposes the newly born premature infant to bright, artificial lights; frequent loud noises; cool, dry temperatures; and gravitational forces that restrict mobility (Als, 1998; White-Traut, Nelson, Burns, & Cunningham, 1994). The premature infant abruptly becomes dependent on an artificial means of survival and is confronted with numerous noxious stimuli (Altimier, 2003; D'Agostino & Clifford, 1998; Graven, Bowen, Brooten, et al., 1992a) (Figure 5-1).

For parents, the NICU is far from the vision that most had when they first learned they were pregnant. The nursery was generally not envisioned as something out of a technodrama and looks little like the living arrangements most parents dreamed about for their child. The environment can be either hostile or comforting for the infant and family, depending on the circumstances and the attention that healthcare professionals provide for them. This dramatic caregiving environment presents the infant and family with many new challenges. This chapter addresses issues and concerns related to traditional NICU environments. Specific information on many of these topics can be found throughout this text. Please consult the table of contents for more in-depth information.

## MEDICAL KNOWLEDGE UNDERPINNING NEONATAL BEHAVIOR

In the past three decades, survival of the premature infant has progressively improved. An infant born at 23 weeks' gestation is considered viable today (Graven, Bowen, Brooten, et al., 1992a; Bagwell, Acree, Karlsen, et al., 2003). The incidence of major handicaps, such as cerebral palsy and mental retardation, has declined (Graven, Bowen, Brooten, et al., 1992a; Vohr & Msall, 1997; Als, 1998; Holditch-Davis, Blackburn, & VandenBerg, 2003). Ventilators have been specifically designed for newborns, and the ability to perform delicate surgical procedures on even the smallest infants have been

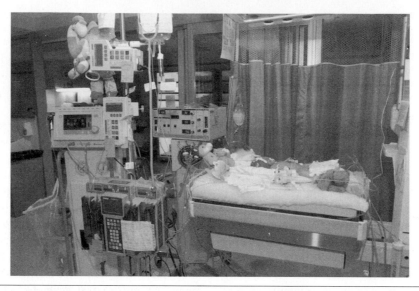

Figure 5-1 Level III neonate who requires high-technology care. (*Courtesy of TriHealth, Cincinnati, OH.*)

perfected. The amount of equipment available for the care of critically ill infants has steadily increased. It has also become more sophisticated, allowing for several different types of physiologic support and monitoring of infants in contemporary NICUs. Devices for continuous monitoring of arterial oxygen saturation, blood pressures, carbon dioxide levels, and even cerebral blood flow have been designed (Gagnon, Leung, & Macnab, 1999; Moniaci & Moniaci, 2003). More and more of these devices are noninvasive to ensure a more positive, gentler monitoring. In addition, more trust has been placed in the data derived from these devices so that longer periods of time for sleep or, at the very least, undisturbed, nonprocedural time is possible for the infants. Nursing care techniques have steadily been developed specifically to address neonatal problems, such as chronic lung disease, and protocols for VLBW infants.

Although there has been much progress in medical interventions for critically ill newborns, the overall number of VLBW infants has not been reduced (Graven, Bowen, Brooten, et al., 1992a; Hack, Taylor, Klein, et al., 1994; Bagwell, Acree, Karlsen, et al., 2003). Complex and chronic health problems of VLBW infants require extended

care in the NICU environment and long-term developmental intervention. Longitudinal follow-up of infants cared for in NICUs has revealed that even infants who appeared normal at discharge might later show signs of school performance problems, social delays, and neurologic abnormalities as they grow older (Hack, Taylor, Klein, et al., 1994; McCarton, Wallace, Divon, & Vaughan, 1996; Holditch-Davis, Blackburn, & VandenBerg, 2003; Hack, Flannery, Schluchter, et al., 2002).

## MEDICAL TERMINOLOGY FOR CARE IN THE NURSERY

Accompanying all of the technologic advances are strange, foreign words that healthcare professionals roll off their tongues with ease. These medical terms are jargon or useful acronyms for the professional; however, parents or caregivers view these as barriers to their understanding and comfort level. Many parents view the words as creating a stratified environment—one of professionals and the other of parents. Use of medical terminology without proper explanation in lay terms places parents and professionals in an adversarial relationship. To combat these problems, health professionals must be aware of how much the parents understand and how to change the medical jargon into understandable language.

## BASIC PRINCIPLES, USES, AND POTENTIAL COMPLICATIONS OF THE NICU EQUIPMENT

The first principle of all neonatal care is thermoregulation. An infant moves from a wet, warm, intrauterine environment to one that is dry and becomes cool, with breezes blowing over a wet body in the delivery room. The infant warmer bed is flat, borderless, and cold compared with the womb. An infant loses heat by:

- Conduction—Direct contact between two surfaces
- Convection—Air circulation around a body or object
- Evaporation—Water changes into a vapor
- Radiation—Heat exchange between two objects not in direct contact (Anderson, 1999; Kenner, 2003)

One goal of neonatal care is providing a neutral thermal environment where the infant is neither gaining nor losing heat at the expense of energy expenditure. The physical environment and its concomitant heat exchange opportunities are the foundation for provision of neonatal care.

## THE PHYSICAL ENVIRONMENT

When a premature infant is born, there is a quick transfer to either an open radiant warmer or an incubator. Although these units provide warmth to maintain the infant's temperature, many of the other fetal regulatory mechanisms are now lost. The diurnal variation of maternal activity and sleep cycles, as well as vestibular-proprioceptive stimulation from the infant's body and movement, are no longer present (Blackburn, 2003a, 2003b; Blackburn, 1998; Holditch-Davis, Blackburn, & VandenBerg, 2003). Visual, auditory, and tactile stimulation suddenly dominate, and care activity occurs with little change in rhythmicities or intensity (White-Traut, Nelson, Silvestri, et al., 1997).

Heavy boards to stabilize intravenous (IV) catheters and tubing from ventilators restrict infant movement. Sleep is frequently interrupted for care. During environmental observations, investigators have reported as many as 234 sleep disruptions within a 24-hour period (Murdoch & Darlow, 1984). These disruptions have held true for the past 20 years, as evidenced by the study by Altimier, Warner, Kenner, and Amlung (1999). They found that stable infants weighing less than 1500 g have been found to be disturbed as many as 23 times in a 24-hour period. Handling of infants seldom occurs for social reasons and is unpredictable and sometimes painful (Blackburn, 1998, 2003a, 2003b). However, from 1984 to 1999, it is obvious that we have learned that sleep is important and that touching an infant just to check the status is not needed. There appear to be fewer times that we now disturb the infant for things other than procedures, but the number is still high and incorporates times that are not necessary for the well-being of the infant.

NICUs generally either have several rooms containing four to six beds or one large room that houses all the sick infants. More units are moving to pods or modular arrangements to decrease noise and increase privacy for families (Figure 5-2). A few units have also moved to a single-room design. There is a variety of equipment within each bedspace; with each infant often requiring several IV pumps, cardiopulmonary and oxygen monitors, and a ventilator. There are many professionals required to care for these infants. These include respiratory therapists, occupational therapists, physical therapists, pharmacists, radiologists, consulting specialists, laboratory technicians, and, of course, several nurses, neonatologists, and, in teaching facilities, residents and students. All of these healthcare workers might at some time during one 24-hour period be handling an individual infant.

Diagnostic tests such as ultrasounds, radiographs, and echocardiograms require additional equipment within the infant's bedspace. All such tests increase the noise, light, and handling of the infant.

The NICU acoustics usually become magnified with telephones, beepers, monitor alarms, and even fan sounds from medication refrigerators, or computer printers and keyboards found at or near the bedside. The most concerning times are usually during medical rounds or when a critical infant is admitted, when noise and light levels are at their peak (Altimier, 2003; Graven, Bowen, Brooten, et al.,

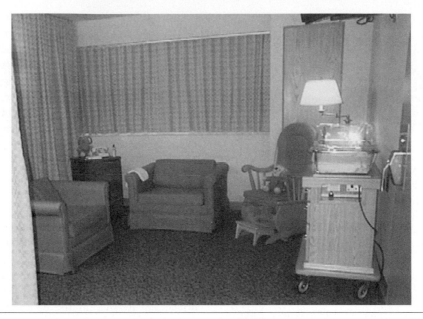

Figure **5-2**  Rooming in. (*Courtesy of TriHealth, Cincinnati, OH.*)

1992b). It is not uncommon for an infant's oxygen saturation to drop during rounds when increased conversation or drumming of fingers on incubator tops occurs.

Human contact is also of concern. Infants who are considered unstable are frequently not held for several days. Speech and conversation is in the environment, but often not directed at the infant during this time (Altimier, 2003; Graven, Bowen, Brooten, et al., 1992b; Holditch-Davis, Blackburn, & VandenBerg, 2003). It might be weeks before infants can breastfeed or have extended contact with their parents. This highly technical, impersonal contact greatly contrasts with the types of experiences of the typical healthy, newborn infant.

The absence of normal parental contact and sensory stimulation, coupled with uncomfortable experiences, stress, and the exposure to the overstimulating environment, is thought to compound the infant's already fragile physical condition and immature organ systems. Even the term *sick infant* is vulnerable to these adverse stimuli. The experiences within the NICU might interfere with the progression of sensory development and integration, and might

affect brain maturation and organization that is vital for future learning and interacting with other human beings (Als, 1998; Holditch-Davis, Blackburn, & VandenBerg, 2003).

## Infection Control and Developmental Outcomes

Infections remain a major source of neonatal morbidity and mortality. The organisms change throughout the years, but the acquisition of perinatal and nosocomial infectious risks do not. The use of cover gowns to protect against infection has been the subject of an age-old argument among infectious-disease personnel and NICU staff. Few systematic studies have been done in the history of NICUs that support their use. Use of isolation rooms for infants who have airborne infections is recommended (White, 2002) and is supported through expert opinion and research. However, when such rooms are used, they should be of sufficient size to promote family-centered care, provide privacy, and be connected by communication devices and monitoring equipment for thorough assessment and access to help (White, 2002).

Hand washing remains the best intervention for decreasing cross contamination. Sinks should be available in each infant-care room, with no bed more than 20 feet away (White, 2002). These sinks should not be of a design that permits standing water that could promote the growth of infectious agents. Entry areas to the unit should provide family and visitors easy access to hand washing, and they should be wheelchair accessible (White, 2002). What does that have to do with developmental care? Infections will slow the progress of infants, prolong their hospital stay, and promote adverse stimuli, such as procedures, medications, excessive handling, and, of course, the disease process itself that might harm the maturing neurologic system. Promotion of an infection-free environment and stay in the NICU increases the chances of a positive developmental outcome.

An area that needs further research is the use of co-wrapping of infants versus co-bedding. This distinction is not often made clear in the literature when co-bedding or co-habiting of infants is done. But some neonatal professionals consider the wrapping together of infants in the same blanket, especially for skin-to-skin contact and co-regulation of vital signs, to be a potential source of infection. Whether it is or not, we need evidence to support or refute the practice. To date, little of the research differentiates the practice of co-bedding (infants placed in the same bed) from co-wrapping.

## MEDICAL COMPLICATIONS: PRIMARY AND IATROGENIC

Infants who have spent considerable time within the NICU environment can contract many sequelae from their early experience. They are prone to upper-respiratory infections and reactive airway disease (Dusick, 1997). Low birthweight infants requiring mechanical ventilation are at higher risk for intraventricular bleeding, chronic lung disease, and retinopathy of prematurity (Als, Lawhon, Duffy, et al., 1994). Some have vision problems such as myopia and strabismus (Dusick, 1997). Many do not reach developmental milestones, even with corrected postconceptional ages. Most infants requiring a NICU stay also require some type of medical care and early intervention during the first

2 years of life. Approximately 50% of the VLBW infants require some form of special education (Hack, Taylor, Klein, et al., 1994). More research and better tools for assessment are necessary to determine the full, long-term impact of a NICU stay and neonatal problems (Majnemer & Rosenblatt, 2000).

More than a decade ago, an individualized approach to neonatal care was developed to support an infant's effort toward self-regulation and enhance clinical outcomes. Als et al. have advocated an individualized approach to providing care that supports the level of infant development. Several research studies have been conducted that compare developmentally supportive care to traditional care and have found increased weight gain, shorter lengths of stay, and shorter time on ventilators (Als, Lawhon, Duffy, et al., 1994; Becker, Grunwald, Moorman, & Stuhr, 1991; Buehler, Als, Duffy, et al., 1995; Fleisher, VandenBerg, Constantinou, et al., 1995; Stevens, Petryshen, Hawkins et al., 1996).

Changing the NICU environment to reduce stress to the infant might help to improve these outcomes (Holditch-Davis, Blackburn, & VandenBerg, 2003; Stevens, Petryshen, Hawkins, et al., 1996). The following areas have been identified as environmental sources of infant stress.

### Sound

All of the equipment within the NICU comes with some type of alarm to alert caregivers. NICUs have constant activity and frequent interactions by healthcare providers. Large pieces of equipment that are routinely brought into the environment, such as portable radiograph machines, compound the continuous background noise.

Blackburn (1998) has identified three major areas of concern regarding NICU sound levels. High intensity sound has the potential to:
- Damage cilia of the cochlea, which results in hearing loss
- Deplete energy reserve and disrupt sleep
- Interact with ototoxic drugs, such as aminoglycosides, increasing susceptibility for hearing loss

NICU sounds have been reported to average from 50 to 90 decibels (dB) (Altimier, 2003; Lotas, 1992). Studies conducted on NICU noise levels have shown:
- Increased infant fatigue
- Irregular sleep-wake states

- Increased heart rate
- Increased intracranial pressure (ICP)
- Hypoxic episodes
- Agitation (DePaul & Chambers, 1995; Holditch-Davis, Blackburn, & VandenBerg, 2003; Lotas, 1992; Zahr & Balian, 1995)

Research findings indicate that peak noise levels can be as high as 120 dB (Thomas, 1995; Altimier, 2003; Holditch-Davis, Blackburn, & VandenBerg, 2003).

According to Occupational Safety and Health Administration (OSHA) regulations, 80 dB is the highest level that does not produce measurable hearing damage (Lotas, 1992). Equipment such as ventilators and IV pumps produces much of the NICU noise. However, the most intense sounds are related to staff activity, conversations, and the opening and closing of doors or drawers (Altimier, 2003; Graven, Bowen, Brooten, et al., 1992a). Although studies have not definitely demonstrated that sensorineural and/or conductive hearing loss is associated with NICU noise, infants at greatest risk for potential damage are those most likely to have the longest exposure to the ambient NICU noise. Continuous background noise has been suggested to interfere with an infant's ability to process auditory stimulation and might be associated with later language delays (Blackburn, 1998, 2003b).

The sleep disruption caused by noise alone has the potential for interfering with the infant's ability to self-regulate and develop progressive sleep-wake patterns (Holditch-Davis, Barham, O'Hale, & Tucker, 1994). The American Academy of Pediatrics (American Academy of Pediatrics [AAP], 1997) has suggested that NICU staff closely monitor noise levels, and sounds greater than 45 dB should be avoided. This recommendation has been supported by White (2002) in the *Recommendations for Newborn ICU Design*.

## Light

The typical NICU lighting levels range from 3.5 to 54 footcandles (ftc) (Bullough, Rea, & Stevens, 1996). In their recommendations on nursery environments, the AAP has additionally indicated that 60 ftc is sufficient illumination to perform most procedures. Design recommendations for new NICUs suggest that 10 to 20 ftc provide adequate ambient light in infant-care areas (White, 2002). Although individual lighting

units and dimmer switches are now available in many units, the most intense illumination tends to occur around the sickest of infants. Supplemental lighting, such as phototherapy lamps, produce more than 300 to 400 ftc. Although eye shielding is usually employed, and treatment lamps range from 200 to 300 ftc, exposing many infants to high levels of light intensity during their stay (Blackburn, 1998; Lotas, 1992) can result in disruption of sleep-wake patterns and, possibly, retinal damage. Continuous light exposure is thought to affect sleep-wake cycles and interrupt the development of diurnal rhythms (Holditch-Davis, Blackburn, & VandenBerg, 2003; Thomas, 1995).

Animal studies have shown retinal damage from high-intensity light exposure in infant primates. Studies conducted on human infants have shown inconsistent results, but there is very little information on specific effects of NICU illumination on sick infants (Lotas, 1992). The effect of light exposure on the incidence of retinopathy of prematurity (ROP) has been investigated in several studies that indicate an interaction between light toxicity and ROP, possibly from free radical oxidative damage. However, a recent multicentered clinical trial examining the use of goggles to decrease light exposure for infants did not alter the incidence of ROP (Reynolds, Hardy, Kennedy, et al., 1998). The relationship between ambient light and ROP remains inconclusive.

Cycled lighting for NICU use has been investigated to decrease constant light exposure. Studies using cycled lighting have found lower heart rates, less infant activity, and more hours of sleep (Grauer, 1989; Miller, White, Whitman, et al., 1995; Holditch-Davis, Blackburn, & VandenBerg, 2003). Although Brandon, Holditch-Davis, and Belyea (2002) used cycled lighting with good results, they did not cycle between bright and darkness. They cycled between low light and darkness. Thus it would appear that the amount of change needed to induce the biorhythms of infants is very low.

## Handling

Many of the descriptive studies addressing the effects of handling in NICUs have consisted of small samples of premature infants but all have resulted in similar findings. They are:

- Decreased oxygen saturation levels following routine procedures (Gorski, Hole, Leonard, & Martin, 1983).

- Increased intracranial pressure
- Increased blood pressure
- Increased agitation
- Episodes of apnea and bradycardia (Evans, 1991; Gagnon, Leung, & Macnab, 1999; Holditch-Davis, Blackburn, & VandenBerg, 2003; Bernert, Siebenthal, Seidi, et al., 1997; Peters, 1998a).

Most infant handling is related to medical or nursing procedures.

Providing tactile stimulation for preterm infants has been explored in several studies showing positive effects for older, stable preterm infants, including increased weight gain and improved tone. However, very young and fragile preterm infants have demonstrated noxious responses to tactile stimulation. The form of tactile stimulation that seems to have the least reported adverse effects is described as gentle touch, when one hand is placed on the infant's head and the other is placed on the infant's lower back (Harrison, 1997). This form of touch is ideal to teach to parents, whose presence is so important to the overall well-being of the child.

## DEVELOPMENTAL INTERVENTIONS

Kangaroo care or skin-to-skin holding began in Columbia in 1981 and consists of mothers holding their infants beneath their clothing, upright on their chest so that there is skin-to-skin contact. In this position, the infants can breastfeed on demand (Anderson, Marks, & Wahlberg, 1986). Randomized clinical trials have been conducted on infants ranging from 26 to 36 weeks' gestation. Although some have examined infants from immediately postbirth, most have been conducted after the acute phase of care is concluded. Infants experiencing Kangaroo care have had fewer episodes of apnea and bradycardia, maintained adequate body temperature, had minimal crying, and had close to twice the amount of sleep of the average infant in the NICU (Bauer, Peyer, Sperling, et al., 1998; Bosque, Brady, Affonso, & Wahlberg, 1995; Holditch-Davis, Blackburn, & VandenBerg, 2003; Mooncey, Giannakoulopoulos, Glover, et al., 1997). The benefits for mothers have been the most notable effects. During Kangaroo care, mothers demonstrated thermal synchrony with their infants as their own body temperature increased or decreased according to the infant's needs. Mothers were inclined to breastfeed their infants longer and produced more milk. They reported feeling closer to their infants and had more confidence in their ability to provide care (see Chapter 15) (Aucott, Donohue, Atkins, et al., 2002; Bauer, Peyer, Sperling, et al., 1998; Chwo, Anderson, Good, et al., 2002).

Another recent innovation is co-bedding of multiples. Co-bedding consists of housing twins or higher multiples in the same incubator or crib to keep them from being separated. Although there have been few formal studies on co-bedding, many units have adopted this practice with no adverse effects reported to date. Confusing the two infants is a concern for nursing care, but most units have adapted quickly, and developed a way to correctly identify the twins, so that events such as medication errors are not seen (Altimier & Lutes, 2001; Kassity, Jones, Kenner, et al., 2003; DellaPorta, Aforismo, & Butler-O'Hara, 1998). Randomized trials are needed to either support or refute the practice of co-bedding. If it is done, it should be with the understanding that there is a lack of evidence to support this intervention. Some would argue that this is really co-mattressing and not co-bedding. Again, our terminology is not always clear; for some institutions, the protocol is to wrap the infants together in the same blanket to promote similar biorhythms. This difference in definition and terminology must be considered when reviewing the literature.

## PARENTS OF CRITICALLY ILL INFANTS

The NICU's physical environment presents several barriers for parents.
- Incubators isolate infants
- Sights and sounds are frightening
- Equipment keeps parents at a distance
- Infants seems more vulnerable due to high-tech needs
- Parents feel helpless because they cannot control the equipment
- Amount of parent involvement varies from unit to unit

The parental image of the infant is influenced greatly by their NICU experience as well as the attitudes of the health professionals. This impression might range from extreme vulnerability to unrealistic views of their infant's medical status. Caring for parents is an important component of neonatal and developmental care. Approaching the care of high-risk infants should be in the context of the family unit. Communication and accurate information are two of the most important factors for parents of sick newborns. Parent care remains underdeveloped and must be a priority in the new millennium.

## RELATIONSHIP OF THE EARLY ENVIRONMENT TO NEONATAL OUTCOMES

The preterm infant is immature in areas of both development and function of most major organ systems. At greatest risk is the neurologic system, with poorly differentiated white matter and synaptic and dendritic organization just beginning to occur within the premature infant's brain (Als, Lawhon, Duffy, et al., 1994). The underdevelopment of cerebral structures prevents inhibition of most stimuli, allowing a preterm infant minimal means of modulating the multitude of stressors from the environment. In addition, the neurosensory system is also immature. Although the tactile, vestibular, and olfactory senses are developed early in gestation, the gustatory, auditory, and visual neuropathways are still forming. Significant damage to hearing and vision might occur due to overexposure to noise and bright lights (Blackburn, 1998, 2003b, Holditch-Davis, Blackburn, & VandenBerg, 2003).

The fetal structure of the germinal matrix is the location where neurons begin their migration, and is still present in the preterm infant. The fragile vessels of this highly vascular area are at risk for rupture and are particularly susceptible to ischemia. Intraventricular hemorrhage and/or periventricular leukomalacia can result (Blackburn, 2003b; Volpe, 2001). Ototoxic drugs such as aminoglycosides can have a synergistic effect when coupled with environmental noise and such conditions as hyperbilirubinemia (Blackburn, 1998, 2003b). Immature vessels of the retina are also susceptible to injury. The smaller the infant is (in terms of

birthweight and gestational age), the higher the incidence of disease (D'Agostino & Clifford, 1998).

## BEHAVIORAL AND DEVELOPMENTAL EFFECTS OF DRUGS IN THE NICU

There are several medications that are routinely used in treatment of the premature infant that might have negative effects on infant growth, physiologic function, and infant behavior. Because maintaining physiologic stability is a priority, monitoring the effects of pharmacologic treatments is extremely important. Although there are many drugs that can be used in the NICU, only a few of the most common are discussed here.

Aminoglucosides, particularly gentamycin, are often used to treat gram-negative bacterial infections. Because the functional maturation of the inner ear occurs during the second half of gestation, premature infants are particularly at risk for ototoxicity when receiving gentamycin (Henley & Rybak, 1993). Even infants that initially have normal hearing screens have later developed conductive hearing loss (Kawashiro, Tsuchihashi, Koga, et al., 1994). Gentamycin can also affect kidney function. Altered glomerular filtration rates and an increase in creatinine levels can lead to nephrotoxicity, particularly when trough levels are consistently high (Uijtendaal, Rademaker, Schobben, et al., 2001). A potentiating effect has been seen when gentamycin is used in conjunction with loop diuretics (Henley, & Rybak, 1993). Because antibiotics for most premature infants are started on the first day of life, routine use of potentially organ-damaging drugs, and future bacterial resistance, are major concerns.

Furosemide (Lasix) is frequently used in premature infants with severe lung disease, and in particular, in cases complicated with patent ductus arteriosus. Electrolyte disturbances often occur, caused by changes in renal tubular absorption. Nephrocalcinosis, or renal calcification, is a side effect of Lasix therapy that causes discomfort, but might reverse at the end of treatment (Narendra, White, Rolton, et al., 2001). Cholelithiasis or gallstones is another adverse effect from the use of Lasix in premature infants. When given in conjunction with parental nutrition, cholestasis might be detected as early as 3 weeks. The development of gallstones is reported to be a longer-term problem (Prandota, 2001). Another issue related to the chronic use of Lasix is the potential for secondary hyperparathyroidism leading to bone demineralization and osteopenia (Prandota, 2001).

Patent ductus arteriosus (PDA) in premature infants can contribute to the development of chronic lung disease. Indomethacin is a drug used to treat symptomatic PDA. Oliguria, increased creatinine values, and retention of urea might result from immature renal system function. Many infants also experience a disruption in feeding while receiving indomethacin treatment, owing to decreased blood flow to the gastrointestinal track and transient thrombocytopenia (Ojala, Ala-Houhala, Ahonen, et al., 2001).

With the survival of very early gestation infants, the use of steroids has become more common in the NICU. Intravenous hydrocortisone is given to premature infants with refractory hypotension, and dexamethazone is commonly used to treat chronic lung changes to improve respiratory function. Glucocorticoids have many potential serious side effects, including hyperglycemia, pituitary and adrenal suppression, bone demineralization, and suppression of the immune system. Many infants receiving steroids have poor weight gain and unstable glucose levels, and some develop rickets (Botas, Kurlat, Young, & Sola, 1995). Disturbance in sleep, which often occurs in adults on glucocorticoids, might affect state regulation in premature infants. In recent years, dexamethasone has been used to assist in weaning from artificial ventilation and to prevent chronic lung disease. One of the most concerning effects has been adrenal suppression and associated electrolyte imbalances (Dusick, 1997). Ironically, Ikeda, Mishima, Yoshikawa, et al. (2002) examined uses of dexamethasone in rats following hypoxic episodes. They found that the steroid improved learning and brain function. This is an animal model and is only one study. Much more research needs to be undertaken. It must also be considered that when steroids are used for a chronic lung condition, they might need to be used long term, and

certainly are not a one-time dose. Other concerns about steroid use are that they interfere with growth, especially brain growth.

Concerns have been raised over several drugs used for sedation of ventilated infants. Lack of experience with these medications and fear of side effects have been obstacles for effective sedation. Most of these drugs require tapering to prevent physiologic withdrawal. Drugs such as midoxalam and valium might lead to hypotension, whereas fentanyl has been related to chest rigidity and increased tolerance to dosing levels (Lago, Benini, Agosto, & Zacchello, 1998). The long-acting nature of these medications and the preterm infant's reduced capacity for hepatic transformation of drugs often lead to prolonged general depression of these infants. Judicious use of these drugs is important for the care of premature infants, because these infants are very sensitive to noxious and painful stimuli, and are capable of mounting stress responses that are consistent with the severity of their illnesses (Barker & Rutter, 1996; Menon, Anand, & McIntosh, 1998).

One of the most commonly used groups of drugs in the NICU are the methylzanthines, particularly theophylline and caffeine. Because many premature infants have apnea of prematurity, these drugs have been used for many years. Tachycardia, sleep disturbances, and gastrointestinal irritation have been reported. Hypothyroidism has also been speculated to result from these drugs, although the studies to date have not proved this relationship (Curzi-Dascalova, Aujard, Gaultier, & Rajguru, 2002). Protecting these infants from inappropriate stimulation and clustering care might help to minimize behavioral effects. Most infants who are monitored within a therapeutic range seem to tolerate these drugs fairly well (Castellanos & Rapoport, 2002).

Another stimulant medication that is under investigation is doxapram. This drug is frequently used when caffeine is not effective in reducing episodes of apnea and bradycardia. Finer and Barrington (2002) and Screenan, Ethces, Demianczuk, et al. (2001) found that very low birthweight infants (less than 1250 g) who received long-term doxapram for apnea, had associated developmental delays. Further research is needed in this area as in all areas regarding stimulants and developmental outcomes.

Premature infants are experiencing rapid development in all areas, particularly physiologic function and neurologic maturation. Their immature organ function affects the distribution, absorption, and excretion of drugs. Infant responsiveness, gastric emptying, and consolabilty are other conditions that might be altered by the many therapies used in the NICU.

## Care Procedures and Development

Although most premature infants survive with little or no disability, the VLBW infant can have up to 50% minor disabilities (Vohr & Msall, 1997). Developmental concerns for the preterm infant population include the areas of cognitive learning ability, behavior difficulties, and mild neuromotor deficits (Koller, Lawson, Rose, et al., 1997; Landry, Denson, & Swank, 1997). Math, reading, language delays, difficulty in logic and impulsive behavior, and poor attention span have all been reported (Blackburn, 2003; Hack, Taylor, Klein, et al., 1994; Holditch-Davis, Blackburn, & VandenBerg, 2003). Hack, Flannery, Schluchter, et al. (2002) conducted a study of VLBW infants who had reached adulthood. They found that difficulties in academic achievement continued even in college. This group, across gender, had neurosensory deficits that were greater than the general population, and their mean IQ was lower than expected.

Many routine nursing practices can cause distress to the premature infant. For example, physical and behavioral responses to energy demands have been demonstrated in many preterm infants during routine bathing (Peters, 1998b). Swaddled bathing is one strategy to decrease this adverse stimulation (Fern, Graves, & L'Huillier, 2002). Other examples of stress-producing activities include suctioning and repositioning. Decreasing the number of routine procedures has been shown to be effective in reducing physiologic distress. Zahr (1998) made observations of noise levels and nursing activities in two different NICUs. One of the units was located in Beirut, Lebanon, and the other was in Los Angeles, California. The Lebanese NICU was less intense and had fewer routine procedures. Infant sleep was interrupted less often, and, for all coded measures, the environment was less invasive than the US intensive care unit (Zahr, 1998). Modifying nursing care by providing standard rest periods for convalescing preterm infants has also resulted in longer bouts of sleep and less quiet awakening (Holditch-Davis et al., 1994, 2003). Measures such as these allow energy conservation and promote development. These observations suggest that a reexamination of current practices is needed, and modifications are planned in the overall approach to neonatal care to prevent demands and energy depletion.

Pain and comfort care are other concerns for the neonate that can be affected by the environment. Anand and Hickey (1987) conducted a classic study demonstrating that intraoperative use of fentanyl mitigated the stress response, as measured by hormonal and chemical indicators. Continuous stress affects infant behavior, places additional physiologic demands on the premature infant, and might affect early synaptic organization of the infant's brain (Gunner & Barr, 1998).

Use of continuous morphine infusions has provided significant stress reduction for ventilated infants and continues to be studied (Quinn, Otoo, Ruserforth, et al., 1992). Grunau, Whitefield, Petrie, et al. (1994) have suggested that the extended NICU stay for infants produces higher somatization in preterm infants. The retention of painful experiences might also contribute to the development of pain syndromes.

Recent pain protocols have included the use of sucrose to reduce discomfort. However, accurate assessment and anticipation of pain is needed to support comfort care (Hummel & Puchalski, 2001).

Alterations in central nervous system (CNS) development might occur from frequent and noxious stimulation experienced by premature infants. Several areas of CNS development occur during the period when preterm infants are in the NICU, including neuron migration, synaptogenesis, and arborization. The patterns of dendrite connections between neurons are critical to cell-to-cell communication. This process might be particularly vulnerable to insults from the environment of the NICU. Fluctuations in oxygen saturation and blood pressure for example, might occur with handling and procedures such as endotracheal suctioning.

The germinal matrix is the site of origin for neurons and glial cells. Migration of cells from this area occurs in the sixth month of gestation to their final location in the CNS. The germinal matrix has fragile and poorly supported blood vessels that receive a large portion of blood flow, making premature infants susceptible to intraventricular hemorrhage (Volpe, 2001).

Another area of the brain that might be affected by environmental stimuli from the NICU is the cerebellum. Because the cerebellum controls muscles and coordination of movement, insults to this area can result in disruption of motor development (Blackburn, 1998).

The traditional environment of the NICU has continued in many centers, even with mounting evidence that the environment is stressful and potentially has negative effects on developmental outcomes (Altimier, 2003; D'Agostino & Clifford, 1998; Holditch-Davis, Blackburn, & VandenBerg, 2003). The premature infant is extremely vulnerable to environmental stress because of neurologic immaturity, physiologic instability, and inability to inhibit stimulation and multiple demands on energy reserve. Most of the stimuli of the NICU environment are inappropriate for adequate sensory development (Blackburn, 1998; White-Traut, Nelson, Silvestri, et al., 1997). Most concerning is the amount of time preterm infants are spending within the NICU. Exposure to the NICU environment increases with decreasing gestational age (Als, Lawhon, Duffy, et al., 1994; Altimier, 2003; Holditch-Davis, Blackburn, & VandenBerg, 2003).

## CONCLUSION

NICUs represent one of the fastest developing areas of technology and treatment intervention in health care today. Numerous techniques, such as surfactant replacement, high-frequency ventilators, and percutaneously inserted central venous catheters have greatly decreased mortality, allowing even infants at early gestations to survive. With innovations such as cardiac surgical techniques and extracorporeal membrane oxygenation (ECMO), critically ill newborns who would have died in the past are now surviving. With all of these medical breakthroughs, however, have come iatrogenic health complications

and developmental delays. The time has come to focus on the quality of life for these infants and their early relationships. For two decades, many have suggested that the environment that was designed to support premature infants' needs has been characteristically inappropriate for supporting normal development and was created more for the convenience of the care providers (Graven, Bowen, Brooten, et al., 1992b).

Full-term infants have been able to mature within the intrauterine environment and are prepared for a variety of sensory experiences and social contacts in the outside world. They have immediate and consistent availability to nurturing parents. Critically ill neonates, however, face additional challenges from overstimulating and invasive environments that isolate them from parents and expose them to multiple caregivers and unpredictable treatments and procedures. Premature infants remain extremely vulnerable to stress. Modifying caregiving practices remains a significant challenge for all who provide care for premature infants, to reduce iatrogenic complications from the environment. Changes in care approaches that emphasize measures to meet neurodevelopment needs and prevent disability are expected to improve long-term outcomes for premature infants.

## REFERENCES

Als, H. (1998). Developmental care in the newborn intensive care unit. *Current Opinion in Pediatrics, 10,* 138-142.

Als, H., Lawhon, G., Duffy, F.H., et al. (1994). Individualized developmental care for the very low-birth-weight preterm infant: Medical and neurofunctional effects. *Journal of the American Medical Association (JAMA), 272*(11), 853-855.

Altimier, L. (2003). Management of the NICU environment (pp. 229-235). In C. Kenner & J.W. Lott (Eds.), *Comprehensive neonatal nursing: A physiologic perspective* (3rd ed.). St. Louis: W.B. Saunders.

Altimier, L., & Lutes, L. (2001). Cobedding multiples. *Newborn and Infant Nursing Reviews, 1*(4), 205-206.

Altimier, L., Warner, B., Kenner, C., & Amlung, S. (1999). Value study. *Neonatal Network, 18*(4), 35-38.

American Academy of Pediatrics (AAP). (1997). Noise: A hazard for the fetus and newborn. *Pediatrics, 100,* 724-726.

Anand, K.J.S., & Hickey, P.R. (1987). Pain and its effects in the human neonate and fetus. *New England Journal of Medicine, 317,* 1321-1329.

Anderson, G., Marks, E.A., & Wahlberg, V. (1986). Kangaroo care for premature infants. *American Journal of Nursing, 86*, 807-809.

Anderson, S. (1999). Thermoregulation. In J. Deacon, & P. O'Neill (Eds.), *Core curriculum for neonatal intensive care nursing* (pp. 63-73). Philadelphia: W.B. Saunders.

Aucott, S., Donohue, P.K., Atkins, E., et al. (2002). Neurodevelopmental care in the NICU. *Mental Retardation and Developmental Disabilities Research, 8*(4), 298-308.

Bagwell, G.A., Acree, C.M., Karlsen, K.A., et al. (2003). Regionalization in Today's Health Care Delivery System (pp. 16-38). In C. Kenner & J.W. Lott (Eds). *Comprehensive neonatal nursing: A physiologic perspective* (3rd ed.). St. Louis: W.B. Saunders.

Barker, D.P., & Rutter, N. (1996). Stress, severity of illness, and outcome in ventilated preterm infants. *Archives of Disease in Childhood Fetal & Neonatal Edition, 75*, F187-F190.

Bauer, K., Peyer, A., Sperling, P., et al. (1998). Effects of gestational and postnatal age on body temperature, oxygen consumption, and activity during early skin-to-skin contact between preterm infants of 25-30 gestation infants and their mothers. *Pediatric Research, 44*, 247-251.

Becker, P., Grunwald, P., Moorman, J., & Stuhr, S. (1991). Outcomes of developmentally supportive nursing care for very low birth weight infants. *Nursing Research, 40*, 150-155.

Bernert, C., Siebenthal, K.V., Seidi, R., et al., (1997). The effect of behavioral states on cerebral oxygenation during endotracheal suctioning of preterm babies. *Neuropediatrics, 28*, 111-115.

Blackburn, S. (1998). Environmental impact of the NICU on developmental outcomes. *Journal of Perinatal Neonatal Nursing, 4*, 42-54.

Blackburn, S.T. (2003a). *Maternal, fetal, & neonatal physiology: A clinical perspective*. St. Louis: W.B. Saunders.

Blackburn, S.T. (2003b). Assessment and management of the neurologic system (pp. 624-660). In C. Kenner & J.W. Lott (Eds.), *Comprehensive neonatal nursing: A physiologic perspective* (3rd ed.). St. Louis: W.B. Saunders.

Bosque, H.M., Brady, J.P., Affonso, D., & Wahlberg, B.W. (1995). Physiological measures of kangaroo vs. incubator care in a tertiary level nursing. *Journal of Obstetric, Gynecologic, and Neonatal Nursing (JOGNN), 24*, 219-226.

Botas, C.M., Kurlat, I., Young, S.M., & Sola, A. (1995). Disseminated candidal infections and intravenous hydrocortisone in preterm infants, *Pediatrics, 95*, 883-887.

Brandon, D.H., Holditch-Davis, D., & Belyea, M. (2002). Preterm infants born at less than 31 weeks' gestation have improved growth in cycled light compared with continuous near darkness. *Journal of Pediatrics, 140*(2), 192-199.

Buehler, D., Als, H., Duffy, F.H., McAnulty, G., & Liederman, J. (1995). Effectiveness of individualized developmental care for low risk preterm infants: Behavioral and electrophysiologic evidence. *Pediatrics, 96*, 923-932.

Bullough, J., Rea, M.S., & Stevens, R.G. (1996). Light and magnetic fields in a neonatal intensive care unit. *Bioelectromagnetics, 17*, 396-405.

Castellanos, F.X., & Rapoport, J.L. (2002). Effects of caffeine on development in infancy and childhood: A review of literature. *Food, Chemical Toxicology, 40*(9), 1235-1242.

Chwo, M.J., Anderson, G.C., Good, M., et al. (2002). A randomized controlled trial of early kangaroo care for preterm infants: Effects on temperature, weight, behavior, and acuity. *Journal of Nursing Research, 10*(2), 129-142.

Curzi-Dascalova, L., Aujard, Y, Gaultier, C. & Rajguru, M. (2002). Sleep organization is unaffected by caffeine in premature infants. *Journal of Pediatrics, 140*, 766-771.

D'Agostino, J.A., & Clifford, P. (1998). Neurodevelopmental consequences associated with the premature neonate. *American Association of Critical Care Nurses (ACCN) Clinical Issues, 9*, 11-24.

DellaPorta, K., Aforismo, D., & Butler-O'Hara, M.J. (1998). Co-bedding of twins in the neonatal intensive care unit. *Pediatric Nursing, 24*, 529-531.

DePaul, P., & Chambers, S.E. (1995). Environmental noise in the neonatal intensive care unit: Implications for nursing practice. *Journal of Perinatal Neonatal Nursing, 8*, 71-76.

Dusick, A.M. (1997). Medical outcomes in preterm infants. *Seminars in Perinatology, 21*, 194-277.

Evans, J.C. (1991). Incidence of hypoxemia associated with care giving in premature infants. *Neonatal Network, 10*, 17-24.

Fern, D., Graves, C., & L'Huillier, M. (2002). Swaddled bathing in the newborn intensive care unit. *Newborn and Infant Nursing Reviews, 2*(1), 3-4.

Finer, N.N., & Barrington, K.J. (2002). Doxapram and neurodevelopment. *Journal of Pediatrics, 141*(2), 296-297.

Fleisher, B., VandenBerg, K., Constantinou, J., et al., (1995). Individualized developmental care for very low birth weight premature infants. *Clinical Pediatrics, 34*, 523-529.

Gagnon, R.E., Leung, A., & Macnab, A.J. (1999). Variations in regional cerebral blood volume in neonates associated with nursery events. *American Journal of Perinatology, 16*, 7-11.

Gorski, P.A., Hole, W.T., Leonard, C.H., & Martin, J.A. (1983). Direct computer recording of premature infants and nursery care: Distress following two interventions. *Pediatrics, 72*, 198-202.

Grauer, T.T. (1989). Environmental lighting, behavioral state, and hormonal response with the newborn. *Scholarly Inquiry for Nursing Practice: An International Journal, 3*, 53-69.

Graven, S.W., Bowen, F.W., Brooten, D., et al. (1992a). The high-risk environment. Part 1. The role of the neonatal intensive care unit in the outcome of high-risk infants. *Journal of Perinatology, XII,* 164-172.

Graven, S.W., Bowen, F.W., Brooten, D., et al. (1992b). The high-risk infant environment. Part 2. The role of the caregiver and the social environment. *Journal of Perinatology, XII,* 267-273.

Grunau, R.V.E., Whitefield, M.F., Petrie, J.H., et al., (1994). Early pain experience, child and family factors, as precursors for somatization: A prospective study of extremely premature and full-term children. *Pain, 56,* 353-359.

Gunner, M.R., & Barr, R.C. (1998). Stress, early brain development and behavior. *Infants and Young Children, 11,* 1-14.

Hack, M., Flannery, D.J., Schluchter, M., et al. (2002). Outcomes in young adulthood for very-low-birth-weight infants. *New England Journal of Medicine, 346*(3), 149-157.

Hack, M., Taylor, G., Klein, N., et al. (1994). School-age outcomes of children with birth weights under 750 g. *New England Journal of Medicine, 331,* 753-759.

Harper, R.G., Rehman, K.U., Sia, C., et al. (2002). Neonatal outcome of infants born at 500 to 800 grams from 1990 through 1998 in a tertiary care center. *Journal of Perinatology, 22*(7), 555-562.

Harrison, L. (1997). Research utilization: Handling preterm infants in the NICU. *Neonatal Network, 16*(3), 65-69.

Henley, C.M., & Rybak, L.P. (1993). Developmental ototoxicity. *Otolaryngologic Clinics of North America, 26,* 857-871.

Holditch-Davis, D., Barham, L.N., O'Hale, A., & Tucker, B. (1994). Effects of standard rest period on convalescent preterm infants. *Journal of Obstetric, Gynecologic, and Neonatal Nursing (JOGNN), 24,* 424-432.

Holditch-Davis, D., Blackburn, S.T., & VandenBerg, K. (2003). Newborn and Infant Neurobehavioral Development (pp. 236-284). In C. Kenner & J.W. Lott (Eds.), *Comprehensive neonatal nursing: A physiologic perspective* (3rd ed.). St. Louis: W.B. Saunders.

Hummel, P., & Puchalski, M. (2001). Assessment and management of pain in infancy. *Newborn and Infant Nursing Reviews, 1*(2), 114-121.

Ikeda, T., Mishima, K, Yoshikawa, T., et al. (2002). Dexamethasone prevents long-lasting learning impairment following neonatal hypoxic-ischemic brain insult in rats. *Behavioral and Brain Research, 136*(1), 161-170.

Kassity, N.A., Jones, J.E., Kenner, C., et al. (2003). Complementary Therapies (pp. 868-875). In C. Kenner & J.W. Lott (Eds.), *Comprehensive neonatal nursing: A physiologic perspective* (3rd ed.). St. Louis: W.B. Saunders.

Kawashiro, M, Tsuchihashi, N., Koga, K., et al. (1994). Idiopathic deafness or hearing loss of unknown etiology following discharge from the NICU. *Acta Oto-Laryngologica, 514,* 81-84.

Kenner, C. (2003). Resuscitation and stabilization of the newborn (pp. 210-227). In C. Kenner & J.W. Lott (Eds.),

*Comprehensive neonatal nursing: A physiologic perspective* (3rd ed.). St. Louis: W.B. Saunders.

Koller, H., Lawson, K., Rose, S.A., Wallace, I., & McCarton, C. (1997). Patterns of cognitive development in very low birth weight children during the first six years of life. *Pediatrics, 99,* 398-399.

Lago, P., Benini, F., Agosto, C., & Zacchello, F. (1998). Randomised controlled trial of low dose fentanyl infusion in preterm infants with hyaline membrane disease. *Archives of Disease in Childhood, Fetal & Neonatal Edition, 79,* F194-F197.

Landry, S.H., Denson, S.E., & Swank, P.R. (1997). Effects of medical risk and socioeconomic status on the rate of change in cognitive and social development for low birth weight children. *Journal of Clinical and Experimental Pediatrics, 19,* 261-274.

Lotas, M. (1992). Effects of light and sound in the NICU on the LBW infant. *Nurses' Association of the American College of Obstetrics and Gynecology's (NAACOG's) Clinical Issues, 5,* 34-45.

Majnemer, A., & Rosenblatt, B. (2000). Prediction of outcome at school age in neonatal intensive care unit graduates using neonatal neurologic tools. *Journal of Child Neurology, 15*(10), 645-651.

McCarton, C.M., Wallace, I.F., Divon, M., & Vaughan, H.G., Jr. (1996). Cognitive and neurologic development of the premature, small for gestational age infant through age 6: Comparison by birth weight and gestational age. *Pediatrics, 98,* 1167-1178.

Menon, G., Anand, K.J., & McIntosh, N. (1998). Practical approach to analgesia and sedation in the neonatal intensive care unit. *Seminars in Perinatology, 22,* 417-424.

Miller, C.L., White, R., Whitman, T.L., et. al. (1995). The effects of cycled versus noncycled lighting, on growth and development in preterm infants. *Infant Behavior and Development, 18,* 87-95.

Moniaci, V., & Moniaci S. (2003). Monitoring neonatal biophysical parameters in a developmentally supportive environment (pp. 285-298). In C. Kenner & J.W. Lott (Eds.), *Comprehensive neonatal nursing: A physiologic perspective* (3rd ed.). St. Louis: W.B. Saunders.

Mooncey, S., Giannakoulopoulos, X., Glover, V., et al. (1997). The effect of mother-infant skin-to-skin contact on plasma cortisol on-endorphin concentrations in preterm newborns. *Infant Behavior and Development, 20,* 553-557.

Murdoch, D.R., & Darlow, B.A. (1984). Handling during neonatal intensive care. *Archives of Diseases of Childhood, 59,* 957-961.

Narendra, A., White, M.P., Rolton, H.A., et. al., (2001). Neprhocalcinosis in preterm babies. *Archives of Diseases in Childhood, Fetal and Neonatal Edition, 85,* F207-F213.

Ojala, R., Ala-Houhala, M. Ahonen, S., et al. (2001). Renal follow up of premature infants with and without perinatal indemethacin exposure. *Archives of Disease in Childhood, Fetal and Neonatal Edition, 84,* F28-F33.

Peters, K.L. (1998a). Neonatal stress, reactivity, and control. *Journal of Perinatal Neonatal Nursing, 11,* 45-59.

Peters, K.L. (1998b). Bathing premature infants: Physiological and behavioral consequences. *Journal of Perinatal and Neonatal Nursing, 7,* 90-100.

Prandota, J. (2001). Clinical pharmaocolgy of furosemide in children: A supplement. *American Journal of Therapeutics, 8*(4), 275-289.

Quinn, M.W., Otoo, J.A., Ruserforth, H.G., et al. (1992). Effects of morphine and pancuronium on the stress response in ventilated preterm infants. *Early Human Development, 30,* 241-248.

Reynolds, K.D., Hardy, R.J., Kennedy, K.A., et. al. (1998). Lack of efficacy of light reduction in preventing retinopathy of prematurity (LIGHTROP) collaborative study. *New England Journal of Medicine, 338,* 1572-1576.

Screenan, C., Ethces, P.C., Demianczuk, N., et al. (2001). Isolated mental developmental delay in very low birth weight infants: Associated with prolonged doxapram therapy for apnea. *Journal of Pediatrics, 139*(6), 832-837.

Stevens, B., Petryshen, P., Hawkins, J., et al., (1996). Developmental versus conventional care: A comparison of clinical outcomes for very low birth weight infants. *Canadian Journal of Nursing Research, 28,* 97-113.

Thomas, K.A. (1995). Biorhythms in infants and role of the care environment. *Journal of Neonatal Nursing, 9,* 61-75.

Uijtendaal, E.V., Rademaker, C.M., Schobben, A.F., et al. (2001). Once-daily versus multiple daily gentamycin in infants and children, *Therapeutic Drug Monitoring, 23,* 505-513.

Vohr, B.R., & Msall, M.E. (1997). Neurophysiological and functional outcomes of very low birth weight infants. *Seminar in Perinatology, 21,* 202-220.

Volpe, J.J. (2001). *Neurology of the newborn* (4th ed.). Philadelphia: W.B. Saunders.

White, R. (2002). *Recommendations for newborn ICU design.* Report of the Fifth Consensus Conference on NICU Design. Available online at *http://www.nd.edu/~kkolberg/DesignStandards.htm.*

White-Traut, R., Nelson, M.W., Burns, K., & Cunningham, N. (1994). Environmental influences on the developing premature infant: Theoretical issues and application to practice. *Journal of Obstetric, Gynecologic, and Neonatal Nursing (JOGNN), 23,* 393-401.

White-Traut, R.C., Nelson, M.N., Silvestri, J.M., et al. (1997). Responses of preterm infants to unimodal and multimodal sensory intervention. *Pediatric Nursing, 23*(2), 169-175, 193.

Zahr, L.K. (1998). Two contrasting NICU environments. *Maternal Child Nursing (MCN), 23,* 28-36.

Zahr, L.K., & Balian, S. (1995). Responses of premature infants to routine nursing interventions and noise in the NICU. *Nursing Research, 44,* 179-185.

# 6 Critical Periods of Development

### Marilyn J. Lotas, Joyce L. King, and Cheryl Ann King

The term "critical periods" in development refers to the concept that, as development occurs, certain events must occur at a particular time or point in the process for the next developmental steps to occur in an appropriate manner. The failure of developmental milestones to occur at a precisely defined point or within a critical period in the development of the embryo/fetus might result in malformation or death. For example, if the fusing of the neural tube does not occur in the critical period of 21 to 23 days postconception, the infant will be born with some degree of spina bifida. The purpose of this chapter is to describe the critical periods of development, including changes occurring in the pregnant woman, and significant points in the developmental process of the embryo/fetus. The final section of the chapter compares the developmental status of the respiratory, cardiovascular, neurologic, skin, and musculoskeletal systems of the preterm infant across conceptional ages from 24 to 36 weeks. Knowledge of the critical periods of development is an essential part of the philosophy of individualized, family-centered, developmental care (IFDC). To minimize iatrogenic environmental hazards of the extrauterine life, one must understand normal fetal development and the stage of development at which the premature infant is born.

## DEVELOPMENT WEEKS 1 TO 8: FERTILIZATION THROUGH THE EMBRYONIC STAGE

The first period of human development begins with fertilization and goes through the development of the zygote (weeks 0 to 2) to the embryonic stage (weeks 2 to 8). This period is characterized by fertilization and early cell division, implantation, the development of the placenta, and the beginning of organogenesis (Moore & Persaud, 2003).

### Stage 1: Fertilization Occurs (1 Day Postovulation)

Zygote size: 0.1 to 0.15 mm

Fertilization begins when one of approximately 3 million sperm penetrates an oocyte and ends with the creation of the zygote (Lott, 2003; Moore & Persaud, 2003). This process takes approximately 24 hours, and occurs in the fallopian tube. A sperm can survive for 48 hours, of which, 10 hours are spent transcending the female reproductive tract to get to the oocyte. The next step is the penetration of the zona pellucida, a tough membrane surrounding the oocyte. Only one sperm needs to bind with the protein receptors in the zona pellucida to trigger an enzyme reaction, allowing the zona to be pierced. Penetration of the zona pellucida takes approximately 20 minutes. Within 11 hours following fertilization, the oocyte has extruded a polar body with its excess chromosomes. The fusion of the oocyte and sperm nuclei marks the creation of the zygote and the end of fertilization.

### Stage 2: Cleavage; First Cell Division (1.5 to 3 Days Postovulation)

Zygote size: 0.1 to 0.2 mm

The zygote now begins to cleave, forming two cells called blastomeres. The zygote's first cell division begins a series of divisions, with each occurring approximately every 20 hours. Each blastomere within the zona pellucida becomes smaller and smaller with each subsequent division. When cell division has produced approximately 16 cells, the zygote becomes morula (the shape of a mulberry). It leaves the fallopian tube and enters the uterine cavity 3 to 4 days after fertilization.

### Stage 3: Early Blastocyst (4 Days Postovulation)

Zygote size: 0.1 to 0.2 mm

The morula enters the uterine cavity approximately 4 days after fertilization. Cell division continues, and a cavity known as a blastocele forms in the center of the morula (Lott, 2003; Moore & Persaud, 2003). Cells flatten and compact on the inside of the cavity while the zona pellicuda remains the same size. With the appearance of the cavity in the center, the organism is now called a blastocyst. The presence of the blastocyst indicates that two cell types are forming: the embryoblast and the trophoblast.

- Embryoblast: Inner cell mass inside of the blastocele
- Trophoblast: The cells on the outside of the blastocele

## Stage 4: Implantation Begins (5 to 6 Days Postovulation)

Zygote size: 0.1 to 0.2 mm

The blastocyst "hatches" from the zona pellicuda on approximately the sixth day after fertilization, as the blastocyst cells secrete an enzyme that erodes the epithelial uterine lining and creates an implantation site for the blastocyst (Lott, 2003; Moore & Persaud, 2003). The ovary is induced to continue producing progesterone; the human chorionic gonadotropin (hCG) is released by the trophoblast cells of the implanting blastocyst in a cyclic process. Endometrial glands in the uterus enlarge in response to the blastocyst, and the implantation site becomes swollen with newcapillaries. Implantation involves three distinct processes: (1) degeneration of the zona pellucida; (2) attachment of the blastocyst to the endometrial endothelium followed by a rapid proliferation of the trophoblast; and (3) erosion of the endometrial epithelium with burrowing of the blastocyst beneath the surface. More research is focusing on the reciprocity of actions between the zygote (a signal from the zygote) and the receptivity of the maternal uterine surface for successful implantation. Many perinatal experts refer to this period as an all or nothing time; meaning that if there is a significant embryologic problem, the implantation might never occur and, in some instances, a woman might have a heavier than usual menstrual flow and never know that a fertilization occurred. If the "error" in the zygotic or embryonic material is not great enough, implantation might occur, but a viable fetus or long-term pregnancy might not happen. More research is needed in this vital area of perinatal/neonatal care.

## Critical Points in Zygotic/Embryonic Development

Two points in this early period are of particular importance in the development of the embryo. The first critical point is that of fertilization itself, and the immediately following cell divisions. It is at this initial point in human development that many chromosomal abnormalities can occur. These might result from more than one sperm fertilizing an egg, resulting in dispermy, or a zygote with extra chromosomes or incomplete mitotic divisions in the early zygotic period. Triploid conceptions account for approximately 20% of chromosomally abnormal abortions. Implantation problems constitute another critical point. Failure of blastocysts to implant might result from a poorly developed endometrium. Early in pregnancy, the corpus luteum increases its hormone production in preparation for implantation of the blastocyst. Degeneration of the corpus luteum is prevented by human chorionic gonadotropin (hCG). Any alterations in hCG production or corpus luteum hormone production can interfere in endometrial development and, therefore, impede implantation.

## Stage 5: Implantation Complete; Placental Circulation System Begins (7 to 12 Days Postovulation)

Zygote size: 0.1 to 0.2 mm

## DEVELOPMENT OF THE PLACENTA

Early in the embryonic period at the point of implantation, the placenta begins to form (Lott, 2003; Moore & Persaud, 2003). The placenta is a temporary fetomaternal organ made of two components—a large fetal portion derived from the chorionic sac and a small maternal portion derived from the endometrium. The placenta forms the intrauterine environment in which the fetus grows and develops. The placenta, together with the umbilical cord, provides the means of transport and exchange of oxygen and nutrients from the mother to the embryo/fetus and carbon dioxide and waste from the embryo/fetus to the mother. The functions of the placenta include:

- Protection of the fetus
- Provision of nutrition
- Oxygen/carbon dioxide exchange

- Waste removal
- Hormone production

## Development of the Placenta and Fetal Membranes

The development of the placenta begins as implantation proceeds. The invasion of the endometrium begins on the seventh day after fertilization and is generally complete by the twelfth day. At this time, the trophoblast begins to differentiate into two layers: the inner cytotrophoblast and the outer syncytiotrophoblast. The cytotrophoblast is a mononucleated layer of cells that forms new trophoblast cells that migrate into the increasing mass of syncytiotrophoblast where they fuse and lose their cell membrane. The syncytiotrophoblast is a rapidly expanding, multinuclear mass, without distinct cell boundaries, that invades the endometrial tissue (capillaries, glands, and connective tissue). As this occurs, the blastocyst becomes imbedded in the endometrium. Proteolytic enzymes produced by the syncytiotrophoblast facilitate this process. The syncytiotrophoblast begins to produce hCG, which maintains the corpus luteum during early pregnancy and forms the basis for pregnancy tests. Eight days after conception, intercommunicating spaces, or lacunae, appear in the syncytiotrophoblast. The lacunae fill with fluid that contains maternal blood from ruptured endometrial capillaries and glandular secretions from eroded uterine glands. The nutrients in this fluid pass to the developing embryo by diffusion. The flow of maternal blood into the lacunar spaces from the maternal capillaries is the beginning of uteroplacental circulation. Both arterial and venous branches of maternal blood vessels communicate with the lacunae, and thereby oxygenated blood enters the lacunae from the spiral arteries and deoxygenated blood is removed from the lacunae from the endometrial veins.

During implantation, the endometrial tissue cells enlarge and accumulate glycogen and lipids. This cellular transformation is referred to as the "decidual reaction," and the altered endometrium is known as the decidua. Consensus is that this reaction protects the myometrium from uncontrolled invasion by the trophoblast. There are three regions of the decidua: (1) the decidua basalis is the part that forms the maternal component of the placenta; (2) the decidua capsularis is the superficial part of the decidua overlying the conceptus; and (3) the decidua parietalis is the remaining part of the decidua.

By the end of the second week following fertilization, there is the appearance of primary chorionic villi. Proliferation of the cytotrophoblast layer produces columns of cells or finger-like projections that grow into the syncytiotrophoblast. A mesenchymal core grows within these projections from which blood vessels will later develop.

As the blastocyst burrows into the endometrium, small spaces appear between the inner cell mass and the cytotrophoblast. This is the early amniotic cavity that gradually enlarges to completely surround the developing fetus. Amnioblasts (amnion forming cells) from the cytotrophoblast form a thin membrane, the amnion, which encloses the amniotic cavity. The epiblast (a type of cell from the embryonic disc) forms the floor of the amniotic cavity.

## Development of the Chorionic Sac

Cells from the yolk sac give rise to a layer of connective tissue, the extraembryonic mesoderm. As changes occur in the trophoblast and endometrium, spaces appear within the extraembryonic mesoderm. These spaces fuse and form a large cavity, the extraembryonic coelom. This cavity surrounds the amnion and yolk sac and splits the extraembryonic mesoderm into the extraembryonic somatic mesoderm, lining the trophoblast and covering the amnion, and the extraembryonic splanchic mesoderm, surrounding the yolk sac. The extraembryonic somatic mesoderm together with the cytotrophoblast and the syncytiotrophoblast, constitutes the chorion. The chorion forms the walls of the gestational sac, within which the connecting stalk suspends the developing embryo and its amniotic sac and yolk sac. Initially chorionic villi cover the entire chorionic sac. As the sac grows, the villi associated with the decidua capsularis are compressed and soon degenerate. This now smooth part of the chorion is called the chorion laeve. The chorionic villi associated with the decidua basalis branch out profusely and enlarge, forming the fetal portion of the placenta, called the chorion frondosum or villus chorion. The mature placenta is established by 4 to 10 weeks after conception but continues to grow in both size and thickness until approximately 20 weeks' gestation. The fully developed placenta covers 15% to 30% of the decidua and weighs approximately one sixth of the total fetus weight.

## Placental Structure

The fetal part of the placenta (chorion frondosum) is attached to the maternal part of placenta (decidua basalis) by anchoring villi (Lott, 2003; Moore & Persaud, 2003). As the chorionic villi invade the decidua basalis, several wedge-shaped areas of decidua are formed, called the placental septa. The placental septa divide the fetal part of the placenta into irregular areas called cotyledons. Each cotyledon consists of two or more main-stem villi and their many branches. The space surrounding the villi contains maternal blood and secretions and is called the intervillous space. Maternal blood enters the intervillous space from the spiral arteries in the decidua basalis and is drained by endometrial veins. The numerous villi are continuously bathed with maternal blood that circulates throughout the intervillous space. This is the site for nutrient transfer and gas exchange. The normal growth and development of the embryo and the fetus is more dependent on the adequate bathing of the villi than on any other factor. Several layers of tissue separate maternal and fetal circulations. These tissues are called the placental membrane. A molecule of oxygen in the maternal blood surrounding the villi must diffuse through four tissue layers in order to reach fetal blood: (1) the syncytiotrophoblast; (2) the cytotrophoblast; (3) the connective tissue of the villus; and (4) the epithelium of the fetal capillaries. This membrane has been called the placental barrier, but it is important to remember that most drugs and other substances in the maternal circulation pass easily through the placental membrane and enter the fetal circulation.

## Fetal-Placental Circulation

Deoxygenated blood leaves the fetus via two umbilical arteries and passes to the placenta. The umbilical arteries, at the site of cord attachment to the placenta, branch into a number of chorionic arteries. The chorionic arteries branch further, forming an extensive arteriovenous system within each villus, bringing fetal blood extremely close to maternal blood. This system provides a large surface area for the exchange of nutrients, gases, and waste products between the maternal and fetal circulation. There is normally no intermingling of maternal and fetal blood, although, occasionally, small quantities of fetal blood might enter maternal circulation through minute defects that might develop in the placental membrane. The veins from each villus converge back into the single umbilical vein at the site of attachment of the umbilical cord. The umbilical vein then carries oxygen-rich blood to the fetus.

Although villous growth continues until term, degenerative changes also begin to occur, such as intervillous thrombi, fibrin deposits, infarcts, and calcification. These degenerative changes can alter gas and nutrient transfer and might result in fetal hypoxia and fetal growth restriction.

## Placental Function

Placental metabolism, specifically, the synthesis of glycogen, cholesterol, and fatty acids, is important early in pregnancy, providing nutrition and energy for the developing embryo/fetus. The transport of substances across the placental membrane occurs as a result of: (1) simple diffusion—in which substances move from areas of higher concentration to lower concentration (e.g., oxygen, carbon dioxide, water, urea, most drugs, and drug metabolites); (2) facilitated diffusion—which requires a carrier to move a substance down a concentration gradient (e.g., glucose); (3) active transport—when substances are transported against a concentration gradient and requires energy expenditure (e.g., amino acids, water-soluble vitamins); and (4) pinocytosis—whereby extracellular fluid containing a particular substance is engulfed by the cells of the plasma membrane (e.g., phospholipids, lipoproteins, maternal antibodies, transferrin).

### Placental Hormones

The endocrine functions of the placenta are critical to maintaining a normal, healthy pregnancy. Utilizing precursors from both the mother and the fetus, the placenta can synthesize protein and steroid hormones. The placenta (syncytiotrophoblast) begins its hormone synthesis as a blasotcyst and continues this function until it is expelled from the uterus at birth. The four major hormones produced by the placenta are hCG; human placental lactogen (hPL), also called human chorionic somatomammotropin (hCS); progesterone; and estrogens.

The primary role of hCG is to maintain the corpus luteum during early pregnancy. Concentrations of hCG in maternal serum double every 1.4 to 2 days until peak values are reached by 2 to 3 months postconception. hCG is the hormone that is the basis for pregnancy testing. hPL promotes fetal growth by altering maternal protein, carbohydrate, and fat metabolism. This hormone is responsible for decreasing maternal insulin sensitivity and glucose usage, thereby increasing the amount of glucose that is available for transport to the fetus. Progesterone has many functions that are essential for the maintenance of pregnancy. It also serves as a substrate for fetal adrenal hormone synthesis. Adequate estrogen is also important for a normal pregnancy. During pregnancy, all three of the major estrogens—estrone, estradiol, and estriol—are markedly increased, although estriol increases the most, at approximately 1000-fold. Placental estrogen synthesis is unique in that it requires precursors from both the fetus and the mother. Approximately 90% of the precursors for estriol are derived from the fetus as well as 60% of the precursors for estrone and estradiol.

## Critical Period of Development

The development of the placenta is a critical point in the development of a pregnancy. Any impairment in the development of the transport system for substances passing between the mother and fetus can result in fetal growth restriction. An impairment in the endocrine function of the placenta (e.g., secretion of hCG, progesterone, estriol) can result in the loss of the pregnancy, because these hormones are necessary for the maintenance of a normal pregnancy. It should be noted that, at this early stage of the pregnancy, environmental factors, such as exposure to cigarette smoke, might result in decreased uterine blood flow, an abnormally small placenta, and resultant intrauterine growth restriction.

## Stage 6: Chorionic Villi Form; Gastrulation (13 Days Postovulation)

Embryonic size: 0.2 mm

This stage, with implantation complete and the placental development in progress, is the beginning of organogenesis. All major organ systems begin to develop at this point—long before many women realize they are pregnant. Chorionic villi "fingers" in the forming placenta now anchor the site to the uterus. The formation of blood and blood vessels of the embryo begin in this stage. The blood system appears first in the area of the "placenta" surrounding the embryo, while the yolk sac begins to produce hematopoietic or nonnucleated blood cells. By the end of the first part of this stage (6a), the embryo is attached by a connecting stalk; this will eventually become part of the umbilical cord to the developing placenta.

Stage 6b begins when a narrow line of cells appears on the surface of the embryonic disc. This primitive streak is the future axis of the embryo and marks the beginning of *gastrulation*, the process that produces the three layers of the embryo—the ectoderm, the mesoderm, and the endoderm.

## Stage 7: Neurulation and Notochordal Process (16 Days Postovulation)

Embryonic size: 1.4 mm

Gastrulation continues with the formation of the audoderm and mesoderm, which develop from the primitive streak, changing the two-layered disc into a three-layered disc (Moore & Persaud, 2003). The cells in the central part of the mesoderm release a chemical causing a dramatic change in the size of the cells in the top layer (ectoderm) of the flat disc-shaped embryo. The ectoderm grows rapidly over the next few days, forming a thickened area. The three layers will eventually give rise to:

1. Endoderm: Form the lining of the lungs, tongue, tonsils, urethra, and associated glands, bladder, and digestive tract.
2. Mesoderm: Form the muscles, bones, lymphatic tissue, spleen, blood cells, heart, lungs, and reproductive and excretory systems.
3. Ectoderm: Form the skin, nails, hair, lens of eye, lining of the internal and external ear, nose sinuses, mouth, anus, tooth enamel, pituitary gland, mammary system, and all parts of the nervous system.

## Stage 8: Primitive Pit, Notochordal Canal, and Neurenteric Canals Form (17 to 19 Days Postovulation)

Embryonic size: 1.0 to 1.5 mm

The embryonic area is not shaped like a pear, and the head region is broader than the tail end. The ectoderm has thickened to form the neural plate. The edges of this plate rise and form a concave area known as the neural groove. This groove is the precursor of the embryo's nervous system and is one of the first organs to develop. The blood cells of the embryo are already developed, and they begin to form channels along the epithelial cells, which form consecutively with the blood cells.

## Stage 9: Somites Appear (19 to 21 Days Postovulation)

Embryonic size: 1.5 to 2.5 mm

The top view of the embryo resembles the sole of a shoe with the head end wider than the tail end, and a slightly narrowed middle. Somites, which are condensations composed of mesoderm, appear on either side of the neural groove. The first pair of somites appear at the tail end and progress to the middle; at this time there are one to three pair of somites. Every ridge, bump, and recess now indicates cellular differentiation. A head fold rises on either side of the primitive streak. The primitive streak runs between one fourth to one third the length of the embryo.

Secondary blood vessels now appear in the chorion/placenta. Hematopoietic cells appear on the yolk sac simultaneously with endothelial cells that will form blood vessels for newly emerging blood cells. Endocardial (muscle) cells begin to fuse and form the two tubes that will become the embryo's heart.

## Stage 10: Neural Fold Begins to Fuse; Heart Tube Fuses (21 to 23 Days Postovulation)

Embryonic size: 1.5 to 3.0 mm

Tremendous growth and change occur as the embryo becomes longer and the yolk sac expands. At this time, on each side of the neural tube, between four and 12 pairs of somites can exist. The cells that become the eyes appear as thickened circles just off the neural folds. The cells of the ears are also present. Neural folds are rising and fusing at several points along the length of the neural tube concomitant with the budding somites, which appear to "zipper" the neural tube closed. Neural crest cells will eventually contribute to the skull and face of the embryo.

The two endocardial tubes fuse to form one single tube derived from the roof of the neural tube; it becomes S-shaped, and makes the primitive heart asymmetric. As the S-shape forms, the cardiac muscle begins to contract.

## Stage 11: Thirteen to Twenty Somite Pairs Have Formed; Rostral Neuropore Closes; Optic Vesicle, Two Pharyngeal Arches Appear (23 to 25 Days Postovulation)

Embryonic size: 2.5 to 3.0 mm

Thirteen to 20 pairs of somites are present and shaped in a modified S curve. The embryo has a bulblike tail and a connecting stalk to the developing placenta. A primitive S-shaped tubal heart is beating, resulting in the rhythmic flow of fluids being propelled throughout the body. However, this is not true circulation, because blood vessel development is still incomplete.

At this stage, the neural tube determines the form of the embryo. Although the primary blood vessels along the central nervous system (CNS) are connecting, the CNS appears to be the most developed system. When 20 somites are present in the embryo, the forebrain is completely closed.

## Stage 12: 21 to 29 Somite Pairs Are Present; Caudal Neuropore Closes; 3 to 4 Pharyngeal Arches Appear; Upper Limb Buds Appear (25 to 27 Days Postovulation)

Embryonic size: 3.0 to 5.0 mm

At this time the embryo has a distinctive C shape. The arches that form the face and neck are now becoming evident under the enlarging forebrain. By the time the neural tube is closed, both the eye and ear will have begun to form. At this stage, the brain and spinal cord together are the largest and most compact tissue of the embryo.

The blood system continues to develop. Blood cells follow the surface of the yolk sac, where they originate, move along the CNS, and move in the chorionic villi and the maternal blood system. Valves and the septa might appear. The digestive epithelium layer begins to differentiate into the future locations of the liver, lungs, stomach, and pancreas. The liver formation begins, with a few cells appearing before the remaining portions of the digestive system develop.

## Stage 13: Four Limb Buds, Lens Disc and Optic Vesicle, 30 to 40 Somite Pairs Can Be Found (Approximately 27 to 29 Days Postovulation)

Embryonic size: 4.0 to 6.0 mm

The brain differentiates into the three main parts: the forebrain, midbrain, and hindbrain. The forebrain consists of lobes that translate input from the senses, and will be responsible for memory formation, thinking, reasoning, and problem solving. The midbrain will serve as a relay station, coordinating messages to their final destination. The hindbrain will be responsible for regulating the heart, breathing, and muscle movements. The thyroid continues to develop, and the lymphatic system, which filters out bacteria, starts to form.

The optic placode invaginates and forms the optic vesicles, which will develop into the structures needed for hearing and maintenance of equilibrium. Retinal discs press outward and touch the surface ectoderm. In response, the ectoderm proliferates, forming the lens disc. Specific parts of the eye, such as the retina, the future pigment of the retina, and the optic stalk are identifiable. The primitive mouth with a tongue is recognizable.

Heart chambers are now filled with plasma and blood cells, making the heart seem distended and prominent. The heart and liver combined are equal in volume to the head at this stage. Blood circulation is well established, although true valves are not yet present. The villous network is in place to accommodate the exchange of blood between the woman and the embryo. Aortic arches 4 and 6 develop and 5 might appear. Lung buds continue to form.

The gall bladder, stomach, intestines, and pancreas continue to form, and the metamorphic bud appears in the chest cavity. The stomach is in the shape of a spindle, and the pancreas can be detected in the intestinal tube. The developing liver receives blood from the placenta via the umbilical cord. The amnion encloses the connecting stalk, helping to fuse it with the longer and more slender umbilical vesicle (the remnant of the yolk sac).

Upper limb buds are now visible as ridges, and the lower limb buds begin to develop. Folding is complete, and the embryo is now three-dimensional and is completely enclosed in the amniotic sac. The somites will be involved in building bones and muscles. The first, thin, surface layer of skin appears, covering the embryo.

## Stage 14: Lens Pit and Optic Cup Appear; Endolymphatic Appendages Are Distinct (4 to 8 Weeks Postfertilization)

Embryonic size: 5.0 to 7.0 mm

### Head and Neck

The brain and head grow rapidly during these periods. The mandibular and hyoid arches are noticeable and form the beginning of the neck and jawbones. Ridges appear that demarcate the three future sections of the brain. The spinal cord wall at this stage contains three zones: the ventricular, the mantle, and the marginal. The ventricular zone will form neurons, glial cells, and ependymal cells; intermediate mantle will form neuron clusters; and the marginal zone will contain processes of neurons. Adenohypophyseal pouch, which will develop into the anterior pituitary, is defined. The lens vesicles open to the surface and are nestled within the optic cup. Optic vesicle increases its size by approximately one fourth, and its endolymphatic appendage is more defined. Nasal plates can be detected by thickened ectoderm.

### Thorax

The esophagus now forms from a groove of tissue that separates from the trachea, which is also visible. Semilunar valves begin to form in the heart. Four major subdivisions of the heart (the trabeculated left and right ventricles, the conus cords, and the truncus arteriosus) are clearly defined during this time. Two sprouts, a ventral one from the aortic sac and a dorsal one from the aorta, form the pulmonary arch. Right and left lung sacs lie on either side of the esophagus.

## Abdominal and Pelvic Regions

Ureteric buds appear. Metanephroi, which will eventually form the permanent kidney, are now developing.

## Limbs: Upper

Upper limbs elongate into cylindrically shaped buds, tapering at the tip to eventually form the hand plate. Nerve distribution and innervation begins in the upper limbs.

## Stage 15: Lens Vesicles, Nasal Pit, and Hand Plate Develop; Trunk Widens; Future Cerebral Hemispheres Are Distinct (6 to 8 Weeks Postfertilization)

Embryonic size: 7.0 to 9.0 mm

## Head and Neck

The brain has increased in size by 33%; it is still larger than the trunk. Rostral neuropore is closed and four pairs of pharyngeal arches are now visible, although the fourth one is still quite small. The maxillary and mandibular prominences of the first arch are clearly delineated. The stomodeum, the depression in the ectoderm, which will develop into the mouth and oral cavity, appears between the prominent forebrain and the fused mandibular prominence. Swellings of the external ear begin to appear on both sides of the head, formed by the mandibular arch. The lens pit has closed, retinal pigment might appear in the external layer of the optic cup, and lens fibers form the lens body. Two symmetrical and separate nasal pits might appear as depressions in the nasal disc.

## Thorax

The esophagus continues to lengthen. Blood flow through the atrioventricular canal is divided into left and right streams, which continue through the outflow tract and aortic sac. The left ventricle is larger than the right and has a thicker wall. Lobar buds appear in the bronchial tree.

## Abdominal and Pelvic Regions

The intestine lengthens. Ureteric buds lengthen, and the tip expands, thus beginning the formation of the final and permanent set of kidneys.

## Limbs: Upper and Lower

Distinct regions of the hand plate, forearm, and arm can now be discerned in the upper limb bud. Lower limb bud begins to round at top, and the tip of its tapering end will eventually form the foot. Innervation, the distribution of nerves, begins in the lower limb buds.

## Spine

The relative width of the trunk increased from the growth of the spinal ganglia, the muscular plate, and the corresponding mesenchymal tissues.

## Stage 16: Growth Spurt (6 to 8 Weeks Postfertilization)

Embryonic size: 9.0 to 11.0 mm

## Head and Neck

The brain is well marked by its cerebral hemispheres. The hindbrain, which is responsible for heart regulation, breathing, and muscle movements, begins to develop. The future lower jaw, the first part of the face to be established, is now visible while the future upper jaw is present, but not demarcated. Mesenchymal cells originating in the primitive streak, the neural crest, and the prechordal plate, continue to form the skull and the face. External retina pigment is visible and the lens pit has grown into a D shape. Nasal pits are still two separate plates, but they rotate to face ventrally as the head widens.

## Thorax

Primary cardiac tubes separate into aortic and pulmonary channels, and the ventricular pouches deepen and enlarge, forming a common wall with their myocardial shells. Mammary gland tissue begins to mature.

## Abdominal and Pelvic Regions

The mesentery, which attached the intestines to the rear abdominal wall, holds them in position, and supplies them with blood, nerves, and lymphatics, is now clearly defined. Ureter, the tube that will convey urine from the kidney to the bladder, continues to lengthen. Proliferation of the coelomic epithelium indicates the gonadal primordium.

## Limbs: Upper and Lower

Hand regions of upper limb bud differentiate further to form a central carpal part and a digital plate. The thigh, leg, and foot areas can be distinguished in the lower limb buds.

## Stage 17: A Four-Chamber Heart and a Sense of Smell (Approximately 41 Days Postovulation)

Embryonic size: 10 to 13 mm

## Head and Neck

Jaw and facial muscles are now developing. The nasofrontal groove becomes distinct and an olfactory bulb forms in the brain. Auricular hillocks become recognizable. The dental laminae or teeth buds begin to form. The pituitary, which is the master gland responsible for growth of hormones that regulate other glands, such as the thyroid, adrenal, and gonads, begins to form. The trachea, the larynx, and the bronchi begin to form.

## Thorax

The heart begins to separate into four chambers. The diaphragm, the tissue that separates the chest cavity from the abdomen, forms.

## Abdominal and Pelvic Regions

Intestines begin to develop within the umbilical cord and will later migrate into the abdomen when the embryo's body is large enough to accommodate them. In the area of the future pelvis, primitive germ cells arrive at the genital area and will respond to genetic instructions, to develop into either female or male genitalia.

## Limbs: Upper and Lower

Digital rays begin to appear in the footplates, and finger rays are more distinct.

## Spine

The trunk becomes straighter.

## Stage 18: Ossification of Skeleton Begins (42 to 46 Days Postovulation)

Embryonic size: 11 to 14 mm

## Head and Neck

Nerve plexuses begin to develop in the region of the scalp. Eyes are pigmented, and eyelids begin to develop and might fold.

## Thorax

Within the heart, the trunk of the pulmonary artery separates from the trunk of the aorta. Nipples appear on the chest. Body appears more like a cube.

## Abdominal and Pelvic Regions

Kidneys begin to produce urine for the first time. The genital tubercle, urogenital membrane, and anal membrane appear.

## Limbs: Upper and Lower

The critical period of arm development ends, and the arms are at their proper location, roughly proportional to the embryo. However, the handplates are not finished, but develop further in the next 2 days. The wrists are clearly visible, and the hands have ridges or notches indicating the future separation of the fingers and the thumbs.

## Spine and Skeleton

Ossification of the skeleton begins.

## Stage 19: Brain Waves and Muscles (Approximately 47 to 48 Days Postovulation)

Embryonic size: 13 to 18 mm

## Head and Neck

The brain has the first detectable brain waves. The head is more erect, and semicircular canals start to form in the inner ear, which will enable a sense of balance and body position.

## Thorax

Septum primum fuses with the septum intermedium in the heart.

## Abdominal and Pelvic Regions

The gonads form. In approximately 1 week, the gender of the embryo will be recognizable in the form of testes or ovaries.

### Limbs: Upper and Lower

Knee and ankle locations are indicated by indentations. Legs are now at their proper location, proportional to the embryo. The critical period for the lower limbs is about to end. Toes are almost completely notched, and toenails begin to appear. Joints grow more distinct.

### Spine, Skeleton, and Muscles

The trunk elongates and straightens, and the bone cartilage begins to form a more solid structure. Muscles develop and get stronger.

## Stage 20: Spontaneous Involuntary Movement (49 to 51 Days Postovulation)

Embryonic size: 19 to 20 mm

### Head and Neck

The brain is now connected to tiny muscles and nerves, enabling the embryo to make spontaneous movements. The scalp plexus is now present. Nasal openings and the tip of the nose are fully formed.

### Limbs: Upper and Lower

The upper limbs become longer and continue to bend at the elbows and extend forward. Skin on the footplate folds down between the future toes, each distinguishable from the other.

## Stage 21: Intestines Begin to Recede into Body Cavity (Approximately 52 Days Postovulation)

Embryonic size: 17 to 21 mm

### Head and Neck

Eyes are well developed, but are still located on the side of the embryonic head. As head development continues, they will migrate forward. External ears are set low on the embryo's head, but will move up as the head enlarges. During the next few days, tongue development is completed.

### Abdominal and Pelvic Regions

Intestines begin migration within the umbilical cord toward the embryo. Liver causes a ventral prominence of the abdomen.

### Limbs: Upper and Lower

Fingers lengthen while distinct grooves form between the fingers, which also lengthen as the hands approach each other across the abdomen. Feet approach each other, but are still fan-shaped, and the toe digits are still webbed.

## Stage 22: Heart Development Ends (53 to 55 Days Postovulation)

Embryonic size: 19 to 24 mm

### Head and Neck

The head is beginning to develop fissures that make it more characteristic of what we recognize as "humanness." Eyelids and external ears are more developed, and the upper lip is fully formed.

### Thorax

The critical period of heart development is completed. The major structures are in place, and the conducting system of the heart has developed.

### Abdominal and Pelvic Regions

In female embryos, the clitoris is beginning to form. The penis will develop from the same tissue.

### Limbs: Upper and Lower

Primary ossification centers appear in the long bones, directing the replacement of cartilage by bone. This process usually begins in the upper limbs. Fingers overlap those of the opposite hand, and the digits of the fingers fully separate. Feet lengthen and become more defined.

### Abdominal and Pelvic Regions

Anal membrane is perforated. Urogenital membranes differentiate in the male and female embryos. Testes or ovaries are distinguishable.

## Stage 23: Essential External and Internal Structures Complete (Approximately 56 to 57 Days Postovulation)

Embryonic size: 23 to 26 mm

### Head and Neck

Head is erect and rounded. External ear is completely developed. The eyes are closed, but the retina of the eye is fully pigmented. The eyelids begin to unite and are only half closed. Taste buds begin to form on the surface of the tongue. The primary teeth are at cap stage. Bones of the palate begin to fuse. Scalp plexus reaches head vertex.

### Abdominal and Pelvic Regions

Intestines begin to migrate from the umbilical cord into the body cavity. The external genitals are still difficult to recognize.

### Limbs: Upper and Lower

Upper and lower limbs are well formed. Fingers get longer, and toes are no longer webbed; all digits are separated and distinct.

### Spine, Skeleton, Muscles, and Skin

A layer of rather flattened cells, the precursor of the surface layer of the skin, replaces the thin ectoderm of the embryo. The tail has disappeared.

*Critical Periods of Development.* At this point, at the end of the eighth week of gestation, the embryonic phase of development is complete as is the period of rapid organogenesis. Although each organ system will continue to develop and mature, the basic structures of each system are in place. It is during this early period that the developing embryo is most vulnerable to the effects of exposure to external substances, such as cigarette smoke, alcohol, and teratogenic drugs that will adversely affect the course of development.

## DEVELOPMENT: WEEKS 9 TO 40: FETAL DEVELOPMENT

Fetal development begins in week 9 and continues through the end of the pregnancy. During this period, organogenesis is complete, the fetus undergoes a period of rapid growth, and critical developmental milestones are reached that allow for the survival of the infant in the extrauterine environment. In this section, we review the sequencing of fetal development and discuss the critical periods in the development of the neurosensory and respiratory systems that impact preterm infant survival.

## Weeks 9 to 11

### Head and Neck

The basic brain structure of the fetus is complete, and brain mass increases rapidly through this period. Sockets for all 20 teeth are formed in gums. The face now has human appearance. Separate folds of the mouth fuse to form the palate, and early facial hair follicles begin to develop.

### Thorax

Vocal cords form in the larynx, and the fetus can make sounds.

### Abdominal and Pelvic Regions

The intestines have migrated into the abdomen from the umbilical cord. Digestive tract muscles are functional and practice contracting. Nutrient-extracting villi line the now folded intestines. The liver and gall bladder are formed, and the liver starts to secrete bile that is stored in the gall bladder. Development of the thyroid, pancreas, and gall bladder is complete, and the pancreas starts to produce insulin. Genitalia continue to develop more differentiated female characteristics (labium minus, argental groove, and labium majoris) and male characteristics (glans penis, urethral groove, scrotum). Neither male nor female genitalia are fully formed.

### Limbs: Upper and Lower

Fingernails begin to grow from nail beds.

### Skin and Muscles

Fetus develops primitive reflexes, and the skin is very sensitive.

## Weeks 12 to 15

The fetus is more flexible, with the ability to move the head, mouth, lips, arms, wrists, hands, legs, feet, and toes, although the mother is likely not able to feel these movements yet.

The somatesthetic system is the first in the fetal sensory developmental system to become functional during this period (Figure 6-1). This includes the sense of touch, pressure, and, probably, pain. Its focus is on the sensory nerve ending of the palms of hands, soles of feet, and perioral and perinasal areas of the face.

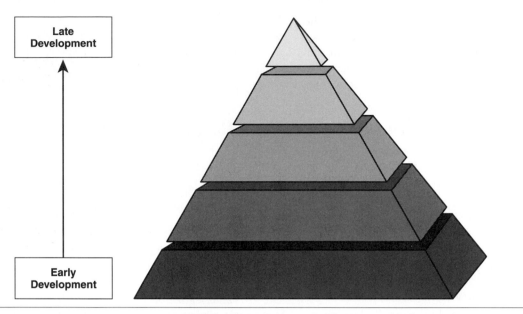

Figure **6-1** Progression of fetal sensory development by system. Top to bottom: Visual, auditory, chemosensory, vestibular, and somatesthetic.

### Head and Neck

The head is approximately 50% of the crown-to-rump length and rests on the well-defined neck instead of shoulders. The developing sucking muscles of the mouth fill out cheeks, tooth buds continue to develop, and salivary glands begin to function. Scalp hair pattern is discernible.

Head and neck are straighter and almost erect as muscles strengthen and additional bone texture forms in the back. Eyes are now oriented in a forward manner, and the ears are close to their final position.

### Thorax

The heartbeat can be detected with external instruments. Lungs develop further as the fetus inhales and exhales amniotic fluid, which is essential for air sacs within the lungs to function properly. The fetal heart pumps approximately 25 quarts of blood per day and increases to 300 quarts per day by the time of delivery.

### Abdominal and Pelvic Regions

Fully functional spleen will assume functions supervised by liver such as removal of old red blood cells and production of antibodies. The fetus' gender can be detected on ultrasound as genitalia become clearly visible.

### Limbs: Upper and Lower

Arms have almost reached final proportion and length, although legs are still quite short relative to the fetus' body. Hands, particularly the thumbs, become functional. Toenails begin to grow from the nail beds.

### Skin, Muscles, and Glands

Muscles function more smoothly. The fetus is more flexible and has advanced movements of head, mouth and lips, arms, wrists, hands, legs, foot, and toes. Fetal positioning, even at this early time, begins to influence later musculoskeletal development. Muscles and nervous system continue to advance. The sweat glands appear, and body hair begins to grow.

### Placenta

By approximately the fourth month (10 to 12 weeks after fertilization), the placenta has achieved its full thickness, with no further development of new cotyledons. Circumferential placental growth continues, with further branching of the villi and growth of the placental capillaries. As a result, the surface area for placental exchange continues to expand until late in gestation, increasing its functional efficiency.

## Weeks 16 to 20

No new structures form after this point, but each system continues to develop in complexity, and the fetus enters into a period of rapid growth.

### Behavior

During this period, the vestibular system is becoming functional. The fetus can now experience changes in position and orientation. The fetus now has phases of sleep and waking and might prefer a favorite sleep position. Also at this point, ultrasound can show the fetus beginning to suck on a thumb or toe. When a family views these pictures, the fetus becomes more "real" to them. Incorporation of the fetus into family life is greatly aided with today's technology.

### Head and Neck

Eyes are in their final position, facing forward, and primitive reflexes, such as blinking, develop. Ears move to their final position and stand out from head. Eyebrows begin to form.

### Abdominal and Pelvic Regions

Meconium begins to form and accumulate in the bowels. Meconium is the product of cell loss, digestive secretion, and swallowed amniotic fluid. Ovaries of female fetuses contain primitive egg cells, all of the eggs a woman will have for her entire life. The uterus of the female fetus is fully formed.

### Limbs: Upper and Lower

Fingertips and toes develop the unique swirls and creases of fingerprints and toe prints.

### Nervous System

The nerve pathways continue to mature and are undergoing myelinization.

### Blood

Fetal circulation is completely functional. The umbilical cord system continues to grow and thicken as blood travels with considerable force through the body to nurture the fetus.

### Skin

Brown fat (colored by capillary growth) coats the neck, chest, and crotch areas around the lymphatic system. The vernix (consisting of dead skin, lanugo cells, and oil from glands) is now clearly formed and visible covering the skin.

### Placenta

Placenta is fully formed and grows in diameter, but not in thickness. The fetus' viability is now dependent on the production of progesterone via the placenta as the corpus luteum is no longer functional. Progestrone is responsible for continued enrichment of the uterine lining and rich vascular support of the pregnancy.

## Weeks 20 to 24

In this period, the infant begins to approach the age of extrauterine viability. The cardiovascular system is functional, and, by 24 weeks, the respiratory system is sufficiently developed to be able to support rudimentary gas exchange. The next sections focus on describing those characteristics of the normally developing fetus that will impact the functioning and care of the preterm infant.

### Behavior

The next fetal sensory system to become functional is the chemosensory system (the senses of smell and taste). This sensory system is not well defined until 24 weeks' gestation. However, the fetus is practicing sucking, swallowing, and breathing, and there are indications from research that the smell and taste of amniotic fluid is similar to that of the mother's breast milk to help with orientation to suckling and breastfeeding. Maternal diet and flavors appear to be part of the amniotic fluid and recognizable after birth (Mennella, Jagnow, & Beauchamp, 2001).

### Head and Neck

At this point, the extremely rapid brain growth begins, which lasts until 5 years after birth. Eyebrows and scalp hair become more visible, and the fetus blinks more often. Lanugo covers the body completely, although it is concentrated around the head, neck, and face. The bones of the ear—hammer, anvil, and stirrup—harden at this point, making sound conduction possible. At this time, the fetus might be aware of maternal sounds such as breathing, heartbeat, digestion, and, possibly, voice. During this period, the fetus also begins to respond to sound originating outside the uterus, resulting in changes in physiologic perimeters. The fetus is also capable of reacting to light. Permanent teeth buds appear high in gums. The nostrils begin to open.

### Respiratory System

The maturation of the lungs has evolved to the canalicular stage. In this stage, the lung tissue is becoming highly vascularized, and the bronchioles are dividing into two or more respiratory bronchioles that will then further divide into three to six alveolar ducts. By 24 weeks conceptional age, extrauterine respiration becomes possible, because some of the primitive alveoli have developed in areas that are sufficiently vascularized to allow an exchange of gas. Surfactant production begins at approximately 20 weeks conceptional age, but in very small amounts. Surfactant production will not reach adequate levels until approximately 28 weeks conceptional age.

### Abdominal and Pelvic Regions

Testes of male fetuses begin descending from the pelvis into the scrotum.

### Limbs: Upper and Lower

Legs approach final length and proportion relative to body. Arms and legs move with more force, as muscles strengthen. The skeleton hardens. Hand strength improves.

Skin—Blood vessels, bones, and organs are visible underneath a thin layer of wrinkled, translucent, pink skin. The fetus is thin with little subcutaneous fat.

## Weeks 24 to 28

### Head and Neck

The forebrain enlarges to cover all other developed brain structures, while still maintaining its hemisphere divisions. Eyes are partially open, and eyelashes are present. Sucking and swallowing improves. Brain wave patterns resemble those of a full-term baby at birth.

### Respiratory System

Lung development now enters the terminal sac period (24 weeks to birth). This stage is characterized by the proliferation of terminal sacs that are the site of gas exchange in the lungs. As the terminal sacs develop, the epithelium becomes thin, and capillaries begin to bulge into the sac to form the intersection for gas exchange. At 24 weeks conceptional age, the sacs are lined primarily with type I alveolar cells also known as squamous epithelial cells. By 28 weeks, the type II alveolar cells will largely replace type I cell. It is the type II cells that secrete pulmonary surfactant. It should be noted that the rate of maturation of the type II cells and the level of surfactant production varies widely among individuals. Full surfactant production is usually present by 38 to 40 weeks conceptional age.

### Nervous System

The brain continues a period of rapid development. As the brain develops, it increases in complexity and in the degree of convolutions. If born, the infant is at the mercy of the environment and unable to habituate or adapt responses to stimuli. The infant cannot shut out noises and is easily overstimulated; stressors are exacerbated by the infants poor muscle tone and control of responses. Interventions during this time should be directed at protecting the infant from the environmental stimulation and might include nesting, positioning with flexion, nonnutritive sucking, and Kangaroo care; however, each intervention must be individually evaluated. Paternal holding is suggested; even when the benefits to the infant are limited, careful consideration of both risks and benefits is recommended.

### Skin and Muscles

During this period of rapid weight gain, the fetus reaches 2% to 3% body fat. Production of red blood cells is entirely taken over by the bone marrow. Physiologic flexion is beginning to develop as the infant continues to grow into the limited space of the womb.

### Abdominal and Pelvic Regions

Testes of male fetuses are completely descended.

## Weeks 28 to 32

It is during this period of development that the auditory system matures, resulting from the maturation of hair cells and their connection through the appropriate ganglion to the auditory cortex. Prior to this period, the response to auditory stimulation is at the brain stem level, affecting physiologic parameters. Subsequent recall or recognition of auditory stimulation can be perceived, and apparently a memory pattern can be established at the cortical level at 32 weeks' gestation. Eyes open during alert times and close during sleep. The fetal brain creates endogenous visual stimuli to the visual cortex during rapid eye movement (REM) sleep; this visual development during REM sleep is essential for normal development of the cortex. The visual sensory system is the last of the primary sensory systems to mature. Also during this period, the fetus begins to develop its own immune system. If born, the infant can be alert for short periods of time; however, periods of deep sleep, when most growth hormone is secreted, might be limited by the environmental stimulation. The infant can suck on a pacifier and can be put to breast for sucking experiences; nutritive sucking abilities are very immature and not recommended. Interventions such as nesting, positioning with flexion, nonnutritive sucking, Kangaroo care, and/or cycled lighting might be beneficial during this time.

### Head and Neck

Rapid brain growth continues, and head size pushes the skull outward creating more surface convolutions. This quick growth increases the number of interconnections between individual nerve cells. The iris is colored, and the pupil reflexes respond to light.

### Limbs: Upper and Lower

Toenails are fully formed. Because of the lack of space in the uterus, the legs are drawn up in what is known as the fetal position.

## Weeks 32 to 36

The placenta is now one sixth of fetal weight. The surface area for placental exchange has continued to expand through the late gestational period, increasing its functional efficiency and continuing

to provide adequate support for the growing fetus. This rate of growth decreases after 34 to 36 weeks; however, cellular hypertrophy continues until term. At term, the average placenta weighs between 500 and 600 g, is 15 to 20 cm in diameter, and is 2 to 3 cm thick. Although villous growth continues until term, degenerative changes, such as intervillous thrombi, fibrin deposits, infarcts, and calcification, begin to occur in the last few weeks of the pregnancy. These degenerative changes might alter gas and nutrient transfer and might result in fetal hypoxia and fetal growth restriction.

### Gastrointestinal System

Gastrointestinal system is very immature and will stay that way until 3 or 4 years after birth. The fetus stores approximately 15% of its weight in fat to keep the body warm. The fetus receives and eliminates nutrition through the umbilical cord. If born, the ability to coordinate nutritive sucking (sucking, swallowing, and breathing) matures between 34 to 36 weeks postconception; the breast or bottle can be offered after this point.

### Respiratory System

The respiratory system continues to develop, increasing the numbers of terminal sacs, continuing to increase vascularization of the area and increasing the percentage of type II alveolar cells and, thus, increasing surfactant production.

### Abdominal and Pelvic Regions

Increased fat stores improve the ability of the fetus to maintain temperature stability.

### Limbs

Upper and lower space limitations continue to restrict fetal movement. Limbs are bent and drawn close to body.

## Weeks 36 to Term

The final weeks of gestational development are devoted to continued, overall growth and maturation of the fetus. The laying down of adipose tissue assists in eventual thermoregulation and insulation of the body. Beyond 36 weeks' gestation, the fetus, if born, is considered term even though a human pregnancy is noted to last 40 weeks. The lung development at 36 weeks and beyond will support life with minimal problems. From a developmental standpoint, a fetus who reaches this point and is born without major illness or congenital anomalies, will generally survive and prosper. The infant's positive development in the extrauterine life is dependent on an appreciation of what has gone before.

## CONCLUSION

In this chapter, we briefly reviewed the critical periods of normal and (to some extent) abnormal embryonic and fetal development. An understanding of in utero development is crucial to the provision of neonatal care that supports positive extrauterine growth and development. Developmental care incorporates the principles of development during both fetal and postnatal life.

## *REFERENCES*

Lott, J.W. (2003). Fetal development: Environmental influences and critical periods (pp. 151-172). In C. Kenner & J.W. Lott (Eds.), *Comprehensive neonatal nursing: A physiologic perspective* (3rd ed.). St. Louis: W.B Saunders.

Mennella, J.A., Jagnow, C.P., & Beauchamp, G.K. (2001). Prenatal and postnatal flavor learning by human infants. *Pediatrics, 107*(6), E88.

Moore, K.L., & Persaud, T.V.N., (2003). *The developing human. Clinically oriented embryology* (7th ed.). St. Louis: Mosby.

# 7 *Neurologic Development*

## Jacqueline M. McGrath

The neurologic system is one of the earliest systems to develop in the embryo; however, it is important to remember that it is not fully matured until adulthood. Early experiences (fetal, neonatal, infancy) will shape later neurobehavioral development (Herschkowitz, 2000). The newborn infant, and, even more so, the preterm infant is employing an immature and fragile system for managing stimuli from both internal and external sources. For example, the neurologic system of the newborn infant is characterized by slow conduction velocity along the nerve fibers and slow synapses potentials with a fair amount of transmission uncertainty (Blackburn, 2003; Volpe, 2001). Nevertheless, an infant's neurologic system is bombarded with the expectation to perform almost from the very moment it begins to develop and even more so on entrance to the extrauterine environment. Responding to stimuli in an organized manner is difficult for the newborn infant. Especially because the amount and type of stimuli in the environment outside the womb can be overwhelming and disorienting even for the mature neurologic system of the adult (Volpe, 2001). For the preterm infant whose system is even more immature and who is often expected to survive in the noxious environment of the newborn intensive care unit (NICU), this overstimulation is more of a problem. Understanding how we can better support the development and maturation of the neurologic system is the basis for individualized, family-centered, developmental care (IFDC) and can be the beginning of helping the newborn infant better manage his world. In this chapter, we examine the early development of the neurologic system, explore the physiologic needs of this system, and describe the functional capacity expected at birth.

## NEUROLOGIC DEVELOPMENT

Neurologic development begins in the third week of gestation with the formation of the neural plate, neural folds, and neural tube during dorsal induction. This first stage of neural development is called primary neurulation. Once the neural tube is formed and becomes a closed system, the different regions of the brain begin to develop. From this point forward, the central nervous system (CNS) development is characterized by five distinct, overlapping processes: neuronal proliferation, migration, formation of synapses, organization, and myelination (Blackburn, 2003). The first areas to develop in the fetal brain are the forebrain, thalamus, hypothalamus, cerebral hemispheres, and basal ganglia (Volpe, 2001). These processes all begin before birth; but are not completely developed until well after birth and even into adulthood.

## Proliferation

Neuronal proliferation begins in the ventricular and subventricular zones at approximately 8 weeks' gestation and peaks between 12 to 18 weeks' gestation. At the peak of production, almost 250,000 neurons are produced every minute (Volpe, 2001). During this time, radial glial cells are also generated that have the distinct purpose of laying down the path for neural cell migration. Within the circuitry of the brain, there are more than 100 trillion glial cells that protect and nourish the neurons. The glial cells also will later facilitate columnar organization of the neurons. Proliferation of neurons continues into infancy. At birth, there are approximately 100 billion developing neurons in the infant brain. This number is twice the number of neurons in an adult brain. The cerebrum and cerebellum are the last areas of the brain for neuronal proliferation to occur. That is why these areas of the brain are extremely susceptible to insult at birth (Blackburn, 2003).

## Migration

Neuronal migration begins to occur shortly after proliferation begins and peaks between 12 and 24 weeks' gestation (Volpe, 2001). Each neuron is genetically programmed to follow a particular radial glial path outward into the cerebral cortex, with the deepest layers forming first, and more superficial layers forming later in development ("inside out" pattern). By 28 weeks' gestation, most neurons have migrated to their distinct permanent place in the cortex. Once the neurons reach the cortex, further differentiation occurs. Although a neuron is programmed to follow a particular path and migrate to a distinct location, interaction between the infant and the environment is believed to shape and "fine-tune" the neuronal connections underlying the brain's functioning (Volpe, 2001; Weisel, 1994). The environment of the fetus and/or young infant provides the ecologic and social setting that decisively supports and cultivates development in much the same way that genetic programming provides the foundation for development.

## Synapses Formation

Synapses formation begins at approximately 8 weeks' gestation and continues in a progression as neurons proliferate, differentiate, and migrate to their appropriate location. As development progresses, both dendrites and axons proliferate with increasing branching, and, thus, the number of possible synapses increases. This organization of connections and transmitters is a prerequisite for interaction to occur within the CNS.

## Organization

Neuronal organization begins with the establishment of layers of neurons in the cortex at approximately 24 to 28 weeks' gestation; however, organization will continue well into childhood. It is during this time that many of the primitive reflexes begin. Swallowing is one of the exceptions that begins as early as 12 weeks' gestation (Gardner & Goldson, 2002). See Table 7-1 for neonatal reflex behaviors.

There are six phases of human brain organization:
- Generation and differentiation of the subplate neurons
- Alignment, orientation, and layering of cortical neurons
- Elaboration of dendrites and axons
- Further establishment of synaptic connections
- Neuronal pruning with cell death and selective elimination of synaptic connections

- Increased proliferation and differentiation of glia cells

During neuronal organization, rhythmic impulse conduction confirms functional operation of the synapses. Experiences of the fetus shape and restructure the synapses as they are developing (Volpe, 2001). There is increasing evidence to support the premise that richer experiences during brain development produce richer brains; however, it is also well known that the natural niche of the human womb appears to be already rich enough to support normal development (Eisenberg, 1999). Those connections between neurons that are used, grow stronger; those that are unused grow weaker, and eventually die. Thus, neuronal activity and experiences determine survivors. This pruning of the neuronal branching occurs well into adulthood and determines the unique patterns of neural structures that enable us to perceive and interact with the environment (Volpe, 2001).

During this pruning process, almost 50% of the neurons in the developing brain die, and the experiences of the fetus have as much influence in this selection process as the original genetic programming of the neurons (Volpe, 2001). This refinement of the neuronal connections allows omission of errors in development and elimination of neurons that have poor connections, or are dislocated (Blackburn, 2003; Volpe, 2001). The plasticity (ability to be shaped) of the developing CNS diminishes as this stage of neurodevelopment concludes in early infancy (Volpe, 2001).

For the fetus, the environment of the uterus supports the input needed for the "normal" early development of these neuronal connections in the brain (Eisenberg, 1995). This environment fosters stimuli that are rich, diverse, and rhythmical (Blackburn, 2003). When the infant is born preterm, however, and enters the highly technical environment of the NICU, that "normal" niche for supporting brain development and organization is altered, and the processes of the brain are modified in an attempt to organize behavior and manage this different environment (Glass, 1999). Therefore, preterm brain development has a different beginning that fosters a different end point. It is not known whether this end point is better or worse for each individual infant. What *is* known is that this end point is different for each infant (Eisenberg, 1995; Glass, 1999).

Table 7-1   NEONATAL REFLEX BEHAVIORS

| Behavior | Begins (in Utero) (Week) | Integrates |
|---|---|---|
| **PROTECTION** | | |
| Morro | 28 | At 6 to 8 months to allow sitting and protective extension of the hands |
| Palmar grasp | 28 | At 5 to 6 months to allow voluntary grasping of objects |
| Plantar grasp | 28 | At 7 to 8 months with foot rubbing on objects; complete at 8 to 9 months for standing and walking |
| Babinski | 28 | (Same as plantar grasp) |
| Tonic neck | 35 | At about 4 months, rolling over and reaching or grasping should occur |
| **GAG*** | 36 | Protects against aspiration—does *not* disappear |
| **BLINK** | 35 | Does *not* disappear |
| **CROSSED EXTENSION** | 38 | Disappears at about 2 months of age |
| **SURVIVAL** | | |
| Rooting* | 28 | At 3 months; decreased response if baby is sleepy or sated |
| Sucking* | 26 to 28 | Not yet synchronized with swallowing |
| Swallowing* | 12 | 32 to 34 weeks—stronger synchronization, with sucking; perfect by 34 to 37 weeks |

From Gardner, S.L., & Goldson, E. (2002). The neonate and the environment: Impact on development. In G.B. Merenstein & S.L. Gardner (eds). *Handbook of neonatal intensive care* (5th ed.; pp. 223). St. Louis: Mosby.

*Although isolated components of feeding behaviors are present before 28 weeks' gestation, they are not effectively coordinated for oral feedings before 32 to 34 weeks gestation (Goldson, 1987; Hack & Fanaroff, 1999; Medoff-Cooper, 1991). Coordination of respiration with sucking and swallowing during bottle feeding is consistently achieved by infants older than 37 weeks' postconception (Arvedson, 1996; Bullough & Rea, 1996).

Glial cell proliferation also occurs during neuronal organization. After migration, glial cell proliferation might occur locally or in the ventricular zones of the brain (Volpe, 2001). These cells are protective and nutritionally supportive to the neural circuitry of the CNS. They have been found to be essential for normal development of neurons in the upper layers of the cortex (Volpe, 2001). Glial cells continue to proliferate in number well into infancy as the energy needs of the developing brain are increasing—then their numbers start to recede.

## Myelination

Myelination is the final developmental stage in the CNS. It begins at about 24 weeks' gestation and continues into adulthood. However, peak development for myelination is from birth to 8 months postbirth (Volpe, 2001). Myelin is a lipoprotein covering that speeds conduction of impulses along nerve fibers. Myelination occurs at different times in different regions of the CNS. In the peripheral nervous system, motor fibers are myelinated first, whereas in the CNS, sensory fibers are myelinated first. Myelination in the CNS and peripheral nervous system corresponds to functional development of these systems. Incomplete myelination does not preclude conduction along the nerve fibers, but it does slow the speed of the impulses (Blackburn, 2003). Inconsistencies in myelination in different areas of the nervous system are the grounds for discrepancies in the integration of sensory and motor activities in the fetus and young infant. Blackburn (2003) summarizes these major stages of human brain development and related defects to give us some clinical examples of alterations in the neurologic system (Table 7-2).

## NEUROLOGIC PHYSIOLOGY

Neurologic physiology consists of two levels, the cellular and functional levels.

### Cellular Level

During early development and well into infancy, the brain requires a generous supply of oxygen and glucose to develop and function optimally. The neonatal brain is highly glucose dependent and is directly affected by hypoglycemia (Volpe, 2001). In the newborn and preterm infant, glycogen stores are, however, minimal or absent. Therefore, both nutrients must be delivered to the brain via the blood supply to the cerebral cavity. If for some reason the perfusion to the brain is compromised, these two components needed to create the energy for neuronal transmission will be unavailable, and the already rudimentary system for responding to stimuli will be even further jeopardized.

The body increases cerebral blood flow to protect the developing brain from gross changes in blood flow in other parts of the body. For example, as pH, oxygen, and glucose decrease in the blood, cerebral blood flow increases to continue to provide adequate supplies of oxygen and nutrients to the brain. However, the degree and duration of hypoglycemia

can have significant long-term and deleterious effects on the brain, and actions must be taken to prevent such insults (Volpe, 2001). Additionally, because of the immature autoregulation of the cerebral blood flow in the preterm infant, hypoxemia and hypercapnia can lead to ischemia and damaged blood vessels, leaving the infant vulnerable to hemorrhagic events with later neurodevelopment effects (Mulvihill, Cahill, & Eicher, 2003; Okumura, Toyota, Hayakawa, et al., 2002; Papile, 1997).

### Functional Level

There are four areas of nervous system function: autonomic, sensory, motor, and state regulation. These areas all begin to develop before birth, but maturation is not attained until well after birth. The basics of fetal neural development can, however, be used to anticipate and support the many developing capabilities of the preterm and term infant (Blackburn, 2003). Much of what is known about the functional development of the neurologic system of the fetus has been learned by studying the development of the preterm infant.

Autonomic function is almost mature at birth and is responsible for the full-term infant's abilities to smoothly transition from intrauterine to extrauterine life. However, the differences in these two environments present major challenges for the infant's neurologic system, including self-regulation of breathing, heart rate, temperature, and nutritional intake (which includes more precise coordination of suck, swallow, and breathing). The infant must adapt and respond to the many changes simultaneously to survive in this new environment (Blackburn, 2003; Volpe, 2001). The infant who is adapting well is noted to have more regular respirations, pink color, and warm skin.

The sensory system begins development before birth, but maturation of each subsystem continues after birth. Generally, the sensory systems develop in utero in a specific order that should remain unaltered. Touch develops first, then smell and vestibular, followed by taste, hearing, and vision. Therefore, myelination of the sensory systems follows this same order. It is important to note that these systems all develop normally in the dark, cushiony, attenuated environment of the womb, and, more

Table **7-2**  Major Stages of Human Brain Development and Related Defects

| Time of Occurrence (Week) | Stage of Human Development | Major Events | | Major Anomalies during Stage |
|---|---|---|---|---|
| 3 to 4 | Neurulation | Notochord | Neural plate | Anencephaly |
| | | | Neural tube | Exencephaly |
| | | | | Meningocele |
| | | | | Meningomyelocele |
| | | | | Myeloschisis |
| | | | Neural tube | |
| | | | Neural crest cells | Arnold-Chiari malformation |
| | | | Brain differentiation of prosencephalon, mesencephalon, and rhombencephalon at 20 days | |
| | | | Spinal cord | |
| | | | Dura | |
| | | Neural crest cells | Dorsal root ganglia | |
| | | | Pia and arachnoid | |
| | | | Schwann cells | |
| | | | Autonomic ganglia | |
| 4 to 7 | Caudal neural-tube formation | Canalization followed by regressive differentiation | | Spina bifida occulta |
| 5 to 6 | Ventral induction (prosencephalon development) | Precordial mesoderm | Face and forebrain | Dermal sinus |
| | | Prosencephalon | | |
| | | | Cleavage of prosencephalon into cerebral vesicles in the form of 2 cerebral hemispheres at 33 days | Faciotele cephalic malformations |
| | | | Differentiation of the hypothalamus | |
| 8 to 16 | Neuronal proliferation | Cellular proliferation in the ventricular and subventricular zones | Optic vesicles | Microencephaly (microencephaly vera and radial microbrain) |
| | | | Olfactory bulbs and tracts | Macroencephaly |
| | | Proliferation of vascular tree, particularly venous | First fibers in internal capsule at 41 days | |
| | | Interkinetic nuclear migration | | |
| | | Neuroblasts | Thalamus and basal ganglia | |
| | | Glioblasts | | |

*Continued*

Table 7-2   Major Stages of Human Brain Development and Related Defects—cont'd

| Time of Occurrence (Week) | Stage of Human Development | Major Events | | Major Anomalies during Stage |
|---|---|---|---|---|
| 12 to 20 | Migration | Cortical lamination | | Schizencephaly |
| | | Radial migration in cerebrum | | Agenesis of the corpus callosum Hirschsprung disease |
| | | Radial tangential migration in the cerebellum | Neuronal migration in the cerebral cortex is completed at about 5 months Neuronal migration in the cerebellum is completed at about 1 year postnatally | |
| 24 to | Organization postnatal | Late neuronal migration in cerebrum and cerebellum | | Mental retardation Down syndrome Perinatal insults |
| | | Alignment, orientation, and layering of cortical neurons | | |
| | | Synaptic contacts | | |
| | | Proliferation of glia and differentiation | | |
| Peak at birth to years postnatal | Myelinization | Bulbospinal tracts | 24 weeks to postnatal | Cerebral white matter hypoplasia |
| | | Motor roots | 24 weeks to postnatal | |
| | | Medial lemniscus | 24 weeks to postnatal | |
| | | Pyramidal tract | 38 weeks to 2 years postnatal | |
| | | Frontopontine tract | 7 to 8 months postnatal to 2 years | |
| | | Corpus callosum | 4 months postnatal to 16 years | |

From Blackburn, S.T. (2003). *Maternal, fetal, and neonatal physiology: A clinical perspective* (2nd ed.; pp. 562-563). St. Louis: W.B. Saunders. Adapted from Hill, A & Volpe, J.J. (1989). *Fetal neurology*. New York: Raven.

importantly, that is where they were meant to develop.

The fetus experiences touch from the walls of the uterus and can respond as early as the second month of gestation. Smell and taste have not been documented in utero; however, the preterm infant responds to odors as early as 26 weeks' gestation, and responses to taste of glucose have been documented at 32 weeks (Blackburn, 2003; Papile, 1997). Mennella, Jagnow, and Beauchamp (2001) found that flavors in the maternal diet were carried by the amniotic fluid to the fetus, who later in infancy seemed to prefer some of these flavors. More research needs to be done in this area before any conclusions can be drawn about this sensory experience and later behaviors. The structures of the inner ear are mature by 20 weeks' gestation, and auditory responses of preterm infants have been noted as early as 25 weeks' gestation. The intrauterine environment is not quiet, and the fetus appears to respond; however, the noises in this environment are attenuated. The visual system is responsive to light between 25 and 30 weeks' gestation. In general,

the uterus is dark. There are some color variations based on light that goes through the abdomen, but, nevertheless, the environment is generally subdued. (For more detail on the development of the sensory system, see Chapter 10.)

When providing stimulation to the preterm or newborn infant, it is important to remember which systems develop first and to provide stimulation to those systems first, because the infant will be more able to receive this stimulation and respond appropriately. Therefore, for the easily overstimulated infant, rocking and holding are generally better tolerated without talking or visual stimulation. Remember, the visual system develops last and, therefore, is the least mature. See Boxes 7-1 and 7-2 and Table 7-3 for more information on the maturation of the auditory, visual, and pain systems.

Even when infants are born at full term, their sensory systems are overloaded. The birth process brings many new experiences to the infant. The ability to receive, modulate, and select stimuli from the environment is poorly developed, and the infant

---

## Box 7-1  Auditory System: Development of Hearing in Preterm and Term Infants

| Age | Anatomic and Functional Development |
|---|---|
| Preterm infants <28 weeks | Fetal hearing begins by 23 to 24 weeks |
| | Threshold ≈65 decibels (dB), with a range of 500 to 100 Hertz (Hz) |
| | Auditory brain stem responses by 26 to 28 weeks |
| Preterm infants 28 to 30 weeks | Rapid maturation of cochlea and auditory nerve |
| | Responses rapidly fatigue |
| | Initial auditory processing by 30 weeks |
| | Threshold 40 dB with an increase in frequency range |
| Preterm infants 32 to 34 weeks | Rapid maturation of cochlea and auditory nerve |
| Preterm infants >34 weeks | Increased speed of conduction |
| | Ossicles and electrophysiology complete by 36 weeks |
| | Hearing threshold 30 dB, with increasing range |
| | Increasing ability to localize and discriminate |
| Term infants | Localize and discriminate sounds |
| | Hearing threshold of 20 dB, with a range of 500 to 4000 Hz |

From Blackburn, S.T. (2003). *Maternal, fetal, and neonatal physiology: A clinical perspective* (2nd ed.; p. 574). St. Louis: W.B. Saunders.

## Box 7-2    Visual System: Development of Vision in Preterm and Term Infants

| Age | Anatomic and Functional Development |
|---|---|
| Preterm infants 24 to 28 weeks | Eyelid; unfuses at 24 to 26 weeks |
| | Lens: cloudy; second of four layers forming |
| | Cornea: hazy until 27 weeks |
| | Retina: rod differentiation and vascularization begin by 25 weeks |
| | Visual cortex: rapid dendritic growth |
| | No papillary response |
| | Eyelids tighten to bright light, but quickly fatigue |
| | Visual evoked response (VER) to bright light quickly fatigues |
| | Very myopic |
| Preterm infants 30 to 34 weeks | Lens: clearing, second layer complete, third forming |
| | Retina: rod complete except for fovea by 32 weeks; cone differentiation begins |
| | Visual cortex: rapid dendritic and synapse development |
| | VER more complex, latency decreases |
| | Bright light causes sustained pupil closure |
| | Abrupt reduction might cause eye opening |
| | Pupil response sluggish, but more mature |
| | Spontaneous eye opening, with brief fixation in low light |
| Preterm infants 34 to 36 weeks | Pupils: complete pupil reflex by 36 weeks |
| | Retina: cone numbers in fovea increase |
| | Blood vessels reach nasal retina |
| | Visual cortex: morphologically similar to term |
| | Increased alertness; less sustained than for a term infant |
| | VER resembles that of term infant with longer latency |
| | Spontaneous orientation toward soft light |
| | Beginning to track and show visual preferences |
| | Less myopic |
| Term infants | Still immature, with much development from birth to 6 months |
| | Retinal vessels reach periphery of temporal retina |
| | Lens transmits more short-wave light than adult |
| | Acuity approximately 20/200 to 20/1600 |
| | Attend to form, object, and face; track horizontally and some vertically |
| | Can see objects to at least $2\frac{1}{2}$ feet; attends best at 8 to 12 inches |

From Blackburn, S.T. (2003). *Maternal, fetal, and neonatal physiology: A clinical perspective* (2nd ed.; p. 575). St. Louis: W.B. Saunders.

Table 7-3   PAIN SYSTEM: ANATOMIC AND FUNCTIONAL DEVELOPMENT OF THE DIFFERENT PARTS OF THE PAIN SYSTEM

| Part of the System | Developmental Event | Weeks |
|---|---|---|
| Nociceptors | Nociceptors appear (starting around the mouth and later developing over the entire body). | 7 to 20 |
| Peripheral afferents | Synapses appear to the spinal cord. | 10 to 30 |
| Spinal cord | Stimulation results in motor movements. | 7.5 |
| | Spinothalamic connections are established. | 20 |
| | Pain pathways myelinized. | 22 |
| | Descending tracts develop. | Postnatal |
| Thalamocortical tracts | First axons appear to the cortical plate. | 20 to 22 |
| | Functional synapse formation of the thalamocortex occurs. | 26 to 34 |
| | Cortical neurons migrate (cortex develops). | 8 to 20 |
| | First electronencephalogram (EEG) burst can be detected. | 20 |
| | Symmetric and synchronic EEG activity appears. | 26 |
| | Sleep and wakefulness patterns become distinguishable on EEG. | 30 |
| | Evoked potential becomes detectable. | 29 |

From Vanhatalo, S., & van Nieuwenhuizen, O. (2000). Fetal pain? *Brain Development, 22,* 146.

might need support to organize and respond appropriately to the environment.

Motor function also begins before birth and is the result of coordination between neuronal and muscle development. With increasing development, the fetus demonstrates increasing movement and tone. Active tone is noted before passive tone, and with increasing gestational age, fewer tremors are noted, movements become smoother, and they are more coordinated (Blackburn, 2003; Volpe, 2001). In addition, with increasing gestational age there is also increasing strength of muscle movements. However, once the infant is born, the forces of gravity make movement more difficult, and the movements of the infant might appear precarious, fragile, or flailing.

Fetal movements demonstrate the development of fetal sleep-wake patterns. Sleep-wake states change with maturation. See Table 7-4 for more information on sleep states. Fetal state can be determined by rhythmicity of heart rate, presence of eye movements, and motor activity. As the fetus matures, these patterns become more regular with both quiet and active sleep patterns noted as early as 32 weeks gestation (Blackburn, 2003; Volpe, 2001). The fetal state cycle is approximately 40 minutes; however, with full-term birth and maturation, the length of the cycle increases. Sleep is necessary for CNS development.

Table 7-4  INFANT STATE CHART (SLEEP AND AWAKE STATES)

| State* | Body Activity | Eye Movements | Facial Movements | Breathing Pattern | Level of Response | Implications for Caregiving |
|---|---|---|---|---|---|---|
| **SLEEP STATES** | | | | | | |
| Quiet (deep) sleep | Nearly still, except for occasional startle or twitch | None | Without facial movements, except for occasional sucking movement at regular intervals | Smooth and regular | Threshold to stimuli very high so that only very intense and disturbing stimuli will arouse | Caregivers trying to feed infants in quiet sleep will probably find the experience frustrating. Infants will be unresponsive, even if caregivers use disturbing stimuli to arouse infants. Infants might arouse only briefly and then become unresponsive as they return to quiet sleep. If caregivers wait until infants move to a higher, more responsive state, feeding or caregiving will be much more pleasant. |
| Active (light) sleep | Some body movements | Rapid eye movement (REM); fluttering of eyesbeneath closed eyelids | Might smile and make brief fussy or crying sounds | Irregular | More responsive to internal and external stimuli; when these stimuli occur, infants might remain in active sleep, return to quiet sleep, or arouse to drowsy | Active sleep makes up the highest proportion of newborn sleep and usually precedes awakening. Because of brief fussy or crying sounds made during this state, caregivers who are not aware that these sounds occur normally might think it is time for feeding and try to feed infants before they are ready to eat. |

Table 7-4  Infant State Chart (Sleep and Awake States)—cont'd

| State* | Body Activity | Eye Movements | Facial Movements | Breathing Pattern | Level of Response | Implications for Caregiving |
|---|---|---|---|---|---|---|
| **AWAKE STATES** | | | | | | |
| Drowsy | Activity level variable, with mild startles interspersed from time to time; movements usually smooth | Eyes open and close occasionally; are heavy-lidded with dull, glazed appearance | Might have some facial movements, but often there are none, and the face appears still | Irregular | Infants react to sensory stimuli, although responses are delayed; state change after stimulation frequently noted | From the drowsy state, infants might return to sleep or awaken further. To awaken, caregivers can provide something for infants to see, hear, or suck, as this might arouse them to a quiet alert state, a more responsive state. Infants who are left alone without stimuli might return to a sleep state. |
| Quiet alert | Minimal | Brightening and widening of eyes | Faces have bright, shining, sparkling looks | Regular | Infants attend most to the environment, focusing attention on any stimuli that are present | Infants in this state provide much pleasure and positive feedback for caregivers. Providing something for infants to see, hear, or suck will often maintain a quiet alert state. In the first few hours after birth, most newborns commonly experience a period of intense alertness before going into a long sleep period. |

*Continued*

Table 7-4   Infant State Chart (Sleep and Awake States)—cont'd

| State* | Body Activity | Eye Movements | Facial Movements | Breathing Pattern | Level of Response | Implications for Caregiving |
|---|---|---|---|---|---|---|
| Active alert | Much body activity; might have periods of fussiness | Eyes open with less brightening | Much facial movement; faces not as bright as in quiet alert state | Irregular | Increasingly sensitive to disturbing stimuli (hunger, fatigue, noise, excessive handling) | Crying is the infant's communication signal. It is a response to unpleasant stimuli from the environment or within infants (e.g., fatigue, hunger, discomfort). Crying says that infants' limits have been reached. Sometimes infants can console themselves and return to lower states. At other times, they need help from caregivers. |
| Crying | Increased motor activity with color changes | Eyes might be tightly closed or open | Grimaces | Irregular | Extremely responsive to unpleasant external or internal stimuli | See note under active alert. Caregivers might need to intervene at this state to console and bring the infant to a lower state. |

From Blackburn, S.T. (2003). *Maternal, fetal, and neonatal physiology: A clinical perspective* (2nd ed.; pp. 584-585). St. Louis: W.B. Saunders. Adapted from Blackburn, S., & Kang, R. (1991). *Early parent-infant relationships* (2nd ed.). White Plains, NY: March of Dimes Birth Defects Foundation.

*State is a group of characteristics that regularly occur together: body activity, eye movements, facial movements, breathing pattern, and level of response to external stimuli (e.g., handling) and internal stimuli (e.g., hunger).

State patterns after birth are individual; however, the infant's attention abilities are reflective of the infant's increasing ability to habituate and adapt to the environment (Gunnar & Barr, 1998). Alertness is often related to feeding and allows more in-depth interaction with the environment. Therefore, alertness should be supported. If the infant is easily overstimulated, alertness might not be available, and stimulation in the environment might need to be decreased for the infant to be responsive. Modulation of sleep-wake states requires excellent neurobehavioral organization and, therefore, can provide an accessible window into the status of the developing brain of the infant.

## CAREGIVING IMPLICATIONS: INDIVIDUALIZED, FAMILY-CENTERED, DEVELOPMENTAL CARE

The maturation of the neurologic system dictates how the neonate will respond to external stimuli. Awareness of infant stress and stability cues is essential to adjusting care accordingly. Watching for signals of distress (yawning, crying, finger splaying, back arching) and of stability (gazing; easy, relaxed posture of all extremities; flexion of arms and legs as a normal posture-not tense; hand-to-mouth self-regulatory behaviors) should be incorporated into routine caregiving. Environmental stimuli, such as excessive light, noise, or even procedural touch, are all areas that can adversely affect the sick or preterm neonate. How they can respond or how much stimulation they can tolerate is dependent on gestational age, maturation of the neurologic system, and the severity of their illness. Chapters in Unit III of this text outline some of the specific aspects of caregiving and research to support these areas as related to the infant's gestational and neurologic maturation. Blackburn (2003) recommends that, as caregivers, we consider the neurologic stage of development and incorporate that into our care; engage parents in our caregiving, and teach them about the infant's ability to respond to stimuli from a neurologic perspective; protect the infant from overstimulation; incorporate our knowledge of states, neonatal reflexes, and neurologic capabilities when assessing the infant and planning care; and modify the macro- and microenvironments to promote positive infant and family development.

## CONCLUSION

As more has been discovered about the developing human brain, the question is not nature or nurture, it is nature and nurture, and what is the balance that bests supports the fragility and plasticity of the developing brain of the infant. Therefore, observing and responding to the individualized neurobehaviors of the infant is an important area of developmental intervention. The family is an essential component of the promotion of positive, continued maturation of the neurologic system when they are treated as partners in caregiving and provided age-appropriate information about the maturation process.

## ACKNOWLEDGMENT

Modified from McGrath, J.M. (2000, October/November). Developmental physiology of the neurological system. In D. Durkin (Ed.), *Central lines: The official publication of the National Association of Neonatal Nurses* (pp. 1-2, 4, 6, 16). Glenview, IL: NANN.

## *REFERENCES*

Blackburn, S.T. (2003). *Maternal, fetal, and neonatal physiology: A clinical perspective* (2nd ed.; pp. 576-593). St. Louis: W.B. Saunders.

Eisenberg, L. (1995). The social construction of the human brain. *American Journal of Psychiatry, 152*(11), 1563-1575.

Eisenberg, L. (1999). Experience, brain, and behavior: The importance of a head start. *Pediatrics, 102,* 1031-1034.

Gardner, S.L., & Goldson, E. (2002). The neonate and the environment: Impact on development (pp. 219-282). In G.B. Merenstein and S.L. Gardner (Eds.), *Handbook of neonatal intensive care* (5th ed.). St. Louis: Mosby.

Glass, P. (1999). The vulnerable neonate and the neonatal intensive care environment. In G.B. Avery, M.A. Fletcher, & M.G. MacDonald (Eds.), *Neonatology-pathophysiology and management* (5th ed.; pp. 91-108). Philadelphia: Williams & Wilkins.

Gunnar, M.R., & Barr, R.G. (1998). Stress, early brain development and behavior. *Infants and Young Children, 11*(1), 1-14.

Herschkowitz, N. (2000). Neurological bases of behavioral development in infancy. *Brain Development, 22*(7), 411-416.

Mennella, J.A., Jagnow, C.P., & Beauchamp, G.K. (2001). Prenatal and postnatal flavor learning by human infants (Editorial). *Pediatrics, 107*(6), E88.

Mulvihill, D., Cahill, J., & Eicher, D. (2003). Biphasic cerebral blood flow velocity patterns in neonatal asphyxia. *Ultrasound & Medical Biology, 29*(5 Suppl), S108-S109.

Okumura, A., Toyota, N., Hayakawa, F., et al. (2002). Cerebral hemodynamics during early neonatal period in preterm infants with periventricular leukomalacia. *Brain Development, 24*(7), 693-697.

Papile, L. (1997). Intracranial hemorrhage. In A.A. Fanaroff, & R.J. Martin (Eds.), *Neonatal-perinatal medicine diseases of the fetus and infant* (6th ed.; pp. 891-899). St. Louis: Mosby.

Volpe, J.J. (2001). *Neurology of the newborn* (4th ed.). Philadelphia: W.B. Saunders.

Weisel. T.N. (1994). Genetics and behavior. *Science, 264*, 1647.

# 8 Motor Development Chronology: A Dynamic Process

## Jane K. Sweeney and Teresa Gutierrez

Neonatal nurses and practitioners (NNPs), as well as other neonatal health professionals, have a unique opportunity to observe early posture and movement in neonates and to collaborate in promoting motor development and preventing or minimizing deformity. In this chapter the chronology of motor development is reviewed in the embryo, fetus, and neonate from the perspectives of musculoskeletal maturation and tone and movement sequences. Continuity and discontinuity are traced in the development of spontaneous movement, posture, and tone. The dynamic process of musculoskeletal shaping is analyzed, with clinical implications outlined for practitioners in neonatal developmental care and follow-up.

## STRUCTURAL DEVELOPMENT

The chronology of musculoskeletal maturation is outlined from the structural perspective of skeletal, joint, and muscle development followed by the functional perspective of posture, tone, and movement. These structural and functional elements create the foundation for coordinated motor behavior.

## Skeleton

The skeletal system in the embryo is derived from mesoderm cells that, near the third week (day 20), form somites, two blocks of mesoderm tissue located close to midline. The somites differentiate into sclerotome (vertebrae, ribs) and dermomyotome (skin, muscle) cells. The sclerotome has loosely organized mesenchymal (mesoderm) cells that further differentiate into the bone, cartilage, and connective tissue components of the skeletal system: fibroblasts, chondroblasts, osteoblasts, or myoblasts.

## Vertebrae and Ribs

The vertebral column is developed during the fourth week when sclerotome cells in the somites migrate medially around the neural tube and notochord forming the cartilaginous structures for the vertebral arches and vertebral bodies. Mesenchymal costal processes on both sides of the thoracic vertebrae develop into the ribs. Cartilaginous vertical bars form on the ends of the ribs, and rib pairs 1 to 7 fuse in midline to form the sternum. Fused vertebrae or ribs, hemivertebrae (Klippel-Feil syndrome), or defects in the vertebral arch (spina bifida) result from disrupted skeletal development in the fourth week of life.

## Limbs

In the fourth week upper (day 26) and lower (day 28), limb buds appear when mesenchymal cells are activated and form a thick apical ectodermal ridge. The flipper-appearing limb buds emerge into flatter hand and foot plates resembling paddles. In the fifth week the limbs elongate with cartilage formation (chrondrification) occurring in the sixth week. By the twelfth week primary ossification centers are present in the long bones, and at term the diaphysis (center shaft) is usually ossified, but the epiphyses (distal end) of bone remain cartilaginous. At secondary ossification centers in the epiphyses, complete ossification varies and can extend through 20 to 30 years of age. Growth in thickness and density of the diaphysis is the most rapid in the prenatal period, with spurts expected at 7 years of age and at puberty (Moore & Persaud, 2003; Sadler & Langman, 2000; Gajdosik & Gajdosik, 2000). During the fourth and fifth week, the following limb anomalies can occur: partial absence of limbs (meromelia; absence of radius); cleft hand or foot; polydactyly; syndactyly; and clubfoot deformities.

Epiphyseal plate demineralization related to rickets and osteopenia of prematurity is reported in 30% of low birthweight (LBW) infants weighing less than 1500 g (Moore & Persaud, 2003). Because of incomplete ossification and decreased bone density, preterm infants are vulnerable to rib fractures during chest physical therapy percussion procedures. The humerus, radius, ulna, and femur (Figure 8-1) are other highly vulnerable sites for fractures in LBW infants with rickets. Immobility for whatever reason, but especially during prolonged periods of sedation such as during mechanical ventilation, might enhance calcium loss and bone demineralization.

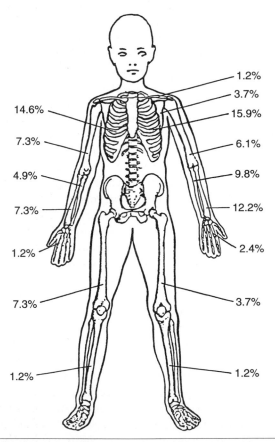

Figure **8-1** Distribution of 82 fracture sites in a sample of 19 low birthweight infants with rickets. (*From Fanaroff, A.A., & Martin, R.J. [2002]. Diseases of the fetus and infants. In Fanaroff, A. A., & Martin, R.J. [Eds.],* Neonatal-perinatal medicine: Diseases of the fetus and infant [*7th ed.*]. *St. Louis: Mosby.*)

In term infants, the clavicle remains the most frequent neonatal fracture (2 to 7 per 1000 live births) from shoulder dystocia during delivery. Lower extremity fractures are less common in term infants and are likely related to underlying neuromuscular disorders limiting joint mobility (e.g., arthrogryposis multiplex congenita) or to bone/connective tissue disorders (e.g., osteogenesis imperfecta) (Butler, 2003). Some of these fractures might be caused inadvertently from stress and torque on bones during handling and positioning when an underlying condition exists such as osteogenesis imperfecta (Jones & Bell, 2002).

## Articular Structures

Derived from mesoderm and mesenchyme, joint structures develop in the sixth through the eighth week postconception when fibrous and cartilaginous connective tissue or synovial membranes develop between bones at articulation points. In joint capsules of extremities, mechanoreceptors are formed to assist in the perception of proprioception and direction and speed of movement. Joint molding is influenced by fetal movement with continued shaping of joints occurring throughout childhood from forces of compression and movement (Butler, 2003; Moore & Persaud, 2003).

Development and alignment of limbs and joints can be altered by intrauterine conditions, including amniotic banding, irregular uterine shape, insufficient amniotic fluid, multiple gestation more than twins, and breech presentation (Butler, 2003). The presence of maturation-related ligamentous laxity and connective tissue elasticity predisposes preterm infants to developing joint effusion or subluxation during vigerous range of motion maneuvers (Sweeney & Swanson, 2001). Respiratory equipment and infusion lines in the neonatal intensive care unit (NICU) restrict variability in positioning fragile neonates, who might experience prolonged pressure and compression of limbs and joints and minimal refinement of mechanoreceptor action. When a variety of recumbent postures are provided within the constraints of neonatal equipment, infants can experience varying forces and pressure through joints and muscles that promote joint and mechanoreceptor development for coordinated movement (de Groot,

Hoek, Hopkins, et al., 1992; Plantinga, Perdock, & de Groot, 1997; Sweeney & Gutierrez, 2002).

## Muscle Tissue

Skeletal muscles emerge from myoblasts differentiated from mesoderm in the myotome area of somites. Myoblasts form elongated, multinucleated myotubes at 5 to 10 weeks and myofilaments (muscle fibers) at 10 to 20 weeks. By 20 weeks postconception, muscle tissue differentiates into slow (type I) and fast (type II) twitch fibers (Moore & Persaud, 2003; Grove, 1989; Sans, 1987). The high oxidative, type I muscle fibers continue to develop while preterm infants are in NICUs, but remain at decreased ratio to the low oxidative type II fibers. Predisposition to muscular fatigue, particularly in respiratory muscles, might be related to this lower ratio of high oxidative type II fibers in preterm neonates. The low postural tone and difficulty sustaining postures might also be related in part to this muscle fiber disparity in preterm compared with term infants. At term gestation, type I and II muscle fibers are expected to be equal in number and to resemble the pattern in adult muscles (Dubowitz, 1965; Dreyfus & Schapira, 1979).

Although overall numbers of muscle fibers continue to grow through the first year of life, muscle growth increases throughout childhood in length and diameter by addition of myofilaments. The eventual size of muscles is influenced by a combination of gender, genetics, nutrition, blood supply, innervation, and exercise (Gajdosik & Gajdosik, 2000).

## PRENATAL MOVEMENT

Observation and assessment of fetal movement and behavior were studied by early investigators who relied primarily on access to aborted fetuses or nonviable preterm newborn infants for analysis and documentation of fetal posture and tone (Gesell, 1945; Saint-Anne Dargassies, 1977; Humphrey, 1978). These early fetal and neonatal movement investigators were challenged by the absence of fetal ultrasound for prenatal observations and limitations of intensive care technology in the 1960s to 1970s for keeping LBW infants alive. The comparatively limited neonatal physiologic support and higher neonatal morbidity and mortality in that era influenced the variability of posture, movement,

and tone in the infants available for study (Prechtl & Nolte, 1984; Towen, 1990; Albers & Jorch, 1994). Current advances in technology have created excellent opportunities for researchers to observe, classify, and document the development of prenatal movement longitudinally (de Vries, Visser, & Prechtl, 1984; de Vries, Wimmers, Ververs, et al., 2001; Prechtl 1984, 1989, 1997b; Kozuma, Okai, Nemoto, et al., 1997; Roodenburg, Wladimiroff, van Es, et al., 1991; Brown, Omar, & O'Regan, 1997).

The earliest movements of the embryo are identified at 7 to 7.5 weeks postconception (Figure 8-2, *A*) and are characterized by slow neck extension. Startles and general movements follow this motor activity. Startles are characterized by fast, phasic contraction of all limbs with secondary involvement of the neck and trunk. General movements follow a distinct, complex pattern of whole-body involvement with fluid movement quality (Milani-Comparetti & Gidoni, 1967). The onset of general movements has been documented in the fetus at 9 weeks postconception (Figure 8-2, *B*), followed by rapid expansion of movement patterns and repertoire. Isolated movement of the extremities appear shortly after 9 weeks postconception, followed by a variety of head movements, including neck rotation and extension. Breathing movements begin between 10 and 12 weeks, accompanied by jaw opening and closing. By 13 weeks, sucking movements begin in rhythmic bursts, followed by swallowing. The rate of sucking and swallowing movements present at 14 weeks is believed to be similar to the rate present in term infants (Prechtl, 1997a; Ianniruberto & Tajani, 1981; deVries, Visser, & Prechtl, 1984). Fetal swallowing has an important functional role in regulating amniotic fluid volume (Prechtl, 1997a).

Fetal movement is well documented during the first half of pregnancy, but few reports review developmental changes in movement during the second half. This disparity is due in part to difficulty with full-body visualization of the fetus during ultrasonography after 20 weeks related to increased growth. Classification methods have been developed to quantify and describe fetal movement, particularly during the second half of pregnancy (Sparling, Van Tol, & Chescheir, 1999; Sparling & Wilhelm, 1993; Kozuma, Okai, Nemoto, et al., 1997). This process of clarifying and describing characteristics of fetal movement might, in the future,

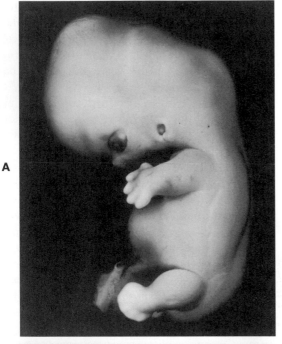

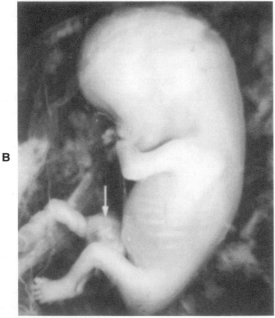

Figure **8-2 A**, Embryo at 7 weeks postconception, when first documented movement of neck extension occurs. **B**, Fetus at 9 weeks, when general movements are detected. (*From Moore, K.L., & Persaud, T.V.N. [2003]. The developing human: Clinically oriented embryology [7th ed.]. St. Louis: Mosby.*)

lead to discrete documentation of fetal movement sequences and assessment of fetal wellness through movement analysis (Sparling & Wilhelm, 1993; Sparling, Van Tol, & Chescheir, 1999; Kozuma, Okai, Nemoto, et al., 1997).

The *continuity* of fetal and neonatal movement from prenatal to postnatal life has been recognized by numerous investigators (Gesell, 1945; de Vries, Visser, & Prechtl, 1984; Saint-Anne Dargassies, 1977; Prechtl, 1984; Hadders-Algra, Klip-Van den Nieuwendijk, Martijn, et al., 1997). Prechtl has led the way with a recent body of research inferring that spontaneous fetal movements are endogenously generated and have recognizable patterns that change over time, with qualitative features highly predictive of brain function (Prechtl, 1997a, 2001; Kakebeeke, von Siebenthal, & Largo, 1998). If, however, the quality of general movements is altered by changes in brain function, the continuity of motor development is disrupted (Prechtl, 1997a, 1997b, 2001; Einspieler, Prechtl, Ferrari, et al., 1997; Cioni, Prechtl, Ferrari, et al., 1997; Ferrari, Cioni, Prechtl, 1990).

The technology used in neonatal intensive care supports survival in preterm infants but also creates vulnerability for disruption in the continuity of motor development. These infants have to cope unexpectedly with the effects of gravity, periods of sedation-related suppression of movement, and postural adaptation to respiratory and infusion equipment. In NICU environments, infant body and extremity alignment and the quantity, frequency, and intensity of spontaneous movement are disrupted intermittently. Early use of developmental care practices in positioning, handling, and environmental modification provide critical support to the *continuity* and quality of movement in neonates during intensive care (see Chapter 16).

## DEVELOPMENT OF POSTURE, MOVEMENT, AND TONE

From the early development and continuity of fetal movement, infants have had an innate repertoire of movement that evolves during a term pregnancy. In the following section, factors that influence the development of muscle tone, posture, and future motor behavior are explored. The movement experience of a term infant is different from that of a preterm infant. The infant born at term has moved within a well-contained and stable environment, receiving a variety of proprioceptive and sensory input under ideal physiologic conditions. The term neonate is equipped with effective muscle power, posture, tone, and movement to respond in dynamic interaction with the extrauterine environment. When birth occurs prematurely, muscle tone, posture, and movement continue to develop, but the infant must now adapt to the influence of gravity and tactile and proprioceptive stimuli from prolonged lying (weight bearing) on a mattress before the musculoskeletal system is equipped to deal with these forces (de Groot, 2000; de Groot, Hopkins, Touwen, 1991; de Groot, Hoek, Hopkins, et al., 1992; de Groot, Hoek, Hopkins, et al., 1993; Prechtl & Nolte, 1984).

Muscle tone is viewed in two ways: passive tone and active or postural tone. Passive tone is measured by the amount of resistance offered in response to passive movement (e.g., traction and recoil). Pronounced, passive flexor tone in term infants is related to the mechanical constraint of uterine-wall resistance during fetal growth in the last trimester. At term, equivalent-age preterm infants do not reach the same level of flexion as infants born at term (Dubowitz & Dubowitz, 1999). The biomechanical advantage of strong "physiologic" flexor tone at birth enhances head control, midline extremity posture, and suck-swallow proficiency.

Postural or active tone involves sustained muscle contraction necessary for maintaining posture against gravity and is fluid, adaptive, and constantly changing in response to movement (Brown, Omar, & O'Regan, 1997; de Groot, 2000). Compared with term infants, decreased postural control in preterm infants might be partly influenced by the decreased proportion of type I (slow-twitch, posture-maintaining) fibers as compared with type II (fast-twitch, easily fatigued) fibers in skeletal muscles.

Development of infant posture and tone has been an ongoing study topic (Gesell, 1945; Amiel-Tison & Grenier, 1983; Saint-Anne Dargassies, 1977; Allen, 1996; Dubowitz & Dubowitz, 1999; Allen & Capute, 1990; de Groot, Hopkins, & Touwen, 1991). Consensus is that preterm infants are hypotonic, and the subsequent development of flexor tone follows a caudad to cephalad progression. Dubowitz and Dubowitz (1999) later reported a longitudinal investigation of

the progression of flexor tone in 57 low-risk, preterm infants at 28 to 35 weeks postconception. They measured passive extremity tone by traction, recoil, and popliteal angles. Earlier assumptions were confirmed on the chronology of passive and active tone, including flexor tone progression in a caudad to cephalad direction. Allen and Capute (1990) documented the beginning of leg flexion at 29 to 32 weeks and arm flexion at 35 to 37 weeks.

In a series of studies headed by de Groot et al. (1991, 1992, 1993), distinction was made between active muscle power and passive tone during examination of posture and movement in preterm infants. The researchers concluded that preterm infants have low muscle tone, measured by resistance to traction or passive movement. Differences in muscle power between preterm and term infants were attributed to differences in weight and muscle mass. They noted that some preterm infants appeared to develop exaggerated, active muscle power expressed by hyperextension of the trunk. Prolonged positioning of preterm infants in supine was hypothesized to be the stimulus (proprioceptive, tactile) for overactivation of neck, trunk, and hip muscles in contact with the supporting surface, causing exaggerated extensor power (better known as "arching behavior"). Overactivation of extensor muscles was considered to be out of synchrony with the level of tone maturation in other muscle groups, creating motor disorganization from a mismatch of intensity and timing between extensor and flexor groups. (de Groot, Hoek, Hopkins, et al., 1992; Plantinga, Perdock, & de Groot, 1997). Placing infants in a variety of positions in the NICU, therefore, becomes an important procedure for providing equal, symmetrical opportunity for tactile and proprioceptive (mechanoreceptor) stimulation and activation of muscle groups.

Key posture and motor competencies expected of preterm infants at term equivalent age (Dubowitz & Dubowitz, 1999) are listed:
- Maintains semiflexed extremity posture in supine and prone positions.
- Moves head side to side in supine and prone positions.
- Lifts head in prone and holds head erect momentarily in supported sitting.
- Head in line with trunk during pull-to-sit maneuver.

- Brings hands toward midline intermittently (e.g., chest; mouth).
- Sustains rhythmic suck, swallow, and breathing sequence.

Demonstrates movements that support behavioral state regulation (e.g., hand to mouth; foot to foot holding).

Although preterm infants might not demonstrate the same level of active, postural tone as term infants at 40 weeks postconception, neonatal caregivers can create supportive environments to help them approach similar postural stability and midline movement.

## CLINICAL IMPLICATIONS FOR NEONATAL CARE

Growth and plasticity of the musculoskeletal system is like a double-edged sword, capable of positive or negative effects. Neonatal healthcare professionals can use the rapid neonatal growth process and joint and tissue laxity not found in later childhood to promote musculoskeletal alignment and motor organization while infants remain in NICUs (Hensinger & Jones, 1981). The rapid growth with inattention to alignment can also contribute to striking positional deformities in the skull and extremities in a remarkably short time.

### Musculoskeletal Shaping

Shaping of the musculoskeletal system occurs during each body position experienced by neonates in the NICU. Supporting skeletal integrity of LBW infants is challenging in the midst of multiple equipment obstacles and limited handling demanded by fluctuating physiologic stability. Skull deformity and extremity malalignment (Table 8-1) from maturation-related hypotonia combined with procedures such as prolonged ventilation or extended reflux wedge positioning, in which symmetric, midline postures are difficult to maintain, are not uncommon. Skull flattening continues to evolve after NICU discharge with overuse of infant seats and limited prone play activities. If strong head-turn preference remains, and asymmetric occipital flattening (plagiocephaly) occurs, a secondary torticollis is likely to emerge (head tilt).

Shoulder-retraction posture (scapular adduction with shoulder elevation and external rotation) can accompany excessive neck and trunk extension posture in preterm neonates. This abnormal upper-extremity position can interfere with later reaching, shoulder stability in prone position, and rolling in the first 18 months of life (Gorga, Stern, Ross, et al. 1988; Georgieff & Bernbaum, 1986). "Out-toeing" gait and excessive tibial tortion were reported in NICU graduates at 3 to 8 years of age and traced to prolonged "frog leg" (excessive hip abduction and external rotation with foot eversion) postures in the NICU (Davis, Robinson, Harris, & Cartlidge, 1993; Katz, Krikler, Wielunsky, & Merlob, 1991). These potential positional deformities disrupt the continuity of musculoskeletal development begun in utero and shaped in the NICU environment but can be minimized during positioning procedures with the following goals:

- Optimize alignment: neutral neck-trunk; semi-flexed, midline extremity posture; neutral foot alignment.
- Support posture and movement *within* "containment boundaries" of rolls, swaddling blanket, or other positioning aids: avoid creating a barrier of immobilization.
- Modify positioning and handling to promote regulation of behavioral states that enhance short-duration interaction and sleep states that promote growth.
- Offer positions that allow controlled, individualized exposure to proprioceptive, tactile, visual, or auditory stimuli: monitor signs of behavioral stress from potential overstimulation.

These goals can be achieved using swaddling, commercial or noncommercial postural devices, and hand support during procedures.

Teaching families principles of optimal musculoskeletal alignment and positioning in the NICU provides them practice under supervision in preparation for continuation during caregiving following discharge. Recommendations for discharge teaching to support skeletal and motor development include the following (Sweeney & Gutierrez, 2002):

- Vary the direction of the head turn for sleeping in supine to prevent plagiocephaly.
- Place the head in midline position with lateral head rolls (extending along side of trunk) in car seats, "bouncy" seats, and swings.

Table **8-1** MUSCULOSKELETAL MALALIGNMENT AND FUNCTIONAL LIMITATIONS IN NEONATES

| Positional Deformity | Consequences | Functional Limitations |
|---|---|---|
| Plagiocephaly | Unilateral, flat, occipital region<br>Head-turn preference<br>High risk for torticollis | Limited visual orientation from asymmetric head position<br>Delayed midline head control |
| Scaphocephaly | Bilateral, flat, parietal and temporal regions | Difficulty developing active midline head control in supine from narrowing of occipital region |
| Hyperextended neck and retracted shoulders | Shortened neck extensor muscles<br>Overstretched neck flexor muscles<br>Excessive cervical lordosis<br>Shortened scapular adductor muscles | Interferes with head centering and midline arm movement in supine<br>Interferes with head control in prone and sitting<br>Limited downward visual gaze |
| "Frog" legs | Shortened hip abductor muscles and iliotibial bands<br>Increased external tibial tortion | Interferes with movement transitions in/out of sitting and prone positions<br>Interferes with hip stability in four-point crawling<br>Prolonged wide-based gait with excessive out-toeing |
| Everted feet | Overstretched ankle invertor muscles<br>Altered foot alignment from muscle imbalance | Pronated foot position on standing<br>Retained immature "foot flat" gait with potential delay in development of "heel to toe" gait pattern from excessive pronation |

Adapted from Sweeney J.K., & Gutierrez, T. (2002). Musculoskeletal implications of preterm infant positioning in the NICU. *Journal of Perinatal and Neonatal Nursing, 16* (1), 58-70.

- Limit the use of the infant seat and replace with play on the floor in prone with a roll under the arms and upper chest to assist head lifting and weight support on arms.
- Discuss the value of the prone play position for strengthening the neck, arms, and trunk in preparation for rolling, sitting, and standing.
- Warn of the injury risk in using infant walkers and the impact on development (Thein, 1997).
- Reinforce the importance of interdisciplinary follow-up for musculoskeletal and neurodevelopmental monitoring.
- Advise expedient follow-up if parents notice signs of head flattening, persistent lateral head

tilt, strong head-turn preference, or asymmetric arm use.

Some infants need specific positioning recommendations from a physical therapist to optimize motor development after discharge (Sweeney & Gutierrez, 2002).

## INTERDISCIPLINARY FOLLOW-UP

Follow-up care at 2, 4, 8, 12, and 18 months minimum, is an essential part of developmental care, to systematically monitor musculoskeletal alignment, growth, and neuromotor maturation through acquisition and refinement of upright posture, manipulative hand skills, movement through basic positions, stance, and ambulation. Refer to Box 8-1 for signs of musculoskeletal or neuromotor abnormality indicating the need for comprehensive examination by a pediatric physical therapist and likely referral for immediate intervention with a strong family teaching component.

Examination of developmental performance in communication and cognitive areas is also critical for early identification of delays so that expedient referral for intervention services will occur. Sensitive management of family concerns and current levels of support (emotional, financial, knowledge) needed for ongoing complex care of their high-risk infant is an important part of the follow-up process.

In addition to routine primary care needs, continuous medical management is required for specific conditions resulting from a preterm birth (e.g., nutrition or feeding difficulty; respiratory or cardiac follow-up).

The interdisciplinary approach using a developmental care team is the ideal way to provide this follow-up for an infant at risk for motor impairment. A pediatrician, nurse practitioner, nurse, physical therapist, and occupational therapist can coordinate the initial care with the family. Consultant services from social work, speech pathology, audiology, psychology, neurology, clinical nutrition, pediatric gastroenterology, and orthopedics might be

---

### Box 8-1   MOTOR IMPAIRMENT "RED FLAGS" DURING NICU FOLLOW-UP

| 2 Months* | 4 Months* | 8 Months* | 12 Months* |
|---|---|---|---|
| Persistent asymmetrical head position; risk for plagiocephaly and torticollis | Poor midline head control in supine position | Inability to sit and roll independently | Inability to pull to stand, 4-point crawl, walk around furniture |
| Jerky or stiff movements of extremities | Difficulty engaging hands at midline and in reaching for dangling toy | Inability to transfer objects between hands | Movement between basic positions |
| Excessive neck or trunk hyperextension in supine position | Persistent fisting of hands | Persistent asymmetry of extremities with differences in muscle tone and motor skill | Persistent asymmetry of control in extremities |
| | Difficulty lifting head and supporting weight on arms in prone position | Hypertonicity of trunk or extremities | |
| | Trunk hypertonicity or hypotonicity | | |
| | Resistance to passive movement in extremities | | |
| | Persistent, dominant asymmetrical tonic neck reflex or tonic labyrinthine reflex in prone position | | |
| | Stiffly extended or "scissored" legs with weight bearing on toes in supported standing | | |

*Ages corrected for prematurity.

indicated. Families are an integral part of the inter-disciplinary team. They might detect functional difficulties in moving or positioning the infant during dressing, bathing, or feeding. The team relies on their concerns and observations to prioritize the case management process.

## CONCLUSION

In this chapter, the chronology and continuity of motor development are discussed in terms of musculoskeletal maturation, prenatal movement sequences, and neonatal posture, tone, and movement competencies. Implications for neonatal care and interdisciplinary monitoring were reviewed for infants with potential musculoskeletal or motor impairment and their families.

As professionals in neonatal care, we have a unique window of opportunity to shape the musculoskeletal system and motor organization of neonates requiring intensive care and to monitor skeletal alignment and motor behavior during the first year of life. We must take advantage of musculoskeletal plasticity through strategic positioning and handling to prevent or minimize deformity in LBW infants, look for early signs of potential movement abnormalities, and advocate for individualized neuromotor, developmental, and family intervention for infants with motor impairment. As members of neonatal developmental care teams, we must make time for creative collaboration on interventions and outcomes to advance, analyze, and refine our practice.

## REFERENCES

Albers, S., & Jorch, G. (1994). Prognostic significance of spontaneous motility in very immature preterm infants under intensive care treatment. *Biology of the Neonate, 66*, 182-187.

Allen, M.C. (1996). Preterm development. In A.J. Capute & P.J. Accardo (Eds.), *Developmental disabilities in infancy and childhood: The spectrum of developmental disabilities* (Vol. 2, 2nd. ed.) (pp. 31-47). Baltimore, MD: Paul H Brookes.

Allen, M.C., & Capute, A.J. (1990). Tone and reflex development before term. *Pediatrics, 85*(3 Pt 2), 393-399.

Amiel-Tison, C., & Grenier, A. (1983). *Neurologic evaluation of the newborn infant.* (J.J. Steichen, P. Steichen-Asch, & C. Paxton Braun, Trans.). New York: Masson Publishing. (Original work published 1980.).

Brown, K.J., Omar, T., & O'Regan, M. (1997). Brain development and the development of tone and movement. In K.J. Connolly & H. Frosberg (Eds.), Neurophysiology & neuropsychology of motor development (pp. 42-53). *Clinics in Developmental Medicine, 143-144.* Cambridge, England: Cambridge Press.

Butler, J.M. (2003). Assessment and management of the musculoskeletal system (pp. 661-672). In C. Kenner & J.W. Lott (Eds.), *Comprehensive neonatal Nursing: A physiologic perspective* (3rd ed.). St. Louis: W.B. Saunders.

Cioni, G., Prechtl, H.F.R., Ferrari, F., et al. (1997). Which better predicts later outcome in fullterm infants: quality of general movements or neurological examination? *Early Human Development, 50*(1), 71-85.

Davis P.M., Robinson R., Harris L., & Cartlidge P.H. (1993). Persistent mild hip deformation in preterm infants. *Archives of Disease in Childhood, 69*(5), 597-598.

de Groot, L. (2000). Posture and motility in preterm infants. Faculty of Human Movement Sciences, Department of Neonatology, Vrije Universiteit, Amsterdam, The Netherlands. *Developmental Medicine and Child Neurology, 43*(1), 65-68.

de Groot, L., Hoek, A.M., Hopkins, B., et al. (1993). Development of muscle power in preterm infants: Individual trajectories after term age. *Neuropediatrics, 24*, 68-73.

de Groot, L., Hoek, A.M., Hopkins, B., et al. (1992). Development of the relationship between active and passive muscle power in preterms after term age. *Neuropediatrics, 23*, 298-305.

de Groot, L., Hopkins, B., & Touwen, B.C.L. (1991). A method to assess development of muscle power in preterms after term age. *Neuropediatrics, 23*, 172-179.

de Vries, J.I.P., Visser, G.H., & Prechtl, H.F.R. (1984). Fetal motility in the first half of pregnancy. In H.F.R. Prechtl (Ed.), *Continuity of neural functions from prenatal to postnatal life* (pp. 46-64). Philadelphia: J.B. Lippincott.

de Vries, J.I., Wimmers, R.H., Ververs, I.A., et al. (2001). Fetal handedness and head position preference: A developmental study. *Developmental Psychobiology, 39*(3), 171-180.

Dreyfus, C.J., & Schapira, F. (1979). Biochemistry of muscle development (pp. 239-252). In U. Stave (Ed.), *Perinatal physiology.* New York: Plenum.

Dubowitz, L.M.S., & Dubowitz, V. (1999). The neurological assessment of the preterm and full-term newborn infant (2nd ed.). *Clinics in Developmental Medicine, 148.* Philadelphia: J.B. Lippincott.

Dubowitz, V. (1965). Enzyme histochemistry of skeletal muscle: Part 1. Developing animal muscle; Part 2. Developing human muscle. *Journal of Neurology, Neurosurgery, & Psychiatry, 28*, 516-524.

Einspieler, C., Prechtl, H.F.R., Ferrari, F., et al. (1997). The qualitative assessment of general movements in preterm, term and young infants—Review of the methodology. *Early Human Development, 50*(1), 47-60.

Ferrari, F., Cioni, G., & Prechtl, H.F.R. (1990). Qualitative changes of general movements in preterm infants with brain lesions. *Early Human Development, 23*, 193-231.

Gajdosik, C.G., & Gajdosik, R.L. (2000). Musculoskeletal development and adaptation (pp. 117-140). In S. Campbell (Ed.), *Physical therapy for children*. Philadelphia: W.B. Saunders.

Georgieff, M.K., & Bernbaum, J.C. (1986). Abnormal shoulder muscle tone in premature infants during their first 18 months of life. *Developmental and Behavioral Pediatrics, 6*, 327-333.

Gesell, A. (1945). The *embryology of behaviour: The beginnings of the human mind*. New York: Harper.

Gorga D., Stern, F.M., Ross G., & Nagler, W. (1988). Neuromotor development of preterm and full-term infants. *Early Human Development, 18*, 137-149.

Grove, B.K. (1989). Muscle differentiation and the origin of muscle fiber diversity. *CRC Critical Reviews in Neurobiology, 4*, 201-234.

Hadders-Algra, M., Klip-Van den Nieuwendijk, A.W., Martijn, A., et al. (1997). Assessment of general movements: Towards a better understanding of a sensitive method to evaluate brain function in young infants. *Developmental Medicine and Child Neurology, 39*(2), 88-98.

Hensinger, R.N., & Jones, E.T. (1981). *Neonatal orthopedics*. New York: Grune & Stratton.

Humphrey, T. (1978). Function of the nervous system during prenatal life. In U. Stave (Ed.), *Physiology of the perinatal period* (Vol. 2; pp. 751-796). New York: Plenum Medical.

Ianniruberto, A., & Tajani, E. (1981). Ultrasonographic study of fetal movements. *Seminars in Perinatology, 5*(2), 175-181.

Jones, S., & Bell, M.J. (2002). Distal radius fracture in a premature infant with osteopenia caused by handling during intravenous cannulation. *Injury, 33*(3), 265-266.

Kakebeeke, T.H., von Siebenthal, K., & Largo, R.H. (1998). Movement quality in preterm infants prior to term. *Biology of the Neonate, 73*, 145-154.

Katz, K., Krikler, R., Wielunsky, E., & Merlob, P. (1991). Effect of neonatal posture on later lower limb rotation and gait in premature infants. *Journal of Pediatric Orthopedics, 11*(4), 520-522.

Kozuma, S., Okai, T., Nemoto, A., et al. (1997). Developmental sequence of human fetal body movements in the second half of pregnancy. *American Journal of Perinatolgy, 14*(3), 165-169.

Milani-Comparetti, A., & Gidoni, E.A. (1967). Pattern analysis of motor development and its disorders. *Developmental Medicine & Child Neurology, 9*(5), 625-630.

Moore, K.L., & Persaud, T.V.N. (2003). *The developing human: Clinically oriented embryology* (7th ed.). St. Louis: Mosby.

Plantinga, Y., Perdock, J., & de Groot, L. (1997). Hand function in low-risk preterm infants: Its relation to muscle power regulation. *Developmental Medicine & Child Neurology, 39*, 6-11.

Prechtl, H.F.R. & Nolte, R. (1984). Motor behavior of preterm infants. In H.F.R. Prechtl (Ed.), *Continuity of neural functions from prenatal to postnatal life* (pp. 79-92). London: Spastics International Medical Publications.

Prechtl, H.F.R. (1984). Continuity and change in early neural development. In H.F.R. Prechtl (Ed.), *Continuity of neural functions from prenatal to postnatal life* (pp. 1-15). London: Spastics International Medical Publications.

Prechtl, H.F.R. (1989). Fetal behavior. In A. Hill & J.J. Volpe (Eds.), *Fetal neurology* (pp. 1-14). International Review of Child Neurology Series. New York: Raven Press.

Prechtl, H.F.R. (1997a). The importance of fetal movements. In K.J. Connolly & H. Frosberg (Eds.), *Neurophysiology and neuropsychology of motor development* (pp. 42-53). Clinics in Developmental Medicine, 143-144. Cambridge, England: Cambridge Press.

Prechtl, H.F.R. (1997b). Editorial: State of the art of a new functional assessment of the young nervous system. An early predictor of cerebral palsy. *Early Human Development, 50*(1), 1-11.

Prechtl, H.R. (2001). General movement assessment as a method of developmental neurology: new paradigms and their consequences. The 1999 Ronnie MacKeith lecture. *Developmental Medicine and Child Neurology, 43*(12), 836-842.

Roodenburg, P.J., Wladimiroff, J.W., van Es, A., & Prechtl, H.F.R. (1991). Classification and quantitative aspects of fetal movements during the second half of normal pregnancy. *Early Human Development, 25*(1), 19-35.

Sadler, T.W., & Langman, J. (2000). *Langman's medical embryology* (8th ed.). Philadelphia: Lippincott, Williams, & Wilkins.

Saint-Anne Dargassies, S. (1977). *Neurological development in the full term and premature neonate*. New York: Excerpta Medica.

Sans, J.R. (1987). Cell lineage and the origin of muscle fiber types. *Trends in Neuroscience, 10*, 119-121.

Sparling, J.W. (Ed.). (1993). Concepts in fetal movement research. *Physical and Occupational Therapy in Pediatrics, 12*(2/3), 1-18.

Sparling, J.W., Van Tol., J., & Chescheir, N.C. (1999). Fetal and neonatal hand movement. *Physical Therapy, 79*(1), 24-39.

Sparling, J.W., & Wilhelm, I.J. (1993). Quantitative measurement of fetal movement: Fetal Posture and Movement

Assessment (F-PAM); Physical Therapy/79 (1); Fetal and Neonatal Hand Movement, *12*(2/3), 97-114.

Sweeney, J.K., & Gutierrez, T. (2002). Musculoskeletal implications of preterm infant positioning in the NICU. *Journal of Perinatal and Neonatal Nursing, 16*(1), 58-70.

Sweeney, J.K., & Swanson, M.W. (2001). Low birth weight infants: neonatal care and follow-up. In D. Umphred (Ed.), *Neurological rehabilitation* (4th ed.; pp. 203-258). St Louis: Mosby.

Thein, M.M. (1997). Infant walker use, injuries, and motor development. *Injury Prevention, 3,* 63-66.

Towen, B.C. (1990). Variability and stereotyping of spontaneous motility as a predictor of neurological development of preterm infants. *Developmental Medicine and Child Neurology, 32*(6), 501-508.

# 9 Factors That Can Influence Fetal Development

## Jacqueline M. McGrath, Carole Kenner, and Kelly A. Amspacher

There are numerous factors that influence fetal development and, therefore, the fetus' and newborn's neurobehavioral development and outcomes. This chapter provides an overview of the most noted factors, according to research and current literature. Individuality is developed at an early stage of intrauterine existence, and the normal growth and development of a fetus is influenced by the integration of several factors. Hereditary factors, as well as the environment of the fetus and the mother, affect the developing infant.

The influences of the prenatal, perinatal, and postnatal periods on fetal/neonatal development are outlined (Figure 9-1). The chapter is categorized by "natal" period, but influences by intrinsic and extrinsic factors on development are also listed. Intrinsic factors are present in all pregnancies. They include maternal age, race, height-weight ratio at conception, height, parity, and gender of the fetus. Extrinsic factors might also be present in pregnancies. Extrinsic factors include: environmental and fetal factors (i.e., multiple births, fetal infections); medical and obstetric complications of pregnancy; and adverse maternal practices (e.g. no or poor prenatal care, cigarette smoking, substance abuse), and genetic/family history. Throughout this chapter, it is imperative that the reader is mindful of individual maternal and fetal differences. From an individualized, family-centered, developmental care (IFDC) philosophy, these fetal influences can affect how the newborn and family respond to the extrauterine environment and to each other. The prenatal period is the beginning and a vital part of the whole picture of developing and implementing IFDC with infants and families.

## PRENATAL INFLUENCES ON FETAL DEVELOPMENT (INTRINSIC FACTORS DURING PREGNANCY)

Prenatal influences on fetal development—the intrinsic factors—comprise the woman's previous pregnancy history as well as age, race, height-weight ratio at conception, height, parity, and the gender of the fetus. For example, did the mother have a previous stillborn? If there was a positive history, the current fetus might be at risk for intrauterine growth restriction (IUGR), prematurity, or another stillborn (usually at term) delivery, possibly related to genetic abnormalities. Was there a history of a premature birth—if so, what was the cause (e.g., incompetent cervix)? This history raises the risk and concern of another premature delivery. A mother who is too young or too old is also at greater risk (Box 9-1). A young mother might have a poorer nutritional status related to her own growth and development, whereas advanced maternal age has been associated with an increase in chromosomal abnormalities, such as Down syndrome (Kinzler, Ananth, Smulian, et al., 2002). It is also known that mothers who were low birthweight (LBW) babies are at increased risk to give birth to lower birthweight infants. Parity is another consideration. A woman who is prima gravida (0) or a multigravida (more than 4) para is suspect for problems. In the first case, there is no previous history of a pregnancy and delivery, and in the latter case, the uterus has been stretched several times, organs have been reshaped, and the woman is older with the current pregnancy than she was with previous. All of these factors can lead to a complication in labor or delivery. Additionally, a short interval between pregnancies and births does not allow the mother's body to rebuild essential nutrients, muscle tissue/tone, and hormonal balance to support another developing

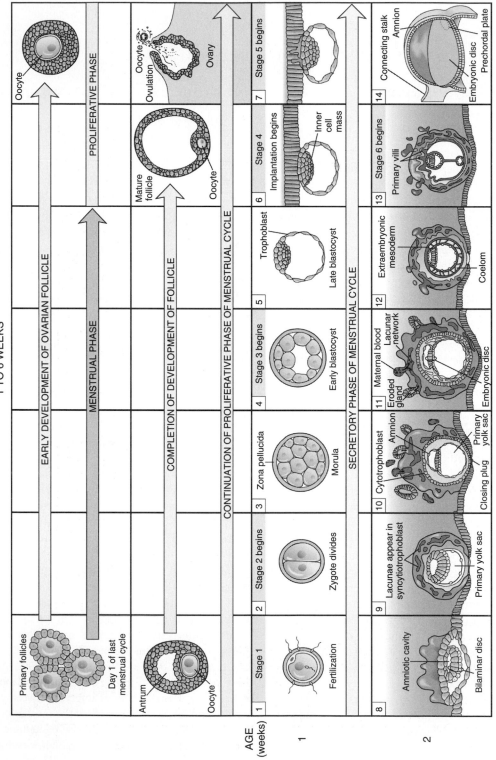

Figure **9–1** Critical periods of development. (*From Moore, K.L., & Persaud, T.V.N. [2003]. Before we are born: Essentials of embryology and birth defects [6th ed.]. St. Louis : W.B. Saunders.*)

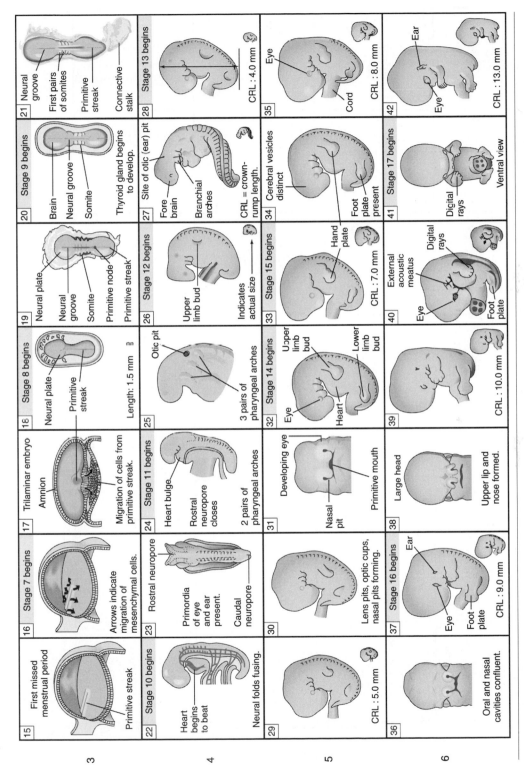

**15** First missed menstrual period — Primitive streak

**16** Stage 7 begins — Arrows indicate migration of mesenchymal cells.

**17** Trilaminar embryo — Amnion — Migration of cells from primitive streak.

**18** Stage 8 begins — Neural plate — Primitive streak — Length: 1.5 mm

**19** Neural plate — Neural groove — Somite — Primitive node — Primitive streak

**20** Stage 9 begins — Brain — Neural groove — Somite — Thyroid gland begins to develop.

**21** Neural groove — First pairs of somites — Primitive streak — Connective stalk

**22** Stage 10 begins — Heart begins to beat — Neural folds fusing.

**23** Rostral neuropore — Primordia of eye and ear present. — Caudal neuropore

**24** Stage 11 begins — Heart bulge — Rostral neuropore closes — 2 pairs of pharyngeal arches

**25** Otic pit — 3 pairs of pharyngeal arches

**26** Stage 12 begins — Upper limb bud — Indicates actual size

**27** Fore brain — Branchial arches — Site of otic (ear) pit — CRL = crown-rump length.

**28** Stage 13 begins — CRL : 4.0 mm

**29** CRL : 5.0 mm

**30**

**31** Developing eye — Nasal pit — Primitive mouth

**32** Stage 14 begins — Eye — Upper limb bud — Lower limb bud — Heart

**33** Stage 15 begins — Hand plate — CRL : 7.0 mm

**34** Cerebral vesicles distinct — Foot plate present

**35** Eye — Cord — CRL : 8.0 mm

**36** Oral and nasal cavities confluent.

**37** Stage 16 begins — Eye — Foot plate — Ear — CRL : 9.0 mm

**38** Large head — Upper lip and nose formed.

**39** CRL : 10.0 mm

**40** Eye — External acoustic meatus — Digital rays — Foot plate

**41** Stage 17 begins — Digital rays — Ventral view

**42** Eye — Ear — CRL : 13.0 mm

3   4   5   6

*Continued*

Figure **9-1** Cont'd.

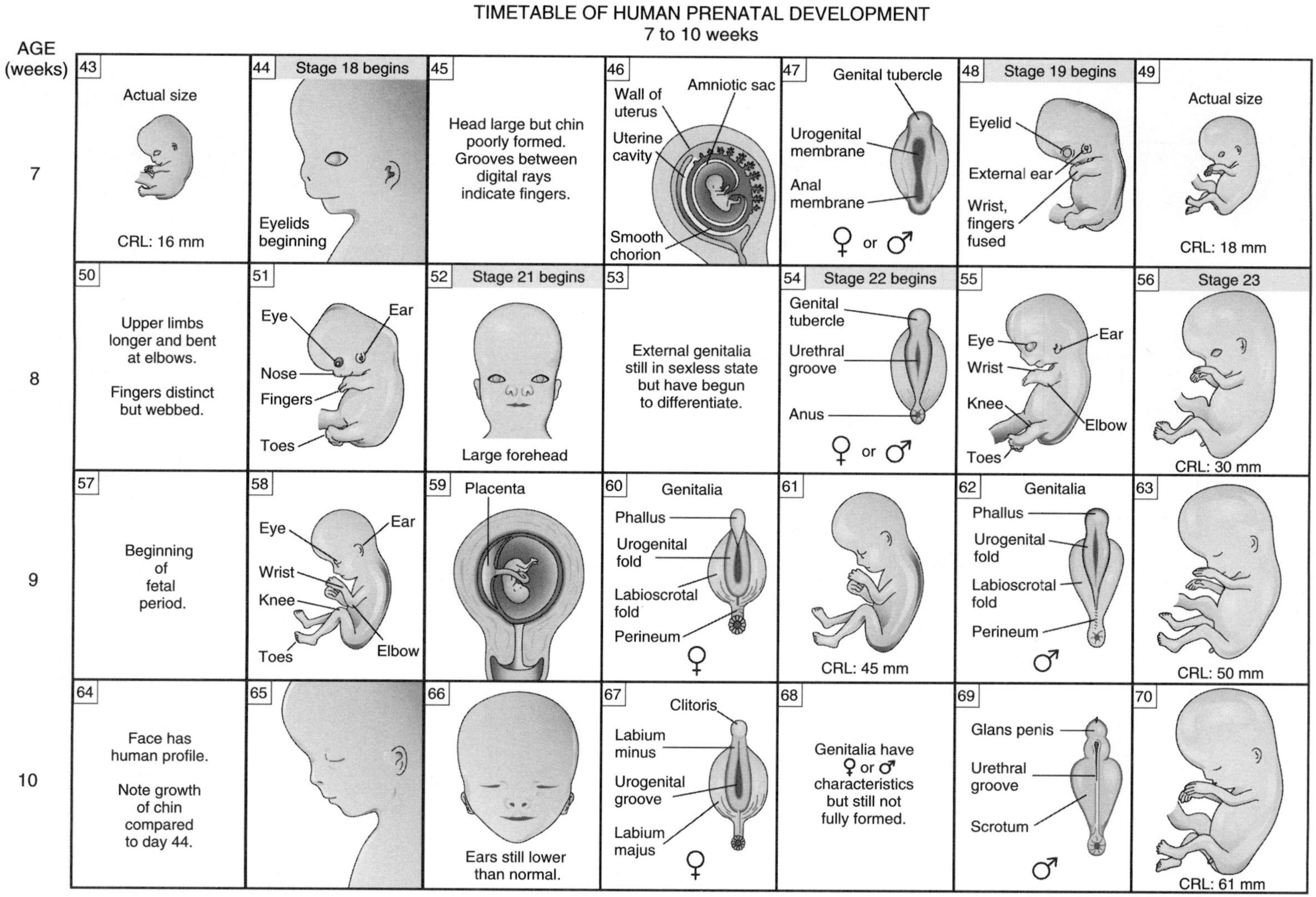

TIMETABLE OF HUMAN PRENATAL DEVELOPMENT
7 to 10 weeks

Figure **9-1** Cont'd.

**Eleventh Week to Full Term**

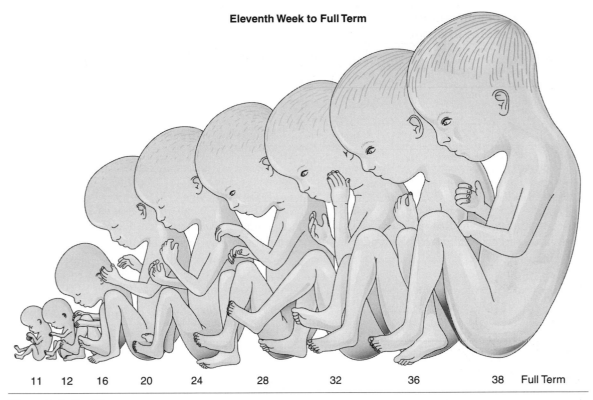

| 11 | 12 | 16 | 20 | 24 | 28 | 32 | 36 | 38 | Full Term |

Figure **9-1**  Cont'd.

Box **9-1**   MATERNAL FACTORS AND INFANT RISK

| Maternal Factor | Fetal/Infant Risks |
|---|---|
| Adolescent age (Kinzler, Ananth, Smulian, et al., 2002) (pregnancy that occurs at the two age extremes [<16 years and 35 years] creates maternal and fetal risks) | • Nutrition (including eating disorders)<br>• Prenatal care<br>• Support system<br>• Socioeconomic system<br>• Preeclampsia<br>• Intrauterine growth restriction<br>• Low birthweight |
| Advanced maternal age issues | • Chronic diseases that affect pregnancy<br>• Increased incidence of chromosomal abnormalities<br>• Pregnancy-related conditions might occur (e.g., diabetes, preeclampsia, vaginal bleeding)<br>• Increased risk for congenital and chromosomal anomalies |
| Small maternal size (weight <100 lbs at conception) | • Intrauterine growth restriction<br>• Increased potential for hypoxia during labor and delivery |
| Large maternal size (weight >200 lbs at conception) | • Increased risk for poor fetal nutrition |

Table 9-1    PROPORTION OF LOW BIRTHWEIGHT AND VERY LOW BIRTHWEIGHT INFANTS
BY RACE/ETHNICITY

| Race/Ethnicity of Infants | Low Birthweight (%) | Very Low Birthweight (%) |
|---|---|---|
| African American | 13.1 | 3.0 |
| Caucasian | 6.8 | 1.2 |
| Native American | 7.3 | 1.3 |
| Asian or Pacific Islander | 7.5 | 1.0 |

Data from Child Trends Databank, 2001.

fetus. Therefore, this period is also a consideration that might adversely affect a neonatal outcome.

Race/ethnicity is another risk factor to consider. Black infants are more likely to be born premature or LBW than are white infants in the United States (Alexander, Kogan, Bader, et al., 2003). However, some researchers are finding that foreign-born blacks have lower infant mortality than native-born blacks—an area that needs further exploration (Rosenberg, Desai, & Kan, 2002). Infants born to black mothers were more than twice as likely to be LBW and nearly three times as likely than infants born to white mothers to be very LBW (VLBW). American-Indian infants were less likely than Asian or Pacific Islander infants to be born LBW, but more likely to be VLBW (Table 9-1). It is also a well known fact that more male fetus's are conceived than female; however, by the end of gestation, these differences are almost completely equal, making the gender of the fetus another issue to consider when other risk factors are being evaluated.

## PRENATAL INFLUENCES ON FETAL DEVELOPMENT (EXTRINSIC FACTORS) DURING PREGNANCY

What are some of the other extrinsic factors that are considered to influence neonatal outcomes and contribute to the differences seen with intrinsic factors and among ethnic groups? Some are marital status; no or poor prenatal care; poor maternal nutrition; maternal disease, including infection history, intake of maternal medications, maternal trauma or surgery, exposure to environmental toxic agents; teratogens; and suspect genetic history. Current researchers are examining the role of genes in mediating prenatal exposures. This research includes

exposures to maternal diseases and medications. Another area of growing research is the perinatal histories of women who are living with chronic conditions and giving birth. Such conditions include sickle cell anemia, cystic fibrosis, congenital heart disease (CHD), and HIV. Until recently, women with these conditions either did not live until childbearing age or were counseled not to conceive or carry a pregnancy to term.

### Maternal Lifestyle

Maternal lifestyle is an important extrinsic factor. Being a single mother with lower socioeconomic status (SES) and educational level (together or separate) are risk factors. These women might live in inadequate housing, and they might not have access to good, consistent prenatal care. Poor prenatal care coupled with these or other risk factors can lead to adverse neonatal outcomes (Vintzileos, Ananth, Smulian, et al., 2002). The nutritional status of these women might be substandard, affecting overall fetal growth and development, placing them at risk for IUGR, LBWs, and, thus, adverse neonatal outcomes (Kramer, 2003).

The nutrition of the mother is one of the major determinants of fetal growth and, therefore, of the weight and health of the infant at birth (Fall, Yajnik, Rao, et al., 2003). Poor diet in the mother places the infant at risk for fetal malnutrition and prematurity (Rondo & Tomkins, 1999). Most LBW infants have small placentas. This finding reflects the fact that placental growth precedes that of the fetus. Research has linked placental size with decreased maternal carbohydrate intake early in the pregnancy and decreased fetal size at birth with decreased protein intake later in the pregnancy (Little, Zadorozhnaja, Hulchiy, et al., 2003).

Box 9-2   DEFICIENCIES IN ESSENTIAL NUTRIENTS DURING PREGNANCY AND NEONATAL OUTCOMES

| Deficient Nutrient | Neonatal Outcomes |
| --- | --- |
| Riboflavin | Poor skeletal formation |
| Pyridoxine | Decreased dendritic arborization and reduced numbers of myelinated axons and synapses, neuromotor complications, less mature reactive and adaptive behavior on the Brazelton Neonatal Assessment Scale, and lower birthweight |
| Vitamin $B_{12}$ | Hydrocephalus |
| Iron | Influences maternal hemoglobin levels, which, in turn, supply oxygen to the fetus |

Deprivation of essential nutrients can lead to stunted growth and various birth abnormalities (Box 9-2). Most of the information available on nutrition for optimal fetal health is based on animal studies and the action of placental hormones (Alejandro, Perez, Pedrana, et al., 2002; Lacroix, Guibourdenche, Frendo, et al., 2002). The first growth phase, hyperplasia, during the first trimester when cells are rapidly dividing and multiplying, requires folic acid and vitamin $B_{12}$, which play a role in the synthesis of nucleic acids. The next fetal growth phase, hypertrophy, occurs during the second and third trimester of pregnancy when the cells increase in size and require amino acids and vitamin $B_{12}$ for protein synthesis.

Much of the current research in this area has come from our knowledge of eating disorders and effects on the maternal organs and, ultimately, fetal growth (Goldman & Koren, 2003a). A low socioeconomic/low educational level is another factor that is linked with an increased incidence of IUGR and LBW (less than 2500 g).

## MATERNAL COMPLICATIONS
### Diabetes

Diabetes in pregnancy has long been recognized as a serious maternal, fetal, and neonatal problem. Due to faulty metabolism of insulin and related risk factors, there are several fetal and neonatal effects. The effects of diabetes on the fetus are directly related to the degree of glucose control before conception and on the presence of maternal vascular complications. The expression of neonatal problems in relationship to maternal disease is linked to the severity of the mother's condition (Bo, Marchisio, Volpiano, et al.,

2003; Catalano, Kirwan, Haugel-De Mouzon, et al., 2003; de Sereday, Damiano, Gonzalez, et al., 2003). Some mothers experience placental insufficiency that can lead to varying degrees of nutritional or hypoxic damage to the fetus resulting in IUGR and oligohydramnios. IUGR has been found to be associated with placental insufficiency in women with class D or higher diabetes and with existing vascular disease before pregnancy.

Congenital defects are four times more likely to occur in diabetic women. Congenital anomalies are directly related to diabetic control in the 3-month period before conception and during the first 2 months of pregnancy, a time when mothers might not be preparing for pregnancy or know they are pregnant. Common fetal anomalies related to diabetes include neural tube defects, cardiac defects, gastrointestinal malformations, and renal anomalies (Chang, Horal, Jain, et al., 2003; Kalter, 2003). Macrosomia is also a common problem related to fetal insulinemia. It occurs in response to elevated maternal glucose that leads to increased growth and fat deposition in the infant. These infants are at increased risk for birth trauma, particularly shoulder dystocia, brachial plexus injuries, facial nerve injuries, and asphyxia, as well as rebound neonatal hypoglycemia related to a sudden decrease in glucose in the blood stream after birth. Infants of diabetic mothers are also at risk for delayed lung maturity. This delay is related to the elevated blood glucose in utero, which appears to interfere with the production of phosphatidyl glycerol (surfactant). Much has been learned about the effects of diabetes on pregnancy, and, with good control, negative outcomes can be limited. Therefore, preconception education and prenatal care in this population is essential.

## Cardiac Disease

The incidence of cardiac disease in the pregnant population is between 0.5% and 2%. Previously the leading cause of cardiac disease, rheumatic fever is responsible for only 50% of cardiac disease in pregnancy. Congenital heart disease (CHD) now plays a more prominent role, because there is better childhood management of CHD. These children are now growing to adulthood and becoming parents (Avila, Rossi, Ramires, et al., 2003; Bianca & Ettore, 2002; Vasapollo, Valensis, Novelli, et al., 2002). If either parent has a congenital heart defect, the fetus has an increased risk for having a congenital cardiac defect. Fetal effects are the result of decreased systemic circulation or decreased oxygenation. When maternal circulation is compromised, uterine blood flow can be severely diminished, leading to such effects as IUGR and CNS hypoxia. Decreases in fetal oxygenation in such cases can also lead to varying degrees of mental retardation and fetal distress. More emphasis is being placed on prenatal screening for cardiac disease and CHD that might otherwise go undetected (Allan, 2003), and on early detection of fetal cardiac problems. Therefore the emphasis can now be directed toward prevention (Suchet, 2003; Zhang, Levi, Alexander, et al., 2002). Additionally, the role of folic acid supplementation is under study as prevention for CHD (McDonald, Ferguson, Tam, et al., 2003). Maternal anemia also has fetal/neonatal implications related to decreased oxygen-carrying capacity that can place the infant at risk for both prematurity and LBW (Bondevik, Lie, Ulstein, 2001; Malhotra, Sharma, Batra, et al., 2002; Rasmussen, 2001). Anemia is defined as:

- <9 g/dL hemoglobin, <29% hematocrit for whites
- <8.2 g/dL hemoglobin, <26% hematocrit for blacks

### Maternal Medications

Drugs, both prescription and over-the-counter, can have a variety of effects on the fetus (Table 9-2). The dose of the agent, timing of exposure, agent synergism, rate of metabolism, and host susceptibility of both mother and fetus play a role in fetal outcome. Polydrug (prescription or street drugs and/or herbals) use further complicates the problem. Problems related to drug use are not just limited to the mother, but

can have an adverse effect on future offspring. In addition, there is a possibility that drugs taken by a man can damage spermatozoa. Abnormal sperma-tozoa can cause congenital malformations.

Common examples of the fetal and neonatal effects of medications and/or drugs include:

- Illicit street drugs such as methamphetamine that can lead to prematurity, IUGR, developmental delays, tremulousness, exaggerated startle reflex, and alterations in visual processing. The quality of alertness in infants can be affected, and frontal-lobe dysfunction can also become apparent later in development (Smith, Yonekura, Wallace, et al., 2003; Won, Bubula, & Heller, 2002).
- Anticoagulants, such as warfarin (Coumadin), can lead to growth and developmental retardation, deafness, and scoliosis when exposure is in the first trimester. When exposure is in the second and third trimester, affects include eye anomalies, hydrocephaly, and other CNS defects, and/or neonatal hemorrhage (Houman, Ksontini-Smida, & Miled, 2002; Srivastava, Gupta, Singh, et al., 2002).
- Anticonvulsants, such as phenytoin (Dilantin), can cause seizure-related hypoxia and acidosis in the embryo/fetus. Intrauterine and extrauterine growth restriction and mental impairment are also not uncommon (Stoler, 2001).
- Antianxiety agents or mood elevators, such as diazepam, have been associated with increased congenital malformations when taken in the first trimester (Iqbal, Sobhan, Aftab, et al., 2002). Trimethadione can cause developmental delay and mental impairment (Azarbaymani & Danielsson, 1998, 2002).
- Antidepressants and psychotropics, such as chlordiazepoxide hydrochloride (Librium), might cause mental retardation, spastic dysplegia, deafness, and microcephaly (Altshuler, Cohen, Szuba, et al., 1997; Einarson, Bonari, Voyer-Lavigne, et al., 2003; Hendrick, Smith, Suri, et al., 2003).

The use of herbal preparations by pregnant women is also growing. Little research outside of animal studies has been done to determine the effects on the developing fetus and the resultant neonate. However, women are asking more questions related

Table **9-2**  DRUGS ASSOCIATED WITH CONGENITAL MALFORMATIONS IN HUMANS

| Drug | Fetal Growth | Postnatal Growth | Mental Retardation | Central Nervous System | Cardiovascular System | Musculo-skeletal System | Uro-genital System | Eyes And Ears | Thyroid Gland |
|---|---|---|---|---|---|---|---|---|---|
| **ANTIMICROBIALS** | | | | | | | | | |
| Tetracycline | | | | | | X | | | |
| Streptomycin | | | | | | | | X | |
| Quinine | | | | | | | | X | |
| **ANTINEOPLASTICS** | | | | | | | | | |
| Methotrexate | X | X | | X | | X | | | |
| Busulfan, chlorambucil, cyclophosphamide | X | X | | X | | X | X | X | |
| **CENTRAL NERVOUS SYSTEM DRUGS** | | | | | | | | | |
| Cocaine | | | | X | X | | | | |
| Lithium | | | | | X | | | | |
| Thalidomide | | | | | | X | | | |
| **ANTICONVULSANTS** | | | | | | | | | |
| Phenytoin | | X | X | | | X | | X | |
| Barbiturates | | X | X | | | x | | | |
| Trimethadione | | X | | | X | X | X | X | |
| Valproic acid | | X | | X | | x | | | |
| Carbamazepine | | | | X | | X | | | |
| **STEROID HORMONES** | | | | | | | | | |
| Androgens | | | | | | | X | | |
| Diethylstilbestrol | | | | | | | X | | |
| Estrogen, progestins | | | | | | | X | | |
| **OTHER** | | | | | | | | | |
| Iodine, propylthiouracil | | | | | | | | | X |
| Warfarin | | X | | | X | X | X | X | |
| Alcohol | | X | X | | | X | | X | |
| Tobacco smoking | X | | | | | | | | |
| Isotretinoin, vitamin A | | | X | X | X | | x | | |

From Blackburn, S.T. (2002). *Maternal, fetal, & neonatal physiology: A clinical perspective* (2nd ed.; p. 200). St. Louis: W.B. Saunders.

to the safety and effects of such products. There are no definitive answers (Goldman & Koren, 2003b), but it is important that the use of herbs, both ingested and topical, be discussed in the maternal history review (Pinn & Pallett, 2002). Some studies have included pregnant women who are using St. John's Wort (Cada, Hansen, LaBorde, et al., 2001; Rayburn, Christensen, & Gonzalez, 2000). Pinn (2001) provides a useful review of herbs used to prevent and treat pregnancy-related issues.

Use of medications such as antibiotics presents a dilemma in that the continued course of prenatal infection might have a worse outcome than the medication's effects on the developing fetus. Examples are: clindamycin to treat bacterial vaginosis might increase the incidence of miscarriage and premature birth (Leitich, Brunbauer, Bodner-Adler, et al., 2003; Ugwumadu, Manonda, Reid, et al., 2003); treatment of group B streptococcus during pregnancy might damage the auditory nerve and lead to deafness (Sanders, Roberts, & Gilbert, 2002); and medications related to toxoplasmosis can have other negative effects (Gilbert & Gras, 2003). The effects of any medications will depend on the critical period of development or stage of fetal development at the time of the exposure (see Table 9-2). The rapidly developing neurologic system is always a concern, even in the last trimester of gestation. See Chapter 6, Critical Periods of Development, and Chapter 7, Neurologic Development, for more information.

## MATERNAL TRAUMA

Trauma is the leading cause of death in women of childbearing years. Unfortunately, a growing trend in our society, globally, is violence against pregnant women (Asling-Monemi, Pena, Ellsberg, et al., 2003; Johnson, Haider, Ellis, et al., 2003). Of the traumatic injuries that occur in pregnant women, 10% occur in the first trimester, 40% in the second trimester, and 50% in the third trimester. The fetus is vulnerable to the affects of maternal trauma, especially blunt or penetrating trauma to the abdomen (Fletcher, Wharfe, & Mitchell, 2003; Naylor & Olson, 2003). Common effects on the fetus caused by violence against pregnant women include: preterm rupture of membranes; premature labor and delivery; occult placental abruption with fetomaternal bleed; fetal

skull injuries, especially when the fetal head is engaged and there is a maternal pelvic fracture; hypoxic compromise secondary to maternal respiratory embarrassment; shock; disseminated intravascular coagulopathy (DIC); thermal injury; or maternal arrest. When trauma occurs, the effects to both the mother and the fetus must be considered.

## MATERNAL SURGERY

Anesthesia management priorities during surgery that must occur during a pregnancy are: maternal safety, avoidance of teratogenic drug use, avoidance of fetal asphyxia, and prevention of premature labor (Al-Fozan & Tulandi, 2002; Goodman, 2002). The following fetal parameters are instrumental in making clinical practice decisions: gestational age of lowest risk for fetus and anesthesia of choice based on surgery and gestational age of the fetus. The most common surgeries during gestation are cholecystectomy; ovarian cystectomy or oophorectomy; appendectomy; and cervical cerclage. Preoperative, intraoperative, and postoperative interventions to monitor for and treat any alteration in maternal tissue perfusion, fetal tissue perfusion, and maternal/fetal dyad health must be a priority in management.

## FETAL COMPLICATIONS

Many other complications can occur during a pregnancy that are not related to the maternal environment or predisposition. These issues are often related to the fetus and intrinsic factors. One example of such complications is hydrops fetalis (Liu, Huang, & Chou, 2002; Meyer, 2003). Hydrops fetalis is generalized subcutaneous edema in a fetus or neonate. It is usually accompanied by ascites and pleural and/or pericardial effusions. In this disease process, maternal alloimmune antibodies cross the placenta and destroy fetal erythrocytes. ABO and Rh incompatibilities with maternal blood types are the most common. Nonimmune hydrops (Henrich, Heeger, Schmider, et al., 2002) occurs for several reasons, including: cardiovascular (most frequent case); hematologic, such as alpha-thalassemia (Sohan, Billington, Pamphilon, et al., 2002); glucose-6-phosphate dehydrogenase deficiency; chronic fetal-maternal or twin-to-twin transfusion; renal; infectious disease (Meyer, 2003), such as syphilis, rubella, cytomegalovirus; pulmonary;

gastrointestinal such as in utero volvulus and meconium peritonitis; and chromosomal, such as achondroplasia, Turner syndrome, trisomy 13, 18, 21, triploidy, and aneuploidy.

## TERATOGENS

Susceptibility of the fetus varies with the developmental stage at the time of exposure. Any of the previously discussed agents—for example, drugs, illegal substances, infections, maternal diseases—can also be considered a teratogen (Blackburn, 2002). Susceptibility also depends on the genetic makeup of the mother and embryo/fetus and the manner in which it responds to environmental factors (Petrini, Damus, Russell, et al., 2002). Pregnant women and, therefore, the fetus are also susceptible to occupational hazards (Box 9-3).

## GENETIC HISTORY

A birth defect is defined as an abnormality of structure, function, or metabolism, whether genetically determined or a result of environmental interference during embryonic life or fetal life. With our growing knowledge of the human genome, we can now identify many of the genes and gene sequences that are involved in congenital anomalies. This is different from a congenital defect that might cause disease from the time of conception through birth or later in life. Autosomal dominant disorders (1218 identified disorders) are the most common. In these disorders, males and females are affected equally, and either parent can pass on the gene to sons or daughters. An affected infant has an affected parent if the mutation is not new. Unaffected offspring of an affected parent will have all normal offspring if the mate is an unaffected person. It can be anticipated that approximately half of the sons and daughters of an affected parent can have the disorder. If both parents are affected, three fourths of the offspring will be affected. Family history of an anomaly indicates a vertical route of transmission through successive generations on one side of the family. Examples of autosomal dominant disorders: myotonic dystrophy, neurofibromatosis, and coronary artery disease.

Autosomal recessive disorders (947 identified disorders) are less common, and, therefore, recessive. Males and females are affected equally. Parents of affected offspring are rarely affected and are usually heterozygous carriers. After the birth of an affected offspring, there is a 25% chance, with each pregnancy, of having another affected offspring and a 50% chance that the offspring will be a carrier. Sometimes in the history there is a distant relative with the disorder. No family history indicates a horizontal route of transmission in the same generation. Examples are: cystic fibrosis, sickle cell anemia, Tay-Sachs disease, and thalassemia major.

The next pattern of inheritance is X-linked dominant disorders. In this pattern, both genders can be affected. Affected males will have all affected daughters and no affected sons. Affected females will transmit the disorder in the same manner as with autosomal dominant patterns. However, in X-linked recessive disorders, only male offspring are affected. Carrier females transmit the disorder. All sons of affected males will be normal. All daughters of affected males will be carriers. Transmission is horizontal among males in the same generation. Examples are: Duchenne's muscular dystrophy, hemophilia, color blindness, and glucose-6-phosphate dehydrogenase deficiency.

## DETECTABLE ANOMALIES

Technology to assess fetal development has become highly sophisticated, and our ability to detect many anomalies before birth is becoming quite precise. Ultrasound is now three-dimensional, and the quality of the pictures is rapidly becoming well defined, thus allowing us to view, anticipate, and prepare for

---

Box **9-3** OCCUPATIONAL HAZARDS THAT MIGHT HAVE FETAL EFFECTS

Ethylene oxide
Halogenated hydrocarbons
Heavy metals
Ionizing radiation
Noise
Organic solvents
Pesticides
Herbicides
Physical energy demands
Waste anesthetic gases
Temperature extremes

the infant with detectable anomalies (Birnbacher, Messerschmidt, & Pollak, 2002; Bromley, Lieberman, Shipp, et al., 2002; Farina, Malone, & Bianchi, 2000; Jaeggi, Sholler, Jones, et al., 2001; Paladini, D'Armiento, Ardovino, et al., 2000; Simpsom, Jones, Callaghan, et al., 2000; Wellesley & Howe, 2001). See Box 9-4 for examples of detectable head anomalies and their causes.

**Box 9-4** EXAMPLES OF DETECTABLE ANOMALIES OF THE HEAD

| Detectible Anomalies of the Head | Causes and Consequences for the Fetus and Infant |
|---|---|
| Anencephaly | • Absent anterior neural tube closure, exposing neural tissue<br>• Malfunction of the first stage of neurologic development, primary neurulation |
| Microcephaly | • Small brain<br>• Occipital frontal circumference (OFC) ≤ third percentile for gestational age<br>• Occurs earlier in utero (most severe microcephaly)<br>• Causes:<br>  • Teratogens: Irradiation; maternal alcoholism or cocaine abuse<br>  • Maternal hyperphenylalaninemia<br>  • Genetic (usually autosomal recessive but can be X-linked)<br>  • TORCH (toxoplasma gondii, rubella, cytomegalovirus [CMV], herpes simplex viruses [HSV-1 and HSV-2], infections)<br>• Outcome dependent on severity and associated with developmental delays |
| Hydrocephalus | • Inadequate cerebrospinal fluid (CSF) absorption secondary to abnormal circulation<br>• Excess ventricular CSF secondary to aqueductal outflow; causes obstructive, noncommunicating hydrocephalus<br>• Causes:<br>  • Aqueductal stenosis<br>  • Dandy-Walker cyst (cystic transformation of fourth ventricle)<br>  • Myelomeningocele with Arnold-Chiari malformation<br>  • Congenital masses and tumors<br>  • Congenital infection (especially toxoplasmosis, cytomegalovirus)<br>• Associated defects:<br>  • Spina bifida<br>  • Encephalocele<br>  • Holoprosencephaly<br>  • Posthemorrhagic hydrocephalus<br>  • Progressive dilation of the ventricles after intraventricular hemorrhage (IVH) caused by injury to the periventricular white matter<br>• Acute:<br>  • Appears rapidly<br>  • Probably occurs secondary to malabsorption of CSF secondary to a blood clot<br>• Subacute:<br>  • Inhibition of CSF flow<br>  • Blood from IVH<br>• Outcome related to initial IVH severity; deficits motor and/or cognitive |

## PERINATAL INFLUENCES ON FETAL DEVELOPMENT (MATERNAL HISTORY, DURING PREGNANCY, INTRINSIC AND EXTRINSIC FACTORS)

The maternal history is a critical component of perinatal/neonatal/infant care. As the list of factors indicates, there are many facets of the mother's background that can impact fetal/neonatal/infant outcomes.

## Maternal Disease

As discussed, maternal disease can adversely influence the development of the fetus. There can be placental dysfunction that is directly related either to a maternal condition or to changes in the placenta or growth itself. Because the placenta is responsible for nourishing the fetus and regulating the oxygen supply as well as toxins, it is understandable that anything that changes the placental growth, surface, or circulation can potentially affect fetal growth. Aspects of the impact of prenatal events are the source of much interest today as we have the technology to follow the fetal and especially the neurofetal development (Scher, 2003). Placental anomalies are associated with poor fetal/neonatal outcomes, including LBW and prematurity (Rhone, Magee, Remple, et al., 2003; Sweet, Hodgman, Pena, et al., 2003).

## Placental Abnormalities

The most common placental abnormality is abruptio placentae. Perinatal mortality for these infants ranges from 15% to 30%. Fetal hypoxia is of real concern in this event. It is caused by uteroplacental insufficiency from separation or decreased perfusion from maternal hypovolemia, uterine hypertonus, or fetal hemorrhage. Total anoxia can develop. Abruptio placentae has been found to be related to preterm labor and delivery, and small for gestational age (SGA) infants. Even if the bleeding stops, decreased placental surface area might not be adequate to meet the increased nutritional needs of the fetus. Therefore, these children are at increased risk for neurologic defects, such as cerebral palsy (CP).

Another placental abnormality is placenta previa. Perinatal mortality is less than 10%; however, these pregnancies will often be subject to premature labor and delivery, and infants might be SGA. It has been noted that SGA most often occurs if the placental exchange is chronically compromised. Risk of CNS, cardiovascular, respiratory, or gastrointestinal tract abnormalities also increases with placenta previa. It should also be noted that anemia in the infant is proportional to maternal blood loss.

## Hypertensive States in Pregnancy

Pregnancy induced hypertension (PIH) affects 5% to 7% of all pregnancies. It can result in placental abruption or other problems for the fetus and neonate (Sheiner, Shoham-Vardi, Hallak, et al., 2003). Due to maternal renal, pulmonary, and hepatic systems affected, fetal complications include LBW, IUGR, and hypoxia. Fetal/neonatal effects may be increased due to prematurity if **h**emolysis, **e**levated **l**iver enzymes, and **l**ow **p**latelets syndrome (HELLP) occurs (2% to 12% of PIH cases). These women are at high risk for acute renal failure (Roberts, Gordon, Porter, et al., 2003).

## Thyroid Disorders

Maternal thyroid disorders have been found to be associated with problems in the fetus (Diehl, 1998). Mothers with hypothyroidism are at greater risk to have infants with mental retardation or congenital anomalies. Mothers with hyperthyroidism have an increased incidence of preterm birth.

## Renal Disease

The renal disease might be due to a maternal anomaly such as polycystic kidney or other genetic disorders or secondary to another condition such as diabetes, HELLP, preeclampsia, systemic lupus erythema, or perinatal infections, including Listeria (Balderas-Pena, Canales-Munoz, Angulo-Vazquez, et al., 2002; Bergmann, Senderek, Sedlacek, et al., 2003; Newman, Robichaux, Stedman, et al., 2003; Rehan, Moddemann, & Casiro, 2002; Tan, Tan, Lee, et al., 2002; Guay-Woodford & Desmond, 2003). These infants are at increased risk for IUGR, and prematurity related to preterm labor (Thorsen & Poole, 2002).

Premature labor is defined as contractions that start the delivery process prior to 37 weeks' gestation. Between 1986 and 1996, the rate of preterm births increased 10% in the United States (from 10% to 11%). Unfortunately, these trends have not changed much in the past few years. Martin, Hamilton, Ventura, et al. (2002) report that preterm birth rates actually increased in 2001. Prematurity/LBW was the second leading cause of infant mortality in 2001; respiratory distress syndrome (RDS) was the fourth leading cause of death. This trend is continuing to rise and is a concern to our nation. Multiple gestations increase the risk of preterm labor. The use of antenatal corticosteriods has increased the survival rate for many babies delivered because of preterm labor. There has been research conducted that serial corticosteriod use and even single use might enhance lung maturation (Sen, Reghu, & Ferguson, 2002). The preferred method of treatment is creating a "steroid window" for delivery of the infant, which is usually done by giving a short series of steroids during the course of 48 hours when delivery appears eminent (Crane, Armson, Brunner, et al., 2003). Prenatal steroid use is not without long-term complications, and the use should be very judicious. The complications of a premature infant are outlined in the postnatal section of this chapter.

## Premature Rupture of Membranes

Premature rupture of membranes (PROM) is linked to approximately 120,000 pregnancies each year (Mercer, 2003). The neonatal outcome is dependent on the gestational age of the fetus at the time of the rupture and the underlying cause. Risks are similar to that of preterm delivery, and chorioamnionitis might be present, adding to the problems for the infant. There might also be a risk of the development of CP (Willoughby & Nelson, 2002). Lee, Carpenter, Heber, et al. (2003) have found no definitive linkage between the occurrence of PROM in one pregnancy and in subsequent pregnancies.

## Maternal Substance Abuse

Maternal substance abuse has increased in the past decade. The drugs used are growing. These drugs include: marijuana, heroin, cocaine, methadone, methylenedioxymethamphetamine (MDMA; ecstasy), and alcohol, (Bada, Das, Bauer, et al., 2002; Cornelius, Goldschmidt, Day, et al., 2002; Dashe, Sheffield, Olscher, et al., 2002; Eustace, Kang, & Coombs, 2003; Ornoy, 2002). See Table 9-2 for examples of illicit drugs and the fetal/neonatal effects. Another aspect of perinatal substance abuse is the continued use after the birth. The developmental outcomes are the focus of current studies examining the effects of drugs, maternal lifestyle, and interaction patterns with infants and children (Coyer, 2003; Johnson, 2001; Kelly, Ritchie, Quate, et al., 2002; Lester, Tronick, LaGasse, et al., 2002; Lyles & Cadet, 2003; Schuler, Nair, & Kettinger, 2003).

We are all aware of the public health issue of substance abuse. However, we often ignore the use of socially acceptable substances along with illicit drugs. These include tobacco and alcohol, which have the addictive effects of other substances. A good maternal history must include all substances to anticipate potential developmental problems. Polydrug use has become common. This might or might not include legal substances. Substance abuse directly affects whether the mother will seek prenatal care, comply with suggested prenatal care, obtain proper nutrition, acquire sexually transmitted infections (STIs), or reside in adequate housing as well as directly affecting the medical well-being of the mother and the fetus. The obstetric complications often associated with substance abuse that affect maternal and fetal well-being include maternal hypertension, urinary tract infections, preeclampsia, premature rupture of membranes, preterm labor and delivery, and low birthweight. One of the overall effects on the fetus is growth restriction and its associated complications. Common effects on the neonates of women who engage in substance abuse include:

- Poor bonding
- Exaggerated startle response
- Generalized growth retardation
- Hypoglycemia
- Intracranial hemorrhage
- IUGR
- LBW
- Meconium aspiration

- Neurobehavioral abnormalities
- Altered sleep patterns
- Irritability
- Jitteriness
- Tremors
- Depressed sucking
- Possible seizures
- RDS
- Small head circumference, or microcephaly

Studies of maternal substances now extend beyond the effects on fetal development to specific neurodevelopmental outcomes, including postnatal environment as a variable. The fetal effects of cocaine, for example, include small head circumference and adverse neurologic outcomes (hypertonia, tremors, and extensor leg posturing). In addition, the long-term consequences include low birthweight, SGA, IUGR, developmental delays, and diminished neurobehavioral development (Behnke, Eyler, Garvan, et al., 2002; Mendola, Selevan, Gutter, et al., 2002; Morrow, Bandstra, Anthony, et al., 2001). Another aspect of substance abuse is the risk for HIV. Perinatal transmission to the fetus has decreased as use of medication cocktails that pass through the placenta has increased. However, HIV infection secondary to substance abuse remains a global problem and one that is still missed in terms of preventive strategies (Peters, Liu, Dominguez, et al., 2003; Soloway, 2003).

## Tobacco

Smoking has decreased in the United States during the past decade. However, many women still smoke during pregnancy. This drug has the potential effect of maternal anemia and vasoconstriction of the placental vessels, leading to less oxygen for mother and fetus, and possible hypoxic episodes. The result is fetal tachycardia, decreased oxygen saturations, polycythemia, or polyglobulia. However, some women still do not comprehend the dangers of their smoking on the developing human (Perry, Jones, Tuten, et al., 2003). Some experts now use the term fetal tobacco syndrome to refer to the fetus exposed in utero to tobacco (Habek, Habek, Ivanisevic, et al., 2002). There is a dose-related impact of smoking on risk of preterm birth. Due to the effect of reduction in uteroplacental blood flow, there is an increased

risk for the fetus to be deprived of oxygen and available nutrients. These infants are at increased risk for LBW, IUGR, prematurity, and neurobehavioral abnormalities.

## Alcohol

Fetal alcohol syndrome (FAS) has several neurobehavioral manifestations (Eustace, Kang, & Coombs, 2003). There is increased irritability, microcephaly, mild-to-moderate mental retardation, poor sucking, IUGR, short palpebral fissures, strabismus, ptosis, and myopia. The IUGR has been found to be linear and lasts a lifetime. Fetal alcohol effects (FAE) might be part of the continuum of FAS and might have related phenotypes (Steinhausen, Willms, Metzke, et al., 2003). Its signs are more neurologic in nature and tend to be found even in the absence of physical symptoms. These deficits are often not detected until preschool or school age (Riley, Mattson, Li, et al., 2003). More emphasis is on the combination of short- and long-term developmental effects as a national prevention agenda is being developed (Weber, Floyd, Riley, et al., 2002).

## Maternal/Fetal Infections

Maternal infections are known potential teratogens. They can adversely affect fetal development. Researchers are currently examining the linkage between perinatal infections and the occurrence of CP (O'Shea & Dammann, 2000). Cytomegalovirus (CMV) is one of the more common infections. Infection is most likely to occur with maternal primary infection. Ninety percent of infected infants are free of symptoms at birth, but 5% to 15% of these might have long-term sequelae. Less then 5% of these infants will have severe involvement at birth, including IUGR, microcephaly, periventricular calcification, encephalopathy, deafness, blindness, chorioretinitis, mental retardation, and hepatosplenomegaly. Chorioamnionitis is one of the most common maternal infections and is often related to premature rupture of membranes and prolonged rupture of membranes, with subsequent premature labor and delivery. These mothers and infants should be monitored closely. Organism-specific antibiotic therapy is recommended for the maternal/fetal dyad and the newborn.

Another maternal infection of concern to the fetus is herpes simplex virus (HSV). There is a mortality rate of 5% to 60% if neonatal exposure is with active primary infection of HSV. Many of these children will exhibit neurologic or ophthalmic sequelae. There will be disseminated infection in 70% of cases with jaundice, RDS, and CNS involvement. Herpes can be transmitted even when the mother's herpes appears inactive; careful assessment is needed, and route of delivery might be a point of discussion. Maternal rubella can also be a danger for the fetus. The fetal infection rate is greatest before 11 weeks and after 35 weeks, but severe sequelae occur with first-trimester infections. Sequelae might include deafness, eye defects, CNS anomalies, and CHD. Toxoplasmosis is another infection that can have fetal effects. Severity varies with gestation (earlier infection results in more severe effects). Fetal effects can include IUGR, hydrocephalus, and microcephaly. Neurologic, ophthalmologic, and co-sequelae are variable. AIDS or HIV are also issues of concern for the fetus. The chance of perinatal transmission continues to drop with new medication combinations; however, screening is mandatory so that treatment is given when needed. New tests allow the detection of the virus very early in an infant's life, but prevention through treatment during pregnancy shows the most promise for the child. Gonorrhea and syphilis infections also have fetal effects including: sepsis or meningitis; stillbirth; IUGR; nonimmune hydrops; or premature labor. Varicella zoster affects 30% to 49% of fetuses born to mothers with active disease. Congenital varicella syndrome includes: IUGR; cataracts; microphthalmos; chorioretinitis; and microcephaly.

Exposure to agents that might be considered teratogens must be included in the maternal history. Whether or not the exposure adversely affects the fetal development in part depends on the interplay between the genotypes of the mother and fetus, along with the environmental exposure. Blackburn (2002) outlines the following principles of teratogenesis:

1. Susceptibility to a teratogenic agent is dependent on the genotype of the embryo and the manner in which the agent interacts with environmental factors.

2. Susceptibility to teratogenic agents is dependent on the timing of the exposure and the developmental stage of the embryo.
3. Teratogenic agents act in specific ways on cells or tissues to cause pathogenesis.
4. The final manifestations of abnormal development are death, malformation, growth retardation, and functional disorders.
5. Access to the embryo by environmental teratogens depends on the nature of the agent.
6. As the dosage increases, manifestations of deviant development increase. The mechanisms of these actions are:
   a. Gene mutation.
   b. Chromosome breaks and nondisjunction.
   c. Mitotic interference and cell death.
   d. Altered nucleic acid integrity or function.
   e. Lack or excess of precursors, substrates, or coenzymes needed for biosynthesis.
   f. Altered energy sources.
   g. Enzyme and growth-factor inhibitions.
   h. Osmolar imbalance.
   i. Altered membrane characteristics.
   j. Altered cell and neuronal migration, or CNS organization.

## POSTNATAL INFLUENCES ON NEONATAL DEVELOPMENT

The results of prenatal influences often result in variations in birthweight and gestational age. The infant must be assessed for neonatal variations. LBW is defined as less than 2500 g. VLBW is weight less than 1500 g. The infant can be average, small, or large for gestational age (AGA, SGA, or LGA), depending on comparisons to normal growth curves for gestational age groups. If the infant's weight is less than expected for the gestational age, then the infant might be considered to be IUGR. This calculation is generally based on the head circumference and length compared with weight. Use of these data help to calculate the risk of problems for the neonate or infant. It is important to classify the infant at birth-by-birth weight and gestational age. SGA infants are smaller than the tenth percentile for weight. Symmetric IUGR is when the weight, length, and head circumference all fall below the tenth percentile. This is often more common in fetuses with congenital infections and anomalies. Asymmetric IUGR is when the head circumference and length are normal, with weight below the tenth percentile. This finding is often related to impaired placental functioning or poor nutrition with sparing of brain growth. Neonatal outcome for these children is variable and is often related to the underlying cause of the growth restriction as well as gestational age at delivery. In the absence of major anomalies, viral infections, or chromosomal abnormalities, growth-restricted newborns might have few complications. Through antenatal testing, absent or reversed end-diastolic flow on Doppler flow studies has been found to be related a high incidence of IUGR and an increased incidence of abnormal neurologic signs in newborns. Head circumference smaller than the tenth percentile at birth and abnormal results from a newborn neurologic examination are associated with poor growth, later microcephaly, and neurologic deficits.

Assessment of gestational age and severity of illness can have many implications for the developing infant. Methods of assessing gestational age include the Dubowitz test and the Ballard Score, which recently has been revised to score infants to 22 weeks' gestation. The Ballard is most often used in the clinical setting because of its ease of use. There are also three severity of illness scoring systems (SISS):

- Score for neonatal acute physiology (SNAP) correlates chronic physiologic instability and neurodevelopmental morbidity.
- Score for neonatal acute physiology–perinatal extension (SNAP + PE). SNAP was extended for use as a mortality risk predictor by inclusion of points for birthweight, SGA, and low Apgars.
- Clinical risk index for babies (CRIB). Six items are weighted according to their risk of mortality. The items include birthweight, gestational age, congenital anomalies, and three physiologic measures: highest and lowest appropriate inspired oxygen and the worst base deficit collected.

## MEDICAL COMPLICATIONS OF NEWBORN

The most common medical complications of the newborn that affect development generally are associated with disturbances in the endocrine, respiratory, and neurologic systems. Theoretically, any system can be affected, but in terms of neurobehavioral development, these are the most common. Some areas that should be considered and questions to be asked as a maternal/neonatal history/assessment is taken are:

1. Hypoglycemia
   a. Occurs in 15% of preterm infants
   b. Occurs in 65% of SGA infants
   c. Can be related to maternal diabetes or over-aggressive intravenous therapy
2. Hyperglycemia
   a. Is common in small infants who are receiving concentrated glucose solutions; also is often an iatrogenic complication of neonatal therapy
3. Seizures (Mustonen, Mustakangas, Uotila, et al., 2003; Sato, Okumura, Kato, et al., 2003).
   a. Is this condition a symptom of neurologic dysfunction?
   b. Is the condition separate from any known neurologic abnormalities?
   c. Is it a result of perinatal infections?
   d. There are five categories of seizure activity.
      1. Metabolic
         a. Decreased production of adenosine triphosphate due to ischemia, hypoxemia, or hypoglycemia.
         b. Hyponatremia or hypernatremia
         c. Hypocalcemia or hypomagnesemia
         d. Errors of metabolism
         e. Pyridoxine dependency
         f. Hyperammonemia
      2. Structural
         a. Intraventricular hemorrhage (IVH)
         b. Cerebral cortical dysgenesis
         c. Hypoxic-ischemic encephalopathy
      3. Intracerebral infections
         a. Group B streptococcus, *Escherichia coli,* or *Listeria monocytogenes*
         b. Nonbacterial infection: TORCH (toxoplasmosis, rubella, cytomegalovirus, and herpes simplex)
      4. Withdrawal from maternal drugs
         a. Onset during the first 3 days of life
         b. From: narcotic-analgesics, sedative-hypnotics, alcohol

5. Familial
   a. Onset within second to third day
   b. Infant appears well between seizures; seizures are self-limiting
   c. Autosomal dominant inheritance
   d. Outcome related to underlying etiology
4. Pneumothorax
   a. Alveolar overdistention and rupture
   b. Occurs as a secondary cause or spontaneously
   c. Outcome depends on underlying lung pathology
   d. Associated with increased incidence of cerebral blood flow interruption
5. RDS
   a. Still very common among premature and sick neonates.
   b. Decreases oxygen circulating to the rapidly developing brain.
   c. Outcomes can be hypoxic episodes leading to neurologic impairment.

## COMPLICATIONS EXPERIENCED BY THE NEWBORN

The complications that are often experienced by a newborn and infant can be anticipated when prenatal and intrapartum exposures are known. The most common complications are listed below with their considerations.

1. Intracranial hemorrhages—some of these can be prevented with newer techniques in intrapartum and neonatal care (Carteaux, Cohen, Check, et al., 2003; Lee, McMillan, Ohlsson, et al., 2003; McLendon, Check, Carteaux, et al., 2003; Paul, Coleman, Leef, et al., 2003). We also must consider the long-term developmental outcomes for these infants as part of our individualized family-centered plans (McGrath & Sullivan, 2002).
   a. Subdural
      1. Usually occurs in term infants.
      2. Tears of cerebral veins over cerebral hemispheres.
      3. If tear or rupture is large, outlook is poor.
      4. Hydrocephalus occasionally develops.
   b. Subarachnoid hemorrhage
      1. Bleeding of venous origin in the subarachnoid space.
      2. Might be precipitated by trauma in term infants and hypoxia in preterm infants.
      3. Outcome is good.
   c. Intracerebellar hemorrhage
      1. Hemorrhages within the cerebellum.
      2. Associations with RDS, hypoxic events, prematurity, and traumatic delivery.
      3. Occurs in 15% to 25% of preterm babies <32 weeks' gestation or weighing <1.5 kg at birth.
      4. Outcome is poor in premature infants.
   d. Periventricular-intraventricular hemorrhages
      1. Associated with infants born <34 weeks' gestation and those who require mechanical ventilation.
      2. Associated with increasing arterial blood pressure and perinatal asphyxia.
      3. Other associated factors:
         • Prematurity
         • Low 5-minute Apgar score
         • Asphyxia
         • LBW
         • Acidosis
         • Hypotension
         • Hypertension
         • Low hematocrit
         • Respiratory distress requiring mechanical ventilation
         • Rapid administration of sodium bicarbonate
         • Rapid volume expansion
         • Infusion of hyperosmolar solution
         • Coagulopathy
         • Pneumothorax
         • Ligation of PDA
         • Transport
      4. Graded on a small to severe scale.
      5. Infants born <28 weeks' have three times higher occurrence than infants born 28 to 31 weeks' gestation
      6. Outcome
         a. Mortality rate is 50% with severe hemorrhage, 15% with moderate hemorrhage, and 5% with small hemorrhage.
         b. Hemorrhage alone does not account for all neurologic deficits.

c. Approximately 25% to 30% of VLBW (<1500 g) infants discharged have a periventricular-intraventricular hemorrhage without major neurodevelopmental sequelae. But, often, follow-up is not continued long enough to definitively determine any minor delays or deficits. More research is needed in this area.

d. Small hemorrhage outcome: neurodevelopmental disability similar to that in premature infants without hemorrhage. Major neurodevelopmental disability is 10%.

e. Moderate hemorrhage outcome: major neurodevelopmental disability is 40% during infancy.

f. Severe hemorrhage outcome: major neurodevelopmental disability is 80%.

2. Hypoxic-ischemic encephalopathy (HIE) still is a common occurrence in the neonatal population. Although the emphasis is on prevention, there are now some specific tests that can be run to trace changes in brain proteins. These tests offer hope to predict those infants who will potentially have adverse neurodevelopmental effects from hypoxemia (Nagdyman, Grimmer, Scholz, et al., 2003). Another area of research is to measure serum concentration levels of thyroid stimulating hormone (TSH), T4, T3, and FT4 to determine if there is an association between HIE and thyroid function. According to Pereira and Procianoy (2003), there appears to be a correlation between thyroid levels and HIE. The common problems associated with HIE are:

a. Hypoxia and anoxia

b. Approximately 60% of VLBW have this defect

c. Timing of defect
   1. Antepartum: 20%
   2. Intrapartum: 30%
   3. Antepartum-intrapartum: 35%
   4. Postpartum occurrence: 10%

d. Three stages
   1. Mild
   2. Moderate
   3. Severe

e. Outcome
   1. Based on severity of brain insult.
   2. Factors associated with poor outcome.
      a. Apgar score
      b. Encephalopathy
      c. Prematurity
      d. Early seizures

3. Periventricular leukomalacia (PVL) (Perrott, Dodds, & Vincer, 2003).

a. Ischemic, necrotic, periventricular white matter

b. Principally ischemic lesion of arterial origin

c. Occurrence secondary to inadequate cerebral perfusion

d. Manifestation of HIE in premature infants 80% to 90% of PVL in premature infants

e. Outcomes
   1. Spastic dysphagia
   2. Motor deficits
   3. Visual impairment
   4. Lower-limb weakness
   5. Based on location and extent of injury
   6. Long-term considerations must be examined, especially beyond the infancy period. School outcomes are beginning to receive attention as more VLBW infants are surviving. The current research is examining those infants that received indomethacin to prevent intraventricular hemorrhage (Vohr, Allan, Westerveld, et al., 2003). They concluded that no effect of indomethacin could be found; however, the home environment and family factors play a role in the developmental outcomes.

4. Meningitis

a. Early onset from vaginal flora.

b. Late-onset from environmental microbes.

c. Outcome dependent on rapidity of detection and initiation of adequate drug therapy.

d. 50% of survivors of bacterial meningitis have significant neurologic sequelae.
   1. Seizures
   2. Sensorineural hearing loss
   3. Visual losses
   4. Mental and motor disabilities

5. RDS
   a. Developmental disorder starting at or soon after birth and occurring most frequently in infants with immature lungs
   b. Inversely related to gestational age
   c. Related complications (Box 9-5)
   d. Infants who weigh more than 1500 g who have mild or moderate RDS have the same developmental outcome as babies of the same gestational age without RDS.
   e. Infants with the most severe developmental outcomes are those who weigh less than 1500 g and have had an IVH.

**Box 9-5**  COMPLICATIONS OF RESPIRATORY DISTRESS SYNDROME

**PULMONARY**
Air leaks
BPD

**CARDIOVASCULAR**
PDA
Systemic hypotension

**RENAL/OLIGURIA**
Most likely after hypoxia, hypotension, shock
Immature renal function with decreased glomerular filtration in VLBW infants.

**METABOLIC**
Acidosis
Hyponatremia or hypernatremia
Hypocalcemia
Hypoglycemia

**HEMATOLOGIC**
Anemia
Disseminated intravascular coagulopathy

**NEUROLOGIC**
Seizures

**OTHER**
Secondary nosocomial infections
Retinopathy of prematurity
Displaced endotracheal tube
Thrombus formation from umbilical catheters

6. Pneumonia
   a. Infection of the fetal or newborn lung that can be intrauterine or neonatal
   b. Intrauterine infection causes
      • Passage of infecting agent by infection of fetal membranes
      • Transplacental transmission
      • Aspiration of meconium or infected fluid during delivery
   c. Neonatal infection
      • Acquired during nursery stay
      • Pathogens are generally different than those acquired in utero
      • Might spread to other newborns
   d. Associated outcomes
      • Meningitis
      • Septic shock
      • DIC
      • Persistent pulmonary hypertension of the newborn (PPHN) (Box 9-6)
        — Caused by right-to-left shunting blood through the fetal shunts at the atrial and ductal levels.
        — It is secondary to persistent elevation of pulmonary vascular resistance and pulmonary artery pressure.
        — The use of nitric oxide has decreased the incidence of severe hypoxia, but the risk is still present (Kinsella, Parker, Ivy, et al., 2003; Sadiq, Mantych, Benawra, et al., 2003).
        — This condition sometimes accompanies other conditions, such as congenital diaphragmatic hernia.
   e. Gram-negative pneumonia: cardiopulmonary complications similar to those of RDS.
      Outcome: prognosis depends on severity, comorbidities of seizures and asphyxia.
7. Bronchopulmonary dysplasia (BPD) can be a result of prenatal events such as poor maternal nutrition, lack of prenatal care, infections, or complications during the intrapartum or postnatal period (Coalson, 2003; Bancalari, Claure, & Sosenko, 2003; Grier & Halliday, 2003; Ogunyemi, Murillo, Jackson, et al., 2003; Reiss, Landmann, Heckmann, et al., 2003). There also seems, for some infants, to be a genetic linkage to

**Box 9-6** COMPLICATIONS: PERSISTENT PULMONARY HYPERTENSION OF THE NEWBORN

**PULMONARY**
Air leaks
Bronchopulmonary dysplasia

**CARDIOVASCULAR**
Systemic hypotension
Congestive heart failure

**RENAL**
Decreased urine output related to asphyxia and hypotension
Kidney damage caused by asphyxia or acute tubular necrosis

**METABOLIC**
Hypoglycemia

**HEMATOLOGIC**
Thrombocytopenia
Disseminated intravascular coagulopathy
Hemorrhage
Neurologic
Central nervous system irritability
Seizures

**IATROGENIC**
Thrombosis formation
Displaced endotracheal tube

lung disease, including BPD (Hallman & Haataja, 2003). BPD is more preventable today owing to advances in maternal steroid use to hasten lung maturation, use of nitric oxide, and fewer days on ventilators. Yet BPD from a developmental standpoint still adversely affects NICU graduates.
a. Chronic lung disease that still requires oxygen at 36 weeks PCA.
b. Complications include:
   • Intermittent bronchospasm
   • Recurrent infections (especially ear infections, pneumonia, upper respiratory infection [URI])
   • Congestive heart failure from cor pulmonale
   • Gastroesophageal reflux disease (GERD)

• Developmental delays—sometimes not found until school age
c. Neurologic and developmental sequelae
   • CP
   • Sensorineural hearing loss
8. Retinopathy of prematurity (ROP). Research is ongoing examining long-term effects of light exposure, especially in the NICU environment, as another factor in the development of ROP (see Chapter 14).
   a. A vasoproliferative retinopathy with five stages.
   b. Normal vasculogenesis process is arrested and followed by rapid, excessive, irregular vascular growth, and shunt formation.
   c. Incidence increases significantly as birthweight and gestational age decrease—47% for 1 to 1.250 kg at birth to 70% for infants born at 750 to 999 g and 90% in infants born at less than 750 g.
   d. Outcome depends on stage. Ninety percent of cases resolve spontaneously.
   e. Laser or cryotherapy has demonstrated a decrease in visual impairment, especially in the presence of zone 1 disease.
9. Hyperbilirubinemia. An old problem that remains a part of neonatal and infant care. Long-term effects can result in neurodevelopmental deficits (Hansen, 2002). Prevention is key (Poland, 2003).
   a. The goal of treating hyperbilirubinemia is to prevent bilirubin toxic effects.
   b. Kernicterus is a neuropathologic finding of yellow staining and neuronal injury in basal ganglia.
   c. Bilirubin encephalopathy is caused by kernicterus and is referred to acute and chronic sequelae of hyperbilirubinemia.
   d. There are four types of hyperbilirubinemia
      1. Physiologic
      2. Breastfeeding
      3. Pathologic
      4. Unconjugated
   e. Management of hyperbilirubinemia in LBW infants is determined by clinical status, age, weight, and history.

## CONCLUSION

This chapter very briefly reviews the factors that influence fetal and neonatal development. Emphasis has been placed on neurodevelopmental outcomes. One critical component of this aspect of developmental care is the role of the home environment and the interaction of the family with the child and with healthcare professionals. The philosophy of developmental care requires that the assessment and plans be holistic, individualized, family-centered, and developmentally supportive. Therefore, the family, not just the maternal history but also the interactions with the infant as part of the environment, is an essential part of the influences on developmental outcomes.

## *REFERENCES*

Alejandro, B., Perez, R., Pedrana, G., et al. (2002). Low maternal nutrition during pregnancy reduces the number of Sertoli cells in the newborn lamb. *Reproduction & Fertility Development, 14*(5-6), 333-337.

Alexander, G.R., Kogan, M., Bader, D., et al. (2003). US birth weight/gestational age-specific neonatal mortality: 1995-1997 rates for whites, Hispanics, and blacks. *Pediatrics, 111*(1), E61-E66.

Al-Fozan, H., & Tulandi, T. (2002). Safety and risks of laparoscopy in pregnancy. *Current Opinions in Obstetrics and Gynecology, 14*(4), 375-379.

Allan, L.D. (2003). Cardiac anatomy screening: What is the best time for screening in pregnancy? *Current Opinion in Obstetrics and Gynecology, 15*(2), 143-146.

Altshuler, L.L., Cohen, L., Szuba, M.P., et al. (1997). Pharmacologic management of psychiatric illness during pregnancy: Dilemmas and guidelines. *American Journal of Psychiatry, 153*(5), 592-606.

Asling-Monemi, K., Pena, R., Ellsberg, M.C., et al. (2003). Violence against women increases the risk of infant and child mortality: A case-referent study in Nicaragua. *Bulletin of World Health Organization, 81*(1), 10-16.

Avila, W.S., Rossi, E.G., Ramires, J.A., et al. (2003). Pregnancy in patients with heart disease: Experience with 1000 cases. *Clinics in Cardiology, 26*(3), 135-142.

Azarbaymani, F., & Danielsson, B.R. (2002). Embryonic arrhythmia by inhibition of HERG channels: A common hypoxia-related teratogenic mechanism for antiepileptic drugs? *Epilepsia, 43*(5), 457-469.

Azarbaymani, F., & Danielsson, B.R. (1998). Pharmacologically induced embryonic dysrhythmia and episodes of hypoxia followed by reoxygenation: A common teratogenic mechanism for antiepileptic drugs? *Teratology, 57*(3), 117-126.

Bada, H.S., Das, A., Bauer, C.R., et al. (2002). Gestational cocaine exposure and intrauterine growth: Maternal lifestyle study. *Obstetrics and Gynecology, 100*(5 Pt 1), 916-924.

Balderas-Pena, L.M., Canales-Munoz, J.L., Angulo-Vazquez, J., et al. (2002). The HELPP syndrome-evidence of a possible systemic inflammatory response in preeclampsia? *Gynecology Obstetrics Mexico, 70*, 328-337.

Bancalari, E., Claure, N, & Sosenko, I.R. (2003). Bronchopulmonary dysplasia: Changes in pathogenesis, epidemiology and definition. *Seminars in Neonatology, 8*(1), 63-71.

Behnke, M., Eyler, F.D., Garvan, C.W., et al. (2002). Cocaine exposure and developmental outcome from birth to 6 months. *Neurotoxicology and Teratology, 24*(3), 283-295.

Bergmann, C., Senderek, J., Sedlacek, B., et al. (2003). Spectrum of mutations in the gene for autosomal recessive polycystic kidney disease (ARPKD/PKHD1). *Journal of the American Society of Nephrology, 14*(1), 76-89.

Bianca, S., & Ettore, G. (2002). Maternal reproductive history and isolated hypoplastic left heart syndrome. *Acta Cardiology, 57*(6), 407-408.

Birnbacher, R., Messerschmidt, A.M., & Pollak, A.P. (2002). Diagnosis and prevention of neural tube defects. *Current Opinions in Urology, 12*(6), 461-464.

Blackburn, S.T (2002). *Maternal, fetal, and neonatal physiology: A clinical perspective* (2nd ed.; p. 200). St. Louis: W.B. Saunders.

Bo, S., Marchisio, B., Volpiano, M., et al. (2003). Maternal low birthweight and gestational hyperglycemia. *Gynecology and Endocrinology, 17*(3), 133-136.

Bondevik, G.T., Lie, R.T., Ulstein, M., et al. (2001). Maternal hematological status and risk of low birth weight and preterm delivery in Nepal. *Acta Obstetric and Gynecology Scandinavia, 80*(50), 402-408.

Bromley, B., Lieberman, E., Shipp, T.D., et al. (2002). Fetal nose bone length: A marker for Down syndrome in the second trimester. *Journal of Ultrasound Medicine, 21*(12), 1387-1394.

Cada, A.M., Hansen, D.K., LaBorde, J.B., et al. (2001). Minimal effects from developmental exposure to St. John's wort (Hypericum perforatum) in Sprague-Dawley rats. *Nutrition-Neuroscience, 4*(2), 135-141.

Carteaux, P. Cohen, H., Check, J., et al. (2003). Evaluation and development of potentially better practices for the prevention of brain hemorrhage and ischemic brain injury in very low birth weight infants. *Pediatrics, 111*(4 Pt 2), E489-E496.

Catalano, P.M., Kirwan, J.P., Haugel-De Mouzon, S., et al. (2003). Gestational diabetes and insulin resistance: Role in short- and long-term implications for mother and fetus. *Journal of Nutrition, 133*(5), 1674S-1683S.

Chang, T.I., Horal, M., Jain, S.K., et al. (2003). Oxidant regulation of gene expression and neural tube development: Insights gained from diabetic pregnancy on molecular causes of neural tube defects. *Diabetologia,* *46*(4), 538-545.

Coalson, J.J. (2003). Pathology of new bronchopulmonary dysplasia. *Seminars in Neonatology, 8*(1), 73-81.

Cornelius, M.D., Goldschmidt, L., Day, N.L., et al. (2002). Alcohol, tobacco and marijuana use among pregnant teenagers: 6-year follow-up of offspring growth effects. *Neurotoxicology and Teratology, 24*(6), 703-710.

Coyer, S.M. (2003). Women in recovery discuss parenting while addicted to cocaine. *MCN: American Journal of Maternal/Child Nursing, 28*(1), 45-49.

Crane, J., Armson, A., Brunner, M., et al. (2003). Antenatal corticosteroid therapy for fetal maturation. *Journal of Obstetrics and Gynecology Canada, 24*(1), 45-52.

Dashe, J.S., Sheffield, J., Olscher, D.A., et al. (2002). Relationship between maternal methadone dosage and neonatal withdrawal. *Obstetrics and Gynecology, 100*(6), 1244-1249.

de Sereday, M.S., Damiano, M.M., Gonzalez, C.D., et al. (2003). Diagnostic criteria for gestational diabetes in relation to pregnancy outcome. *Journal of Diabetes Complications, 17*(3), 115-119.

Diehl, K. (1998). Thyroid dysfunction in pregnancy. *Journal of Perinatal and Neonatal Nursing, 11*(4), 1-12.

Einarson, A., Bonari, L., Voyer-Lavigne, S., et al. (2003). A multicentre prospective controlled study to determine the safety of trazodeon and nefazoldeon use during pregnancy. *Canadian Journal of Psychiatry, 48*(2), 106-110.

Eustace, L.W., Kang, D.H., & Coombs, D. (2003). Fetal alcohol syndrome: A growing concern for health care professionals. *Journal of Obstetric, Gynecologic, and Neonatal Nursing (JOGNN), 32*(2), 215-221.

Fall, C.H., Yajnik, C.S., Rao, S., et al. (2003). Micronutrients and fetal growth. *Journal of Nutrition, 133*(5), 1747S-1756S.

Farina, A., Malone, F.D., & Bianchi, D.W. (2000). Fetal sonographic findings: Analysis of the most frequent patterns and their specificity of association. *American Journal of Medical Genetics, 91*(5), 331-339.

Fletcher, H.M., Wharfe, G.H., & Mitchell, S.Y. (2003). Placental separation from a seat belt injury due to severe turbulence during aeroplane travel. *Journal of Obstetric, Gynecologic, and Neonatal Nursing (JOGNN), 23*(1), 72-74.

Gilbert, R., Gras, L. (2003). European multicentre study on congenital toxoplasmosis. *British Journal of Obstetrics and Gynecology, 110*(2), 112-120.

Goldman, R.D., & Koren, G. (2003a). Anorexia nervosa during pregnancy. *Canadian Family Physician, 49,* 425-426.

Goldman, R.D., & Koren, G. (2003b). Taking St. John's wort during pregnancy. *Canadian Family Physician, 49,* 29-30.

Goodman, S. (2002). Anesthesia for nonobstetric surgery in the pregnant patient. *Seminars in Perinatology, 26*(2), 136-145.

Grier, D.G., & Halliday, H.L. (2003). Corticosteroids in the prevention and management of bronchopulmonary dysplasia. *Seminars in Neonatology, 8*(1), 83-91.

Guay-Woodford, L.M., & Desmond, R.A. (2003). Autosomal recessive polycystic kidney disease: The clinical experience in North America. *Pediatrics, 111*(5 Pt 1), 1072-1080.

Habek, D., Habek, J.C., Ivanisevic, M., et al. (2002). Fetal tobacco syndrome and perinatal outcome. *Fetal Diagnosis and Therapy, 17*(6), 367-371.

Hallman, M., & Haataja, R. (2003). Genetic influences and neonatal lung disease. *Seminars in Neonatology, 8*(1), 1-27.

Hansen, T.W. (2002). Mechanisms of bilirubin toxicity: Clinical implications. *Clinics in Perinatology, 29*(4), 765-778, viii.

Hendrick, V., Smith, L.M., Suri, R., et al. (2003). Birth outcomes after prenatal exposure to antidepressant medication. *American Journal of Obstetrics and Gynecology, 188*(3), 812-815.

Henrich, W., Heeger, J., Schmider, A., et al. (2002). Complete spontaneous resolution of severe nonimmunological hydrops fetalis with unknown etiology in the second trimester—A case report. *Journal of Perinatal Medicine, 30*(6), 5722-5727.

Houman, M.H., Ksontini-Smida, I., & Miled, M. (2002). Heparin use during pregnancy. *Tunis Medicine, 80*(6), 297-305.

Iqbal, M.M., Sobhan, T., Aftab, S.R., et al. (2002). Diazepam use during pregnancy: A review of the literature. *Developmental Medicine Journal, 74*(3), 127-135.

Jaeggi, E.T., Sholler, G.F., Jones, O.D., et al. (2001). Comparative analysis of pattern, management and outcome of pre- versus postnatally diagnosed major congenital heart disease: A population-based study. *Ultrasound of Obstetrics and Gynecology, 17*(5), 380-385.

Johnson, J.K., Haider, F., Ellis, K., et al. (2003). The prevalence of domestic violence in pregnant women. *British Journal of Obstetrics and Gynecology, 110*(3), 272-275.

Johnson, M.O. (2001). Mother infant interaction and maternal substance use/abuse: An integrative review of research literature in the 1990s. *Online Journal of Knowledge Synthesis Nursing, 8,* 2.

Kalter, H. (2003). Maternal diabetes mellitus and infant malformations. *Obstetrics and Gynecology, 101*(4), 815-816.

Kelly, P.A., Ritchie, I.M., Quate, L., et al. (2002). Functional consequences of perinatal exposure to 3,4-methylenedioxymethamphetamine in rat brain. *British Journal of Pharmacology, 137*(7), 963-970.

Kinsella, J.P., Parker, T.A., Ivy, D.D., et al. (2003). Noninvasive delivery of inhaled nitric oxide therapy for late pulmonary hypertension in newborn infants with congenital diaphragmatic hernia. *Journal of Pediatrics, 142*(4), 397-401.

Kinzler, W.L., Ananth, C.V., Smulian, J.C., & Vintzileos, A.M. (2002). Parental age difference and adverse perinatal outcomes in the United States. *Paediatrics and Perinatal Epidemiology, 16*(4), 320-327.

Kramer, M.S. (2003). The epidemiology of adverse pregnancy outcomes: An overview. *Journal of Nutrition, 133*(5), 1592S-1596S.

Lacroix, M.C., Guibourdenche, J., Frendo, J.L., et al. (2002). Placental growth hormones. *Endocrine, 19*(1), 73-79.

Lee, S.K, McMillan, D.D., Ohlsson, A., et al. (2003). The benefit of preterm birth at tertiary care centers is related to gestational age. *American Journal of Obstetrics and Gynecology, 188*(3), 617-622.

Lee, T., Carpenter, M.W., Heber, W.W., et al. (2003). Preterm premature rupture of membranes: Risks of recurrent complications in the next pregnancy among a population-based sample gravid women. *American Journal of Obstetrics and Gynecology, 188*(1), 209-213.

Leitich, H., Brunbauer, M., Bodner-Adler, B., et al. (2003). Antibiotic treatment of bacterial vaginosis in pregnancy: A meta-analysis. *American Journal of Obstetrics and Gynecology, 188*(3), 752-758.

Lester, B.M., Tronick, E.Z, LaGasse, L., et al. (2002). The maternal lifestyle study: Effects of substance exposure during pregnancy on neurodevelomental outcome in 1-month-old infants. *Pediatrics, 1110*(6), 1182-1192.

Little, R.E., Zadorozhnaja, T.D., Hulchiy, O.P., et al. (2003). Placental weight and its ratio to birthweight in a Ukrainian city. *Early Human Development, 71*(2), 117-127.

Liu, C.A., Huang, H.C., & Chou, Y.Y. (2002). Retrospective analysis of 17 liveborn neonates with hydrops fetalis. *Chang Gung Medical Journal, 25*(12), 826-831.

Lyles, J., & Cadet, J.L. (2003). Methylenedioxymethamphetamine (MDMA, ecstasy) neurotoxicity: Cellular and molecular mechanisms. *Brain Research and Brain Research Reviews, 42*(2), 155-168.

Malhotra, M., Sharma, J.B., Batra, S., et al. (2002). Maternal and perinatal outcome in varying degrees of anemia. *International Journal of Gynecology and Obstetrics, 79*(2), 93-100.

Martin, J.A., Hamilton, B.E., Ventura, S.J., et al. (2002). Births: Final data for 2001. *National Vital Statistics Report, 51*(2), 101-102.

McDonald, S.D., Ferguson, S., Tam, L., et al. (2003). The prevention of congenital anomalies with periconceptional folic acid supplementation. *Journal of Obstetrics and Gynecology Canada, 25*(2), 115-121.

McGrath, M., & Sullivan, M. (2002). Birth weight, neonatal morbidities, and school age outcomes in full-term and preterm infants. *Issues Comprehensive Pediatric Nursing, 25*(4), 231-254.

McLendon, D., Check, J., Carteaux, P., et al. (2003). Implementation of potentially better practices for the prevention of brain hemorrhage and ischemic brain injury in very low birth weight infants. *Pediatrics, 111*(4 Pt 2), E497-E503.

Mendola, P., Selevan, S.G., Gutter, S., et al. (2002). Environmental factors associated with a spectrum of neurodevelopmental deficits. *Mental Retardation and Developmental Disabilities Research Reviews, 8*(3), 188-197.

Mercer, B.M. (2003). Preterm premature rupture of the membranes. *Obstetrics and Gynecology, 101*(1), 178-192.

Meyer, O. (2003). Parvovirus B19 and autoimmune diseases. *Joint Bone Sine, 70*(1), 6-11.

Morrow, C.E., Bandstra, E.S., Anthony, J.C., et al. (2001). Influence of prenatal cocaine exposure on full-term infant neurobehavioral functioning. *Neurotoxicol Teratol, 23*(6), 533-544.

Mustonen, K., Mustakangas, P., Uotila, L, et al. (2003). Viral infections in neonates with seizures. *Journal of Perinatal Medicine, 31*(10), 75-80.

Nagdyman, N., Grimmer, I., Scholz, T., et al. (2003). Predictive value of brain-specific proteins in serum for neurodevelopmental outcome after birth asphyxia. *Pediatric Research,* no pages listed yet. (In press).

Naylor, D.F., Jr., & Olson, M.M. (2003). Critical care obstetrics and gynecology. *Critical Care Clinics, 19*(1), 127-149.

Newman, M.G., Robichaux, A.G., Stedman, C.M., et al. (2003). Perinatal outcomes in preeclampsia that is complicated by massive proteinuria. *American Journal of Obstetricians and Gynecology, 188*(1), 264-268.

Ogunyemi, D., Murillo, M., Jackson, U., et al. (2003). The relationship between placental histopathology findings and perinatal outcome in preterm infants. *Journal of Maternal, Fetal, and Neonatal Medicine, 13*(2), 102-109.

Ornoy, A. (2002). The effects of alcohol and illicit drugs on the human embryo and fetus. *Israeli Journal of Psychiatry and Relational Science, 29*(2), 120-132.

O'Shea, T.M., & Dammann, O. (2000). Antecedents of cerebral palsy in very low-birth weight infants. *Clinical Perinatology, 27*(2), 285-302.

Paladini, D., D'Armiento, M., Ardovino, I., et al. (2000). Prenatal diagnosis of the cerebro-oculo-facio-skeletal (COFS) syndrome. *Ultrasound Obstetrics and Gynecology, 16*(1), 91-93.

Paul, D.A., Coleman, M.M., Leef, K.H., et al. (2003). Maternal antibiotics and decreased periventricular leukomalacia in very low-birth-weight infants. *Archives of Pediatric Adolescent Medicine, 157*(2), 145-149.

Pereira, D.N., & Procianoy, R.S. (2003). Effect of perinatal asphyxia on thyroid-stimulating hormone and thyroid hormone levels. *Acta Paediatrics, 92*(3), 339-345.

Perrott, S., Dodds, L., & Vincer, M. (2003). A population-based study of prognostic factors related to major disability in very preterm survivors. *Journal of Perinatology, 23*(2), 111-116.

Perry, B.L., Jones, H., Tuten, M., et al. (2003). Assessing maternal perceptions of harmful effects of drug use during pregnancy. *Journal of Addictions Disease, 22*(1), 1-9.

Peters, V., Liu, K.L., Dominguez, K., et al. (2003). Missed opportunities for perinatal HIV prevention among

HIV-exposed infants born 1996–2000, pediatric spectrum of HIV disease cohort. *Pediatrics, 111*(5 Part 2), 1186-1191.

Petrini, J., Damus, K., Russell, R., et al. (2002). Contribution of birth defects to infant mortality in the United States. *Teratology, 66*(Suppl 1), S3-S6.

Pinn, G. (2001). Herbs used in obstetrics and gynecology. *Austrailian Family Physician, 30*(4), 351-354, 356.

Pinn, G., & Pallett, L. (2002). Herbal medicine in pregnancy. *Complementary Therapy and Nurse Midwifery, 8*(2), 77-80.

Poland, R.L. (2003). How to avoid kernicterus. *Journal of Pediatrics, 142*(20), 213-214.

Rasmussen, K. (2001). Is there a causal relationship between iron deficiency or iron-deficiency anemia and weight at birth, length of gestation and perinatal mortality? *Journal of Nutrition, 131*(2S-2), 590S-601S.

Rayburn, W.F., Christensen, H.D., & Gonzalez, C.L. (2000). Effect of antenatal exposure to Saint John's wort (Hypercum) on neurobehavior of developing mice. *American Journal of Obstetrics and Gynecology, 183*(5), 1225-1231.

Rehan, V.K., Moddemann, D., & Casiro, O.G. (2002). Outcome of very-low-birth-weight (<1,500 grams) infants born to mothers with diabetes. *Clinics in Pediatrics, 41*(7), 481-491.

Reiss, I., Landmann, E., Heckmann, M., Misselwitz, B., & Gortner, L. (April 8, 2003). Increased risk of bronchopulmonary dysplasia and increased mortality in very preterm infants being small for gestational age. *Archives of Gynecology and Obstetrics*, pages unknown.

Rhone, S.A., Magee, F., Remple, V., et al. (2003). The association of placental abnormalities with maternal and neonatal clinical findings: A retrospective cohort study. *Journal of Obstetrics and Gynecology Canada, 25*(2), 123-128.

Riley, E.P., Mattson, S.N., Li, T.K., et al. (2003). Neurobehavioral consequences of prenatal alcohol exposure: An international perspective. *Alcohol Clinical Experimental Research, 27*(2), 362-373.

Roberts, G., Gordon, M.M., Porter, D., et al. (2003). Acute renal failure complicating HELLP syndrome, SLE and anti-phospholipid syndrome: Successful outcome using plasma exchange therapy. *Lupus, 12*(4), 251-257.

Rondo, P.H., & Tomkins, A.M. (1999). Maternal and neonatal anthropometry. *Annals of Tropical Paediatrics, 19*(4), 349-356.

Rosenberg, K.D, Desai, R.A., & Kan, J. (2002). Why do foreign-born blacks have lower infant mortality than native-born blacks? New directions in African-American infant mortality research. *Journal of National Medical Association, 94*(9), 770-778.

Sadiq, H.F., Mantych, G., Benawra, R.S., et al. (2003). Inhaled nitric oxide in the treatment of moderate persistent pulmonary hypertension of the newborn: A randomized controlled, multicenter trial. *Journal of Perinatology, 23*(2), 98-103.

Sanders, T.R., Roberts, C.L., & Gilbert, G.L. (2002). Compliance with a protocol for intrapartum antibiotic prophylaxis against neonatal group B streptococcal sepsis in women with clinical risk factors. *Infectious Disease in Obstetrics and Gynecology, 10*(4), 223-229.

Sato, Y., Okumura, A., Kato, T., et al. (2003). Hypoxic ischemic encephalopathy associated with neonatal seizures without other neurological abnormalities. *Brain Development, 25*(30), 215-219.

Scher, M.S. (2003). Fetal and neonatal neurologic case histories: Assessment of brain disorders in the context of fetal-maternal-placental disease. Part 1: Fetal neurologic consultations in the context of antepartum events and prenatal brain development. *Journal of Child Neurology, 18*(2), 85-92.

Schuler, M.E., Nair, P., & Kettinger, L. (2003). Drug-exposed infants and developmental outcome: Effects of a home intervention and ongoing maternal drug use. *Archives of Pediatric and Adolescent Medicine, 157*(20), 133-138.

Sen, S., Reghu, A., & Ferguson, S.D. (2002). Efficacy of a single dose of antenatal steroid in surfactant-treated babies under 21 weeks' gestation. *Journal of Maternal & Fetal Neonatal Medicine, 12*(5), 298-303.

Sheiner, E., Shoham-Vardi, I., Hallak, M., et al. (2003). Placental abruption in term pregnancies: Clinical significance and obstetric risk factors. *Journal of Maternal, Fetal and Neonatal Medicine, 13*(1), 45-49.

Simpsom, J.M., Jones, A., Callaghan, N., et al. (2000). Accuracy and limitations of transabdominal fetal echocardiography at 12-15 weeks of gestation in a population at high risk for congenital heart disease. *British Journal of Obstetrics and Gynecology, 107*(12), 1492-1497.

Smith, L., Yonekura, M.L., Wallace, T., et al. (2003). Effects of prenatal methamphetamine exposure on fetal growth and drug withdrawal symptoms in infants born at term. *Journal of Developmental and Behavioral Pediatrics, 24*(1), 17-23.

Sohan, K., Billington, M., Pamphilon, D., et al. (2002). Normal growth and development following in utero diagnosis and treatment of monozygous alpha-thalassaemia. *British Journal of Obstetrics and Gynecology, 109*(11), 1308-1310.

Soloway, B. (2003). Report from the Tenth Retrovirus Conference. Perinatal transmission. *AIDS Clinical Care, 15*(4), 38-39.

Srivastava, A.K., Gupta, A.K., Singh, A.V., et al. (2002). Effect of oral anticoagulant during pregnancy with prosthetic heart valve. *Asian Cardiovascular and Thoracic Annals, 10*(4), 306-309.

Steinhausen, H.C., Willms, J., Metzke, C.W., et al. (2003). Behavioral phenotype in fetal alcohol syndrome and fetal alcohol effects. *Developmental Medicine and Child Neurology, 45*(3), 179-182.

Stoler, J.M. (2001). Maternal antiepileptic drug use and effects on fetal development. *Current Opinion in Pediatrics, 13*(6), 566-571.

Suchet, I. (2003). Fetal echocardiography—Beyond the four-chamber view into the next millennium. *Canadian Association of Radiology Journal, 54*(1), 56-60.

Sweet, M.P., Hodgman, J.E., Pena, I., et al. (2003). Two-year outcome of infants weighing 600 grams or less at birth and born 1994 through 1998. *Obstetrics and Gynecology, 101*(1), 18-23.

Tan, L.K., Tan, H.K., Lee, C.T., et al. (2002). Outcome of pregnancy in Asian women with systemic lupus erythematosus: Experience of a single perinatal center in Singapore. *Annals of Academic Medicine in Singapore, 31*(3), 290-295.

Thorsen, M.S., & Poole, J.H. (2002). Renal disease in pregnancy. *Journal of Perinatal and Neonatal Nursing, 15*(4), 13-26.

Ugwumadu, A., Manonda, I., Reid, F., et al. (2003). Effect of early oral clindamycin on late miscarriage and preterm delivery in asymptomatic women with abnormal vaginal flora and bacterial vaginosis: A randomised controlled trial. *Lancet, 341*(9362), 983-988.

Vasapollo, B., Valensis, H., Novelli, G.P., et al. (2002). Abnormal maternal cardiac function and morphology in pregnancies complicated by intrauterine fetal growth restriction. *Ultrasound Obstetrics and Gynecology, 20*(5), 452-457.

Vintzileos, A., Ananth, C.V., Smulian, J.C., et al. (2002). The impact of prenatal care on postneonatal deaths in the presence and absences of antenatal high-risk conditions. *American Journal of Obstetrics and Gynecology, 187*(5), 1258-1262.

Vohr, B.R., Allan, W.C, Westerveld, M., et al. (2003). School-age outcomes of very low birth weight infants in the indomethacin intraventricular hemorrhage prevention trial. *Pediatrics, 111*(4 Pt 1), E340-E346.

Weber, M.K., Floyd, R.L, Riley, E.P., et al. (2002). National Task Force on Fetal Alcohol Syndrome and Fetal Alcohol Effect: Defining the national agenda for fetal alcohol syndrome and other prenatal alcohol-related effects. *Morbidity & Mortality Weekly Report, Recommendations Report, 51*(RR-12), 9-12.

Wellesley, D., & Howe, D.T. (2001). Fetal renal anomalies and genetic syndromes. *Prenatal Diagnosis, 21*(11), 992-1003.

Willoughby, R.E, Jr., & Nelson, K.B. (2002). Chorioamnionitis and brain injury. *Clinics in Perinatology, 29*(4), 603-621.

Won, L., Bubula, N., & Heller, A. (2002). Fetal exposure to methamphetamine in utero stimulates development of serotonergic neurons in three-dimensional reaggregate tissue culture. *Synapse, 43*(2), 139-144.

Zhang, W.H., Levi, S., Alexander, S., et al. (2002). Sensitivity of ultrasound screening for congenital anomalies in unselected pregnancies. *Review of Epidemiology Sante Publique, 50*(6), 571-580.

# 10 The NICU Experience and Its Relationship to Sensory Integration

## Linda M. Lutes, Chrysty D. Graves, and Katherine M. Jorgensen

The preterm infant in the neonatal intensive care unit (NICU) is unfortunately exposed to an abnormal world that is not always nurturing and protecting, as the womb is. The preterm infant is abruptly thrust into an unfamiliar NICU world full of noxious stimuli. Noise, lights, and equipment become everyday experiences for the developing infant. Instead of the warmth and comfort of the mother's womb, which provides boundaries and tactile stimulation, the newborn preterm infant is exposed to a multitude of painful stimuli, including routine procedures such as heel pricks, intravenous (IV) sticks, eye examinations, blood pressure checks, and, possibly, intubation. Gone is the gentle, fluid uterine environment. Instead, forces of gravity exerted by the attached equipment complicate movement and handling.

With the integration of the concept of individualized, family-centered, developmental care (IFDC), caregivers are challenged to reevaluate the NICU environment, procedures, and tasks as they relate to the preterm infant responses both physiologic and behavioral. Developmental care has refocused our approach to caregiving and refined caregiving standards so that the family is a priority for the professional and is, in many ways, treated equally with the needs of the infant. Relationship-based care is becoming the accepted standard of care rather than the traditional model that focused on performance of tasks. The NICU should be a gentle, kind, family-centered environment. There is evidence to support the positive effect of such care (Peters, 1999). Research indicates that an infant who receives developmentally supportive care experiences fewer ventilator days, earlier discharge, and improved developmental outcomes (Hendricks-Munoz, Predergast, Caprio, et al., 2002).

We are challenged to explore additional ways to improve our efforts as caregivers to facilitate better infant outcomes. What more can we do to improve our care, and how can we measure outcomes? The issues of the long-term effects of the NICU are something families, follow-up nurses, clinicians, therapists, educators, and NICU graduates have been coping with for many years. As follow-up and community care providers have developed a heightened awareness to assess and evaluate high-risk infants and children for sensitivity to the environment and sensory defensiveness by infants; this information is being passed on to care providers in the NICU. Sensory integration dysfunction is a life-long issue for some of these infants and their families. Not all infants who have a NICU stay experience long-term sensory dysfunction. However, we must anticipate that it might occur. What the caregiver does, and does not do, with the infant, can have lasting, irreversible effects. Sensory integration (the organizing of information) brought in by our senses is an additional phenomenon to consider in gaining a comprehensive perspective regarding development. Using this information to make caregiving decisions might improve long-term developmental outcomes. If we understand what sensory integration is to the developing human being, this knowledge might provide clarity about how the NICU's macro- and microenvironments contribute to the developmental capacities of the infant. Reviewing neurosensory development, physiology, and function provides a foundational understanding of sensory integration. As caregivers, we can continue to make changes and adaptations to facilitate the development of happy, integrated children. This chapter defines sensory integration and common sensory dysfunction. In addition, it will review the development of the brain, central nervous system (CNS), and peripheral sensory nervous system. A case is presented to demonstrate sensory integration as related to neonatal care.

## SENSORY INTEGRATION

The term "integration" is defined by *Webster's Dictionary* (Merriam-Webster, 1999) as "bringing together and organizing parts into a whole." A. Jean Ayers, PhD, defines

1. Sensory integration as . . .
   a. The process by which the brain organizes sensory information for appropriate use.
   b. The interaction or coordination of two or more neural functions or sensory processes in a manner that enhances the adaptability of the brain's response.
   c. The organizing and processing of sensory information from the different sensory channels and the ability to relate input from one channel to another to emit an adaptive response. The greatest development of sensory integration occurs during an adaptive response to the environment. An adaptive response is a purposeful, goal-directed response to sensory experience. A baby sees a rattle and reaches for it. Reaching is an adaptive response. Merely waving the hands about aimlessly is not adaptive. A more complex adaptive response occurs when the child perceives that the rattle is too far away and crawls to get it. In an adaptive response, we master a challenge and learn something new—the formation of an adaptive response helps the brain develop and organize itself. A child, parent, or teacher cannot tell the brain to organize itself.
   d. The process of organizing sensory inputs so that the brain produces a useful body response and also useful perceptions, emotions, and thoughts.
2. If all sensory stimuli that is received by the CNS were allowed to bombard the higher levels, the individual would be utterly ineffective. It is the brain's function to filter, organize, and integrate a mass of stimulation so it can be used for the development and execution of the brain's functions.
3. Sensory integration sorts, orders, and eventually puts all the individual sensory inputs together into an integrated brain function that uses all the capacities available in the CNS. When the functions of the brain are whole and balanced, body movements are highly adaptive, learning is easy, and good behavior is a natural outcome. Sensory integration provides us information about the physical conditions of our body and the environment around us (Ayers, 1981, pp. 6-8). The brain must organize all of these sensations, flowing in a well-organized or integrated manner. Sensory integration puts it all together or makes a whole from all the parts, which are often greater than the sum of these parts.

Sensory integration begins in the womb and continues through approximately the next 7 years of life. Moving, talking, and playing are the primary goals that provide the groundwork for more complex sensory integration, such as reading, writing, and behavior. Sensory integration function develops in a natural order, and each child follows the same basic sequence. The infant takes in information and puts it all together to make an "adaptive response" (Ayers, 1981).

Understanding two simple words, "sensory" and "motor," will provide a foundation for understanding sensory integration. Sensory implies the perception of a stimulus. When we smell something burning, we perceive a stimulus. The odor that reaches our olfactory sense tells us something. How we interpret the odor depends on past experiences stored in higher levels of the nervous system. We react to the stimulus by doing something, and this reaction is a motor response to a simple stimulus. Notice that the stimulus must precede the motor response, not vice versa.

The nervous system has three ways of perceiving sensations. First, the nervous system detects or picks up sensations from the external skin surface (touch, temperature, and pain) or via the other sensory systems—visual, auditory, olfactory, gustatory, or vestibular—and reacts to any changes that these systems perceive. Those stimuli that are picked up by receptors "outside of us" are called exteroceptors, meaning exterior receptors, such as cutaneous sensations, which are heard, seen, or smelled, for example. Therefore, the exteroceptors are groups of general and specialized receptors that receive stimuli from the periphery of our bodies. These receptors only react to change.

Second, there are stimuli that are interior and are picked up by receptors called "interoceptors." These receptors recognize hunger, nausea, cold, heat, pain, and so on. These can also be referred to as "visceral receptors" or "receptors of visceral stimuli."

Third, there are receptors concerned with movement and posture. These receptors are neither visceral nor external, but lie in an intermediate position, around joints and ligaments, in muscles and tendons, in the pads of our hands and feet, and in our inner ear. There are also specialized receptors that are associated with muscle tendons, joints, and fascia. These are called "proprioceptors"—that is, receptors of "one's own" ("proprius" = "one's own"). The word "property" is from the same Latin word. Certainly, among the greatest properties humans have are the muscles and tendons, which endow us with the ability to move, communicate, express ideas, create, and survive. One can argue that our intellectual capacity is our greatest asset when compared with other animals. However, this is of no value unless we have the means whereby to carry out our thoughts, ideas, and feelings. Without muscles and proprioceptive sensation from muscles and allied structures, we cannot write, speak intelligently, see or hear normally, or communicate in any known way. Therefore, perhaps our greatest endowment is our ability to move and to use this movement effectively to carry out the necessities of life and express our intelligence.

Muscles for movement's sake are valueless, unless we somehow know at all times what a muscle is doing. For muscles to work smoothly, maintain posture and position sense, move, walk, or shove, we must have a sensory mechanism that initially perceives a stimulus as well as a sensory "feedback system" from our muscles, tendons, and ligaments to tell us what is going on at every moment. This is the purpose of the proprioceptors. They send sensations to the nervous system to keep it continually informed so that we can use the muscles or muscle groups as needed. Unless these proprioceptors are intact, our muscles are, for all essential purposes, of little or no value to us.

In summary, a sensory stimulation is needed to activate the nervous system. In turn, the nervous system reacts by moving muscles. The reaction is the motor response to the stimulus. That stimulus is the trigger, which sets into motion some recordable responses, and movements results. This series of events cannot work in reverse—motor first, stimulus last. All movement, therefore, is the motor result of preceding stimuli. Within the tactile system, an example of an adaptive infant response would be to touch the lips with the reciprocal rooting reflex or the withdrawal of a limb when skin is punctured with a needle. The response is dependent on the integration of sensory stimuli.

## SENSORY SYSTEMS AND EXAMPLES OF ADAPTIVE BEHAVIOR

Before giving examples of adaptive behaviors as a result of sensory stimulation, some definitions of the various sensory systems are needed. These definitions include:

1. Vestibular (gravity and balance) system—The system responsible for a sense of balance. It is one of the first sensory systems to develop in utero.
2. Proprioception (muscle and joint sensations)—The infant's sense of movement and positioning.
3. Gustatory (taste) system—The part of the sensory system responsible for an infant's sense of taste.
4. Olfactory (smell) system—The receptors responsible for the infant's sense of smell.
5. Tactile (touch) system—The sensory system that is responsible for an infant's ability to respond to any form of touch.
6. Auditory (sound) system—The portion of the sensory system responsible for hearing. This system develops later in gestation compared with the previously mentioned sensory systems.
7. Visual (sight) system—The last sensory system to develop in utero. It is responsible for sight.

All of these systems and their adaptive responses are dependent on the infant's gestational age, severity of illness, and extent of exposure to multiple stimuli. The vestibular system responds to changes in gravity or position. If the infant is pushed to the side, there will be an attempt to right the position. There is an emergence of righting reactions with movements as the infant matures. For the proprioceptor system, the adaptive responses that are often seen in the NICU are a withdrawal of a leg related to a heel stick. Therefore, part of this system is also responsible for pain responses. This is also an example of a response to tactile stimuli. Another example is use of facilitated tuck to calm an infant who is upset—again, touch is also involved, but this time with creating boundaries for the touch. Stimulation of the gustatory system results in adaptive responses that are seen when the infant is given a drop of breast milk; the tongue protrudes, and a licking motion occurs. The olfactory system, or sense of smell, is shown when an infant is exposed to a noxious odor and turns away toward his/her mother's smell. The auditory system's adaptive response is demonstrated by the infant's startle to sharp noises or the turning toward his/her mother's voice. The visual response occurs when an infant is exposed to sudden light changes and closes the eyes or opens them within a dim environment.

Figure 10-1 shows the correlation between sensory development and NICU sensory exposure. Box 10-1 outlines the development of hearing in the preterm and term infant. The development of vision was outlined in Box 7-2.

## SENSORY INTEGRATIVE DYSFUNCTION

Sensory integrative dysfunction occurs when the brain is not processing or organizing the flow of sensory impulses in a manner that provides the individual the precise information about himself/herself or the world. The word "dysfunction" is synonymous with "malfunction"; therefore, sensory integration dysfunction is a malfunction, not an absence, of function (Ayers, 1981).

The brain does not organize the incoming sensory information in an efficient way, and learning becomes difficult; often the individual cannot cope with ordinary demands of life and stress.

The symptoms of sensory integrative dysfunction might include muscle tone and coordination difficulties; hyperactivity and distractibility; speech and language delays; behavior problems; and difficulty learning, with problems in reading, writing, and arithmetic, or with higher learning and organization. Not all infants/children will display all the symptoms or have the same problems with integration. There is often much individualization in how or when the symptoms are exhibited. Sensory impairment or dysfunction is an area

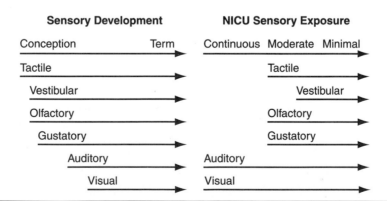

Figure **10-1** Comparison of sensory development to sensory experienced in the NICU. (*From Kenner, C., & Lott, J.W. [Eds.],* Comprehensive neonatal nursing: A physiologic perspective *[3rd ed.; p. 243]. St. Louis: W.B. Saunders; and White-Traut, R., Nelson, M.N., Burns, K., et al. [1994]. Environmental influences on the developing premature infant: Theoretical issues and applications to practice.* Journal of Obstetric, Gynecologic, and Neonatal Nursing *[JOGNN], 23[5], 393-401.*)

Box **10-1**   DEVELOPMENT OF HEARING IN PRETERM AND TERM INFANTS

| Age | Anatomic and Functional Development |
|---|---|
| Preterm infants <28 weeks | Fetal hearing begins by 23 to 24 weeks |
| | Threshold approximately 65 decibels (dBs), 500 to 1000 Hertz (Hz) |
| | Auditory brain stem responses by 26 to 28 weeks |
| Preterm infants 28 to 30 weeks | Rapid maturation of cochlea and auditory nerve |
| | Responses rapidly fatigue |
| | Initial auditory processing by 30 weeks |
| | Threshold 40 dB with an increased frequency range |
| Preterm infants 32 to 34 weeks | Outer hair cells mature by 32 weeks |
| | Rapid maturation of cochlea and auditory nerve |
| Preterm infants >34 weeks | Increased speed of conduction |
| | Ossicles and electrophysiology complete by 36 weeks |
| | Hearing threshold 30 dB, increasing range |
| | Increasing ability to localize and discriminate |
| Term infants | Ability to localize and discriminate sounds |
| | Hearing threshold 25 dB |
| | Range 50 to 4000 Hz |

From Holditch-Davis, D., Blackburn, S.T., & VandenBerg, K. (2003). Newborn and infant neurobehavioral development (pp. 236-284). In C. Kenner & J.W. Lott (Eds.), *Comprehensive neonatal nursing: A physiologic perspective* (3rd. ed.; p. 247). St. Louis: W.B. Saunders.

of growing research as technologic advances have increased the survival of the most immature infant (Allen, 2002).

Given the immaturity of the developing CNS in the human infant and the multitude of noxious stimuli in the NICU, the integration of normal sensory development can be disrupted, resulting in inappropriate sensory development that will then affect the development of sensory integration and may lead to sensory integrative dysfunction. Abnormal sensory input experienced by the NICU infant can cause sensory integrative dysfunction. However, this is a new concept, and much of what we know at this time is untested theory because longitudinal research is difficult to conduct.

If the infant suffers from CNS events such as hypoxia, intraventricular hemorrhage (IVH), or cerebral vascular insult, sensory integration will likely be affected. Premature infants are at risk for these events, as well as potential interruption of the development of the sensory systems due to abnormal stimuli or sensory input related to the environment of the NICU and the severity of the child's illness.

Hellerud and Storm (2002) examined exposure to repeated tactile and painful stimuli in preterm and term infants. They found that repeated exposure to certain nociceptive stimuli, such as heel sticks and routine tasks requiring touch, in preterm (compared with term infants), evoked adaptive responses. In the preterm infant, even repeated tactile stimulation resulted in equal or greater signs of physiologic stress than seen with the initial painful stimuli. They speculated that these tactile exposures "rewire" the infant's response to pain. Most of the neonatal sensory research has used the animal model to determine what happens when there is neurologic impairment, exposure to medications, and overstimulation of the sensory system (Couper & Brujes, 2003; Szoke, Czeh, Szolesanyi, et al., 2002). What is the significance of this work? The concerns raised are related to the long-term effects of negative sensory stimuli and the lack or dysfunction of sensory integration.

As the child matures, the long-term end products of sensory integration are as follows: the ability to concentrate, the ability to organize oneself, positive self-esteem, good self-control, self-confidence, academic learning ability, capacity for abstract thought and reasoning, and specialization of each side of the body and the brain. Therefore, if there is a dysfunction of these systems, the child is at risk for many behavioral and learning problems.

To understand what might cause sensory integrative dysfunction, we must first review aspects of neurologic development followed by a discussion of the sensory systems. The sensory systems include: tactile (touch), vestibular (gravity and balance), proprioception (muscle and joint sensations), gustatory (taste), olfactory (smell), auditory (sound), and visual (sight). Sensory integration dysfunction is related to neurologic and sensory development. Some researchers have theorized that treating these aspects separately will render sensory integration dysfunction easier to understand, making it possible to avoid problems in one or the other. Some health professionals believe that if they provide care in a "positive" way, the infant will not have these sensory integration dysfunction issues. This is not true. Even repeated tactile stimuli that are not painful can overload the newborn's system and result in sensory integration dysfunction. Sensory integration dysfunction is often a result of brain insults. These insults can be linked to macro- and microenvironment, caregiving, and handling, but the bottom line for alterations is the effect on the brain. Thus, the neurologic system and the sensory system must be considered together—not as separate entities. Together they constitute the neurobehavioral-sensory development of the infant.

## ASPECTS OF NEUROLOGY

The brain is molded by experience: every sight, sound, and thought imprints specific neural circuits, alters the way potential sights, sounds, and thoughts will be recorded. Brain hardware is living, active tissue that is constantly meeting the sensory, motor, emotional, and intellectual demands at hand. From the first cell division, brain development is a delicate relationship between genetic predisposition and environment. By understanding each of the subtle interactions, we can understand the degree to which heredity and experience makes each human being unique (Liebman, 1991).

Significant improvements in technology allow us to visualize every part of the living brain in action—from the largest circuits down to the tiny gap between neurons and synapses; to recording electrical activity from single molecules in the brain; to retrieving human DNA; and identifying single genes involved in early neural development, mental retardation, and senile dementia. Researchers have devised other ingenious ways to probe babies' emerging sensory, emotional, and cognitive abilities through objective observation of infant behaviors. These technologies, together with the rapidly expanding knowledge of brain function and development, give us a far better understanding of "what is going on" in an infant's mind than ever before (Harris, 1998).

Upon entering the world, the infant's brain is equipped with a variety of mental skills, predispositions, and abilities to meet the critical needs of early life. Their brains are small and still developing. The nervous system matures in a programmed sequence from caudad to cephalad. When born full-term, the spinal column and the brain stem are almost fully developed and are largely responsible for meeting the newborn's essential needs—to survive, grow, and bond with the caregiver/parents.

After birth, this sequence of development continues, as higher-brain areas progressively take control of an infant's mental well-being. These areas include the cerebellum and basal ganglia, which are involved in movement; the limbic system that controls emotion and memory; and the cerebral cortex that controls willed behavior, conscious experience, and rational abilities. The cerebral cortex remains the most markedly underdeveloped at birth. As the cortex gradually matures during the first months and years of life, a child grows steadily more capable and aware of his own existence.

Genes program the sequence of neural development. This genetic influence has been explored in relationship to brain development and malformation (Tanaka & Gleeson, 2000). Genetic linkages with sensory aspects are growing as the human genome is nearing completion of its mapping. In addition to genetic influences, however, the quality of that development is shaped by environmental factors. In the earliest stages, embryonic cells respond to a slight gradient in the concentration of particular molecules, which direct them to become cephalad or caudad, vertebral column, or cerebellum. Later, a pattern of electrical excitation subtly alters some cerebral cortex synapses. These innumerable, intricate interactions take place in the brain at the molecular level. The brain is a chain of communication cells and is inescapably linked to the world. Every touch, movement, and emotion is translated into electrical and chemical activity that affects development, subtly modifying the way a child's brain is wired together.

Genes and environment are both significant; we can do very little at this time to alter our genes, and a great deal to alter the environment. It is, therefore, very important that we examine genetic predisposition for problems in relationship to the environment. When little genetic history is available, it is even more important that we assess the impact the environment has on the baby's continued development. It is important that we have a good understanding of each sensory system of the brain and how it develops, and the degree to which genes and environment are known to influence the system's formation. In the womb, we need to fully understand the degree of sensory and motor development and, thus, the abilities of the newborn. In addition to the womb, after birth all the higher mental functions explain how and why a child's various mental abilities emerge.

The basic processes of brain development consist of how the remarkably complex brain emerges— how its many crucial circuits become "wired up" through the dual influence of genes and experience. The same biologic principles hold for every sensory, motor, and higher system in the brain. The focus on the development of each sensory system is roughly the order in which they mature—tactile, vestibular, olfactory, gustatory, auditory, and visual. This principle of development serves as a foundation and is relevant for understanding the long-term effect of the NICU experience. A child's emotional, memory, language, and other cognitive skills emerge and evolve through the interaction of programmed brain maturation and early experience.

The brain is our most fascinating organ. Parents, physicians, nurses, therapists, educators, and society as a whole have tremendous power to shape the hills and valleys inside each child's head, and, with it, the kind of person he or she will turn out to be. We owe it to our children, and the children that we work with every day, to help them grow the best brains possible.

## BRAIN DEVELOPMENT BY 24 WEEKS' GESTATION

By 24 weeks' gestation, the fetus is typically 14 inches long and capable, in the direst circumstances, of surviving outside the womb. The lungs can exchange air, if necessary, but the small alveolar sacs are not fully formed. The brain stem, the regulator of vital functions, such as breathing, is capable of directing rhythmic breathing movements. The cerebral cortex is still not functional, which is reflected in its immature structure: its surface is still mostly smooth, the major sulci, the valleys of the brain, are just beginning to develop. These fissures allow the growing brain to fold in on itself, thus increasing its surface area. The elevated regions between the sulci are called gyri, and it is within these mounds of gray matter that the most sophisticated processing in the brain takes place.

Cortical sulci come in three sizes: primary, secondary, and tertiary. The large primary sulci, similar to the central sulcus that separates the frontal parietal lobes, are typically well defined by the seventh month gestation. Secondary sulci demonstrate more variation. The smallest or tertiary sulci vary greatly among individuals, signifying they are not solely genetically determined. Tertiary sulci initiate development in the last month of gestation and are not fully formed until the baby's first birthday. Although certain gyri and sulci are present in almost every human brain, no two brains, or even hemispheres of the same brain, have exactly the same pattern of gyri and sulci. Two grooves, the lateral fissures and the central sulcus, help divide each hemisphere into four main areas, or lobes. The frontal lobe is anterior to the central sulcus, and the parietal lobe is posterior to it. Lying below the lateral fissure is the temporal lobe, and an imaginary line drawn down from the parieto-occipital fissure separates the parietal lobe from the occipital lobe. Each lobe has its specific areas and gyri. In the frontal lobe, the precentral gyrus, lying just anterior to the central sulcus, is the motor center that initiates impulses to the voluntary muscles. The most anterior area, the frontal lobe, is the seat of personality. Injuries here often result in alterations of personality. The function of the cerebral cortex is to process information within columns of neurons that run perpendicular to its surface; each column contains thousands of cells that function as a distinct processing unit. The larger the surface area of the cortex, the more processing units it can hold. The number, depth, and cortical convolutions also significantly expand during the infant's development, beginning in the late fetal period and continuing into the first year of life. This maturation and increasing complexity of the cerebral cortex allows the infant to respond to external stimuli in a more integrated manner. Brain maturation and development, especially of the cerebral cortex, continues through the first year. The brain practically triples in size, growing from approximately one quarter to nearly three quarters of its adult weight. From a functional point of view, these postnatal changes are as dramatic as the elaborate processes of prenatal brain formation. The difference is they take place at the microscopic level. From the surface, the appearance of the brain changes very little after birth, but there is a profound growth and differentiation of the billions of tiny cells within.

The brain comprises billions of nerve cells, or neurons, each of which is shaped much like a tree. Therefore, a mature neuron has an extensive root system, comprised of the dendrites, that receives input from other neurons, and a trunk, or axon, that can be extremely long and ultimately branches out to relay information to the next neurons in its circuit.

In between these two branched systems lies an enlarged area, the cell body, which contains the nucleus and oversees the basic metabolic functions of the cell. Within each neuron, information is transmitted electrically by brief impulses called action potentials; but when the impulse arrives at the end of each axon branch, the information must cross a gap, the synapse, to be transmitted to the next neuron in the circuit. The gap is traversed by the release of a chemical messenger, or neurotransmitter, from the presynaptic terminal of the axon. Neurotransmitter molecules then diffuse the short distance across the synapse, where they bind the special receptors on the postsynaptic neuron's dendrites, triggering electrical responses in each receiving neuron. This same sequence of electrical and chemical transmission repeats itself through every cell and synapse of the circuit.

There are two different types of cells in the nervous system: neurons, which are connected to each other in the process just described and form information-processing circuits; and glia, which are supporting cells that provide the structural framework and metabolic sustenance for the neurons (Figure 10-2). Glia are important in both the development and the functioning of the nervous system; they outnumber neurons 10 to 50 times, but neurons are where the action is, mentally speaking.

Neurogenesis begins as soon as the neural tube forms (third week of development), reaches a peak in the seventh week, and is largely completed by 18 weeks. To a very small extent, some neurons continue to be products in the latter parts of fetal life and on into the first few postnatal months. The glia cells, however, continue to be products at a low rate throughout life. But, for the most part, these basic building blocks of our brains are all formed by just 4 months gestation (when the fetus is approximately 9 in long and weighs 9 oz). Most of these neurons will survive a lifetime. The brain is unlike other body systems (such as the liver, blood, and bones) whose cells can continue to divide, generating new cells throughout life. Neurons are terminally differentiated, meaning the cell division that produces them is the last they will undergo. This difference is why brain damage is often much more devastating than damage to other tissues: once the

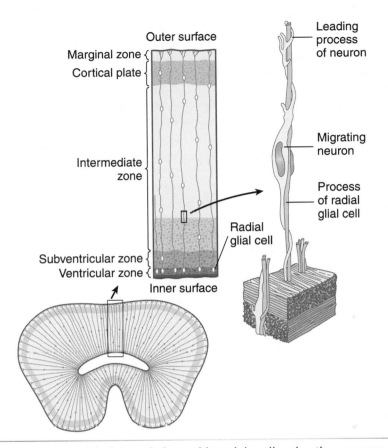

Figure **10-2** Radial glial cells and their associations with peripherally migrating neurons during the development of the brain. (*From Blackburn, S.T. [2003]. Maternal, fetal, & neonatal physiology: A clinical perspective [2nd ed.; p. 571]. St. Louis: W.B. Saunders. Based on Rakic, P. [1975].* Birth defects original article series XI, 7, *95-129.*)

cells comprising a particular neural circuit are lost, they can never be replaced. Although stem cells and other genetic methods of growing new neural cells might prove to be valuable in the future, our knowledge and technology is not yet there. However, the brain has other compensatory mechanisms that can somewhat lessen the impact of brain injury.

The speed of neurogenesis is amazing. To ensure that the 100 billion neurons in the brain are produced, they must develop at a rate of 250,000/min, averaged over the 9 months of gestation. Because most neurons are developed by the midpoint of gestation, the actual rate is more than 500,000/min. When the infant is born prematurely, these neurons

might not yet have developed, leading to a decrease in the body's ability to transmit signals through the system. This massive neural cell division provides the initial formation of different brain regions. The remaining and most intricate part of brain sculpting is accomplished by neural cell migration. As the cells develop on the ventricular walls, new neurons—strong, elongated glial cells called radial glia—migrate outward, away from the ventricle, along tracks made by individual glial cells. New neurons, which consist of only an oblong cell body with two hairlike processes extending from either end, jump onto the radial glia, and, following various molecular cues, make their way along to a predestined zone in the thickening brain. In the cerebral cortex, composed of six layers of neurons, this migration proceeds in an inside-out sequence. The first cells to migrate stop in a layer closest to the ventricle, and each of five subsequent waves of neurons pass by the earlier cells to settle in progressively higher spots.

As the neurons develop, migration is initiated. By the end of neurogenesis, halfway through gestation, most have taken up their final position, and all the major brain structures are in place. This is just the beginning of brain development. Because the neurons are held in place with only a tiny axon, a few short dendritic branches, and practically no synaptic connections, they cannot communicate effectively.

Synaptogenesis begins in the vertebral column by the fifth week of embryogenesis and, in the cortex, around 7 weeks' gestation. In the cerebral cortex, 100 billion cells form their synapses later than any other part of the brain. Synaptogenesis continues throughout gestation, through much of the first year, and, in some regions of the brain, well into the second year of postnatal life. At its peak, some 15,000 synapses are produced on every cortical neuron, which corresponds to a rate of 1.8 million new synapses per second between 2 months gestation and 2 years after birth.

The synapse is a communication point between two cells, and to accommodate this massive synapse formation, neurons must vastly expand their dendritic surfaces. Initially, synapses form directly on the smooth surface of new dendrite branches. But before long, this contact coaxes the branch to produce a nubbin, called a "dendritic spine." Dendritic spines measure just one thousandth of a millimeter in diameter, but they profoundly affect the way electrical signals are processed by the postsynaptic neuron. Spines dot the entire length of mature dendrites, their number closely paralleling the spine (and later pruning), leading to an increased number of synapses.

About 83% of total dendritic growth occurs after birth, to accommodate the enormous influx of new synapses. During this period, the cerebral cortex triples in thickness during the first year of life. This thickening is a result of this enormous dendritic growth. Each neuron manages to grow both its axon and dendritic branches to precisely the right position, aligning its input and output connections so

that the end result is coherent circuits for vision, language, movement, and the like.

Brain wiring involves an intricate dance between nature and nurture. Genes direct the growth of axons and dendrites to their correct approximate locations, but once these fibers start linking together and actually functioning, experience takes over, reshaping and refining these crude circuits to customize each child's hardware to his or her unique environment. There is just not enough genetic material to guide all the functioning that is to occur.

Brain wiring begins with the outgrowth of axons. Once the neurons have migrated, with its body in a permanent position, a fine axon begins to develop with an enlarged tip known as a growth cone. At the end of each growth cone are approximately a dozen long tentacles that shoot out in all directions and pick up a variety of different signals. They seek out the best-textured surfaces, locate chemical cues, and use tiny electrical fields to help the axon arrive at its appropriate targets. The axons grow very long; development starts very early in the embryonic stage, when the distance between any two parts of the embryo is still comparatively short. Axons are guided by specific chemical attractants and by potential target neurons to attract synaptic mates over relatively long distances. Led by their own genetically coded receptor molecules, these axons elongate in the direction of an increasing concentration of the attractant molecules until they reach its source, the target neurons with matching chemical identity.

Once an axon completes its journey, it branches out expansively, contacting hundreds of possible neurons that have released the same chemical identity. Contact enables synapse formation, but these initial connections are extravagant: both numerous and unselective. During infancy and early childhood, the cerebral cortex overproduces synapses, approximately twice as many as it will need. This initial wiring scheme is diffuse, with a lot of overlap making information transfer inaccurate and disorganized.

With an overproduction of synapses, the brain is forcing competition, allowing the most electrical-activity synapses to survive. Synapses that are highly active, receiving more electrical impulses and releasing greater amounts of neurotransmitter, are the most selective in stimulating their postsynaptic target. This heightened electrical activity triggers molecular changes that stabilize the synapse, thus cementing it in place. The less active synapses that do not evoke enough electrical activity to support themselves regress and atrophy. This synaptic pruning is an extremely efficient way of adapting each organism's neural circuits to the exact demands imposed by its environment.

Everything an infant sees, touches, hears, feels, tastes, and thinks render an electrical activity in a subset of his or her synapses, tipping the balance for long-term resilience and/or resistance of channels for informational transfer.

Coinciding with the extended period of dendritic growth and synapse refinement is one more critical event in neural development, called myelination. One important function of myelination is to increase the transmission of electrical signals. Neurons transmit electrical signals not by the flow of electrons, but by the flow of ions—dissolved salts like sodium, calcium, and potassium (which carry a positive charge) and chloride (which carries a negative charge). Unfortunately, nerve cell membranes are leaky. As electrical signals race along the length of an axon, some of these ions leak out, reducing the efficiency of transmission. Myelination seals the leaks. Before myelination, many fibers are incapable of transmitting impulses all the way to their end point synapses, because they lose too much ionic current along the way. Unmyelinated axons cannot fire successive action potentials fast enough to meaningfully transmit information. Even when neurons have grown their branches and formed the synapses that complete the fundamental brain circuits, these circuits do not work efficiently until the axons are myelinated, but they do work to some degree.

Myelination initiates in the nerve fibers of the spinal cord at 5 months gestation, and the ninth prenatal month in the brain. It is a very slow process, progressing through several stages, allowing the myelin wrapping to get progressively thicker as it changes to a mature composition. Different areas of the brain are distinctly uneven in myelination. Together with the rise in synapse formation, the development of myelination is critically important for the manifestation of a particular region's function, and the rate of myelination controls the speed at which that function progresses. This is particularly evident in the emergence of different motor skills.

The order of myelination in different regions of the brain is largely genetically controlled and follows a roughly phylogenetic sequence: axonal fibers in older brain regions, controlling basic vegetative and reflexive functions, tend to get myelinated well before fibers in higher areas, which control more sophisticated mental abilities. However, although genes control the timing of myelination, environmental factors, such as malnutrition, have been found to adversely affect the degree of myelination, that is, the thickness of the wrapping around individual axons.

Myelin is composed of about 80% lipid, including approximately 15% cholesterol together with about 20% protein, produced by special types of glial cells, the number of which is related to the quality of nutrition in early life.

The nervous system matures from caudad to cephalad. The spinal cord and brain stem are almost fully organized and myelinated by birth; the midbrain and cerebellum begin myelinating just after birth; subcortical parts of the forebrain (including the thalamus, basal ganglia, and parts of the limbic system) follow in the first year. The cerebral cortex, which is both the slowest and most uneven of all brain structures to mature, is last. Sensory areas of the cerebral cortex mature relatively quickly, followed by motor areas.

## FUNCTION: TACTILE SYSTEM (TOUCH)

Touch comprises four different sensory abilities, each with distinct neural pathways. Cutaneous is the feeling that part of your skin is contacting another being or object. The somatosensory system directs the sensations of temperature, pain, and proprioception—the senses of position and movement. Touch, temperature, and pain are initiated in the skin, where dedicated receptors for each modality can be found. Proprioception uses information from the skin and signals from the muscles and joints to update the brain at any given instant about where limbs are positioned.

How the brain assimilates this information can easily be described and explained. You reach out with your right hand and grab something cold. The pressure of the cold object stimulates the touch receptors in your fingers, the end points of touch—sensitive sensory neurons. The special receptors interpret mechanical pressure into long-distance electrical signals—action potentials—that spread along the sensory neurons' axons from your finger, up your arm, into the right side of your spinal cord, and up to your brain stem. When reaching the brain stem, these primary-touch neurons synapse on their first set of relay cells, neurons whose axons cross to the other side of the brain stem and terminate up into your left thalamus. (The thalamus dispatches virtually all types of sensory information.) When action potentials in these relay neurons reach the thalamus, they activate the touch-communicating neurons, whose axons reach the left somatosensory region of the cerebral cortex, a vertical strip comprising the frontal most portion of the parietal lobe. It is here in the somatosensory cortex, where the neurons that allow us to perceive the feeling of the cold object are found.

Corresponding with the sensation of pressure, the cold object stimulates cold receptors in our right hand. These receptors have their own set of sensory and relay neurons, crossing over in the spinal cord, synapsing in the thalamus, and then projecting up to the left somatosensory cortex. When the neural excitation reaches this "touch center" in the cortex, the two sensations—pressure and cold—combine, giving us the conscious perception of a cold object. The difference between pressure and cold is that they travel up to the brain along different pathways. The same is true for pain and proprioception receptors and pathways.

The ability to feel lies within the two strips of somatosensory cortex, one on each side of the brain. Each strip contains one systematic pathway of the body's surface area: neurons activated by touch to the leg are adjacent to neurons activated by a touch to the trunk; arm areas are next to the hand and face areas, with lips, mouth, and tongue grouped together. The somatosensory pathway is orderly, but not a perfect replica of the surface area of our body. It is divided into halves; the sensory pathways cross the middle of the body on their ascent, sensations on the right side of the body trigger activity in the left strip of somatosensory cortex, and vice versa.

Each strip contains a pathway of half the body—the opposite half. These pathways do not accurately duplicate the surface of the body; there is distortion. Lips and fingertips, which are more sensitive, have an increased amount of cortical space. Our bodies are programmed to develop more sensory receptors in regions that need greater sensitivity to perform all the delicate manipulations at which we are so adept. More sensory receptors mean more relay paths reaching the cortex. The more sensory fibers of a particular type, the more they impinge on the cortical territory. Establishment of the pathways in the somatosensory cortex depends on electrical activity in the incoming sensory fibers. Different body parts, based on the relative amount of sensory experience, determine the cortical pathway (Figure 10-3).

Our early touch experiences determine the extent of possible tactile sensitivity. Anything that increases a baby's variety of touch stimulation is likely to enhance many aspects of brain and mental development. Touch sensitivity develops from cephalad to caudad. The mouth is the first region to become sensitive and is used by babies to explore everything.

Touch establishes identity and security within the environment. It is a protective as well as a discriminatory system. Protection that goes awry could lead to tactile defensiveness, which is an overactive protective response. As an infant, touch sensations are most important as a source of emotional satisfaction. For example, the sensations from a wet diaper make the infant uncomfortable. Touch can also create emotions that are positive, such as the touch between the infant and the mother, necessary to create a bond. Because skin is the largest system, touch is the largest sensory system and plays a vital role in our physical and mental well-being. The tactile system is the first to develop, and when touch is provided in a negative or abnormal way, the nervous system tends to become unbalanced. For more information on "touch" research, see Chapter 14.

## SENSORY INTEGRATION DYSFUNCTION

Sensory integration dysfunction to date has been based on Ayers's (1981) writings and mostly clinical observations. Systematic research is needed in this area. At this time, we must recognize the level of

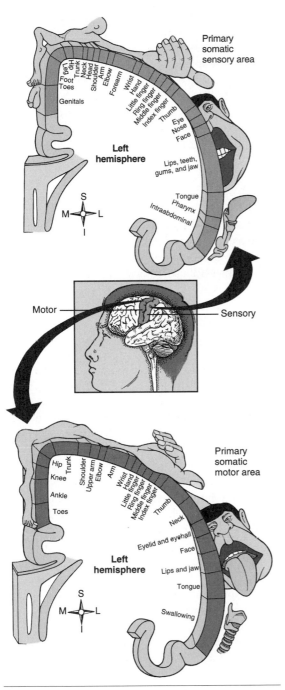

Figure **10-3** Picture of the brain with areas along cortex where sensation of each body part occurs. (*From McCance, K.L., & Huether, S.E. [2002]. Pathophysiology: The biologic basis for disease in adults and children [4th ed.; p. 372]. St. Louis: Mosby.*)

evidence (expert opinion) that underlies most of what we know about sensory integration dysfunction. More research has been done in the areas of learning, developmental disabilities, and neurologic impairment in older children than has been done in the newborn or infant from a medical or nursing perspective. So what do we "know" about sensory integration dysfunction? What we have observed is that sensory integration dysfunction can occur within or among any parts of the overall sensory system. Within the tactile system, it manifests as behaviors that can be exhibited as aggressiveness, avoidance, withdrawal, and intolerance of daily routines—defensive behaviors. Simple tasks, such as combing or shampooing hair, cutting fingernails, or brushing teeth, can be exhausting and difficult for families of children who react defensively with acting-out behaviors or tantrums. Other children might cope by being rigid and demanding with insistence on certain textures of clothing, cutting all tags and labels out of clothing, or displaying extremely limited choices of food because of intolerance to textures. Social skills can be very limited if the child withdraws or hits as a result of unexpected touch. Children with tactile disorders often are less affectionate. Even if a parent provides hugs and kisses, the stimulus might not satisfy the infant's needs if the brain does not integrate the information efficiently. Children with regulatory disorders often have difficulty establishing appropriate sleeping and eating patterns, are unable to calm or console themselves, and might overreact to environmental stimuli.

The developing fetus is at risk for sensory integrative dysfunction as is the neonate in the NICU. Certainly, it appears that sensory integrative dysfunction can be exacerbated by adverse stimuli in the NICU environment. To relate this to the NICU, further evaluation and long-term studies are necessary. Sensory integrative testing might be indicated for those infants who exhibit signs or symptoms in any one or more of the sensory systems. We should examine our practice within the NICU, look at each procedure and task, and provide the optimal experience for the developing infant. What we do as caregivers obviously has a long-term impact. Further research is necessary to document this relationship.

## Vestibular System (Gravity, Balance, and Motion)

The vestibular system functions below the level of the cerebral cortex, and is crucial for our ability to maintain head and body posture, and to move most parts of our body, especially our eyes. When sensing the direction of gravity and motion, we alter our position, maintaining balance and smoothness of action.

The vestibular system is named for the hollow opening in the skull, the vestibule. This space houses the inner ear, a complicated set of chambers and ducts that includes both the hearing organ, or cochlea, and two kinds of vestibular organs: the semicircular canals, which detect head turns, and the otolith organs, which detect linear movements, head tilts, and the body's position with respect to gravity. There are three semicircular canals, each filled with fluid and oriented in each of the three perpendicular planes of space, enabling this organ to sense any conceivable rotational movement. Of the two otolith organs, one, the saccule, detects linear movements, both side to side and up and down, whereas the other, the utricle, is activated any time the position of the head changes with respect to gravity, as when you lie down or tilt your head in any direction.

In spite of their differences, each of the vestibular organs converts movement to electrical signals in a similar way. Within each structure lie thousands of tiny receptor cells, called hair cells, or cilia. In the semicircular canals, these cilia sit in fluid, but in the otolith organs, they are embedded in a gelatinous mass containing tiny crystals. When jumping up and down, the movement imbeds the cilia in all the vestibular organs, especially in the saccule. Depending on whether one is going up or down, this bending either opens or closes tiny ion channels in the membranes of the saccule hair cells, decreasing or increasing their voltage and, thereby, translating motion into electrical information.

Hair cells form synapses onto the first neurons in the vestibular pathway, some 20,000 cells whose axons extend from the ear into the brain stem, forming the vestibular nerve. In the brain stem, these vestibular nerve fibers synapse on several groups of neurons that serve as a juncture, sharing informa-

tion about balance and motion into many places: to the eyes, which automatically move in compensation for a change in head position; to motor neurons down in the spinal cord, that control overall posture and the position of arms and legs; to the cerebellum, which integrates vestibular information with vision and touch (proprioceptive) input, thereby coordinating sense of balance. Some vestibular fibers also travel directly from the ear to the cerebellum, without stopping at the brain stem, illustrating just how important the role of vestibular input is in the cerebellum's job of coordinating movements.

The vestibular nerve is the first fiber tract in the entire brain to begin myelinating, approximately the last week of the first trimester. By 5 months gestation, the vestibular structure has reached its full size and shape. The vestibular pathways to the eyes and spinal cord have begun to myelinate, and the entire vestibular system is functioning. Some other vestibular pathways progress at a very slow pace, up to puberty. A mature vestibular system is what allows a fetus to sense his orientation with respect to gravity and to turn in the proper position (head down) in the weeks or days before birth. Indeed, babies born with defects in their vestibular system have a much greater chance of being in a breech position, presumably because they cannot adequately discern the difference between up and down.

The vestibular function enables the postural reflexes that are tested when assessing a newborn's neurologic health. Premature babies exhibit asymmetrical tonic neck reflex by 35 weeks' gestation. This reflex is well established in a term infant in the first month after birth, and by 7 months, it can no longer be elicited by turning the infant's head. Although this reflex never completely disappears, adults spontaneously adopt opposing flexion and extension to stabilize their posture during a sudden position change, as when falling or jumping.

The vestibular system overcompensates during infancy, reaching its highest sensitivity between 6 and 12 months, and declining rapidly until $2\frac{1}{2}$ years, and more gradually until puberty. This oversensitivity explains why infants and toddlers are unsteady on their feet, although this phenomenon might be useful for understanding other aspects of neurologic development. The slow maturation of vestibular sensitivity is known to result from gradual modification in the synaptic strength and dendritic growth of neurons in the brain stem and higher neural centers, as opposed to any changes in the inner ear.

Maturation of the vestibular system is also important for the development of a child's postural abilities. Maintaining balance is no easy task for a young toddler, depending on the vestibular, visual proprioceptive, and motor skills. Researchers have been able to separate these different sources of postural cues and have found that the contribution of the vestibular system to maintaining balance does not fully mature until at least age 7, and perhaps not until puberty (Ayers, 1981). This gradual vestibular maturation is necessary to keep up with the child's steadily expanding range of movement, and might be orchestrated by the very slow myelination of certain vestibular tracts.

The vestibular senses play a surprisingly important role in mental and neurologic development. One study found a large proportion of young children with a deficient nystagmus response were delayed in their motor development; nearly half were not walking by 18 months, and some walked as late as 4 years of age (Forssberg & Nashner, 1982).

It is easy to see how the sense of balance might influence the development of motor skills, but vestibular deficits are also frequently found among children with emotional problems, perceptual or attention deficits, learning disabilities, language disorders, and autism (Hirabayashi & Iwasaki, 1995). Although it is unlikely that vestibular dysfunction is totally responsible for this range of disorders, these findings suggest that the sense of balance and motion is more important than is commonly realized (Hirabayashi & Iwasaki, 1995).

Mental development is highly cumulative. As one of the earliest senses to mature, the vestibular system provides a large share of a baby's earliest sensory experiences. These experiences probably play a critical role in organizing other sensory and motor abilities, which, in turn, influence the development of higher emotional and cognitive abilities.

Vestibular stimulation can have a profound impact on a baby's overall behavioral state. Young babies tend to go through periods when they are "disorganized"—flailing extremities, tensing hands and face, and insistent, high-pitched crying. Parents will do just about anything to stop the crying, holding the infant up, over the shoulder, and gently jiggling, so that the infant stops crying, his body relaxes, and, for a brief time, he is highly alert, looking intently. Infants who are comforted through vestibular stimulation show greater visual alertness than babies comforted in other ways (Korner & Thoman, 1972).

The fetus's vestibular system is stimulated throughout most of the pregnancy by the mother's movements. Motion and position changes can be overstimulated to the infant in the NICU. Caregivers should re-evaluate handling, position changes, and motions experienced by the infant, to determine overstimulation to this system. Daily tasks should be examined, and each task analyzed to provide smooth movements and motion to the developing infant. Abnormal stimulation might include "flipping" the infant from back to front or lifting the buttocks to change the diaper. These routine interventions might, in fact, be noxious to the vestibular system (Ayers, 1981).

Sensory integration dysfunction within the vestibular system manifests as defensiveness to intolerance to movement or unstable surfaces with fearfulness, avoidance, or motion sickness. The child might be afraid to go down steps or to ride an escalator. Some will not step up a few inches on a floor mat or refuse to step up a curb. Some are reported to be so sensitive to motion in the car that expressways have to be avoided. Social skills might be limited if the child is unable to participate in playground activities such as swinging, using monkey bars, riding a teeter-totter, or going down a slide.

## PROPRIOCEPTION (MUSCLE AND JOINTS)

The sensation of muscles and joints is necessary for later motor development. The word proprioception refers to the sensory information caused by contraction and stretching of muscles and by bending, straightening, pulling, and compression of the joints between bones. Proprioceptive input to the developing infant might be perceived as positive or negative, and again, as caregivers, we should evaluate our handling skills. Tugging, pulling, or stretching of limbs or joints that can occur when locating a vein for an IV should be avoided. Appropriate input for the developing infant might include facilitated tuck with gently cupping of hands around the infant to improve behavioral organization. The purpose of appropriate and available boundaries is positioning to provide a surface for tactile input with a response to brace hands and/or feet, thereby facilitating flexion. (For more information, see Chapter 16.)

Proprioception helps us move. There are three different sensations—proprioception, fine touch, and vibratory senses. Proprioception is the sense that enables one to know exactly and at all times where the parts of the body are in space and in relation to each other. Thus, it enables a person, with eyes closed, to bring up the hands and touch the tip of the nose with the index finger. Fine touch enables the child to discriminate between two points when being touched by both points simultaneously. One might consider the effects of multiple caregivers bombarding the infants' sensory systems during certain procedures. Examining common tasks and decreasing overstimulation might prove to be beneficial for the outcome of the infant. Vibratory sense is, as its name implies, the sensation of vibrating objects. (Some units use vibration devices for chest physiotherapy.) Without proprioception, one would have a hard time with daily motor tasks, such as buttoning a shirt, walking down steps, or playing sports.

One type of poor coordination that is the result of sensory integrative dysfunction is a deficit in motor planning. Motor planning is the ability to plan and carry out an unfamiliar action. A child who experiences difficulty with motor planning might be referred to as "dyspraxic." "Dyspraxia" refers to a neurologic dysfunction that results in clumsiness or uncoordinated movements. The dyspraxic child is slow and inefficient; if on a bicycle, the child might find it difficult to pedal or pedal backwards. This motor planning can also affect speech in the form of apraxia. "Apraxia" refers to a neurologic disorder of dysfunctional speech patterns, articulation, or incoordination of the action of speech. For example, the child will not know where to put his feet on the bicycle or what to do with them (dyspraxia) or be able to articulate his/her ideas (apraxia). Movement disorders (includ-ing those of speech) manifest in many ways and require evaluation and treatment by sensory integrative therapists. Sensory integration therapy is carried out by occupational, physical, speech-language, and educational therapists, who specialize in sensory integration.

## Gustatory (Taste) Development

Gustatory is the system of taste, known as "chemical sense," in which the nervous system detects specific molecules in the environment and converts this information into distinct electrical signals. Taste is straightforward; our taste buds detect only four basic categories—sweet, salty, bitter, and sour. By 20 weeks gestational age, the taste buds are emerging, and by birth, 7000 taste buds have developed; therefore, infants have a high level of discriminatory taste. The taste buds are mostly distributed over the perimeter of the tongue—approximately 4500 on the tip, sides and back; some are on the soft palate area and the upper throat. Each taste bud contains approximately 40 taste-receptor cells, whose hairlike microvilli wave around in the pore, perfectly binding to one of the four basic types of food stimuli that are floating by the receptor.

Within the taste receptor cells, chemical information is converted into neural, or electrical, signals. Each of the four categories of food molecules activates a different kind of molecular receptor located in the microvilli; a change in the taste cell's voltage triggers its release of neurotransmitter-stimulating small dendtritic buds in the first neurons, in the gustatory pathway. These primary taste neurons transmit their action potentials along axons that run through the base of the skull and into the first relay station for taste in the CNS, located in the lower brain stem, or medulla.

Taste input significantly impacts the medulla. It triggers several brainstem reflexes that are necessary for feeding, including salivation, swallowing, and tongue movements. The medulla also transfers taste information to the upper brain stem, or pons, and thalamus. From the pons, taste input is relayed to several limbic structures, to the amygdala and hypothalamus, which control our motivation to eat and drink, and to the limbic cortex, where the hedonic, or pleasurable, aspects of taste are received. From the thalamus, taste input is relayed up to the cerebral cortex to where tastes are consciously perceived.

The conscious awareness of taste is controlled by a relatively small area of the cerebral cortex, located at the border between the frontal and temporal lobes, underneath the area that receives touch input from the tongue. This proximity possibly makes it easier to access information regarding taste and integrate it with information about food texture, helping to identify different foods. However, the flavor distinctions depend on the integration of taste and smell that occurs in the cortex, possibly in the orbitofrontal regions that are responsible for olfactory perception.

Taste buds mature at the end of the first trimester, when the fetus begins to suck and swallow. These actions increase the flow of chemicals over the taste buds, stimulating them, and influence the formation of their synaptic connections. Early taste function might critically control the development of taste perception.

Amniotic fluid is rich with chemicals that excite taste cells: sugars, such as glucose and fructose, stimulate sweet receptors; acids, such as citrate and lactate, stimulate sour receptors; and various salts, such as potassium and sodium, activate fetal salt receptors. Amniotic fluid is constantly changing due to strong flavors in the mother's diet, and with the fetus' own urination, which provides an ever-varying mix of stimuli to activate receptors and their emerging neural pathways.

The fact that babies begin to taste before birth has important developmental consequences. The formation of taste pathways and preferences before birth helps babies recognize and find comfort with their mothers, after birth, because many of the same flavors in amniotic fluid will also be present in her breast milk.

From 24 weeks' gestational age to term, the fetus will suck and swallow, in utero, an average of 1 liter of amniotic fluid daily. Although this is a normal gustatory development for the fetus, the preterm infant misses out on this practice, and, therefore, the coordination of suck, swallow, and breathing becomes a challenge. The infant in the NICU might experience abnormal tastes, such as medications, vitamins, or the taste of a glove! The sense of taste encourages an important developmental skill, which encourages oral play, hand to mouth, mouth exploration, and midline activities.

A sensory-integrated dysfunction that might be observed within this system include oral-motor or feeding disorders. Feeding disorders might also include intolerance to textures or temperatures of food. In extreme cases, children might not feed by mouth and exhibit severe oral-motor delay with refusal to eat. These children might eventually require gastrostomy tubes to provide nutritional support. Sensory-based dysphagia (difficult swallowing) might also be evident among infants with sensory-integrated dysfunction. Infants with sensory issues might also find trips to the dentist or brushing teeth very difficult (Ayers, 1981).

## Function: Olfactory (Smell)

The olfactory system is the system of smell. We are typically unaware of the influence of smell in our lives. Odor is an important factor, and the sense of smell is quite useful. Smell is known as a "chemical" sense, initiated by neural excitation in response to specific molecules in the immediate surroundings. Phylogenetically, it is a primitive sense. Smell is unique in that its information is transmitted directly from the nose to the cerebral cortex. The primary olfactory areas are better developed by birth than the cortex. Although smell is one of our less vital senses, newborns most likely depend on it more heavily than later in life.

### Olfactory or Smell Physiology

Molecules are dissolved into a mucus layer deep inside the nostrils. The watery mucus layer contains the hairlike cilia of olfactory epithelial cells, which are the first neurons in the chain of odor perception. Cilia trap the odorous molecules, binding them to specific protein receptors that convert their chemical information into electrical signals, or action potentials. Each olfactory epithelial cell is thought to respond to one or a few specific chemicals. The number of action potentials generated rates the strength of an odor.

Once activated, olfactory epithelia send their action potentials along short axons that travel straight up through pores in the skull. Synapse occurs in the olfactory bulb, the first relay point with the brain. This oblong structure lies underneath the frontal lobe, above the nasal cavity. The olfactory bulb contains a small network of neurons that integrate information from all the epithelial receptor cells. The mitral cells send their long axons along the base of the frontal lobe, known as the olfactory tract, to different areas in the primary olfactory cortex, located at the bottom, innermost bulges of the temporal lobe. Included among the several direct targets of olfactory bulb neurons are portions of the limbic system.

Within the brain, different regions use olfactory information for different purposes. For example, one set of mitral cells is projected to a limbic area known as the entorhinal cortex, responsible for learning and remembering odors and their associations. Another limbic target, the amygdala, uses direct olfactory input to control feeding and certain aspects of social and reproductive behavior in animals. From the primary olfactory cortex, odor information is transferred to brainstem centers that control motor reactions, such as salivation, head turning, facial expressions, and sucking. Eventually, olfactory information reaches the higher regions of the cerebral cortex. Neurons in the primary olfactory cortex project both directly and via the thalamus to the orbitofrontal cortex, also located on the underside of the frontal lobe, close to the olfactory bulb, where the conscious perception and discrimination of odors, takes place. This region might also be responsible for the integrations of smell and taste senses, which give us the perception of flavors.

## Olfactory Development

At 5 weeks' gestation, a nasal pit appears in the primitive face, gradually deepening and dividing to form true nostrils by 7 weeks' gestation. The olfactory epithelial cells begin to form, taking their place along the lining of the nasal cavity. These oval-shaped cells send a thick dendrite down toward the nasal surface, terminating in the ciliated tuft that would bind odor molecules; then, from their top end, growing a long, thin axon piercing the nasal boundary, forming the olfactory nerve, which advances to the brain. By 11 weeks' gestation, the olfactory epithelia are plentiful and outwardly quite mature. They do not begin to function until several

months later, when more subtle aspects of their biochemical development are complete.

The olfactory epithelial cells are the only neurons known to continually generate throughout life. When the olfactory cells die, they are replaced approximately every 60 days, progressing through the same sequence of cilia growth, axon projection, and synapse formation in the olfactory bulb.

As the axons of the olfactory epithelia occupy the brain, they start the development of neurons in the olfactory bulb. This begins taking form in the eighth week of gestation, with its main output neurons, and the mitral cells, first forming in the tenth week. At 13 weeks, the olfactory bulb becomes walled off from the nasal cavity by an emerging bony plate, perforated with holes through which the various branches of the olfactory nerve pass. The olfactory bulb appears fully mature by 20 weeks' gestation. The primary olfactory tracts are myelinated before birth, confirming that the structures underlying smell are well developed in newborns.

## Womb Smell

The fetus experiences many of the same odors and flavors that the mother does while pregnant. This exposure influences postnatal taste experiences (Mennella, Jagnow, & Beauchamp, 2001). The ability to smell is initiated at approximately 28 weeks' gestation. Although the olfactory neurons develop earlier, they do not exhibit the final biochemical specializations that make them capable of detecting odors until this point.

Premature babies begin to respond to strong odors at 28 weeks' gestation. They respond by sucking, grimacing, or moving their heads.

Olfactory abilities rapidly improve during the third trimester, and the fetus's olfactory life is amazingly stimulated. The sense of smell is not impeded by amniotic fluid, because odor molecules normally enter a liquid phase—the nasal mucus—before binding to their olfactory receptors. In fact, a fluid environment might actually enhance the diffusion of certain odor molecules to their receptors, as do the fetus's own swallowing and breathing movements, which become quite active in the third trimester and help circulate odors to the nasal detectors. Along with the fetus's improving olfactory sense, the placenta becomes increasingly permeable during the third trimester, letting more molecules from the outer world reach the amniotic fluid.

Amniotic odors are both appealing and comforting to newborn babies. There is evidence that unwashed babies are more successful than washed babies at bringing their hand to their mouth in the first hour after birth, an important method of self-calming. Their mother's milk and other bodily secretions, such as sweat and saliva, contain some of the same odors as the amniotic fluid, because they are imprinted by the same dietary, environmental, and genetic factors. As long as a newborn stays close to the mother, the familiar olfactory environment will be maintained.

The sense of smell is primordial, both developmentally and as are neural pathways that process it. Smell provides babies with many of their first impressions about their social and physical surroundings and can be a strong source of sensory stimulation. Given the importance of smell to bonding and emotional security, parents and other caregivers should try to make the newborn's olfactory environment as pleasant, stable, and comforting as possible.

Infants might react with approach or withdrawal to olfactory stimuli. An approach response can be observed as an infant turns toward the smell of his mother's breast milk. A withdrawal behavior might be witnessed as the infant grimaces or exhibits a physiologic response to the smell of an alcohol, such as desaturation or increase or even a decrease in heart rate. Hypoxia can affect smell, and, thus, affect feeding interest.

Sensory-integration dysfunction within the system of smell manifests as olfactory defensiveness. In humans, the sense of smell can trigger memories, various emotions, and their related reflexes. For example, the smell of unspoiled food causes pleasure and salivation, whereas that of rotten eggs causes disgust, nausea, and even vomiting. Odors might elicit long-forgotten memories. A well-known case in literature is cited in Proust, Scott-Moncrieff, & Kilmartin (1982). Intolerance to odors can cause gagging or other symptoms of distress and are noted with certain smells, which others do not seem to notice or mind. An example is a deli where the odor might cause someone to feel sick, but not affect others.

## Auditory (Sound)

The neural structures essential for hearing develop early in utero and begin functioning prior to the end of gestation. At birth, babies have about 12 week's worth of actual listening experience, and have become quite discriminating concerning what they like to hear. Mother's voice is the favorite, especially when she speaks in the higher-pitched, singsong style known as "parentese."

Hearing is initiated early and matures gradually. Babies hear quite well at birth. Their auditory skills continue improving into school age. Hearing evolves gradually, in parallel with a child's eventual mastery of language. Hearing influences the quality of auditory development, the listening that occurs from the third trimester on, and shapes the way brains become wired to process and understand different sounds. Children's early experience with speech and music are tremendously important in shaping many higher aspects of brain function, including emotion, language, and other cognitive abilities.

Hearing begins in the ear, where the auditory information passes through numerous brainstem sites before making its way to the auditory cortex. All these structures are known as the auditory system, which receives sound waves, translates them into electrical signals, and then discriminates these different signals according to all the familiar sounds.

Sound waves are produced when a physically vibrating source creates an alternating pressure change in the surrounding medium (air or water). Its amplitude, the height of its peaks, and its frequency, the number of times the wave crests per second, characterize a sound wave. The amplitude of a sound wave corresponds to its loudness, and the frequency to its pitch. The human ear is sensitive to pressure waves ranging from about 20 to 20,000 vibrations per second, or Hz. Lower numbers correspond to deeper tones. Loudness, or sound pressure, is quantified into units of decibels (dB), which is a logarithmic scale. Therefore, a 20-dB increase in loudness actually corresponds to a tenfold increase in sound intensity; 40 dB corresponds to a hundred-fold increase; and so on.

The ear is divided into three sections: outer, middle, and inner. When sound waves strike the outer ear, or pinna, they are funneled into the ear canal until they strike the eardrum, or tympanic membrane. Sound waves set up a vibration in this elastic membrane, making the three bones in the middle ear oscillate. The bones, malleus, incus, and stapes (Latin for hammer, anvil, and stirrup), amplify the vibration and transmit it to the oval window, a second membrane that marks the edge of the inner ear. Usually, both the outer and the middle ear are filled with air, and the inner ear with fluid. With an otitis media (ear infection), the middle ear is filled with fluid.

The cochlea is the auditory organ in the inner ear, converting vibration into electrical signals. The cochlea has a likeness to a snail's shell, as it is a long, coiled tube, divided into three, lengthwise compartments. In the middle compartment sit hair cells very similar to those in the vestibular system. Sound-induced vibrations bend the fine cilia that sit on top of the hair cells; these tiny movements (a billionth of an inch) stretch open ion pores in the cell's outer membrane. Charged sodium and potassium ions hurry through these briefly opened pores, changing the electrical potential of the hair cells. This depolarization sets off a chain of synaptic excitation, transmitting auditory information to the brain.

Sound discrimination begins in the cochlea and is attributable to well-evolved properties of the basilar membrane, a long sheet of tissue that the hair cells sit on. The width and flexibility of the basilar membrane change continuously along the length of the cochlea. Near the oval window, the membrane is narrow and stiff, at its far end, deep inside the coil; it is wide and very flexible. The basilar membrane moves, or resonates, better to different-frequency sound waves. High-pitched sounds deform the membrane at its narrow end; low-pitched sounds deform it at its widest end. It is the movement of the basilar membrane that actually causes hair-cell cilia to bend, meaning different sounds are translated into electrical excitement in different portions of the cochlea. To increase this frequency segregation, hair cells also differ progressively along the length of the cochlea. Those nearest the oval window have shorter, stiffer cilia, responding best to higher frequencies;

those at the far end have long, flexible cilia that are more responsive to low-frequency sounds.

The cochlea differentiates different sounds by separating them in space, a transformation known as "tonotopy." Similar tone maps are repeated at every step of auditory processing in the brain, including the cerebral cortex.

The cochlear hair cells synapse causing the sound impulses to make their way into the primary auditory neurons, which are cells whose axons travel from the inner ear, through the auditory nerve, to reach the cochlear nucleus in the lower brain. From the cochlear nucleus, auditory fibers travel up to a higher brainstem site, the superior olive, which localizes sounds in space that, in turn, travel to the midbrain, in an area called the inferior colliculus, located below the visual system's superior colliculus. The last stop before the cortex is the thalamus, in a region called the medial geniculate nucleus (MGN), which is adjacent to the visual system's lateral geniculate nucleus. Finally, fibers from the MGN travel to the primary auditory region of the cerebral cortex, located on the upper ridge of the temporal lobe. Higher-order auditory areas surround this primary auditory cortex. They are also located within the upper part of the temporal lobe.

The auditory information passes in succession through all the brainstem relay stations before reaching the cortex. Information from the two ears does not remain segregated. As soon as it leaves the cochlear nucleus, auditory information is parceled out to both sides of the brain stem, comparing or combining input from the opposite ear. The first point that input from both ears merges is in the superior olive. Based on very small differences in the timing or intensity of input from each ear, neurons in the superior olive can compute where sounds are located in space. Each relay station above the olive also processes sound information entering both ears.

A great deal of auditory processing is carried out by the brain stem and thalamus, but not until auditory input reaches the temporal lobe of the cortex does the child consciously perceive it. Auditory information is processed for its pitch, loudness, and location, and then interpreted by higher areas of the auditory cortex as music, talking, or a loud noise.

After 4 weeks' gestation, two fireplug-shaped structures emerge on either side of the embryonic head: the primordial otocysts, out of which both the cochlea and the vestibular organs will evolve. Between 5 and 10 weeks' gestation, the vestibular canals branch out of the top of the otocysts, two cochlear tubes elongated out of their bottoms, coiling as they grow. By 11 weeks, the cochleas have completed all their turns and look similar to snail shells, continuing to grow in girth until midgestation. Between 10 and 20 weeks' gestation, the roughly 16,000 hair cells (in each cochlea) mature, sprouting their characteristic cilia and forming synapses with the first neurons in the auditory system. Hair cells do not emerge simultaneously along the cochlea but in a gradient, beginning at the base and finishing at the apex, or coiled end. This gradient presents somewhat of a contradiction, because fetuses can first hear only in the low-frequency range, the part of the sound spectrum that is normally sensed by hair cells at the apex. The inconsistency is explained by the fact that individual hair cells actually change their frequency response during development. Cells near the base, which mature first, initially respond to lower frequencies, as the properties of the basilar membrane change. These cells become sensitive to higher and higher tones, while hair cells farther out in the cochlea, just beginning to mature, take over the job of sensing low frequencies. Therefore, there is a gradual shift in the tonotopic map during development, with lower tones moving out to progressively more distant cochlear locations.

Before the cochleas are fully formed, auditory neurons begin emerging in the embryonic brain stem. The earliest auditory neurons appear at just 3 weeks of development. By 6 weeks, the auditory nerve, the cochlear nuclei, and the superior olive are all clearly distinguishable. Higher brainstem auditory centers are obvious by 13 weeks, and the MGN begins to show its adult-like subdivisions at 17 weeks' gestation. Cortical neurons emerge later, although the auditory cortex matures earlier than any other part of the cerebral cortex, with the exception of areas involved in touch perception. In all parts of the auditory system, synapses form shortly after growing axons reach their targets, although there is an extended period of synaptic refinement during which the tonotopic maps become more precisely defined.

The speed of auditory development is exposed by its pattern of myelination. Similar to other tracts in the brain stem, the first several projections in the auditory system start to myelinate very early in development. By 24 weeks' gestation, all of the relays between the ear and the inferior colliculus have begun myelinating, and by birth, they are nearing completion. The higher relay tracts in the auditory system myelinate only gradually. The thalamic auditory fibers are still undergoing this process and will not be fully myelinated for at least 2 more years.

Noise damage in fetal and preterm babies' ears can occur. There is one cautionary note about prenatal hearing. Because we know fetuses can hear, and sounds reach them through the mother's body, some researchers have raised concerns about the dangers of excessive noise exposure during pregnancy (AAP, 1997). Animal experiments by Philbin, Ballweg, and Gray (1994) have demonstrated that loud noise can damage cochlear hair cells, leading to some degree of permanent hearing loss. The hair cells are especially vulnerable in infant animals just after the onset of hearing. For humans, the period of greatest sensitivity to noise damage begins at 6 months of gestation and extends through a few months after birth. The danger of noise-induced hearing loss is the greatest for premature babies. Preterm infants lack the protection of their mother's body during this critical period, often housed in noisy incubators (60 to 80 dB) and subjected to the many alarms and other loud sounds of a NICU. Hearing loss is especially prevalent among children born preterm, although many other factors are involved. Reducing noise exposure in NICUs should improve their auditory prospects (Anagnostakis, Petmezakis, Papazissis, et al., 1982; Bergman, Hirsch, Fria, et al., 1985; Brookhouser, Worthington, & Kelly, 1992; Ciesielski, Kopka, & Kidawa, 1980; Nzama, Nolte, & Dorfling, 1995).

There is some evidence that fetuses exposed to high levels of noise in the womb suffer a higher-than-normal rate of permanent hearing loss (AAP, 1997; Gerhardt & Abrams, 2000).

Hopefully, awareness of the noise sensitivity of the young auditory system will lead to improved safety standards for premature babies and pregnant women in the near future. There are a growing number of recommendations in this area. The AAP (1997) recommended that incubator noise be kept below 45 dB. Researchers further recommend that pregnant women not be exposed to occupational noise levels greater than 85 dB.

The auditory system is the sense of hearing. Although the sensory systems develop interdependently, the auditory and vestibular systems work closely together. Preterm infants have a limited ability to habituate, making the auditory system very sensitive. Hearing is important for attention and learning; essential for recognition; motivating for alerting and orientation behaviors; and essential and basic for language development. The infant is sometimes exposed to abnormal or excessive decibels in the NICU environment. Monitors, ventilators, and human voices all are a challenge to keep within the recommended range. Stress cues, physiologic, behavioral, and adverse effects on auditory development, are associated with increased sound levels within the incubator or NICU itself (Graven, 1997, 2000; Johnson, 2001; Kent, Tan, Clarke, et al., 2002).

Sensory-integration dysfunction within the auditory system might manifest later as attention problems (Ayers, 1981). These children might lack the ability to attend to a task that depends on the ability to screen out, or inhibit, nonessential sensory information, background noises, or visual information. The child with sensory integration dysfunction might frequently respond to or register sensory information without this screening ability and is considered distractable, hyperactive, or uninhibited. These children are always "on the alert" and constantly asking about or orienting to sensory input that others ignore, such as a refrigerator motor, heater fan, distant airplane. Other children might fail to register unique sensory input and are unresponsive to stimuli; for example, they might not turn around or respond when their name is called. Additional auditory problems might include auditory memory, comprehension, and additional auditory-language disorders. A speech and language pathologist is often necessary to evaluate and treat children with these disorders (Ayers, 1981).

## Visual (Sight)

Vision begins when light passes through the cornea. The transparent outer coating is focused by the lens, striking the retina, a three-layered blanket of neurons that covers the entire back surface of the eyeball. This stimulus travels through the nervous system, where it converts light information into electrical signals, identifying color and intensity at each point in the visual field. It must also interpret what the eyes see, deciding which array of dots corresponds to a single object, what the object is, where it is located in three-dimensional space, the direction and speed at which it might be moving, and a multitude of other judgments.

The extraction of visual information begins at the very first level of visual processing, within the retina. When you look at an object, light reflects from it and strikes two different types of photoreceptors in the retina—rods and cones. Photoreceptors and specialized nerve cells that contain pigment molecules are capable of capturing a single light particle, or photon, and converting its energy into a chemical reaction. The resulting chemical surge produces an electrical signal, beginning the process of neural transmission in the visual system.

Rods contain more pigment molecules than cones; consequently, they are more sensitive to light and are especially useful for seeing in low-light conditions, such as nighttime. Rods also play a dominant role in peripheral vision, because they are mostly located away from the center of the retina. Cones are less sensitive to light overall, and can detect colors. They are responsible for our most acute vision, because they are densely packed in the centermost part of the retina, called the "fovea."

Three different types of cones contain three different types of pigment molecules. One absorbs blue light best; one green light; and one red light. By comparing the degree of activation of these three classes of cones, the nervous system can differentiate all the different colors of the spectrum.

Both rods and cones synapse on the next layer of retinal neurons, called bipolar cells. Bipolar cells, in turn, synapse on the third layer of retinal neurons, the ganglion cells. Ganglion cells put out extremely long axons that constitute the main output fibers from the eye, and they divide themselves into two different pathways. One pathway goes to the brain stem, where visual information is used to control eye movements and reflexes. The other pathway projects to the visual area of the thalamus, known as the "lateral geniculate nucleus" (LGN), which sends visual information to the cerebral cortex. Of the two pathways, the brain stem, or subcortical route, targets an area of the midbrain called the "superior colliculus," largely responsible for a baby's vision until about 2 months after birth. Although capable of visual tasks, this subcortical pathway operates on a subconscious level and is not responsible for what we commonly think of as "seeing."

It is the second pathway that creates visual perception. A million ganglion cells from each retina send their long axons through each optic nerve to form synapses in the LGN. LGN neurons send their axons to the occipital lobe of the cerebral cortex, to an area called the primary visual cortex (VC). Inside the VC, thalamic axons synapse on the first set of visual cortical neurons, initiating the intense cortical processing that underlies our most sophisticated visual abilities.

Compared with the other senses, the sense of vision is still primitive at the time of birth. Newborn babies cannot adjust their focus and are unable to make out any kind of detail in the visual world. Before the eighth month, the preterm exhibits an immature iris sphincter response to increased light. The preterm infant's fixed focal length is 10 to 14 inches.

With the rapid wiring of neurons in the VC, the sense of vision will dramatically improve within a few short months. By 6 months of age, the primary visual abilities have emerged: depth perception, color vision, fine acuity, and well-controlled eye movements. By 1 year of age, the visual system is fully developed, revealing a colorful, three-dimensional world.

With the visual system, the right amount at the right time is essential for the proper development of the brain circuits underlying vision. Vision is the only system that receives no stimulation in the womb; therefore, it is not surprising that it is poorly developed at birth.

The brain devotes more of its territory to vision than to all the other senses combined. In view of its great size and complexity, it is not surprising that the visual system takes more time to develop and organize during a baby's development. Visual development begins in the fourth week of embryonic life, with the initial formation of the eye. Proceeding in a sequence from outside in: neurons and synapse form first in the retina, followed by subcortical visual areas, followed by the VC, followed by the higher visual centers in the temporal and parietal lobes. It is not until many months after birth that the whole system is functional, and years more before all of its pathways are firmly stabilized.

The first optic tissue emerges 22 days after fertilization, with the formation of two large bubbles at the front of the neural tube. By 5 weeks, these bubbles have bowed into two cup-shaped structures and differentiate to include both the retina and the lens. Each eyecup is attached to the brain by a short, broad stalk taking up a large proportion of the space inside the primitive head. From the outside, they appear as two small spots, facing out sideways, similar to dolphins' eyes. The upper and lower eyelid folds form and fuse shut, until late in the second trimester.

The retina is entirely derived from neural ectoderm and, consequently, develops like a "minibrain." Its neurons divide and migrate to successive layers, taking up functions distinct to their layer. Ganglion cells are the first layers of the neurons to emerge, between approximately 6 and 20 weeks' gestation. They immediately sprout axons; as early as 8 weeks' gestation, immature fibers are emerging from the eyestalk, beginning to form the optic nerves.

The retina matures slower, progressing from the fovea out toward its most peripheral regions. The foveal cells are formed by 14 weeks' gestation; some rods and bipolar cells in the most peripheral parts of the retina are still emerging several months after birth. This slow development of the peripheral retina is surprising, because a newborn's vision is actually better toward the edge than in the center of his visual field. Foveal vision improves dramatically in the first several months after birth due to a specialized change in the cone photoreceptors.

The second trimester is a period of massive growth in the visual cortex. The 100 million neurons in the primary visual cortex are formed between 14 and 28 weeks of gestation. In the fifth month, synapses begin forming in the VC, which is only the beginning of a process that continues for nearly another full year, at the amazing rate of some 10 billion new synapses per day.

As the emergence of cells and synapses progresses inward from the eye, to the LGN, to the VC, to a higher cortical area, myelination of visual axons proceed along a similar gradient. The optic nerves begin to myelinate 2 months before birth, continuing until 7 months postnatally. LGN neurons do not begin to myelinate until 7 weeks after birth, and continue until about 8 months of age. Within the VC, cells from different layers myelinate according to the same sequence in which their synapses formed; higher visual areas myelinate even later than the VC, some continuing until midchildhood.

The purpose of the visual system is recognition, investigation, and learning discrimination. Sensory integration dysfunction within the visual system manifests as visual defensiveness, which can occur with hypersensitivity to light or avoidance or gaze.

Long-term developmental outcomes for these children might indicate visual perceptual deficits. Because the VC is one of the last systems to develop or become myelinated, therefore, higher levels of perception do not occur until later in the child's development—for example, visual spatial relationship (puzzle pieces knowing where it goes and proper placement); visual motor coordination (reaching for the object); visual memory (concentration card game, Simon electronic game); and figure ground (*Where's Waldo?*, hidden pictures). With a lesion in the posterior parietal area, the child has no difficulty identifying an object that is being looked at, but rather, it is very difficult for the child to pick it up. These children are lacking the function that will allow them to guide their hand to the right place or use the appropriate motion to grasp it. However, with temporal lobe damage, one can accurately track a moving object or pick it up off the table, but cannot identify visually where it is. Temporal lobe visual deficits can be very specific, such as an inability to recognize colors, animals, or familiar faces. These disorders are often identified later, usually during kindergarten screening.

## Case Study of Sensory Integration Dysfunction

Josh, who is currently 15 months old, born at 24 weeks' gestation, spent the first 6 months of life in a level III NICU. He suffers from no neurologic problems, with MRI, CT scan, and neurosonogram of his brain all within normal limits.

His motor skills are currently on target for his age; however, his parents think that Josh is not a normal little boy. His day consists of three structured meals with a therapeutic approach due to sensory-based dysphagia. Josh does not tolerate touch to lips or gums and gags at the sight of food. He screams when placed in his high chair. Modified barium swallow results indicate normal swallow for the pharyngeal phase with no signs of GERD. He receives nutritional support via a gastrostomy tube. In addition to his feeding program, his parents take Josh to occupational and speech therapy three times per week. His therapists report many sensory integrative problems in the area of touch, taste, visual-motor, and feeding. His parents will tell you, tearfully, that although Josh is a beautiful boy, their lives are not normal, by any means.

We celebrate the discharge of our NICU graduates. We hold reunions to celebrate life. However, as caregivers, we do not understand fully what our parents face once they leave the hospital with their infant. In some ways, their journey has just begun. Although the issues that Josh might face might seem minor to us, his parents will tell you differently.

## CONCLUSION

Is there a correlation between the NICU experience and sensory integrative dysfunction? Can we impact outcome? Our challenge is to investigate these issues further. Researchers are challenged to examine the infant who receives developmental care and determine if sensory integration is affected with long-term case studies and standardized sensory integration testing. We cannot be satisfied with a checklist of normal motor skills, but rather, we need to look further into the additional issues that the family of a NICU infant must face. We must realize that not all NICU graduates will experience long-term sensory integration dysfunction. But we do know that the NICU environment impacts neonatal development, including the sensory system that is often developing in the environment of the NICU. Integration of sensory stimuli in a positive manner can be enhanced through use of IFDC. Use of relationship-based care that forces us to "read" the infant's cues and act accordingly affords us the opportunity to promote positive sensory integration and potentially avoid dysfunction. Recommendations for how this can best be accomplished must be formulated based on "evidence." In the meantime, use of IFDC is a step toward promotion of optimal sensory integration.

## REFERENCES

Allen, M.C. (2002). Preterm outcomes research: A critical component of neonatal intensive care. *Mental Retardation & Developmental Disabilities Research Reviews, 8*(4), 221-233.

American Academy of Pediatrics (AAP). (1997). Noise: A hazard for the fetus and newborn. American Academy of Pediatrics, Committee on Environmental Health. *Pediatrics, 100*(4), 724-727.

Anagnostakis, D., Petmezakis, J., Papazissis, G., et al. (1982). Hearing loss in low-birthweight infants. *American Journal of Diseases in Children, 136*, 602-604.

Ayers, A.J. (1981). *Sensory integration and the child* (pp. 6-8). Los Angeles, CA: Western Psychological Services.

Bergman, I., Hirsch, R.P., Fria, T.J., et al. (1985). Cause of hearing loss in the high-risk premature infant. *Journal of Pediatrics, 106*, 95-101.

Brookhouser, P.E., Worthington, D.W., & Kelly, W.J. (1992). Noise-induced hearing loss in children. *Laryngoscope, 102*, 645-655.

Ciesielski, S., Kopka, J., & Kidawa, B. (1980). Incubator noise and vibration: possible iatrogenic influence on neonate. *International Journal of Pediatric Otorhinolaryngology, 1*, 309-316.

Couper, L.J.M., & Brujes, P.C. (2003). Neonatal focal denervation of the rat olfactory bulb alters cell structure and survival: A Golgi, Nissl, and confocal study. *Brain Research & Developing Brain Research, 140*(2), 277-286.

Forssberg, H., & Nashner L.M. (1982). Otogenetic development of postural control in man: Adaptation to altered support and visual conditions during stance. *Journal of Neuroscience, 2*(5), 545-552.

Gerhardt, K.J., & Abrams, R.M. (2000). Fetal exposures to sound and vibroacoustic stimulation. *Journal of Perinatology, 20*(8 Pt 2), S21-S30.

Graven, S.N. (2000). Sound and the developing infant in the NICU: Conclusions and recommendations for care. *Journal of Perinatology, 20*(8)(Pt 2), S88-S93.

Graven, S.N. (1997). Clinical research data illuminating the relationship between the physical environment and patient medical outcomes. *Journal of Healthcare, 9*, 15-19, 21-24.

Harris, J. R. (1998). *The nurture assumption: Why children turn out the way they do.* New York: Free Press.

Hellerud, B.C., & Storm, H. (2002). Skin conductance and behaviour during sensory stimulation of preterm and term infants. *Early Human Development, 70*(1-2), 35-46.

Hendricks-Munoz, K.D., Predergast, C.C., Caprio M.C., et al. (2002). Developmental care: The impact of Wee Care® developmental training on short-term infant outcome and hospital costs. *Newborn and Infant Nursing Reviews, 2*(1), 39-45.

Hirabayashi, S., & Iwasaki, Y. (1995). Developmental perspective of sensory organization on postural control. *Brain and Development, 17*, 111-113.

Johnson, A.N. (2001). Neonatal response to control of noise inside the incubator. *Pediatric Nursing, 27*(6), 600-605.

Kent, W.D., Tan, A.K., Clarke, M.C., et al. (2002). Excessive noise levels in the neonatal ICU: Potential effects on auditory system development. *Journal of Otolaryngology, 31*(6), 355-360.

Korner, A.F., & Thoman, E.B. (1972). The relative efficacy of contact and vestibular-proprioceptive stimulation in soothing neonates. *Child Development, 43*(2), 443-453.

Liebman, M. (1991). *Neuroanatomy made easy and understandable* (4th ed.). Gaithersburg, MD: Aspen.

Mennella, J.A., Jagnow, C.P., & Beauchamp, G.K. (2001). Prenatal and postnatal flavor learning by human infants. *Pediatrics, 107*(6), E88.

Merriam-Webster, Inc. (1999). *Merriam-Webster's collegiate dictionary.* Springfield, MA: Merriam-Webster.

Nzama, N.P., Nolte, A.G., & Dorfling, C.S. (1995). Noise in a neonatal unit: Guidelines for the reduction or prevention of noise. *Curationis, 18*, 16-21.

Peters, K.L. (1999). Handling in the NICU: Does developmental care make a difference? An evaluative review of the literature. *Journal of Perinatal Neonatal Nursing, 13*(3), 83-109.

Philbin, M.K., Ballweg, D.D, & Gray, L. (1994). The effect of an intensive care unit sound environment on the development of habituation in healthy avian neonates. *Development Psychobiology, 27*, 11-21.

Proust, M., Scott-Moncrieff, C.K., & Kilmartin, T. (1982). *Remembrance of things past.* New York: Knopf.

Szoke, E., Czeh, G., Szolesanyi, J., et al. (2002). Neonatal anadamide treatment results in prolonged mitochondrial damage in the vanilloid receptor type 1-immunoreactive B-type neurons of rat trigeminal ganglion. *Neuroscience, 115*(3), 805-814.

Tanaka, T., & Gleeson, J.G. (2000). Genetics of brain development and malformation syndromes. *Current Opinions in Pediatrics, 12*(6), 523-528.

# 11 *Infant Sleep Position Protocols*

Terrie Lockridge and Lauren T. Taquino

Caregivers striving to provide developmentally supportive care for high-risk newborns face many challenges during the course of each child's hospitalization. Regardless of gestational age, many physiologically compromised infants benefit from strategies such as prone placement and supportive positioning. This positioning is typically in the form of bedding "nested" around the infants to provide containment. Such interventions are integral to the basic nursing care of critically ill infants. Therefore, it can be daunting for both healthcare providers and family members to consider introducing the American Academy of Pediatrics (AAP) recommendations for healthy infant sleep into the realm of the neonatal critical care setting (AAP, 2000).

The AAP recommendations advocate supine sleep on firm surfaces without soft or loose bedding (AAP, 2000). Because these recommendations are clearly identified for healthy infants within the first year of life, it might seem logical to disregard them until the infant is considered healthy enough for hospital discharge. It is important to recognize that regardless of how the critically ill infant is positioned for sleep in the neonatal intensive care unit (NICU), upon discharge, this same infant will be expected to sleep supine without supportive containment once at home. Therefore, it is reasonable to prepare, before discharge, for the sleep situations that will be expected of NICU graduates in their home setting. New parents will be especially grateful for an infant who has acclimated to supine sleep without comforting containment before the first night home.

In this chapter, we consider the issues associated with integrating AAP recommendations for infant sleep and developmentally supportive care. Sudden infant death syndrome (SIDS) is defined, and the relationship between SIDS and infant sleep position is examined. Because some healthcare providers have questioned the safety and efficacy of supine sleep positioning, historical background is provided to highlight the gradual implementation of supine sleep positioning for healthy infants and its impact on SIDS incidence. Safety concerns and potentially adverse outcomes associated with supine sleep are addressed. Current AAP recommendations are reviewed, with particular focus on potentially modifiable risk factors for SIDS that should be included in family discharge teaching. Integration of these recommendations into the NICU setting are discussed, with a focus on the apparent contradictions between the intended "healthy infant" population and the NICU population. Appropriate opportunities to transition infants to supine positioning are identified. The transition process is interpreted in the framework of a developmental continuum, with the infant progressing from "ill" status to "healthy" status, and from prone, supported positioning to supine, unsupported positioning. Protocol development and implementation are discussed, as well as strategies to enhance implementation. Family education is addressed throughout the chapter, so that NICU care providers can present families with the information needed to reduce the risk of SIDS for their child.

## DEFINITION OF SUDDEN INFANT DEATH SYNDROME

Sudden infant death syndrome is the leading cause of infant death after the neonatal period (National Institute of Child Health and Human Development, 2002). It is defined as "the sudden death of an infant younger than 1 year of age, which remains unexplained after a thorough case investigation, including performance of a complete autopsy, examination of the death scene, and review of the clinical history" (Willinger, James, & Catz, 1991). SIDS rarely occurs during the first month of life, with peak incidence noted between 2 and 4 months of age (National Institute of Child Health and Human Development, 2002). Documented as far back as the biblical era, " . . . and this woman's child died during the night, because she overlaid it" (I Kings 3:19-20), SIDS was historically believed to be the result of accidental overlying.

## SUDDEN INFANT DEATH SYNDROME AND INFANT SLEEP POSITION: THE INTERNATIONAL EXPERIENCE

The subject of considerable scrutiny during the past five decades, the cause of SIDS remains unknown. Researchers have long speculated that infant sleep positions might be involved (Bayes, 1974; Carpenter & Shaddick, 1965), and numerous studies exploring the link between SIDS and sleep positions have been published since the mid-1960s. The Dutch experience also pointed to a strong association between SIDS and infant sleep position. The incidence of SIDS in the Netherlands, traditionally fairly low, nearly tripled in the late 1980s following a media campaign that advocated a change from supine to prone sleep positioning. The SIDS rate declined accordingly after a subsequent campaign discouraged prone sleep positioning (AAP 1992; DeJonge, Engleberts, Koomen-Lieftig, & Kostense, 1989; Guntheroth & Spiers, 1992).

Nearly all of the early studies examining the association between SIDS and infant sleep were conducted outside the United States, and received little attention from the North American medical community (Myerberg, 1993). However, researchers abroad carefully evaluated the growing body of evidence linking prone sleep with SIDS, and campaigns against prone sleep positioning were successfully initiated in areas of Europe, Scandinavia, Australia, and the United Kingdom (DeJonge, Engleberts, Koomen-Lieftig, & Kostense, 1989; Markestad, 1993; Mitchell, Aley, & Eastwood, 1992; Stewart, Mitchell, Tipene-Leach, & Fleming, 1993). By the early 1990s, those countries with declining prevalence of prone sleep were also reporting 50% or greater reduction in SIDS incidence. No increase in adverse outcomes, such as aspiration or acute life-threatening events, were noted in conjunction with the change from predominantly prone sleep (Willinger, Hoffman, & Hartford, 1994).

## SUDDEN INFANT DEATH SYNDROME AND INFANT SLEEP POSITION: THE AMERICAN EXPERIENCE

In 1992, the AAP Task Force on Infant Sleep Position and SIDS released its first statement recommending that healthy infants younger than 1 year of age be positioned for sleep on either their sides or backs. Potential exceptions to supine or sidelying positions were identified, including preterm infants with respiratory distress, infants with symptomatic gastroesophageal reflux (GER), and those with craniofacial anomalies or upper airway obstructions. Before releasing the recommendations, approximately 25 studies examining the association between sleep position and SIDS were reviewed. Many of these studies were quickly eliminated from consideration because they failed to meet task-force criteria for suitable SIDS definition, comparable control groups, and statistically significant data. The remaining 11 studies all indicated a higher incidence of SIDS among infants positioned prone for sleep (AAP, 1992). Although the Task Force acknowledged the limitations of the existing studies, as well as the significant differences in cultural factors and infant care customs, they concluded that, "taken as a group the studies are convincing" (AAP, 1992; p. 1120).

The AAP statement noted that prone positioning does not cause SIDS, and that even when positioned prone, the actual probability of SIDS is still relatively low. Although the studies reviewed by the Task Force did not identify prone sleep as the *cause* of SIDS, they suggested an *association* between the two. Several hypotheses were identified that might explain this link. One possible mechanism was airway obstruction, thought to be more likely to occur when infants were positioned prone. A second potential mechanism was rebreathing of exhaled gases, especially when infants were placed prone on soft sleep surfaces that might permit gas-trapping and the development of potentially noxious microclimates. Yet another potential mechanism was thermal stress, in which overheated infants were thought to be less effective at dissipating heat when positioned prone versus supine (AAP, 1992).

The initial AAP statement was met with a flurry of controversy, and compliance within the United States was inconsistent during the next few years. Concerns were raised about the quality of the data and its relevance to the American population, as well as the potential risks of supine sleep (Freed, Steinschneider, Glassman, et al., 1994; Hunt & Shannon, 1992; Hudak, O'Donnell, & Mazyrka, 1995). Because initial compliance was variable, it was difficult to determine whether SIDS rates in the United States had been impacted by recommended changes in sleep position. However, the incidence of SIDS was dropping significantly elsewhere in the world in response to campaigns against prone sleep, with no serious adverse effects observed. By 1994, the international experience with SIDS and prone sleep positions was impressive enough that several U.S. federal agencies and the AAP joined forces to implement "Back to Sleep," an aggressive public health campaign against prone sleep positioning during infancy (Willinger, Hoffman, & Hartford, 1994). The AAP reaffirmed its previous recommendations, and, consistent with a safety alert published that same year by the Consumer Product Safety Commission, discouraged soft surfaces and gas-trapping objects within the sleep environment (AAP, 1994; Willinger, Hoffman, & Hartford, 1994).

The incidence of SIDS in the United States had fallen 15% to 20% by 1996. At this time, the Task Force updated its recommendations to clarify different aspects and to incorporate the latest international research. Overseas data suggested that the risk of SIDS was slightly higher among infants who were positioned on their sides rather than supine, possibly because the sidelying position was less stable and might permit an infant to accidentally roll prone. The AAP noted that both sidelying and supine positioning reduced the risk of SIDS, but that supine positioning afforded the lowest risk and was preferable. The Task Force also clarified areas of confusion over the exceptions to prone positioning, specifically in reference to preterm infants. The updated recommendations were more clearly directed toward healthy infants, regardless of gestational age, and provided specific directives to minimize complications of supine sleep such as positional plagiocephaly (flattened heads) (AAP, 1996).

## CURRENT AMERICAN ASSOCIATION OF PEDIATRICS RECOMMENDATIONS

As of this writing, the most recent AAP statement on SIDS and infant sleep was released in 2000 (AAP, 2000). Readers are encouraged to review the literature for any updates that might have subsequently occurred. The latest statement was intended to consolidate and replace earlier commentaries by the Task Force. At this point in time, it was noted that during the previous 8 years, the prevalence of prone sleep among U.S. infants had declined from more than 70% to approximately 20%, and the incidence of SIDS had dropped by more than 40% (Figure 11-1); (AAP, 2000). The change from predominantly prone to predominantly supine sleep positions was considered responsible for saving approximately 2000 lives yearly (Kattwinkel, 2000). As successful as the "Back to Sleep" campaign had been, the Task Force observed that some modifiable risk factors remained that warranted greater attention by healthcare providers and parents. Proposed mechanisms of SIDS, independent risk factors, and complications of prone sleep were also addressed by the Task Force in this latest revision (AAP, 2000).

### Proposed Etiology of Sudden Infant Death Syndrome

Despite the progress made in reducing the incidence of SIDS, the AAP Task Force observed that the cause of SIDS is still uncertain. Numerous etiologies have been proposed and studied, and most investigators now agree that SIDS might be due to a variety of causes of death rather than a single physiologic entity. There is evidence that some defensive responses (such as protective airway reflexes) to life-threatening stimuli are diminished in prone versus supine sleep, and, thus, might play a role in some SIDS cases (AAP, 2000). Another leading theory is that a large percentage of SIDS cases are related to delayed and/or abnormal development of arousal or cardiorespiratory control in the brain. For some infants, the region of the brain stem (arcuate nucleus) involved in hypercapnic ventilatory reactions, chemosensitivity, and blood pressure responses, fails to develop properly. When physiologically compromised during sleep, these infants might not arouse enough to avoid

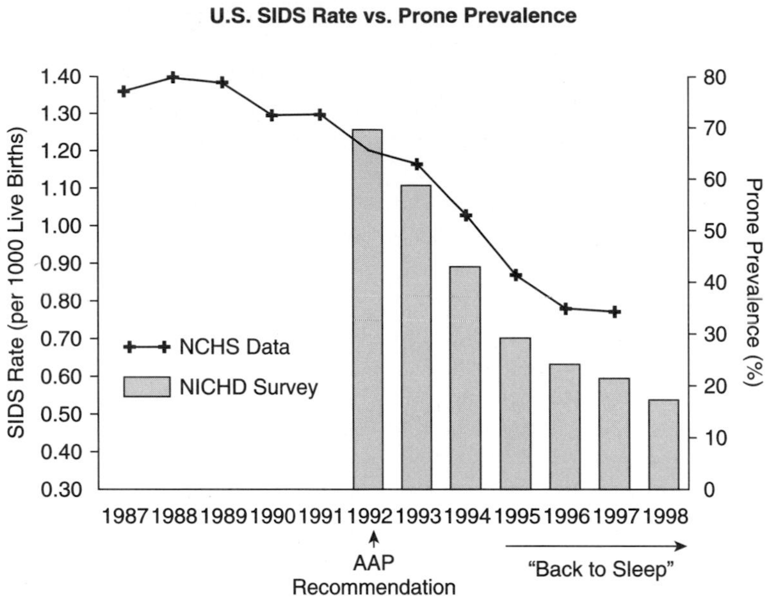

**U.S. SIDS Rate vs. Prone Prevalence**

Figure **11-1** Sudden infant death syndrome rate in the United States (*line*) from National Center for Health Statistics (NCHS) data and prone positioning rate from National Institute for Child Health and Human Development (NICHD) surveys (*bars*). (*From AAP Task Force on Infant Positioning and Sudden Infant Death Syndrome [SIDS]. [2000]. Changing concepts of sudden infant death syndrome: Implications for infant sleeping environment and sleep position. Pediatrics, 105, 651.*)

potentially lethal insults (AAP, 2000; National Institute of Child Health and Human Development, 2000). These noxious insults might include rebreathing and hyperthermia, which are more likely to occur when infants are positioned prone for sleep on soft surfaces or if the head is accidentally covered by loose bedding (AAP, 2000).

## INDEPENDENT RISK FACTORS FOR SUDDEN INFANT DEATH SYNDROME

The AAP statement identified numerous independent risk factors for SIDS, including: prone sleep position, soft sleep surfaces, overheating, maternal smoking during pregnancy, late or no prenatal care, younger mothers, prematurity and/or low birthweight. Ethnicity also played a role, with Native American and African American populations having an incidence of SIDS two to three times higher than the national average (AAP, 2000). Persistent prone sleep positioning might

also play a role in some of these SIDS deaths, because evidence suggests that black infants are twice as likely to be placed prone for sleep as white infants (AAP, 2000; Hauck, Merrick-Moore, Herman, et al., 2002). Although minority outreach had always been part of the "Back to Sleep" campaign, an additional component was added to the existing program to reduce the disparity in SIDS rates among African Americans, and extra effort should be targeted toward this population by healthcare providers (U.S. Department of Health and Human Services, 1999).

Although many of the risk factors associated with SIDS cannot be readily modified, there are some that can be easily eliminated by parents and caregivers. The Task Force focused its recommendations on these modifiable risk factors, most of which involved infant sleep position and environment: prone sleep positioning, overheating, soft sleep surfaces, and inappropriate sleep environments. The various aspects of infant positioning and sleep environment all have direct implication to nursing practice in terms of parent teaching. Neonatal nurses are in an excellent position to role model and educate families about modifiable risk factors. Because SIDS might occur when others are providing care (such as daycare providers or grandparents), parents should be encouraged to share this information with anyone who might temporarily assume responsibility for a sleeping infant (AAP, 2000). This is especially important because the risk of SIDS is higher when infants who usually sleep supine are subsequently positioned prone for sleep (Mitchell et al., 1999).

## Modifiable Risk Factors: Prone Sleep

Prone sleep position has emerged as a significant risk factor for SIDS. In the United States and abroad, declining prevalence of prone sleep positioning has been accompanied by a substantial reduction in the incidence of SIDS. Current AAP recommendations advocate non-prone positions for healthy infant sleep. Supine sleep is associated with the lowest risk of SIDS and is preferable. Although side sleeping is safer than prone sleep, it is not as safe as supine sleep because, as mentioned, the instability of this position might allow the infant to accidentally roll prone. If a sidelying position is chosen, the dependent arm should be brought forward to reduce the risk of the infant rolling prone. Positioning aids designed to maintain sidelying sleep positions are available commercially, but are discouraged because they have not been adequately tested for safety or efficacy (AAP, 2000).

## Modifiable Risk Factors: Overheating

The incidence of SIDS has historically shown a noticeable seasonal pattern, with more deaths occurring during winter months in temperate climates such as the United States. The risk of SIDS appears to be related somehow to environmental factors, such as season and room temperature, as well as the amount of clothing or bedding. The risk is especially high when overheated infants are positioned prone, less so when positioned supine. Although the mechanism is unclear, falling rates of both prone sleep and SIDS have been accompanied by a considerable decline in seasonal association

with SIDS. Current AAP recommendations discourage overbundling and overheating, and note that the infant should not feel hot to the touch. The Task Force suggests that the infant be lightly clothed for sleep in a room that feels comfortable in terms of temperature for a lightly clothed adult (AAP, 2000).

## Modifiable Risk Factors: Soft Sleep Surfaces

Soft sleep surfaces, such as polystyrene bead-filled pillows (i.e., beanbags), pillows, sheepskins, quilts, duvets, and comforters have all been associated with increased risk of SIDS. Although polystyrene bead-filled pillows were removed from the market in 1992, many soft-bedding options remain available to parents and caregivers. This bedding is considered especially dangerous when placed under a sleeping infant (AAP, 2000; U.S. Consumer Product Safety Commission, 1999). Loose bedding is similarly hazardous, even for infants who are positioned supine (AAP, 2000; Franco, Lipshutz, Valente, et al., 2002).

Current AAP recommendations are to avoid soft mattresses and soft materials under a sleeping infant or within the infant's sleep environment. Gas-trapping objects, such as stuffed toys or animals, should not be permitted in the sleep setting. Blankets and sheets might become loose and can also be considered dangerous. If a blanket is used, it should be tucked under the mattress in such a manner that it reaches no further than the level of the infant's chest (Figure 11-2). Another option is to clothe the infant in a sleeper without additional bedding (AAP, 2000).

## Modifiable Risk Factors: Inappropriate Sleep Environments

Appropriate sleep environments for infants are defined further by the Task Force. Cribs should conform to safety standards established by federal agencies such as the Consumer Product Safety Commission (U.S. Consumer Product Safety Commission, 2003). Safety standards have not yet been established for many cradles and bassinets. Sleep surfaces intended for adults pose the threat of entrapment between the mattress, bed components (such as head boards), or wall, and are not considered a safe option. In addition to avoiding adult beds, infants should not be allowed to sleep on

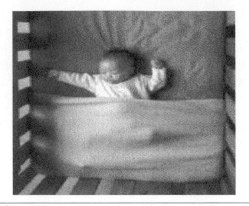

Figure **11-2** If you use a blanket, place the baby with his or her feet at the foot of the crib. The blanket should reach no higher than the baby's chest, and the ends of the blanket should be tucked under the crib mattress. (*From National Institute of Child Health and Human Development:* SIDS: Back to sleep campaign. *[2002]. Available online at* www.nichd.nih.gov/new/releases/sidsbrainstem. cfm?from=sids.)

waterbeds or soft sofas. Bed sharing can be dangerous for infants, especially when tobacco, drugs, or alcohol have been consumed by parents, or if multiple family members share the same adult bed (AAP, 2000). There have been numerous cases of infant suffocation reported during bed sharing. Soft sleep surfaces, overlying, entrapment, or the possibility of rolling prone might play a part in these deaths. Most of the overlying deaths involved infants younger than 3 months of age. Infants who suffocated as a result of wedging (often between a bed and a wall) tended to be slightly older (3 to 6 months) with some motor skills that allowed them to move about the bed (Drago & Dannenberg, 1999). Bed railings are not intended for use in infants younger than 1 year of age due to the risk of entrapment between the bed rail and mattress, which could compress the neck and culminate in mechanical asphyxia (Nakamura, Wind, & Danello, 1999).

The Task Force recognized the dangers involved in bed sharing but acknowledged that many parents choose to bed share to enhance breast-feeding. They noted that, "it was the consensus of the Task Force that there are insufficient data to conclude that bed sharing under carefully controlled conditions is clearly hazardous or clearly safe" (AAP, 2000, p. 654). Rather than bed share, the Task Force recommended placing the infant's crib closer to the parent's bed to facilitate breast-feeding. If a mother chooses to bed share with her infant for breastfeeding, it was recommended that careful attention be directed to each of the Task Force recommendations. Entrapment risks should be carefully evaluated and eliminated. Bed sharing should be limited to parents and infant, and parents should not use alcohol or drugs that might alter their own level of consciousness. Because the risk of SIDS is considerably higher among bed sharing infants of smokers, parents should be advised of this additional risk (AAP, 2000).

## Safety Concerns and Adverse Outcomes

Although prone sleep has been clearly linked with a higher risk of SIDS, there are many healthcare providers and parents who have been reluctant to embrace supine sleep positioning. Concerns have been expressed since the initial AAP statement about adverse outcomes such as aspiration, gastroesophageal reflux (GER), positional plagiocephaly, and developmental delay (AAP, 1992, 2000). Many of these issues have been addressed in the latest AAP statement (AAP, 2000). The most common objection involved the increased potential for aspiration. Conventional wisdom in both the lay and medical communities dictated that aspiration risks were greater among supine infants, and the North American practice of prone sleeping might well have emerged from the fear that sleeping infants might vomit and then aspirate (Lockridge, 1997). This view was never supported in the literature, and there were never any data to validate the theory that aspiration was more likely to occur among supine infants than among prone infants (AAP, 1992; 2000). Aspiration deaths among Dutch infants actually declined following the shift back to supine sleep (Guntheroth & Spiers, 1992). In the years following the transition to supine sleep patterns, there has been no evidence of an increase in aspiration (AAP, 2000; Byard & Beal, 2000; Malloy, 2002).

There is actually some evidence to support the concept that vomiting infants are at greater risk of aspiration when they are positioned prone for sleep (AAP, 2000).

Another frequently voiced concern involves gastroesophageal reflux (GER). Although the initial statement did not apply to infants with diagnosed GER, critics worried about infants with undiagnosed GER whose reflux was being inadvertently minimized by prone sleep positioning. Some feared that these infants might become unexpectedly symptomatic once placed supine for sleep, and thus at risk for apparent life-threatening events associated with GER (AAP, 1992; Orenstein et al., 1993). There is no evidence to substantiate this in populations that have changed from mostly prone to primarily supine positioning (AAP, 2000; National Institute of Child Health & Human Development, 2002). The current AAP statement does not specifically exempt infants with GER from the supine sleep recommendation, but suggests that "individual medical conditions [might] warrant a physician to recommend otherwise, after weighing the relative risks and benefits" (AAP, 2000, p. 653).

An increased incidence of occipital plagiocephaly (flattening of the head) has been observed since full implementation of the AAP recommendations (AAP, 2000). Because most infants with positional plagiocephaly do not have true synostosis, they can often be managed by nonsurgical means, such as helmet therapy (Pollack et al., 1997). Although helmet therapy is a good, nonsurgical option, it can be difficult and expensive for families to comply with (Kane, Mitchell, Craven, & Marsh, 1996). Infants with flattening in the occipital area tend to position themselves preferentially on that side, which might lead to contracture of the neck muscles and torticollis (Raco et al., 1999). Some children with positional plagiocephaly have shown evidence of restricted neck motion, requiring physical therapy to improve range of motion (Kane, Mitchell, Craven, & Marsh, 1996). Both occipital plagiocephaly and acquired torticollis are obviously best managed by preventive measures. Current AAP recommendations advocate "Back to Sleep" for sleep periods and supervised

"Tummy Time" while awake. Specific strategies to avoid positional plagiocephaly by changing head position during sleep are suggested, including positioning of the infant's head to one side for a week or so, then alternating to the other side for a similar period of time (AAP, 2000). More frequent position changes might be considered, such as alternating head position from right to left sides for supine sleep (Hunter & Malloy, 2002). The Task Force also suggested that parents occasionally move the crib to change the infant's orientation to outside activity (i.e., the bedroom door). Because positional plagiocephaly and accompanying muscular changes can be avoided by incorporating these simple tactics into daily routines, appropriate parent teaching is essential (AAP, 2000; Hunter & Malloy, 2002).

Potential for developmental delay has also been identified as an adverse outcome of supine sleep positioning. Infants who are placed supine for sleep tend to reach gross motor milestones slightly later than those infants who are positioned prone for sleep; however, this disparity is transient and not measurable by 18 months of age (Davis et al., 1998; Dewey, Fleming, & Golding, 1998). While these motor differences appear to resolve with time, such delays should be avoided because they can affect an infant's ability to explore his environment, and thus impact cognitive learning (Hunter & Malloy, 2002). Again, current AAP recommendations encouraging prone positioning for play can help minimize these differences (AAP, 2000; Pontius, Aretz, Griebel, et al., 2001).

## APPLICATION IN THE NICU SETTING

The population of patients cared for in the NICU setting present a dilemma with regard to AAP recommendations and SIDS-prevention positioning. On the surface, it would be easy to accept the premise that NICU patients are different from healthy, term infants, and, therefore, the information does not apply. Infants in the NICU are usually attached to physiologic monitors and life-support devices. They might be premature, have major congenital anomalies, or require surgical intervention, any or all of which could preclude the recommendation for supine sleeping. Currently, these patients are not indicated for inclusion in the AAP recommendations.

These contradictions are further strengthened by the benefits of prone position in the promotion of physiologic stability. Premature infants, in particular, show improvements in respiratory and cardiovascular stability when nursed in the prone position (Martin, Herrell, Rubin, & Fanaroff, 1979; Heimler, Langlois, Hodel, et al., 1992; Kurlak, Ruggins, & Stephenson, 1994). Impact of infant position on gastrointestinal function and tolerance of feedings has been long debated (Blumenthal, Ebel, & Pildes, 1979; Blumenthal & Lealman, 1982). Common nursing practices are based on the belief that digestion is enhanced when the infant is supported in a prone or right, sidelying position. There are also differences in need for thermal support in the prone position. Infants in incubators might experience more thermal stability in the prone position (Blackburn, DePaul, Loan, et al., 2001). Neuromotor and neurobehavioral stability of preterm infants are overarching goals of ongoing care and development. These are commonly supported through careful positioning—often prone and with motoric support described as containment. These important components of nursing care for premature and ill infants have been lessons hard won with neonatal nurses. At first glance, it seems counterproductive to introduce mandates that are in conflict with them.

Nesting, bedding, and positioning devices serve a twofold function for the neonatal nurse, infant, and, ultimately, the family. The application of soft bedding supports the aforementioned goals of promoting motoric support for behavioral calming, organization, and appropriate development (Taquino & Lockridge, 1999). Another primary outcome of supported positioning is the achievement of flexion and midline extremity alignment, thus minimizing the risk of joint and muscular malformation and promoting normal strength development (Downs, Edwards, McCormick, et al., 1991; Fay, 1988; Mouradian & Als, 1994). In addition, the use of soft blankets, rolls, and supports, promotes some psychologic benefit for the nurse and family of the evidence of infant comfort. The caregiver can influence an element of control over the environment, and ultimately to individualize the care provided to the needs of the infant. This individualized care, as described previously, and throughout this text, is the central premise of providing developmentally supportive care.

It is clear that the AAP guidelines are designed for healthy infants and, thus, most NICU patients are distinctly exempt from the recommendations. However, the NICU patient is not always ill, or preterm, and it is the responsibility of the care providers in the NICU to prepare the infant and family for ongoing care in the home setting. This preparation for discharge includes minimizing known risks for SIDS. In our opinion, the key is development of applicable criteria, and, ideally, a protocol for transition from exempt to inclusion status with regard to the AAP recommendations.

## DEVELOPMENTAL CONTINUUM

The framework of a developmental continuum might be useful in this setting. Caregivers are accustomed to providing care to the preterm and ill term infant in conjunction with clinical status changes, with increases in gestational maturity and within the context of emerging physiologic and neurobehavioral competence. This represents an approach that individualizes care rather than applying rigid standardized practices. Nursing staff and families can benefit from recognition of cues or triggers that signal the need for a change in thinking and, thus, caregiving approaches. When infants reach a point at which the benefits of supportive bedding and prone positioning are outweighed by the risks, it is essential that the staff shifts the focus from intensive intervention to achieving competence that can support discharge to home. Nurses and family members must begin to think of the infant within the framework of convalescing toward health. The best timing for SIDS prevention positioning is obviously individual. One strategy might be to use a standard weight criteria such as 1500 g. However, such arbitrary criteria will not have equal application for small for gestational age (SGA) infants or those who have an ongoing physiologic need for prone or supported sleep positions. Competencies such as transition to a crib, or achieving full oral feedings might be better approximations for determining readiness for SIDS prevention positioning. These competencies both occur at or around a particular gestational age, or more precisely, maturity.

## PROTOCOL DEVELOPMENT: TRANSITION TO SUPINE SLEEP POSITION

Development of a unit or facility protocol for transitioning to AAP recommendations is a pivotal element to providing nurses with the information and reminders needed to successfully implement the practices. An example of such a protocol is available in the literature, and can be adapted to meet the unique needs of different neonatal care settings (Lockridge, Taquino, & Knight, 1999). Gracey (2001) describes several critical components of a protocol. These include a consensus-driven definition for medical stability; targeting an appropriate gestational and/or chronologic age for initiation of supine sleep position in the hospital; and criteria to assess an individual infant's tolerance of the position (e.g., changes in oxygen saturation, apnea, feeding intolerance, or sleep/wake cycle). Guidelines for supine sleep positioning of preterm or previously ill infants in the hospital should also include clear exception criteria. Uniform application of a protocol is desired; however, among the neonatal intensive care patient population, there will nearly always be patients who are not yet ready or might never meet criteria for supine positioning. Clear identification of potential exceptions to the protocol will promote successful application of practice changes for most patients as they transition from fragile to competent status in terms of sleep position. Exceptions might include: symptomatic preterm infants with signs of respiratory distress, for whom prone positioning is clearly beneficial clinically; infants with known or suspected airway obstruction (such as Pierre Robin sequence); infants on assisted ventilation; infants receiving phototherapy; infants with severe GER, who respond positively to prone positioning, and infants with birth defects (i.e., neural tube defects) for whom the supine position would be contraindicated (Lockridge, Taquino, & Knight, 1999). These infants should receive care in a closely monitored setting, typically with continuous physiologic and comprehensive physical assessment as a baseline. Preparation for transition to a less

acute or home setting should be the impetus for a reevaluation of clinical and developmental status with regard to possible inclusion at that time.

## PROTOCOL DEVELOPMENT: BEDDING AND SLEEP SURFACES

Once it has been identified that an infant meets criteria for transition to supine sleeping, the recommendations regarding prevention of microclimates and rebreathing should also be initiated. These include placement on a firm, flat mattress covered with a single sheet, and removal of additional bedding, linen, nesting, and positioning supports. Swaddling and wrapping of the infant may be continued, with careful attention to limit swaddling to below the nipple line. Some supportive positioning devices might still be required to support the infant's development. If deemed necessary, foot supports should be immobile, and side supports should be tightly rolled and maintained below the level of the shoulder. The infant should be dressed for warmth, although this might be difficult to achieve in the hospital setting with intravenous tubing, electrodes, and other required medical devices. A light blanket can be used for cover, but should extend no higher than the chest. Hospitalized infants who have dermatologic, musculoskeletal, or other conditions requiring specialized sleep surfaces should be identified as exceptions to the policy for bedding and reevaluated accordingly.

Transitioning an infant from fully supported sleep position and bedding to healthy sleep expectations is best achieved gradually to encourage the infant to adapt to the changes. The competencies of self-regulation in prone sleep position are not achieved immediately; therefore, it can be expected that the transition to supine sleep position without benefit of supportive bedding and positioning aids will take some time as well. One strategy for the nurse is to begin by placing the infant in a sidelying position for sleep before ultimately transitioning to supine. Similarly, removal of bedding elements periodically over a few days might minimize stress to the infant and enhance the success of the transition. Creating a smooth and effective transition implies that the process occurs early enough before discharge that the infant has time to regain competence with the new sleep position. It is less than optimal to transition the infant at the time of discharge. The addition of a foreign sleep pattern is likely to cause sleep disturbances that will result in increased stress for the infant and family.

## PROTOCOL DEVELOPMENT: PRONE FOR PLAY

In addition to education and role modeling of supine sleep positioning and appropriate bedding, nurses should ensure that families understand the importance of encouraging their infant to spend time in the prone position. Specific, concise information from nurses about the development of upper body strength, normal progression to optimal fine and gross motor skills, and timely cognitive development will help parents understand the value of supervised prone positioning (Hunter & Malloy, 2002). This concept should be integrated into hospital practices, protocols, and education. As described earlier, this time is commonly referred to as "Tummy Time," whereby the infant is placed prone during nonsleeping periods. It can also be conceptualized as "Supine for Sleep" and "Prone for Play." The infant is meant to be awake and alert; there is supervision and interaction provided by the parent or caregiver. The duration of time can be varied in accordance with the infant's tolerance of the position, how the parent feels about the interaction, and other factors. The key is to regularly give the infant the opportunity for prone experiences. This can and should be a part of any transition within the hospital setting. Gracey (2001) and Hunter and Malloy (2002) provide practical parent-teaching guides to supervised "tummy time."

## PROTOCOL IMPLEMENTATION STRATEGIES

The development of a perfect protocol or set of guidelines would be useless without strategies to ensure successful implementation among nursing staff, especially those practicing in the NICU or Special Care Nursery setting. Nursing opinion has been shown to be a significant barrier to implementation of the AAP Guidelines among healthy infants cared for in hospital nurseries (Delzell, Phillips, Schnitzer, & Ewigman, 2001; Peeke,

Hershberger, Kuehn, & Levett, 1999). Years after the introduction of the "Back to Sleep" campaign, many nurses in Iowa hospitals were still placing infants in sidelying sleeping positions in the hospital. The researchers proposed that parents were confused about optimal home practices based on their observations of sidelying sleep positions in the hospital (Hein & Pettit, 2001). If nurses caring for healthy infants are reluctant to fully adopt the AAP recommendation that supine sleep offers the lowest risk of SIDS and is preferable to sidelying sleep, it can be assumed that those working in intensive care settings might be even less likely to do so. Despite the evidence supporting supine positioning, some nurses clearly remain hesitant to position infants supine and choose the sidelying position as a "safer option." Because parents are likely to mimic hospital practices at home, they should be made aware that the risk of SIDS is higher for those infants placed sidelying rather than supine.

Changing nursing practice and individual behaviors can be a daunting task, especially when the practices are well ingrained, have been practiced over time, have personal application (e.g., their own infants were cared for in prone positions), or are complex to integrate into existing practices. The first step to changing nursing practice is often the provision and acceptance of information, ideally a scientific or conceptual rationale to support the change. In the case of SIDS risk reduction, the information is available, but many NICU care providers are not yet engaged or open to the information. The "Back to Sleep" campaign has been targeted at families and lay public rather than at healthcare providers. Additionally, the inherent ambiguities in recommendations for preterm and ill infants have not provided a solid base of convincing evidence for NICU staff members. Information dispelling the myths of supine positioning risks, evidence of SIDS rate reduction with AAP recommended practices, and local or regional SIDS rates are examples of content that should be directed toward NICU caregivers to provide the basis for bringing about practice changes. In conjunction with the dissemination of information, nurses and NICU care providers need to identify benefits to their patients, and finally accept accountability for integrating the recommendations into their practice.

Upon achievement of consensus, it might be valuable to simplify the content of protocols or policies to address the needs most applicable to the unit or NICU care setting. If a unit has a largely homogeneous population, the inclusion criteria might be simpler than if there are numerous patients with valid exceptions to the guidelines, posters, and visual aids. Showing techniques to achieve appropriate positioning support can be helpful for initial education and for ongoing reference to reinforce the desired practices. Reminders of goals for sleep versus play positions, and patient exception criteria can also be highlighted to assist staff with integration of the information. Nurses might be helped by the use of reminder cards placed either on the crib or in the unit, or other means of quickly cueing in that an infant meets criteria for transition, or is in the process of transitioning to healthy sleep behaviors. It is also often helpful to identify an "idea champion" or member of the staff that takes on the role of observing and reinforcing the change. The use of peer support to reward the appropriate behaviors and gently remind the staff of the expectations can be invaluable in solidifying the change and in preventing reversion to old ways. Some units or staff groups might respond better to a stringent policy and implementation with a firm hand. Others might have a culture that supports a more gradual approach with emphasis on positive reinforcement. Techniques and approaches should be tailored to obtain the desired effect of practice change.

## FAMILY EDUCATION

Family education is obviously critical to the effective reduction of SIDS risk. Families and extended families might have already integrated the recommendations for sleep position in older children. If this is the case, efforts should be targeted at explaining why or how the preterm or ill infant is different, with attention to when and how the transition to supine sleeping should occur. The importance of the message should be easy to convey; no parent will want to risk the safety of their infant if they understand the risks and rationale for the recommendations. There are abundant materials for families describing the AAP recommendations, many of which are easily available from Internet sources. The "Back to Sleep" campaign has been successful at transcending most U.S. population groups, although there are still groups such as African Americans showing lower rates of acceptance. The modifiable risk factors, as identified by the AAP 2000 statement, should be central content for addressing education to parents and families of hospitalized infants. The target areas should include: prone sleep, overheating, soft sleep surfaces, and inappropriate sleep environments. The importance of encouraging "Tummy Time" should be integrated into parent education strategies.

In addition to providing families with information and education, the expected behaviors must be consistently established and reinforced in the hospital setting. The nurse, physician, or other healthcare provider is truly the model for the parent, with significant impact on parent beliefs and behaviors. Despite apparent contrasts with published or presented information such as "Back to Sleep" recommendations, families will continue to demonstrate behaviors and techniques seen in the hospital setting (Hein & Pettit, 2001). It is important for families to be aware that the differences in sleep practices for hospitalized ill infants might be only temporary. Information about timing and techniques for transition should be shared with families early on and throughout the infant's hospital stay. Families need encouragement from trusted individuals that their infant is progressing along the developmental continuum, and meets criteria to transition to healthy sleep behaviors and eventual discharge. Achievement of healthy sleep position should be considered a developmental milestone in line with achieving full oral feedings and weaning from other medical devices.

Neonatal nurses and caregivers have a critical impact on the outcomes of their patients in all aspects of care. Reducing the risk of SIDS and the promotion of healthy sleep behaviors are no exception. Role modeling of safe sleep positioning and sleep environments are critical elements of discharge preparation. Family teaching must include accurate information about modifiable risk factors for SIDS so that parents are capable of making informed decisions about infant sleep position and environment in the home setting. NICU caregivers should acknowledge the safety and efficacy of supine sleep positions in terms of reducing the risk of SIDS, and must be willing to incorporate AAP recommendations into their daily practice when appropriate. With careful consensus building, integrated protocol development, and the employment of implementation strategies, caregivers can easily achieve successful application of the AAP guidelines in even the most critically ill patient populations. The use of a developmental continuum as a framework for introduction and application of the recommendations not only achieves the goals set forth by the AAP, but also resolves the perceived conflict between "Back to Sleep" and principles of developmentally supportive care. Successful transitioning of high risk, critically ill, and premature infants to acceptable sleep positions and behaviors is an expectation of care. Accountability for achieving the ultimate outcome of healthier infants and SIDS reduction is shared among professionals, families, and the community at large.

## CONCLUSION

The issues associated with integrating AAP recommendations for infant sleep and developmentally supportive care have been identified and discussed throughout the chapter. Neonatal healthcare providers must rise to the challenges created by these recommendations during the infant's hospitalization so that the risk of SIDS is minimized once the infant is discharged to home.

## *REFERENCES*

American Academy of Pediatrics Task Force on Infant Positioning and SIDS (Kattwinkel, J., Brooks, J., & Myerburg, D.). (1992). Positioning and SIDS. *Pediatrics, 89*(6), 1120-1126.

American Academy of Pediatrics Task Force on Infant Positioning and SIDS. (Kattwinkel, J., Brooks, J., Keenan, M., et al.). (1994). Infant sleep position and sudden infant death syndrome (SIDS) in the United States: Joint commentary from the American Academy of Pediatrics and Selected Agencies of the Federal Government. *Pediatrics, 93*(5), 820.

American Academy of Pediatrics Task Force on Infant Positioning and SIDS, 1996-1997. (Kattwinkel, J., Brooks, J., Keenan, M., et al.). (1996). Positioning and sudden infant death syndrome (SIDS) update. *Pediatrics, 98,* 1216-1218.

American Academy of Pediatrics Task Force on Infant Positioning and Sudden Infant Death Syndrome (SIDS). (2000). Changing concepts of sudden infant death syndrome: implications for infant sleeping environment and sleep position. *Pediatrics, 105,* 650-656.

Bayes, B.J. (1974). Prone infants and SIDS. *New England Journal of Medicine, 290,* 693-694.

Blackburn, S., DePaul, D., Loan, L.A., Marbut, K., Taquino, L.T., Thomas, K.A., & Wilson, S.K. (2001). Neonatal thermal care, part III: The effect of infant position and temperature probe placement. *Neonatal Network—Journal of Neonatal Nursing, 20*(3), 19-23.

Blumenthal, I., Ebel, A., & Pildes, R.S. (1979). Effect of posture on the pattern of stomach emptying in the newborn. *Pediatrics, 63,* 532-536.

Blumenthal, I., & Lealman, G.T. (1982). Effect of posture on gastro-esophageal reflux in the newborn. *Archives of Disease in Childhood, 57,* 555-556.

Byard, R.W., & Beal, S.M. (2000). Gastric aspiration and sleeping position in infancy and early childhood. *Journal of Pediatric Child Health, 36,* 403-405.

Carpenter, R.G., & Shaddick, C.W. (1965). Role of infection, suffocation, and bottle feeding in cot death. *British Journal of Preventive Social Medicine, 19,* 1-7.

Davis, B.E., Moon, R.Y., Sachs, H.C., & Ottolini, M.C. (1998). Effects of sleep position on infant motor development. *Pediatrics, 102,* 1135-1140.

DeJonge, G.A., Engleberts, A.C., Koomen-Lieftig, A.J.M., & Kostense, P.J. (1989). Cot death and prone sleeping position in the Netherlands. (Department of Paediatrics, Free University Hospital, Amsterdam, The Netherlands.). *British Medical Journal, 298*(6675), 722.

Delzell, J.E., Phillips, R.L., Schnitzer, P.G., & Ewigman, B. (2001). Sleeping position: Change in practice, advice, and opinion in the newborn nursery. *Journal of Family Practice, 50*(5), 448.

Dewey, C., Fleming, P., & Golding, J. (1998). Does the supine sleeping position have any adverse effects on the child? II. Development in the first 18 months. (ALSPAC Study Team.). *Pediatrics, 101*(1), E5.

Downs, J.A., Edwards, A.D., McCormick, D.C, Roth, S.C., et al. (1991). Effect of intervention on development of hip posture in very preterm babies. *Archives of Disease in Childhood, 66,* 797-801 (special section).

Drago, D. A., & Dannenberg, A. L. (1999). Infant mechanical suffocation deaths in the United States, 1980-1997. *Pediatrics, 103*(5), e59

Fay, M.J. (1988). The positive effects of positioning. *Neonatal Network, 6,* 23-28.

Franco, P., Lipshutz, W., Valente, F., Adams, S., Scaillet, S., & Kahn, A. (2002). Decreased arousals in infants who sleep with the face covered by bedclothes. *Pediatrics, 109*(6), 1112-1117.

Freed, G.E., Steinschneider, A., Glassman, M., et al. (1994). Sudden infant death syndrome: Prevention and understanding of selected clinical issues. *Pediatric Clinics of North America, 41*(5), 967-990.

Gracey, K. (2001). Ensuring safe sleep. *Advances in Neonatal Care, 1*(2), 107-114.

Guntheroth, W.G., & Spiers, P.S. (1992). Sleeping prone and the risk of sudden infant death syndrome. *Journal of the American Medical Association, (JAMA) 267*(17), 2359-2362.

Hauck, F.R., Merrick-Moore, C., Herman, S.M., et al. (2002). The contribution of prone sleeping position to the racial disparity in sudden infant death syndrome: The Chicago infant mortality study. *Pediatrics, 110*(4), 772-780.

Heimler, R., Langlois, J., Hodel, D.J., et al. (1992). Effect of positioning on the breathing pattern of preterm infants. *Archives of Disease in Childhood, 67*, 312-314.

Hein, H.A., & Pettit, S.F. (2001). Back to sleep: Good advice for parents but not for hospitals? *Pediatrics, 107*, 537-539.

Hudak, B.B., O'Donnell, J., & Mazyrka, N. (1995). Infant sleep position: Pediatricians advice to parents. *Pediatrics, 95*(1), 55-58.

Hunt, C.E. & Shannon, D.C. (1992). Sudden infant death syndrome and sleeping positions. *Pediatrics, 90*(1)(Pt 1), 115-118.

Hunter, J.G, & Malloy, M.H. (2002). Effect of sleep and play position on infant development: Reconciling developmental concerns with SIDS prevention. *Newborn and Infant Nursing Reviews, 2*(1), 9 16.

Kane, A., Mitchell, L, Craven, K., & Marsh, J. (1996). Observations on a recent increase in plagiocephaly without synostosis. *Pediatrics, 97*, 877-885.

Kattwinkel, J. (2000). *AAP news release—SIDS rate: Decrease seen, but more can be done.* Available online at *www.aap.org/advocacy/archives/marsids.htm.*

Kurlak, L.O., Ruggins, N.R., & Stephenson, T.J. (1994). Effect of nursing position on incidence, type, and duration of clinically significant apnea in preterm infants. *Archives of Disease in Childhood, 71*, F16-F19.

Lockridge, T. (1997). Now I lay me down to sleep: SIDS and infant sleep positions. *Neonatal Network, 16*(7), 25-31.

Lockridge, T., Taquino, L.T., & Knight, A. (1999). Back to sleep: Is there room in that crib for both AAP recommendations and developmentally supportive care? *Neonatal Network, 18*(5), 29-33.

Malloy, M. (2002). Trends in postneonatal aspiration deaths and reclassification of sudden infant death syndrome: Impact of the "Back to Sleep" program. *Pediatrics, 109*(4), 661-665.

Markestad, T. (1993). Information about sudden infant death syndrome for the general public. *Acta Paediatrica Supplement, 389*, 124-125.

Martin, R.J., Herrell, N., Rubin, D., & Fanaroff, A. (1979). Effect of supine and prone positions on arterial oxygen tension in the preterm infant. *Pediatrics, 63*, 528-531.

Mitchell, E.A., Aley, P., & Eastwood, J. (1992). The national cot death prevention program in New Zealand. *Australian Journal of Public Health, 16*, 158-161.

Mitchell, E.A., Thach, B.T., Thompson, J., & Williams, S. (1999). Changing infants' sleep position increases risk of sudden infant death syndrome. *Archives of Pediatrics and Adolescent Medicine, 153*(11), 1136-1141.

Mouradian, L.E., & Als, H. (1994). The influence of neonatal intensive care unit caregiving practices on motor functioning of preterm infants. *American Journal of Occupational Therapy, 48*, 527-533.

Myerberg, D.Z. (1993). Sleep positioning and sudden infant death syndrome. *Western Journal of Medicine, 158*(2), 181-182.

Nakamura, S., Wind, M., & Danello, M.A. (1999). Review of hazards associated with children placed in adult beds. *Archives of Pediatric and Adolescent Medicine, 153*, 1019-1023.

National Institute of Child Health and Human Development. (2000). *NIH news alert—NICHD funded researchers uncover abnormal brain pathways in SIDS victims.* Available online at *www.nichd.nih.gov/sids/sleep_risk.htm.*

National Institute of Child Health and Human Development. (2002). *SIDS: Back to Sleep Campaign.* Available online at *www.nichd.nih.gov/new/releases/sids-brainstem.cfm?from=sids.*

Orenstein, S.R., Mitchell, A.A., & Davidson W.S. (1993). Concerning the American Academy of Pediatrics recommendations on sleep position for infants (commentary). *Pediatrics, 91*(2), 497-499.

Peeke, K., Hershberger, C.M., Kuehn, D., & Levett, J. (1999). Infant sleep position: Nursing practice and knowledge. *MCN: American Journal of Maternal Child Nursing, 24*, 301-304.

Pollack, I., Losken, H., & Fasick, P. (1997). Diagnosis and management of posterior plagiocephaly. *Pediatrics, 99*, 180-185.

Pontius, K., Aretz, M., Griebel, C., Jacobs, C., LaRock, K., and members of OT-PT Baby Team. (2001). PM & R update: Back to sleep—Tummy time to play. *Newsletter of the Children's Hospital Physical Medicine and Rehabilitation, Denver, Colorado, 4*(4), 1-3.

Raco, A., Raimondi, A.J., De Ponte, F.S., et al. (1999). Congenital torticollis in association with craniosyncstosis. *Child's Nervous System, 15*, 163-169.

Stewart, A., Mitchell, E.A., Tipene-Leach, D., & Fleming, P. (1993). Lessons from the New Zealand and UK cot death campaigns. *Acta Paediatrica Supplement, 389*, 119-123.

Taquino, L.T., & Lockridge, T. (1999). Caring for critically ill infants: Strategies to promote physiological stability and improve developmental outcomes. *Critical Care Nurse, 19*(6), 64-79.

U.S. Consumer Product Safety Commission. (1999). *News from CPSC: Recommendations revised to prevent infant deaths from soft bedding.* Available online at *www.cpsc.gov/cpscpub/prerel/prhtml99/99091.html.*

U.S. Consumer Product Safety Commission. (2003). *Recommendations revised to prevent infant deaths from soft bedding.* Available online at *www.cpsc.gov.*

U.S. Department of Health & Human Services. (1999). *"Back to Sleep" campaign seeks to reduce incidence of SIDS in African American populations.* Available online at *www.hhs.gov/news/press/1999pres/991026.html? from=sids.*

Willinger, M., Hoffman, H.J., & Hartford, R.B. (1994). *Infant sleep position and risk for sudden infant death syndrome.* (Report of a meeting held January 13 and 14, 1994, National Institutes of Health, Bethesda, MD). *Pediatrics, 93*(5), 814-819.

Willinger, M., James, L.S., & Catz, C. (1991). Defining the sudden infant death syndrome (SIDS): Deliberations of an expert panel convened by the National Institute of Child Health and Human Development. *Pediatric Pathology, 11*(5), 677-684.

# 12 Pain Management

## Marlene Walden and Katherine M. Jorgensen

Pain is assessed and managed inadequately in a large proportion of neonates, despite the ready availability of assessment instruments and safe and effective pharmacologic and nonpharmacologic interventions (Anand, Selanikio, & SOPAIN, 1996; Bauchner, May, & Coates, 1992). A prospective study of analgesic and sedation practices in 109 neonatal intensive care units (NICUs) that included 1068 preterm neonates demonstrated that procedural pain was not routinely treated with either pharmacologic or nonpharmacologic interventions (Anand, Selanikio, & SOPAIN, 1996). Many questions must be answered if we are to anticipate pain and manage it effectively. Some of these questions are: What do we know about neonatal pain? What do we do to minimize or alleviate pain? How do we know these interventions are working appropriately? How does it relate to palliative or end-of-life (EOL) care? What is the relationship to individualized, developmental care? In this chapter, we explore pain as a physiologic phenomenon, what we know and do not know, how we can objectively measure pain, and strategies for effectively anticipating, preventing, and managing pain.

## STANDARDS OF PRACTICE

Recognition of the widespread inadequacy of pain management promoted various professional and accrediting organizations to issue position statements and clinical recommendations in an effort to promote effective pain management in undertreated populations. The first, and perhaps most comprehensive, clinical practice guideline was issued in 1992 by the Agency for Health Care Policy and Research (currently known as the Agency for Healthcare Research and Quality [AHRQ]). It addresses acute pain management for operative or medical procedures and trauma in adults, infants, children, and adolescents (U.S. Department of Health and Human Services, 1992). Position statements by the National Association of Neonatal Nurses (NANN) (1999;

2001), the Association for Women's Health, Obstetrics, and Neonatal Nursing (AWHONN, 1995), and the American Academy of Pediatrics/Canadian Paediatric Society (AAP/CPS, 2000) also support the importance of optimal pain assessment and management in hospitalized neonates. The standards currently receiving the most widespread attention are those of the Joint Commission on Accreditation of Healthcare Organizations (JCAHO, 1999) that were implemented in 2001. These standards are being used to evaluate pain management practices in hospitals and other clinical agencies providing inpatient and outpatient healthcare services. There is considerable consistency in the recommendations set by these various professional and accrediting organizations. A summary of these professional and accrediting organization guidelines and standards are provided in Box 12-1. The various guidelines have provided momentum for institutions to reexamine their philosophy and practices of pain management. The clinical challenge remains on how to implement these standards in various institutional settings based on patient types, frequently occurring clinical procedures performed, and current staffing patterns.

## PHYSIOLOGY OF PAIN

The theory of nociception divides the pain system into three components: peripheral pain system, dorsal horns, and supraspinal centers. The peripheral pain system registers the initial noxious stimuli; initiates local pain reactions (vasomotor, inflammatory); and conducts the nociceptive input to the central nervous system (Deshpande & Anand, 1996). Transmission of nociceptive impulses occurs along two types of afferent sensory fibers. A-delta fibers are thinly myelinated, rapid-conducting fibers associated with acute pain or "first pain" (e.g., sharp, localized, pricking). C fibers are polymodal, unmyelinated, slow-conducting fibers associated with aching, burning, throbbing, poorly localized, chronic or "second pain." It is notable that nociceptive impulses are carried through unmyelinated

**Box 12-1**   SUMMARY OF RECOMMENDATIONS ON PAIN BY PROFESSIONAL AND ACCREDITING
ORGANIZATIONS

| Standards | References |
| --- | --- |
| Education and competency in pain assessment and management should be conducted during orientation and at regularly defined intervals throughout employment for all nurses delivering care to neonates and young infants. | AAP/CPS, 2000; IASP, 2000; JCAHO, 1999; NANN, 1999 |
| Pain is assessed and reassessed at regular intervals throughout the infant's hospitalization. A valid and reliable multidimensional pain assessment instrument should be used. | AAP/CPS, 2000; AHCPR, 1992; ASA, 1995; AWHONN, 1995; IASP, 2000; JCAHO, 1999; NANN, 1999 |
| Use both nonpharmacologic and pharmacologic therapies to control and/or prevent pain. | AAP/CPS, 2000; AHCPR, 1992; IASP, 2000; NANN, 1999 |
| A collaborative, interdisciplinary approach to pain control should be used, including input from all members of the healthcare team and the infant's family, when appropriate. | AAP, 1992; AHCPR, 1992; AWHONN, 1995; IASP, 2000; JCAHO, 1999; NANN, 1999 |
| Pain assessment and management practices should be documented in a manner that facilitates regular reassessment and follow-up intervention. | ASA, 1995; IASP, 2000; JCAHO, 1999 |
| Institutions should establish policies and procedures that support and promote optimal pain assessment and management practices. | AAP/CPS, 2000; AHCPR, 1992; JCAHO, 1999 |
| Institutions should collect data to monitor the appropriateness and effectiveness of pain-management practices. | AHCPR, 1992; IASP, 2000; JCAHO, 1999 |

From Carrier, C.T., & Walden, M. (2001). Integrating research and standards to improve pain management practices for newborns and infants. *Newborn and Infant Nursing Reviews, 1*(2), 122-131.

*AAP/CPS*, American Academy of Pediatrics/Canadian Paediatric Society; *AHCPR*, Agency for Health Care Policy and Research (currently known as Agency for Healthcare Research and Quality; *ASA*, American Society of Anesthesiologists Pain Management Task Force; *AWHONN*, Association for Women's Health, Obstetrics, and Neonatal Nursing; *IASP*, International Association for the Study of Pain; *JCAHO*, Joint Commission on Accreditation of Healthcare Organizations; *NANN*, National Association of Neonatal Nurses.

and thinly myelinated fibers even in adult peripheral nerves (Anand, Phil, & Hickey, 1987).

The dorsal horns of the spinal cord integrate pain and other sensory stimuli and modulate pain perception (Deshpande & Anand, 1996). According to the gate-control theory (Melzack & Wall, 1965), neural mechanisms in the dorsal horns of the spinal cord act like a gate that alters the flow of nerve impulses from afferent fibers in the periphery to the spinal cord cells that project to the brain. Somatic input is, therefore, subjected to the modulating influence of the spinal gating mechanism in the substantia gelatinosa before it evokes pain perception and response. The theory suggests that large-diameter fibers inhibit ("close the gate"), whereas small-diameter fibers tend to facilitate transmission ("open the gate") of nerve impulses. The selective central processes in the brain, by way of large-diameter, rapidly conducting descending fibers, also influence spinal gating mechanisms. A characteristic pattern of pain behavior and response occurs when the capacities of neural mechanisms are exceeded by nerve impulses arriving in the dorsal horns (Melzack & Wall, 1965).

Transmission of nociceptive impulses through the dorsal horns is mediated through the release of excitatory neurotransmitters such as substance P, glutamate, calcitonin-gene-related peptide (CGRP), vasoactive intestinal polypeptide (VIP), neuropeptide Y, and somatostatin (Deshpande & Anand, 1996). Modulation of nociceptive transmission occurs by the release of metenkephalin from local interneurons, as well as dopamine, norepinephrine, and serotonin from descending inhibitory axons (Deshpande & Anand, 1996). This is important in considering interventions to alter the pain response of neonates. Nonnutritive sucking (NNS) and sucrose are thought to modulate transmission or processing of nociception through mediation by the endogenous opioid and nonopioid systems (Blass, Fitzgerald, & Kehoe, 1987; Gunnar, Connors, Isensee, & Wall, 1988). A nonpharmacologic intervention, hand swaddling, is thought to block the processing of nociception by stimulating sensory afferent neurons from peripheral touch receptors (Mackenna & Callander, 1990).

Supraspinal centers (thalamus, cerebral cortex) integrate and process pain information, elaborately modifying the cascade of neurochemical events triggered by nociception. Supraspinal centers are also involved in memory and learning from nociceptive experiences, and produce systemic responses to pain including cardiovascular, respiratory, hormonal, metabolic, and immune adaptations and alterations (Deshpande & Anand, 1996).

## SIGNIFICANCE OF PAIN RESPONSE IN NEONATES

Repetitive, unrelieved pain can lead to serious and adverse consequences for neonates (Anand & Hickey, 1992; Anand, Phil, & Hickey, 1987; Evans, 2001; Fitzgerald & Shortland, 1988). Short-term consequences of painful procedures include decreased oxygen saturations and increased heart rates that can place increased demands on the cardiorespiratory systems (Craig, Whitfield, Grunau, et al., 1993; McIntosh, Van Veen, & Brameyer, 1994; Stevens & Johnston, 1994; Stevens, Johnston, & Horton, 1993). In addition, pain can cause elevation in intracranial pressure, thereby increasing risk for intraventricular hemorrhage in preterm neonates (Stevens & Johnston, 1994; Stevens, Johnston, & Horton, 1993; Anand, Barton, McIntosh, et al., 1999; Evans, 2001).

Long-term consequences of repeated painful procedures include decreased sensitivity to the commonplace pain of childhood, higher incidence of somatic complaints and somatization of unspecified origin, and long-term structural changes in the brain and spinal cord (Evans, 2001; Fitzgerald & Shortland, 1988; Grunau et al., 1991; Grunau, Whitfield, & Petrie, 1994; Grunau et al., 1994).

## DEFINITION OF PAIN

Pain is a multidimensional phenomenon that is dependent on an individual's sensory and emotional perception of its existence (Melzack & Wall, 1965). The International Association for the Study of Pain (IASP), which comprises specialists in anesthesia, dentistry, neurology, neurosurgery, neurophysiology, psychiatry, and psychology, has defined pain as "unpleasant sensory and emotional experience associated with actual or potential tissue damage, or described in terms of such damage" (p. 250; 1979). Pain has been defined further as a subjective experience that is best communicated and represented through self-reports. Verbal communication and self-report are considered the "gold standard" for pain assessment. The IASP definition implies that the meaning of pain must be learned through experience and articulated within the context of verbal language. This conceptualization of pain perpetuates the misconceptions that infants, who lack linguistic skills, do not experience pain (Anand & Craig, 1996). Therefore, for infants who are not capable of verbal communication, other means of pain assessment are required. In neonates, responses to painful stimuli include immediate physiological, behavioral, and hormonal indicators that provide objective and quantifiable information about the location, intensity, and duration of painful stimuli. Although these responses are not specific to pain, they can be used in conjunction with other contextual indicators to infer the existence of pain. Furthermore, because pain is a multidimensional phenomenon, a composite measure that incorporates both physiologic and behavioral indicators should be used for its assessment.

## CLINICAL PROCEDURES CAUSING PAIN

Immediately after birth, infants are subject to painful procedures such as instrumental deliveries, intramuscular (IM) injections of vitamin K, and, possibly, circumcisions. Infants born prematurely or acutely ill are exposed to many more painful procedures than their healthy counterparts. The most frequently occurring painful procedures include endotracheal suctioning and intubation, peripheral venous catheter insertion, and heel sticks. Barker and Rutter (1995) reported that the frequency of invasive procedures is inversely related to gestational age and acuity of medical illness. Therefore, the smaller and sicker neonates are those who are subject to the largest numbers of most painful procedures. In Barker and Rutter's study, one 23-weeks' gestation, 560-g infant had 488 painful, intrusive procedures performed during her hospital stay. Stevens, Johnston, Franck, et al. (1999) found that infants born between 27 and 31 weeks' gestation received on average a mean of 134 painful procedures within the first 2 weeks of life, and approximately 10% of the youngest or sickest infants received more than 300 painful procedures.

Porter, Wolf, and Miller (1999) found that infants experienced varying numbers of painful procedures immediately following birth. Suspected intensity of pain associated with the procedures was directly related to gestational age and severity of illness, with the most immature and vulnerable infants experiencing the most intrusive procedures. Preterm infants experienced, on average, more than 700 painful procedures during their hospitalization. These procedures were characterized as mildly (e.g., insertion of gavage tube, umbilical arterial catheter

insertion), moderately (e.g., heel sticks, venipunctures), or highly invasive (e.g., lumbar punctures, circumcision). However, no research has systematically and objectively evaluated pain intensity associated with commonly performed procedures in the NICU for establishing assessment guidelines or individualized nonpharmacologic interventions.

## PAIN ASSESSMENT

Pain research on neonates has produced several instruments with acceptable measurement properties, including the CRIES (**C**rying, **R**equires Oxygen Saturation, **I**ncreased Vital Signs, **E**xpression, **S**leeplessness) Neonatal Postoperative Pain Measurement Score (Krechel & Bildner, 1995); the Premature Infant Pain Profile (PIPP) (Stevens, Johnston, Petryshen, et al., 1996); the Neonatal Infant Pain Scale (NIPS) (Lawrence, Alcock, McGrath, et al., 1993); and, more recently, the Neonatal Pain, Agitation, and Sedation Scale (N-PASS) (Hummel & Puchalski, 2002). The CRIES (Table 12-1) is a postoperative pain measure validated in infants 32 to 60 weeks' gestational age. The PIPP (Table 12-2) has been routinely used with preterm infants from 28 weeks' gestational age through 40 weeks' gestational age. The PIPP includes a recommended scoring adjustment for use with neonates of varying gestational ages and behavioral states observed immediately before the clinical procedure. Both gestational age and behavioral state

**Table 12-1    CRIES: Neonatal Postoperative Pain Assessment Score**

| Indicator | 0 | 1 | 2 |
|---|---|---|---|
| Crying | No | High-pitched | Inconsolable |
| Requires oxygen for saturation >95% | No | <30% | >30% |
| Increased vital signs | Heart rate and blood pressure within 10% of preoperative value | Heart rate and blood pressure 11% to 20% higher than preoperative value | Heart rate and blood pressure 21% or more higher than preoperative value |
| Expression | None | Grimace | Grimace/grunt |
| Sleepless | No | Wakes at frequent intervals | Constantly awake |

From Krechel, S., & Bildner, J. (1995). From "CRIES: A new neonatal post-operative pain measurement score: Initial testing of validity and reliability. *Paediatric Anaesthesia, 5*(1), 53-61.

Table **12-2**   PREMATURE INFANT PAIN PROFILE (PIPP)

| Process | Indicator | 0 | 1 | 2 | 3 | Score |
|---|---|---|---|---|---|---|
| Chart | Gestational age | 36 weeks and more | 32 to 35 weeks, 6 days | 28 to 31 weeks, 6 days | Less than 28 weeks | |
| Score 15 sec immediately before event | Behavioral state | Active/awake Eyes open Facial movements | Quiet/awake Eyes open No facial movements | Active/sleep Eyes closed Facial movements | | |
| Record baseline heart rate ____ | Maximum heart rate | 0 to 4 beats/minute increase | 5 to 14 beats/minute increase | 15 to 24 beats/minute increase | 25 beats/minute or more increase | |
| Observe infant 30 seconds immediately following event | | | | | | |
| Record baseline oxygen saturation ____ | Minimum oxygen saturation | 0% to 2.4% decrease | 2.5% to 4.9% decrease | 5.0% to 7.4% decrease | 7.5% or more decrease | |
| Observe infant 30 seconds immediately following event | | | | | | |
| Observe infant 30 seconds immediately following event | Brow bulge | None 0% to 9% of time | Minimum 10% to 39% of time | Moderate 40% to 69% of time | Maximum 70% of time or more | |
| Observe infant 30 seconds immediately following event | Eye squeeze | None 0% to 9% of time | Minimum 10% to 39% of time | Moderate 40% to 69% of time | Maximum 70% of time or more | |
| Observe infant 30 seconds immediately following event | Nasolabial furrow | None 0% to 9% of time | Minimum 10% to 39% of time | Moderate 40% to 69% of time | Maximum 70% of time or more | |
| | | | | | **Total** | **Score** ____ |

From Stevens, B., Johnston, C., Petryshen, P., & Taddio, A. (1996). Premature infant pain profile: Development and initial validation. *Clinical Journal of Pain, 12*, 13-22.

are known to modify pain expression in preterm neonates (Craig, Whitfield, Grunau, et al., 1993; Grunau & Craig, 1987; Johnston, Stevens, Franck, et al., 1999; Stevens & Johnston, 1994; Stevens, Johnston, & Horton, 1994). Similar to the PIPP, the N-PASS (see Appendix F) also includes a recommended scoring adjustment for use with neonates of varying gestational ages. The N-PASS is unique in that the instrument also incorporates a separate scoring system to assess the level of sedation, a useful adjunct for infants receiving opioid therapy. The NIPS (Figure 12-1) has been used in both preterm and term infants in evaluating procedural pain. This instrument provides particular clinical utility in monitoring pain in healthy newborns, as the instrument does not require an infant to be attached to a cardiac monitor or pulse oximeter as assessment parameters.

| | Before Time | | During Time | | | | | After Time | | |
|---|---|---|---|---|---|---|---|---|---|---|
| | 1 | 2 | 1 | 2 | 3 | 4 | 5 | 1 | 2 | 3 |
| **Facial expression**<br>0-Relaxed<br>1-Grimace | | | | | | | | | | |
| **Cry**<br>0-No cry<br>1-Whimper<br>2-Vigorous | | | | | | | | | | |
| **Breathing patterns**<br>0-Relaxed<br>1-Change in breathing | | | | | | | | | | |
| **Arms**<br>0-Relaxed/restrained<br>1-Flexed/extended | | | | | | | | | | |
| **Legs**<br>0-Relaxed/restrained<br>1-Flexed/extended | | | | | | | | | | |
| **State of arousal**<br>0-Sleeping/awake<br>1-Fussy | | | | | | | | | | |
| **Total** | | | | | | | | | | |

Time is measured in 1-minute intervals.

Figure **12-1** Neonatal Infant Pain Scale. (*From Lawrence, J., Alcock, D., McGrath, P., et al. [1993]. The development of a tool to assess neonatal pain.* Neonatal Network, 12*[6], 59-66.*)

## CONTEXTUAL FACTORS MODIFYING NEONATAL PAIN RESPONSES

Pain expression is altered by the contextual factors surrounding the pain event. Behavioral state has been shown to act as a moderator of behavioral pain responses in both full-term and preterm infants. Infants in awake or alert states demonstrate a more robust reaction to painful stimuli than infants in sleep states (Grunau & Craig; 1987; Stevens & Johnston, 1994; Stevens, Johnston, Taddio, et al., 1996; Johnston, Stevens, Franck, et al., 1999).

Research examining facial and body activity has demonstrated that the magnitude of infant's observable behavioral response to pain is less vigorous and less robust when the infant is of a less mature postconceptional age (Craig, Whitfield, Grunau, et al., 1993; Johnston, Stevens, Yang, & Horton, 1995; Johnston, Stevens, Franck, et al., 1999). These observations, however, are contrary to data that suggest that more immature preterm infants have a lower threshold and are hypersensitive to painful stimuli compared with older preterm neonates (Andrews & Fitzgerald, 1994; Fitzgerald, Millard, & McIntosh, 1989). Craig, Whitfield, Grunau, et al. (1993) suggested that the less vigorous behavioral responses demonstrated by younger preterm infants "should be interpreted in the context of the energy resources available to respond and the relative immaturity of the musculoskeletal system" (p. 296). In addition, many preterm infants do not cry in response to a noxious stimulus (Johnston, Stevens, Yang, & Horton, 1995; Stevens, Johnston, & Horton, 1993; Stevens, Johnston, & Horton, 1994; Johnston, Stevens, Franck, et al., 1999). The absence of response might only indicate the depletion of response capability and not lack of pain perception (Walden & Franck, 2003).

Emerging evidence suggests that NICU experience might produce altered behavioral responses to noxious stimuli. Johnston, Stevens, Franck, et al. (1999) found that time since last painful procedure predicted subsequent response to a heel-stick procedure in preterm neonates. Johnston and Stevens (1996) reported a decreased behavioral response to heel stick with a higher number of invasive procedures over 4 weeks in the NICU. Therefore, the postconception age of the infant, the total num-

ber of painful procedures, and the time since the last painful procedure are important assessment parameters to know when preparing an infant for another painful event. Specific recommendations related to pain assessment can be found in Box 12-2.

## NONPHARMACOLOGIC INTERVENTIONS FOR CLINICAL PROCEDURES CAUSING MINOR PAIN

Painful procedures in the NICU are unavoidable; therefore, it is vital that caregivers investigate strategies to assist infants to cope with and recover from necessary but painful clinical procedures. Nonpharmacologic strategies have been shown to be important accompaniments to clinical procedures to help minimize neonatal pain and stress while maximizing the infant's own regulatory and coping abilities. This is particularly true for preterm infants who have less capacity for recovery after acute procedure-induced pain than do term, healthy infants (Beaver, 1987; Owens & Todt, 1984; Walden, Penticuff, Stevens, et al., 2001).

Although it is beyond the scope of this chapter to discuss the pharmacologic management of pain in neonates in depth, it is important to recognize when pharmacologic interventions are indicated for relief of pain in the NICU. Analgesics should be used when severe or prolonged pain is assessed or anticipated (U.S. Department of Health and Human Services, 1992). Although sedatives might have an adjunctive role to opioids in managing pain, it is important to remember that they blunt behavioral responses to noxious stimuli without providing pain relief and should only be used when pain has been ruled out (Hartley, Franck, & Lundergan, 1989). Franck and Miaskowski (1998) performed an excellent research critique of the use of opioids to provide analgesia in critically ill, premature neonates.

The evidence base for pain management is presented within a developmentally supportive care framework. The components of developmental care can be divided into those related to the total nursery environment (macroenvironment) and those related to the individual infant's environment or care experiences (microenvironment).

Box **12-2**    Recommendations for Pain Assessment

- Use physiologic measures to assess pain in infants who are paralyzed for mechanical ventilation or who are severely neurologically impaired.
- Preterm infants responses "should be interpreted in the context of the energy resources available to respond and the relative immaturity of the musculoskeletal system" (Craig, Whitfield, Grunau, 1993, p. 296).
- Developmental maturity, health status, and environmental factors can all contribute to an inconsistent, less robust pattern of pain responses between infants and even within the same infant over time and situations (Craig, Whitfield, Grunau, et al., 1993; Johnston, Stevens, Craig, & Grunau, 1993; Shapiro, 1993). Therefore, contextual factors that have been demonstrated to modify the pain experience must be considered when assessing for the presence of pain in neonates.
- Based on psychometric data available, there is fair research-based evidence to support the use of the CRIES (**C**rying, **R**equires Oxygen Saturation, **I**ncreased Vital Signs, **E**xpression, **S**leeplessness) (Krechel & Bildner, 1995); The Premature Infant Pain Profile (Stevens, Johnston, Petryshen, et al., 1996); and the Neonatal Infant Pain Scale (Lawrence, Alcock, McGrath, et al., 1993) to assess pain in hospitalized neonates. An emerging tool that shows promise is the Neonatal Pain, Agitation, and Sedation Scale (Hummel & Puchalski, 2002). With further psychometric testing, other pain instruments might emerge as valid and reliable instruments to measure pain in the neonatal population.
- Hospital policy or individual nursing preference might determine which instrument is selected to measure pain in hospitalized neonates. However, to promote consistency in pain assessment and management over a period of time, the same instrument should be used to assess pain in an infant from admission to discharge or until a more age-appropriate tool is needed.
- A clinical challenge in the use of most pain instruments is how to determine the infant's baseline values. For example, the Premature Infant Pain Profile (PIPP) scales for physiologic indicators reflect increasing amounts of change from baseline. In procedural pain, the baseline is 30 seconds prior to the clinical procedure. For postoperative patients and patients with presumed or known painful clinical conditions such as necrotizing enterocolitis, epidermalysis bullosa, and so on, the baseline value is less evident. As no data exist to guide practice, nurses must use clinical judgment in determining baseline values for these infants.
- Because previous painful experiences might modify pain expression, further research is needed to develop and test an instrument to assess chronic pain in the infant requiring prolonged hospitalization who has been subjected to multiple painful clinical procedures.

## Macroenvironment

Components of the macroenvironment include reducing the total noxious load to which the infant is exposed, streamlining procedural techniques, and restructuring the physical environment to reduce light and noise levels. Box 12-3 provides recommendations for support of the infant's macroenvironment.

Prevention is the first step in reducing the infant's exposure to noxious stimuli. Therefore, strategies to prevent pain should be employed whenever possible. All diagnostic and therapeutic procedures should be examined daily in caregiver rounds to determine

medical necessity (Franck & Lawhon, 1998). Laboratory studies that will not be acted on should be discontinued. Care procedures should also be examined, such as frequency of endotracheal suctioning (ETS). Routine orders for ETS should be avoided and should instead be performed only when clinically indicated, by physical examination findings or deteriorating blood gas values. Other examples of caregiving strategies to prevent or limit the noxious load to which an infant might be exposed includes grouping blood draws to minimize the number of venipunctures per day, establishing central vessel

## Box 12-3   RECOMMENDATIONS FOR THE MACROENVIRONMENT

- Automated incision devices should be used when heel-stick procedures are performed.
- Venipuncture might be preferable to the heel-stick procedure in minimizing procedural-related pain in term neonates. No data are available to make recommendations regarding method of blood sampling in the preterm population.
- Only trained laboratory, medical, and nursing personnel should be used to perform venipuncture or heel-stick procedures. Each neonatal intensive care unit (NICU) has a responsibility to monitor the competency level of personnel performing these procedures on hospitalized neonates.
- Reduce environmental sources of stress by lowering light and sound levels in the NICU.

access to minimize vein and artery punctures, and limiting adhesive tape and gentle removal of tape to minimize epidermal stripping.

The pain experience by hospitalized patients is often affected by the manner in which procedures are approached. The International Evidenced-Based Group for Neonatal Pain provides guidelines for preventing and treating neonatal procedural pain (Anand & International Evidence-Based Group for Neonatal Pain, 2001). Strategies for the management of diagnostic, therapeutic, and surgical procedures commonly performed in the NICU are summarized in Table 12-3.

Heel sticks account for more than 50% of painful clinical procedures performed in the NICU (Barker & Rutter, 1995). Evidence supports that the use of automated lancets results in decreased bruising, fewer repeat lance punctures, and fewer behavioral and physiologic distress responses compared with heel-stick procedures performed using manual lancets (Harpin & Rutter, 1995; McIntosh, Van Veen, & Brameyer, 1994; Burns, 1989). Research suggests that the heel squeeze might be the most painful part of the heel-stick procedure (Grunau & Craig, 1987).

In addition, facilitated tucking (discussed later) in preterm neonates and the use of sucrose pacifiers decrease pain responses associated with the heel-stick procedure (Corff, Seideman, Venkataraman, et al., 1995; Stevens & Ohlsson, 1998; Ramenghi, Griffith, Wood, et al., 1996; Stevens, Taddio, Ohlsson, & Einarson, 1997; Skogsdal, Eriksson, & Schollin, 1997). A meta-analysis on venipuncture versus heel lance for blood sampling in term neonates reported that venipuncture, when performed by a trained phlebotomist, was associated with less pain and appears to be the method of choice for blood sampling in term neonates (Shah & Ohlsson, 1999; Shah, Taddio, Bennett, & Speidel, 1997; Larsson, Tannefeldt, Lagercrantz, & Olsson, 1998).

Virtually no research has been done to systematically document the effects of sound and ambient light levels on pain responses in preterm infants. However, it is known that excessive and unpredictable sound levels (Long, Lucey, & Philips, 1980; Gorski, 1983) and bright and/or continuous lighting levels (Shiroiwa, Kamiya, & Uchibori, 1986) have been associated with increased physiologic and behavioral stress in preterm neonates in the NICU. Although no research has been done to systematically document the effects of sound and lighting levels on pain responses in preterm neonates, clinical experience would suggest that light and sound levels should be minimized during painful clinical procedures. Research is needed in this area to validate these assumptions.

### Microenvironment

Microenvironmental components include organization of caregiving, containment/positioning strategies, nonnutritive sucking with or without sucrose, and integration of the infant's family. Box 12-4 provides specific recommendations to support the infant's microenvironment.

Caregiving activities should be organized to provide periods of rest and recovery for the infant. Emerging evidence suggests that following exposure to a painful stimulus, pain sensitivity of preterm neonates is accentuated by an increased excitability of nociceptive neurons in the dorsal horn of the spinal cord. This sensory hypersensitivity, referred to as the windup phenomenon, has been

Table **12-3**  SUGGESTED MANAGEMENT OF PAINFUL PROCEDURES COMMONLY PERFORMED IN THE NICU

| Procedures | Pacifier with Sucrose | Swaddling, Containment or Facilitated Tucking | EMLA Cream | Subcutaneous Infiltration of Lidocaine | Opioids | Other |
|---|---|---|---|---|---|---|
| **DIAGNOSTIC PROCEDURES** | | | | | | |
| Arterial puncture | X | X | X | X | | Consider venipuncture; skin-to-skin contact with mother; mechanical spring-loaded lance |
| Heel lancing | X | X | | | | Use careful physical handling |
| Lumbar puncture | X | | X | X | | |
| Venipuncture | X | X | X | X | X | |
| **THERAPEUTIC PROCEDURES** | | | | | | |
| Central venous line placement | X | X | X | X | X | Consider general anesthesia |
| Chest tube insertion | X | X | | X | X | Anticipate need for intubation and ventilation in neonates spontaneously breathing; consider short acting anesthetic agents; avoid midazolam |
| Gavage tube insertion | X | X | | | | Gentle technique and appropriate lubrication |
| Intramuscular injection | X | X | X | | | |
| Peripherally inserted central catheter placement | X | X | X | | X | Give drugs intravenously, whenever possible |

| | | | | Comments |
|---|---|---|---|---|
| Endotracheal intubation | | | X | Various combinations of atropine, ketamine, thiopental sodium, succinylcholine chloride, morphine, fentanyl, nondepolarizing muscle relaxant; consider topical lidocaine spray |
| Endotracheal suction | Sucrose optional | X | X | |
| **SURGICAL PROCEDURES** | | | | |
| Circumcision | X | | X | Mogen clamp preferred over Gomco clamp; dorsal penile nerve block, ring block, or caudal block using plain or buffered lidocaine; consider acetaminophen for postoperative pain |

From Walden, M., & Franck, L. (2003). Identification, management, and prevention of newborn/infant pain. In C. Kenner & J.W. Lott (Eds.), *Comprehensive neonatal nursing: A physiologic perspective* (3rd ed.). St Louis: W.B. Saunders.

## Box **12**-4   Recommendations for Microenvironment

- Avoid clustering care around painful procedures.
- Although no research data exist on how long caregiving should be postponed following painful clinical procedures, it seems reasonable to recommend that the infant's stress cues be used to determine when the infant has returned to baseline activity and to guide decisions regarding the timing of future caregiving episodes.
- Decrease physiologic/behavioral destabilization associated with procedural handling.
- Ensure that developmentally supportive techniques are used to position infants prior to painful clinical procedures.
- Limit unnecessary handling prior to painful clinical procedures.
- Containment strategies, such as facilitated tucking or swaddling, might be more effective if instituted prior to the painful clinical procedure rather than instituted during the recovery phase, especially for younger preterm infants.
- Containment strategies, such as facilitated tucking or swaddling, should be instituted before and maintained throughout the procedure and into the recovery period until the infant's physiologic and behavioral cues stabilize and return to baseline.
- In evaluating the scientific evidence, there is good research-based evidence to support the recommendation of nonnutritive sucking as a nonpharmacologic pain relief intervention in neonates.
- Use single doses of sucrose as a nonpharmacologic pain intervention in neonates. Not enough evidence exists regarding the safety of implementing sucrose interventions in preterm neonates to recommend its widespread use for repeated painful procedures in the NICU. When providing sucrose interventions, ensure that safe administration practice is used to avoid aspiration.
- Discuss openly and honestly with parents the acute and chronic pain associated with medical diseases as well as pain associated with operative, diagnostic, and therapeutic procedures.
- Give parents accurate and unbiased information about the risks, benefits, and alternatives so that they can make informed treatment choices about analgesia and anesthesia.
- Encourage parents to exercise their right to seek another medical opinion or to refuse the burdensome course of therapy altogether.
- Involve parents as much as they are willing and able in providing nonpharmacologic comfort measures for their infant. For example, parents might be used to provide facilitated tucking or to hold their infant's pacifier in place, thus providing an increased opportunity for the infant to engage in nonnutritive sucking during a painful clinical procedure.
- Document the degree of parent satisfaction with the pain management approach that their infant is receiving while in the hospital (U.S. Department of Health and Human Services, 1992).

documented in immature rat pups compared with adult rats (Fitzgerald, Shaw, & MacIntosh, 1988; Fitzgerald, Millard, & MacIntosh, 1989). This finding suggests that in preterm infants, for prolonged periods after a painful stimulus, other, nonnoxious stimuli (handling, physical examination, nursing procedures, etc.) might cause heightened activity in nociceptive pathways, leading to the systemic physiologic responses to stress. Therefore, it seems reasonable to recommend that adequate rest periods be provided following painful clinical procedures. It would also be reasonable to consider doing the least

noxious stimuli first in a caregiving cluster and the most noxious last so that the stress of the caregiving is not unnecessarily heightened for the infant.

Porter, Miller, Cole, et al. (1991) demonstrated that preterm neonates observed prior to and during lumbar punctures showed as much heightened arousal from the time they were positioned to the start of the lumbar puncture, as they did during the lumbar puncture itself. In a subsequent study, Porter, Wolf, and Miller (1998) reported that healthy, preterm, and full-term newborn infants who experienced a series of handling and immobilization manipulations before a routine heel stick exhibited significantly more physiologic responses and behavioral arousal to the heel stick compared with infants who had not been handled.

*Hand swaddling* is a broad term that includes use of hands to encompass or position infants to provide a "nest." These positioning procedures facilitate the infant's self-regulatory development. Containment is thought to reduce pain by providing gentle stimulation across the proprioceptive, thermal, and tactile sensory systems. Two studies have been conducted in the preterm population using different methods of swaddling. A hand swaddling technique known as "facilitated tucking" (holding the infant's extremities flexed and contained close to the trunk), implemented prior to the heel-stick procedure, was shown to reduce pain responses in preterm neonates as young as 25 weeks' gestational age (Corff, Seideman, Venkataraman, et al., 1995). In that study, preterm infants in the post–heel-stick recovery phase demonstrated significantly reduced heart rates and crying, and more stability in sleep-wake cycles in the hand-swaddled position.

A similar containment study conducted by Fearon, Kisilevsky, Hains, et al. (1997) used blanket swaddling for nesting. The researchers examined the effectiveness of blanket swaddling after a heel lance in younger (younger than 31 weeks postconceptual age [PCA]) and older (at or older than 31 weeks' PCA) preterm infants. Trends were noted; swaddling was effective in reducing heart rate and negative facial displays in the post–heel-stick phase for the older infants, and oxygen saturation levels were higher for younger infants in the swaddled condition.

Nonnutritive sucking is the provision of a pacifier into the mouth to promote sucking without the provision of breast milk or formula for nutrition. Franck (1987) found that pacifiers were ranked by NICUs as the first choice of pain intervention. Although NNS has been used for generations, it has only recently been rigorously examined as a nonpharmacologic intervention. NNS is thought to produce analgesia through stimulation of orotactile and mechanoreceptors when a pacifier is introduced into the infant's mouth. NNS is hypothesized to modulate transmission or processing of nociception through mediation by the endogenous nonopioid

system (Blass, Fitzgerald, & Kehoe, 1987; Gunnar, Connors, Isensee, & Wall, 1988).

Nonnutritive sucking has been shown to reduce behavioral pain responses in term infants during immunizations (Blass, 1997) and heel lances in term and preterm infants (Blass & Shide, 1994; Miller & Anderson, 1993). One study found that NNS reduced composite pain responses in preterm infants during heel lances (Stevens, Johnston, Franck, et al., 1999). However, pain relief was greater in infants who received both NNS and sucrose. Compared with blanket swaddling (Campos, 1989) or rocking (Campos, 1994) during painful procedures, NNS reduced duration of cry and soothed infants more rapidly. Unlike blanket swaddling, however, there was a rebound in distress when the NNS pacifier was removed from the infants' mouth. The efficacy of NNS is immediate but appears to terminate almost immediately upon cessation of sucking.

Sucrose with and without NNS has been the most widely studied intervention for infant pain management. Sucrose is a disaccharide consisting of fructose and glucose. A systematic review and meta-analysis of four studies of term infants, plus one study of preterm infants ($n = 271$) on the efficacy of sucrose for relieving pain revealed that sucrose is associated with statistically and clinically significant reductions in crying after a painful stimulus. The pain reduction response is particularly evident when 2 ml of sucrose are administered approximately 2 minutes before the painful stimulus (Stevens, Taddio, Ohlsson, et al., 1997). This 2-minute time interval appears to coincide with endogenous opioid release triggered by the sweet taste of sucrose (Stevens, Johnston, Franck, et al., 1999). In a second systematic review, smaller doses of sucrose (as little as 0.05 ml) are shown effective in decreasing the occurrence of facial expressions of pain when administered in either single or triple oral applications to preterm neonates between 25 and 34 weeks' gestation (Johnston, Stremler, Stevens, & Horton, 1997; Stevens & Ohlsson, 1998).

A critical role for care providers in the NICU is to support family integration into care from admission to discharge. It is important that parents and caregivers work together to help minimize pain and support infants in coping with commonly performed painful clinical procedures. To watch or know your child is in pain is one of the hardest experiences possible. Box 12-4 details specific strategies to assist caregivers to support family participation in providing care to their infant.

## END-OF-LIFE CARE

Palliative and end-of-life (EOL) care are areas in which neonatal care has lagged behind other specialties. Today we recognize the need for symptom management (palliative care) and EOL in even the most immature infant and family. Pain management is a cornerstone of this aspect of care. It requires application of excellent assessment skills and anticipation of pain as related to the dying process. Families should be involved in EOL care, including pain management strategies. (For specific information on this topic, see Chapter 13.)

## DEVELOPMENTALLY SUPPORTIVE CARE: PAIN

How do we implement effective pain management in this vulnerable population? Two examples of evidence-based protocols for either the elimination or reduction of pain are provided. These are the protocols by Hummel and Puchalski (2002) on neonatal pain and sedation assessment and management, and by Geyer, Ellsbury, Kleiber, et al. (2002) provide an evidence-based multidisciplinary protocol for neonatal circumcision pain management. Both use a combination of nonpharmacologic and pharmacologic interventions. (See the protocols in Boxes 12-5, 12-6, 12-7, 12-8, and 12-9.) Walden and Carrier (2003) summarize strategies to prevent and manage irritability. This

---

**Box 12-5  PROTOCOL FOR NEONATAL CIRCUMCISION: EVIDENCE-BASED**

- Administer 10 to 16 mg/kg acetaminophen within 1 hour before the procedure and every 4 to 6 hours for 24 hours after the procedure.
- Administer dorsal penile nerve block with buffered lidocaine (preservative free and without epinephrine, prepared daily by pharmacy) no less than 5 minutes before the circumcision, using a 30-gauge needle.
- Offer a sucrose-dipped pacifier to the newborn before the block and during the circumcision procedure.
- Swaddle the newborn's upper body during the circumcision.
- Pad the circumcision restrain board with blankets.
- Modify the environment, by dimming the lighting and playing soft music via tape recorder during the procedure.

From Geyer, J., Ellsbury, D., Kleiber, C., et al. (2002). An evidence-based multidisciplinary protocol for neonatal circumcision pain management. *Journal of Obstetric, Gynecologic, and Neonatal Nursing (JOGNN), 31*(4), 403-410.

---

is another good example of using developmental care and neurobehavioral support to anticipate, assess, and manage irritability as a manifestation of pain (Table 12-4). They link people, environmental, and infant factors in a fishbone diagram along with drugs, equipment, procedures, treatment, technology, system, process, and communication with irritability (Figure 12-2).

---

**Box 12-6  PROTOCOLS AND GUIDELINES FOR ASSESSMENT AND MANAGEMENT OF PAIN**

**UNIVERSITY OF ILLINOIS MEDICAL CENTER AT CHICAGO CLINICAL CARE GUIDELINE**

**Subject: Neonatal Pain Assessment and Documentation**

**Objective**

To assess neonates and infants for pain, provide for the relief of the pain and discomfort, and document the response to pharmacologic and nonpharmacologic interventions.

**Definition**

For the purpose of this guideline, the following definitions apply.

Pain—Pain is an unpleasant sensory and emotional experience, associated with actual or potential tissue damage, or described in terms of such damage. Pain is always subjective.

International Society for the Study of Pain

## Box 12-6  PROTOCOLS AND GUIDELINES FOR ASSESSMENT AND MANAGEMENT OF PAIN—CONT'D

**Position Statements**

Neonates might exhibit pain responses differently than older children or adults and often require higher doses of analgesics and anesthetics. The sensory nerve tracts appear in the perioral area during the seventh week of gestation, and connections between sensory neurons and spinal cord dorsal horn cells are completed by the second trimester. Neonates have more cutaneous nerve endings than adults and have an increased sensitivity to pain. The cortical perception of pain is complete prior to 24 weeks gestation. Continued stimulation of the pain tract leads to hyperalgesia and leads to the experience of chronic pain. The hormonal and behavioral stress responses to pain might persist during later infancy, resulting in touch aversion, feeding difficulties, impaired parental interaction, and failure to thrive. The sum total effect can lead to permanent affect neuronal and synaptic brain organization.

**Procedure**

1. Each infant admitted to the neonatal intensive care or intermediate care nursery should be assessed for evidence of pain or discomfort minimally each time the vital signs are assessed using the Premature Infant Pain Profile (PIPP)
2. The PIPP should be scored for each infant and recorded on a blank column on the nursing-care section of the NICU/ICN flow sheet. The column should be marked "Pain Assessment" or "PIPP."
3. Using the PIPP, a score of 6 usually indicates no pain and a score of more than 12 reflects moderate to severe pain.
4. The infant's response to both pharmacologic and nonpharmacologic therapy should be noted within 30 minutes of administration or intervention.
5. Infants on continuous analgesic therapy should be assessed for pain with every performance of vital signs and/or with any nursing care.
6. Narrative notes (PIPP) may also be written in the medical record.
7. Physiologic manifestations of pain responses in the neonate are:

| Increased | | Decreased |
|---|---|---|
| Heart rate | Skin blood flow | Oxygen saturation |
| Respiratory rate | Skin color | Arterial oxygen concentration |
| Blood pressure | Mean airway pressure | Skin temperature |
| Intracranial pressure | Palmar sweating | Heart rate variability |

8. Behavioral manifestations of pain responses in a neonate include:

| Vocalization | State Changes | Facial Expression |
|---|---|---|
| Cry pitch, length, number | Wakefulness | Grimacing |
| Whimpering | Fussiness/irritability | Eye squeeze |
| Moaning | Difficult to comfort | Brow bulge |
| Hiccoughs | Feeding difficulties | Quivering chin |
| Gasps | Listlessness/lethargy | Taut tongue |
| Gagging | | Open lips |
| | | Pursed lips |

| Muscle Tone | Body Movements | Skin Color |
|---|---|---|
| Fist/toe clenching | Fisting | |
| | Finger splaying | |
| Hypertonicity | Diffuse squirming | Pallor |
| Knee/leg flexion | Restlessness | Flushing |
| Hypotonicity/flaccidity | Rigidity/extension | |
| | Trunk arching | |
| | Thrashing | |
| | Kicking | |

*Continued*

**Box 12-6**　PROTOCOLS AND GUIDELINES FOR ASSESSMENT AND MANAGEMENT OF PAIN—CONT'D

9. Biochemical responses to pain include:

| **Increased** | | **Decreased** |
|---|---|---|
| Cortisol | Growth hormone | Insulin |
| Epinephrine | Glucagon | |
| Norepinephrine | Aldosterone | |

10. Pharmacologic intervention for pain is morphine or fentanyl, which attenuate the hemodynamic, hormonal, and metabolic responses to pain stress.
    a. Doses are calculated by weight and titrated to clinical response.
    b. Long-term use can result in tolerance, requiring higher doses to achieve similar clinical response.
    c. Physiologic dependency can occur, requiring weaning after long-term use.
    d. Pain associated with surgery should be assessed every 2 to 4 hours with continuous infusions of analgesics for the first 24 hours and additional boluses as needed.
11. Sedation with lorazepam or chloral hydrate does not provide pain relief.
12. Nonpharmacologic interventions attempt to prevent behavioral disorganization by promoting organizing behaviors and include:

| **Environmental Modifications** | **Behavioral Interventions** | **Sensory Stimulation** |
|---|---|---|
| Lower light levels | Nesting | Rocking |
| Turning down monitor alarm | Swaddling | Talking |
| Limit telephone ringing | Flexed positioning | Massage |
| Close incubator doors gently | Boundaries | Soft music |
| Limit storage on top of incubator | Facilitated tucking | Nonnutritive sucking |
| Cover incubator | Minimal-handling protocol | Clustering of care |
| | | Rounds away from bedside |

13. All procedures should be explained to parents including a discussion of the plan for the relief of pain.
14. Inform parents of the current medications used for the relief of pain.
15. Guide parents in how they can touch and interact with their infant.
16. Teach parents to understand their infant's manifestations of stress/discomfort or pain.

International Association for the Study of Pain. (1998). IASP pain terminology. International Association for the Study of Pain. Available online at *halcyon.co/iasp/termsp.html*. From University of Illinois Medical Center at Chicago Women's and Children's Nursing Services. Used with permission by Dharmapuri Vidyasagar, MD, Catherine Theorell, RNC, MSN, NNP, and Beena Peters, RN, MS.

*NICU/ICN*, Neonatal intensive care nursery/intensive care nursery.

**Box 12-7**　NICU PAIN AND SEDATION ASSESSMENT AND NURSING MANAGEMENT GUIDELINES

**Purpose**

To outline pain and sedation assessment and nursing management of the infant who is in pain or being sedated.

**Background Information**

Addressing pain is an ethical duty for healthcare professionals, and a primary focus of nursing care. Neonates, both term and preterm, perceive and respond to pain. Untreated pain, whether intermittent or continual, can result in adverse sequelae. Assessment of neonatal pain is difficult, owing to the neonate's limited verbal and neurologic repertoire. It is difficult to distinguish pain from agitation, distress, or even hunger. Pain should be presumed in neonates in all situations that are usually painful for adults and children. Pain treatment should be instituted in all cases in which pain is a possibility. Side effects of this treatment should be monitored for and treated as needed. It is also important to assess infants for sedation. Sedation might be the goal for an infant, or babies might become sedated in response to the administration of analgesics. The desired level of sedation will vary, depending on the clinical goal or situation.

**Procedure**

**Pain Assessment**

1. Identify actual or potential sources of pain for the neonate: surgical procedures, invasive/indwelling tubes, heel sticks, suctioning, peritonitis, fractures, renal stones, noxious environment.
2. Pain assessment is the fifth vital sign. Assessment for pain should be included with every vital-sign measurement.
3. More frequent pain assessments should be performed in the following situations:
   a. Invasive tubes or lines other than IVs or feeding tubes: every 2-4 hours.
   b. Receiving analgesics and/or sedatives: every 2-4 hours.
   c. One hour after an analgesic is given for pain behaviors: to assess response to medication.
   d. Postoperative: every 2 hours for 24 to 48 hours, then every 4 hours until off medications.
4. The N-PASS (Neonatal Pain, Agitation, and Sedation Scale) will be used to assess pain and sedation—see attached N-PASS scale (see Figure 12-1)
5. Points are added to the premature infant's pain score, based on gestational age to compensate for their limited ability to behaviorally or physiologically communicate pain.
6. Treatment/interventions should usually be initiated for scores of more than 3. Some older infants might have a higher baseline score; interventions should then be instituted for consistent elevation in scores. Infants being weaned from opioids might also have a higher baseline score. A SCORE SHOULD ALWAYS BE EVALUATED WITHIN THE CONTEXT OF THE CLINICAL SITUTATION.
7. This treatment or intervention can be pharmacologic and/or nonpharmacologic, depending on the clinical situation.
8. The goal of pain treatment/intervention should be a score of 3 or less, or a decrease in the pain score.
9. Pain and sedation scores are recorded separately.

**Sedation Assessment**

1. Sedation is scored to assess the infant's response to stimuli.
2. Sedation does not need to be assessed with every pain score.
3. Sedation assessment should occur with "hands-on" vitals and more frequently as needed. Sedation assessment requires an assessment of response to stimuli; the baby should not be stimulated unnecessarily to accomplish this.
4. The N-PASS is useful when sedation of the infant is the goal, as well as when assessing for oversedation related to sedative/opioid administration.
   a. Levels of sedation are noted as negative scores
   b. Desired levels of sedation vary according to the situation
   c. Deep sedation: goal is -10 to -5
   d. Light sedation: goal is -5 to -2
5. Deep sedation is not recommended unless an infant is receiving ventilator support, related to the high potential for apnea and hypoventilation.
6. A negative score without the administration of opioids/sedatives:
   a. Indicates neurologic depression, sepsis, or other pathology.
   b. A premature infant who has experienced prolonged untreated pain and/or stress may also appear sedated, as these infants have been observed to become lethargic and "shut down" in response to their unrelenting pain.
7. Pavulon/paralysis:
   a. It is impossible to clinically or behaviorally evaluate a paralyzed infant for pain.
   b. Analgesics should be administered continuously by drip or around-the-clock dosing

*Continued*

Box 12-7   NICU Pain and Sedation Assessment and Nursing
            Management Guidelines—cont'd

c. Higher, more frequent dosing might be required if the infant has had surgery, has a chest tube, or has other pathology (such as NEC) that would normally cause pain.

d. Increases in heart rate and blood pressure might be the only indicator of a need for more analgesia.

e. Opioid doses should be increased by 10% every 3 to 5 days as tolerance occurs without symptoms of inadequate pain relief.

**Pain Management**

1. If the N-PASS score is more than 3, or more than the baby's usual baseline score, pain management interventions should be instituted. Pain management interventions can be instituted with lower scores, as clinically appropriate.

2. Implement nonpharmacologic comfort measures first if the infant has no identifiable cause for pain.

   a. Developmental positioning (knees flexed, arms close to body, hands to mouth), swaddling, nesting, pacifier, reducing environmental stressors (light, noise, handling). Older babies might respond to rocking, holding.

   b. Optimize ventilation: babies become agitated when they are not being adequately ventilated. This should be corrected by optimizing ventilation (suctioning, adjusting ventilator settings).

   c. These measures should always be instituted along with analgesics if the infant has an identifiable pain source: i.e., postoperative, chest tube, etc.

3. Administer analgesics or sedatives to provide relief of pain in the least painful route possible.

   a. Sedatives do not provide pain relief, but enhance the effects of opioids. Therefore, sedatives should rarely be given alone because it is usually not possible to distinguish between pain and agitation in the neonate.

   b. Sedatives are not recommended for use in preterm infants. Seizure-like myoclonic movements have been observed in preterm infants receiving sedatives. Adverse neurologic outcomes have been associated with sedative use in preterm infants.

4. Treat anticipated procedure-related pain prophylactically.

   a. Invasive procedures such as chest tubes and abdominal drains, should include premedication.

   b. Brief, less invasive procedures, such as IV starts and heel sticks, usually do not require premedication.

   c. Sucrose water attenuates the pain response and should be considered as an adjunctive measure before and during any procedure.

   d. All babies will tolerate procedures better if swaddled, or contained by parents or other staff members.

   e. Efforts should be made to calm the baby before and after the procedure.

5. Provide continuous cardiorespiratory monitoring and continual pulse oximetry when using opioids or sedatives for pain relief or to achieve sedation.

6. Correct detrimental side effects of the medications.

7. Evaluate effectiveness of pain medication 30 minutes to 1 hour after administration.

8. If pain score is not falling as expected, additional medications and nonpharmacologic measures should be instituted, and the baby should be reevaluated for additional causes of pain and agitation.

**Parent/Caregiver Education**

1. A letter outlining the unit's efforts in pain assessment and management is included in the admission booklet (Box 12-9).

2. Parents should be taught infant pain behaviors and be included in the assessment and treatment of the infant's pain.

**Documentation**

1. N-PASS score will be documented on the appropriate column on the NICU flow sheet.

2. This column is slashed: the top area will be used for pain assessments, and the bottom area will be used to document the sedation score.

Box **12-7**   NICU Pain and Sedation Assessment and Nursing
                    Management Guidelines—cont'd

3. If management is changed in response to a score: (i.e., pain medication, comfort measures, increase or decrease in medication), a response to this intervention is documented in the same column in the next hourly space. This indicates response to the intervention 30 to 60 minutes after the intervention.

**Pain Assessment with Painful Procedures**
1. Short-lived painful procedures, such as heel sticks, venipuncture, and arterial punctures, do not necessitate pain assessment scores before, during, and after the procedure.
2. Bedside surgical procedures, such as chest tube, abdominal drain insertion, and circumcision, should have pain assessment scores before and during the procedure. Postprocedure scoring: continue to assess pain with each vital sign assessment, as infants will need more frequent vital signs following these procedures.
3. Assessments will be documented on the NICU flow sheet.

Developed by Patricia Hummel, MA, RNC, NNP, PNP, & Mary Pulchaski, MS, RNC. Used with permission from Loyola Medical Center, Maywood, Illinois.

*NICU*, Neonatal intensive care unit.

Box **12-8**   Opioid Weaning Guidelines: Neonatal Intensive Care Unit

**Purpose**
To provide guidelines for weaning opioids following intrauterine exposure or NICU dependence.

**Background Information**
At least 50% of infants exposed to heroin and/or methadone intrauterine exhibit signs of neonatal abstinence syndrome (NAS). In addition, infants in the NICU who received opioids around the clock or as a continual drip for more than 1 week or so will develop tolerance, become dependent, and exhibit signs of NAS when the medication is abruptly discontinued. Gradual weaning of the opioid is outlined to minimize withdrawal symptoms.

**Procedure**
**Weaning Fentanyl Drip**
1. Fentanyl is associated with a higher and more rapid rate of withdrawal compared with morphine. Use of fentanyl for more than 5 days has been associated with a more than 50% chance for opiate withdrawal, and a 100% chance in infants receiving it for more than 9 days.
2. Weaning of the opiod drip should start when the infant is stable and the pain source is eliminated. Few or no analgesic effects are present during weaning.
3. The Finnegan scoring system should be initiated when weaning begins to assess withdrawal and therefore determine the patient's ability or inability to tolerate weaning. The scoring should be done every 3 or 4 hours, depending on how often the baby is "hands-on."
4. Weaning guidelines:

| Duration of Drip | Guidelines |
| --- | --- |
| Less than 3 days | Stop infusion without weaning or decrease by 50% for 12 to 24 hours and then discontinue |
| 3 to 7 days | Decrease drip 25% every 12 to 24 hours |
| 8 to 14 days | Decrease drip 10% every 12 to 24 hours |
| More than 14 days | Decrease drip 10% daily, every other day, or less |

*Continued*

Box **12-8**   OPIOID WEANING GUIDELINES: NEONATAL INTENSIVE CARE UNIT—CONT'D

5.  Weaning should be guided by Finnegan scores:
    a.  In general, Finnegan scores of more than 8 are considered indicative of withdrawal; however, less than 8 to 11 is generally acceptable for attempting weaning, if the patient is otherwise stable.
    b.  If the average of scores over 24 hours is 8 or less, the infusion can be weaned.
    c.  If the patient's infusion has been weaned, and subsequent Finnegan scores are more than 11 for 3 consecutive scoring periods, increase the infusion back to the previous rate.
    d.  The goal is not to have a Finnegan score of 0. Babies have to be gently pushed off the opioid.
6.  Conversion from opioid drips to morphine boluses:

| When to Discontinue Infusion | Conversion Dose of Intermittent Morphine |
|---|---|
| Fentanyl drip 0.5 $\mu$g/kg/hour | Morphine 0.1 mg/kg IV every 4 hours* around the clock |
| Morphine drip 0.02 mg/kg/hour | Morphine 0.1 mg/kg IV every 4 hours* around the clock |

*Scheduling of is morphine 0.075 mg/kg every 3 hours is acceptable if this is compatible with the baby's feeding or "hands-on" schedule.

7.  If fentanyl drip is being discontinued, give the first morphine bolus 30 minutes before stopping infusion. If morphine drip, give the first morphine bolus does at the time the drip is stopped.
8.  Morphine dose should not be weaned for 24 hours after discontinuance of opioid infusion.
9.  If after 24 hours the Finnegan scores are lower than 8 and the patient is stable, the morphine should be weaned every day or every other day.
10. Weaning morphine boluses:

**Step 1:**

Wean **dose** by 50% as tolerated, based on Finnegan scores. Continue same interval (every 3 or 4 hours)

IV: Morphine 0.1 mg/kg 0.05 $\rightarrow$ mg/kg $\rightarrow$ 0.025 mg/kg
PO: Morphine 0.3 mg/kg $\rightarrow$ 0.15 mg/kg $\rightarrow$ 0.075 mg/kg

**Step 2:**

Wean dosing **interval** when morphine has been weaned to:
IV: 0.025 mg/kg/dose; or
PO: 0.05 to 0.075 mg/kg/dose

IV: 0.025 mg/kg/dose every 3 or 4 hours $\rightarrow$ every 6 hours $\rightarrow$ every 8 hours $\rightarrow$ every 12 hours
PO: 0.075 mg/kg/dose every 4 or 4 hours $\rightarrow$ every 6 hours $\rightarrow$ every 8 hours $\rightarrow$ every 12 hours
Weaning is determined by Finnegan scores

**Step 3:**

Once weaned to morphine:
0.025 mg/kg IV every 8 or 12 hours; or 0.05 to 0.075 mg/kg PO every 8 or 12 hours **and** if Finnegan scores are stable

Discontinue morphine.
Continue Finnegan scoring for 48 hours after morphine is discontinued for any rebound withdrawal symptoms.

11. Keep in mind that this process may take a few days or several weeks. In general, the longer the baby has been on the medication, the longer it will take to get him or her off.

### Changing Morphine Boluses from IV to PO

1.  The baby should be changed from IV or oral morphine as soon as is feasible, depending on the baby's condition and feeding status. ORAL MORPHINE DOSES ARE THREE TO FIVE TIMES THAT OF IV DOSES. At Loyola, we use three times the IV dose (i.e., morphine 0.1 mg/kg IV = 0.3 mg/kg PO).
2.  Oral morphine is obtained from the pharmacy diluted to a 1 mg/ml concentration.

### Opioid Overdose

1.  It is difficult to overdose a baby that is so tolerant that they are showing abstinence signs, but it can happen. Remember that the goal is not to have Finnegan scores of 0. Let the baby have

## Box **12-8** Opioid Weaning Guidelines: Neonatal Intensive Care Unit—cont'd

tolerable withdrawal; generally Finnegan scores of less that 8 are acceptable. Gently push these infants off the medication.

2. Avoid naloxone use if the tolerant/dependent baby is experiencing severe side effects from the opioid. This can cause severe withdrawal and possibly seizures. Supportive treatment is indicated until the medication is excreted.

3. Apnea should be rare. You will first see that the baby is sleepy and lethargic, with very low Finnegan scores. This would indicate that a dose or more should be held and the dose decreased.

4. If necessary, Naloxone 0.01 mg/kg in repeated doses can be administered.

5. Seizures known to be due to opioid withdrawal should be treated with morphine or fentanyl. Phenobarbitol can be added for seizures.

**Discharge of Patient**

1. The baby should be weaned off morphine before discharge, if possible.

2. If this is not possible, the baby can be discharged on oral morphine with a weaning plan.
   a. Oral morphine needs to be diluted, however, so this should be obtained only from Loyola's Mulcahy outpatient pharmacy.
   b. Discharge on paregoric is not desirable, because it contains a large amount of preservatives and alcohol. However, paregoric is already diluted to a usable concentration. The paregoric dose (in ml) is equal to what the baby is receiving of the morphine 1 mg/ml dilution. (Example: If the baby is receiving 0.6 ml of $MSO_4$ 1 mg/ml, the paregoric dose would be 0.6 ml.)
   c. Parents/caretakers should be educated about withdrawal signs and the weaning plan.
   d. The baby should be followed by a home care nurse and be scheduled in the neonatal follow-up clinic approximately 1 month after discharge.

Developed by Patricia Hummel, MA, RNC, NNP, PNP, & Mary Pulchaski, MS, RNC. Used with permission from Loyola Medical Center, Maywood, Illinois.

## Box **12-9** Parent Letter Regarding Pain Management and Assessment

To the parents of our NICU infants,

About pain . . .

We realize that your infant will have some painful experiences while in our unit. We are continually trying to make everything less painful. This is very important to us, and, we are sure, important to you. Please let the nurses or doctors know if you think that your baby's pain is not being treated.

It can be difficult to tell if a baby is having pain. Sometimes babies, especially premature infants, cannot let us know when they are having pain and how bad it is. Signs that your baby might be in pain are: crying, lack of deep sleep, a worried face with a grimace or frown, tightly fisted hands and feet, a rigid or tense body, and higher than normal heart rate and blood pressure. The oxygen levels might fall rapidly when the baby is touched or handled. Of course, a hungry baby will cry, tense up, and have a high heart rate, but this stops when he/she is fed or given a pacifier. We are using a method of assessing your infant's pain called the N-PASS (Neonatal Pain, Agitation, and Sedation Scale). You can discuss this with your nurse if you want more information.

Some of the things that cause pain are procedures such as a heel stick, IV, or chest tube placement. Surgeries, of course, cause pain. Also, being on a ventilator seems to be uncomfortable for some infants, but not all babies need medications for this.

In addition to medications, there are many other things that can be done by you or the nurses to relieve your baby's pain. Keeping the area as dark and quiet as possible will be helpful. Some babies like to be rocked, talked to, massaged, or given a pacifier. Some babies like to be wrapped snugly.

*Continued*

Box **12-9**    Parent Letter Regarding Pain Management and Assessment—cont'd

Some babies like to be left alone—they cannot handle any stimulation at that time. Your baby's nurse will help you decide what works best for your infant.

Some babies who have been on pain medications for a long time (more than 5 to 7 days) need to be weaned slowly from them. Taking them away too quickly can be bad for your baby. This does not mean that your baby is addicted to the medicine—his or her body has just gotten used to them.

Please be assured that we are doing all we can to keep your infant from being in pain. Your presence at the bedside can be very comforting to your infant. We look forward to working with you.

The NICU staff

Developed by Patricia Hummel, MA, RNC, NNP, PNP, & Mary Pulchaski, MS, RNC. Used with permission from Loyola Medical Center, Maywood, Illinois.

*NICU*, Neonatal intensive care unit.

Table **12-4**    Strategies to Prevent and Manage Irritability

| Category | Strategies |
| --- | --- |
| Assessment | See Figure 12-2, the fishbone diagram. |
| Philosophy of care | Provide relationship-based neurobehavioral support. |
| | Implement individualized family-centered and developmentally supportive care. |
| | Provide predictable routines and people who are familiar, by reducing number of caregivers or establishing limited number using primary team. |
| | Establish familiarity with infant and parents. |
| Environmental | Reduce noxious stimuli. |
| | Decrease light and/or encourage development of day/night rhythms. |
| | Minimize personnel and equipment noise. |
| | Determine tolerable caregiving events based on infant's thresholds and sensitivity. |
| | Implement handling and positioning techniques appropriate to infant's age, condition, and tolerance. |
| | Limit painful procedures or therapies to those that are essential. |
| Behavioral | Consistently respect infant's cues; allow infant opportunities to set pace of interactions. |
| | Provide opportunities for infant to interact with people before objects or toys. |
| | Avoid abrupt disruption of activity or sleep, by letting infant know that an interaction is about to take place by voice and then touch. |
| | Utilize flexible care times based on behavioral state. |
| | Develop predictable routines that include time for sleep/rest and interaction as indicated. |
| | Implement individualized therapeutic touch and positioning. |
| | Provide sensory stimulation in addition to and not associated with routine care such as therapeutic touch (e.g., gentle containment, skin-to-skin [kangaroo] holding, conventional cuddling, massage), gentle side-to-side movement or rocking, face-to-face interaction with or without talking, music as tolerated, age-appropriate visual stimuli, and nonnutritive sucking. |
| | Normalize routine care and sensory experiences to foster enjoyment (e.g., tube feeding with accompanying sensations of being held and sucking a pacifier). |
| | Provide planned multisensory opportunities, pacing the interaction to allow the infant to be an active participant. |
| | Offer age-appropriate activities that include both familiarity and variety and change based on infant readiness. |

**Table 12-4** STRATEGIES TO PREVENT AND MANAGE IRRITABILITY—CONT'D

| Category | Strategies |
|---|---|
| Procedural techniques | Use a variety of positions, seating, and locations (e.g., floor mat) to promote exploration and motor development appropriate for age and condition. |
| | Respond promptly, appropriately, and consistently to crying and cues. |
| | Follow recommendations and plans consistently and evaluate and update frequently or as indicated. |
| | Use experienced practitioners. |
| | Use equipment that is reliable and least painful. |
| | Support infant during and after procedures. |
| | Comfort infant after handling and procedures. |
| Consultation | Refer infants as indicated to appropriate experts, such as physical, occupational, or child-life specialist; developmental specialist; and child psychologist. |

From Walden, M., & Carrier, C.T. (2003). Sleeping beauties: The impact of sedation on neonatal development. *Journal of Obstetric, Gynecologic, & Neonatal Nursing (JOGNN), 32*(3), 396. Based on data from Franck, L.S., & Lawhon, G. (1998). Environmental and behavioral strategies to prevent and manage neonatal pain. *Seminars in Perinatology, 22*(5), 434-443 and Goldberger, J. (1990). Lengthy or repeated hospitalization in infancy. *Clinics in Perinatology, 17*(1), 197-206.

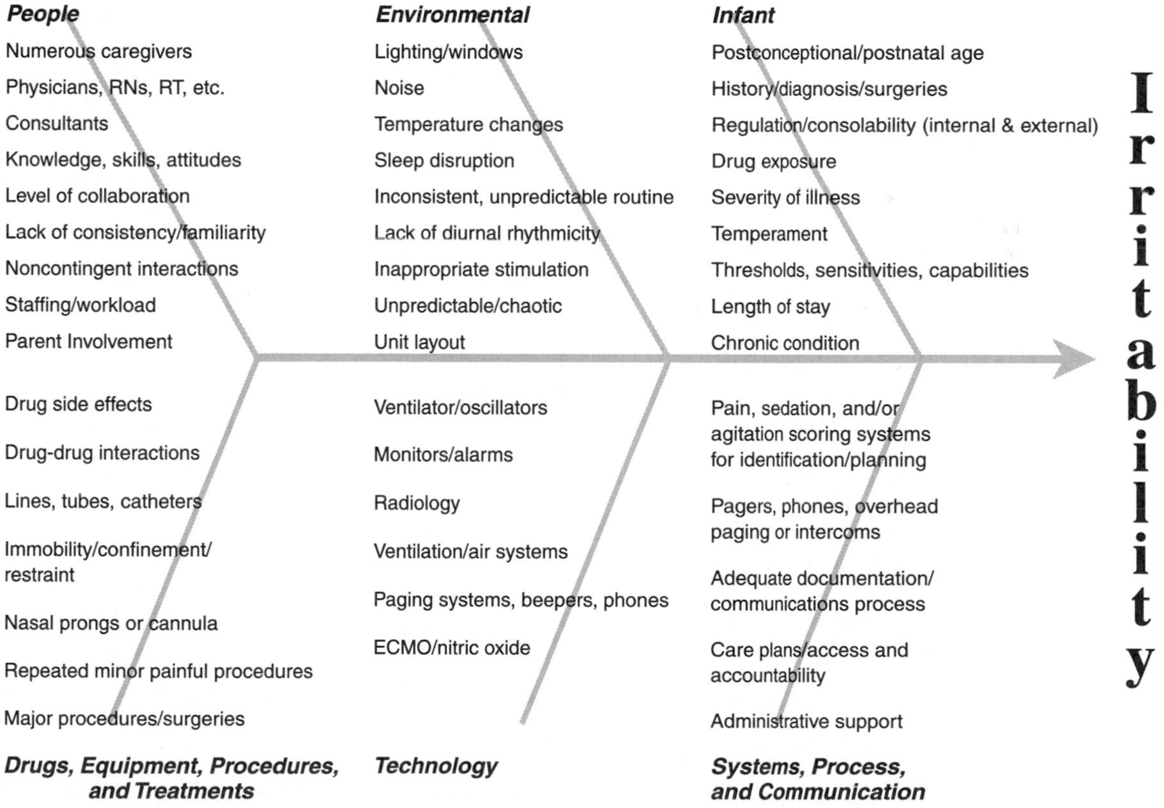

Figure **12-2** Fishbone diagram of factors influencing irritability. (*From Walden, M., & Carrier, C.T. [2003]. Sleeping beauties: The impact of sedation on neonatal development.* Journal of Obstetric, Gynecologic, & Neonatal Nursing [JOGNN], *32[3], 394.*)

## CONCLUSION

Nurses play an important role in facilitating optimal pain assessment and management care practices in the NICU. Nurses are in an optimal position to observe infant responses to painful procedures or clinical conditions using valid and reliable pain instruments. Nurses can use these assessment data to effectively implement nonpharmacologic approaches to caregiving and to advocate more effectively for the use of analgesia when deemed clinically necessary. Neurobehavioral support is essential to pain assessment and management.

## *REFERENCES*

Agency for Health Care Policy and Research (currently known as Agency for Healthcare Research and Quality). (1992). *Position statement* (No. 92-0020). Rockville, MD: Public Health Service, U.S. Department of Health and Human Services. Available online at *www.nann.org/files/public/3019.doc.*

American Academy of Pediatrics/Canadian Paediatric Society. (2000). Prevention and management of pain and stress in the neonate. *Pediatrics, 105,* 454-461.

American Society of Anesthesiologists Pain Management Task Force. (1995). Practice guidelines for acute pain management in the perioperative setting: A report by the American Society of Anesthesiologists Task Force on Pain Management, Acute Pain Section. *Anesthesiology, 82*(4), 1071-1081.

Anand, K., Barton, B.A., McIntosh, N., et al. (1999). Analgesia and sedation in preterm neonates who require ventilatory support: Results from the NOPAIN trial. *Archives of Pediatrics & Adolescent Medicine, 153*(4), 331-338.

Anand, K., & Craig, K. (1996). New perspectives on the definition of pain, *Pain, 67*(1), 3-6.

Anand, K., & Hickey, P. (1992). Halothane-morphine compared with high-dose sufentanil for anesthesia and postoperative analgesia in neonatal cardiac surgery. *New England Journal of Medicine, 326*(1), 1-9.

Anand, K. & the International Evidence-Based Group for Neonatal Pain. (2001). Consensus statement for the prevention and management of pain in the newborn. *Archives of Pediatric Adolescent Medicine, 155*(2), 173-180.

Anand, K., Phil, D., & Hickey, P. (1987). Pain and its effects in the human neonate and fetus. *New England Journal of Medicine, 317*(21), 1321-1329.

Anand, K., Selanikio, J., & SOPAIN Study Group. (1996). Routine analgesic practices in 109 neonatal intensive care units (NICUs). *Pediatric Research, 39,* 192A.

Andrews, K., & Fitzgerald, M. (1994). The cutaneous withdrawal reflex in human neonates: Sensitization, receptive fields, and the effects of contralateral stimulation. *Pain, 56*(1), 95-101.

Association of Women's Health, Obstetric, and Neonatal Nurses (AWHONN). (1995). *Clinical commentary: Pain in neonates.* New Brunswick, NJ: Johnson and Johnson Consumer Products.

Barker, D., & Rutter, N. (1995). Exposure to invasive procedures in newborn intensive care unit admissions. *Archives of Disease in Childhood, 72*(1), F47-F48.

Bauchner, H., May, A., & Coates, E. (1992). Use of analgesic agents for invasive medical procedures in pediatric and neonatal intensive care units. *Journal of Pediatrics, 121*(4), 647-649.

Beaver, P. (1987). Premature infants' response to touch and pain: Can nurses make a difference? *Neonatal Network, 6*(3), 13-17.

Blass, E. (1997). Milk-induced hypoalgesia in human newborns. *Pediatrics, 99*(6), 825-829.

Blass, E., Fitzgerald, E., & Kehoe, P. (1987). Interactions between sucrose, pain, and isolation distress. *Pharmacology, Biochemistry & Behavior, 26*(3), 483-489.

Blass, E., & Shide, D. (1994). Some comparisons among the calming and pain relieving effects of sucrose, glucose, fructose and lactose in infant rats. *Chemical Senses, 19*(3), 239-249.

Burns, E. (1989). The effects of stress during the brain growth spurt. In J. Fitzpatrick & H. Werley (Eds.). *Research in nursing practice* (pp. 57-82). Philadelphia: W.B. Saunders.

Campos, R. (1989). Soothing-pain-elicited distress in infants with swaddling and pacifiers. *Child Development, 60*(4), 781-792.

Campos, R.G. (1994). Rocking and pacifiers: Two comforting interventions for heelstick pain. *Research in Nursing & Health, 17*(5), 321-331.

Corff, K., Seideman, R., Venkataraman, P., et al. (1995). Facilitated tucking: A nonpharmacologic comfort measure for pain in preterm neonates. *Journal of Obstetric, Gynecologic, and Neonatal Nursing (JOGNN), 24*(2), 143-147.

Craig, K., Whitfield, M., Grunau, R., et al. (1993). Pain in the preterm neonate: Behavioral and physiological indices. *Pain, 52*(3), 287-299.

Deshpande, J., & Anand, K.J.S. (1996). Basic aspects of acute pediatric pain and sedation. In J. Deshpande and J. Tobias (Eds.), *The pediatric pain handbook* (pp. 1-48). St. Louis: Mosby.

Evans, J.C. (2001). Physiology of acute pain in preterm infants. *Newborn and Infant Nursing Reviews, 1*(2), 75-84.

Fearon, I., Kisilevsky, B.S., Hains S.M., et al. (1997). Swaddling after heel lance: age-specific effects on behavioral recovery in preterm infants. *Journal of Developmental and Behavioral Pediatrics, 18*(4), 222-232.

Fitzgerald, M., Millard, C., & McIntosh, N. (1989). Cutaneous hypersensitivity following peripheral tissue damage in newborn infants and its reversal with topical anaesthesia. *Pain, 39*(1), 31-36.

Fitzgerald, M., Shaw, A., & MacIntosh, N. (1988). Postnatal development of the cutaneous flexor reflex: A comparative study in premature infants and newborn rat pups. *Developmental Medicine and Child Neurology, 30*(4), 520-526.

Fitzgerald, M., & Shortland, P. (1988). The effect of neonatal peripheral nerve section on the somadendritic growth of sensory projection cells in the rat spinal cord. *Developmental Brain Research, 470*(1), 129-136.

Franck, L. (1987). A national survey of the assessment and treatment of pain and agitation in the neonatal intensive care unit. *Journal of Obstetric, Gynecologic, and Neonatal Nursing (JOGNN), 16*(6), 387-393.

Franck, L., & Lawhon, G. (1998). Environmental and behavioral strategies to prevent and manage neonatal pain. *Seminars in Perinatology, 22*(5), 434-443.

Franck, L., & Miaskowski, C. (1998). The use of intravenous opioids to provide analgesia in critically ill, premature neonates: A research critique. *Journal of Pain and Symptom Management, 15*(1), 41-69.

Geyer, J., Ellsbury, D., Kleiber, C., Litwiller, D., Hinton, A., & Yankowitz, J. (2002). An evidence-based multidisciplinary protocol for neonatal circumcision pain management. *Journal of Obstetric, Gynecologic, and Neonatal Nursing (JOGNN), 32*(1), 10.

Gorski, P. (1983). Premature infants' behavioral and physiological responses to care-giving interventions in the intensive care nursery. In J. Call, E. Gallenson, & R. Tyson (Eds.), *Frontiers of infant psychiatry* (pp. 256-263). New York: Basic Books.

Grunau, R., & Craig, K. (1987). Pain expression in neonates: Facial action and cry. *Pain, 28*(3), 395-410.

Grunau, R., et al. (1991). Pain sensitivity in toddlers of birthweight < 1000 grams compared with heavier preterm and full birth weight toddlers. *Pediatric Research, 29*, 256A.

Grunau, R., Whitfield, M., & Petrie, J. (1994). Pain sensitivity and temperament in extremely low-birthweight premature toddlers and preterm and full-term controls. *Pain, 58*(3), 341-346.

Grunau, R., Whitfield, M., Petrie, J., et al. (1994). Early pain experience, child and family factors, as precursors of somatization: A prospective study of extremely premature and fullterm children. *Pain, 56*(3), 353-359.

Gunnar, M., Connors, J., Isensee, J., & Wall, L. (1988). Adrenocortical activity and behavioral distress in human newborns. *Developmental Psychobiology, 21*(4), 297-310.

Harpin, V., & Rutter, N. (1995). Pain-reducing properties of sucrose in human newborns. *Childhood, 58*, 226-228.

Hartley, S., Franck., L., & Lundergan, R. (1989). Maintenance sedation of agitated infants in the NICU with chloral hydrate: New concerns. *Journal of Perinatology, 2*(2), 162-164.

Hummel, P., & Puchalski, M. (2002, June 23-25). *Establishing initial reliability & validity of the N-PASS: Neonatal Pain, Agitation, and Sedation Scale.* Poster presentation at Association for Women's Health, Obstetric, and Neonatal Nursing (AWHONN) 2002 National Convention, Boston, MA.

International Association for the Study of Pain. (IASP). (2000). Outline curriculum on pain for schools of nursing. Available online at *www.halcyon.com/iasp/nursing_toc.html.*

International Association for the Study of Pain Subcommittee on Taxonomy. (1979). Pain terms: A list with definitions and notes on usage. *Pain, 6*(3), 249-252.

Johnston, C., & Stevens, B. (1996). Experience in a neonatal intensive care unit affects pain response. *Pediatrics, 98*(5), 925-930.

Johnston, C., Stevens, B., Craig, K.D., & Grunau, R.V. (1993). Developmental changes in pain expression in premature, full-term, two- and four-month-old infants. *Pain, 52*(2), 201-208.

Johnston, C., Stevens, B., Franck, L., et al. (1999). Factors explaining lack of response to heel stick in preterm newborns. *Journal of Obstetric, Gynecologic, and Neonatal Nursing (JOGNN), 28*(6), 587-594.

Johnston, C., Stevens, B., Yang, F., & Horton, L. (1995). Differential response to pain by very premature neonates. *Pain, 61*(3), 471-479.

Johnston, C., Stevens, B., Yang, F., et al. (1996). Developmental changes in response to heelstick by premature infants: A prospective cohort study. *Developmental Medicine and Child Neurology, 38*(5), 438-445.

Johnston, C., Stremler, R., Horton, L., & Friedman, A. (1999). Effect of repeated doses of sucrose during heel stick procedure in preterm neonates. *Biology of the Neonate, 75*(3), 160-166.

Johnston, C., Stremler, R., Stevens, B., & Horton, L. (1997). Effectiveness of oral sucrose and simulated rocking on pain response in preterm neonates. *Pain, 72*(1-2), 193-199.

Joint Commission on Accreditation of Healthcare Organizations. (1999). Pain management standards for 2001. Available online at *www.jcaho.org.*

Krechel, S., & Bildner, J. (1995). CRIES: A new neonatal post-operative pain measurement score: Initial testing of validity and reliability. *Paediatric Anaesthesia, 5*(1), 53-61.

Larsson, B., Tannefeldt, G., Lagercrantz, H., & Olsson, G.L. (1998). Venipuncture is more effective and less painful than heel lancing for blood tests in neonates. *Pediatrics, 101*(5), 882-886.

Lawrence, J., Alcock, D., McGrath, P., et al. (1993). The development of a tool to assess neonatal pain. *Neonatal Network, 12*(6), 59-66.

Long, J., Lucey, J., & Philips, A. (1980). Noise and hypoxemia in the intensive care nursery. *Pediatrics, 65*(1), 143-145.

Mackenna, B.R. & Callander, R. (1990). Central nervous system locomotor system. In *Illustrated physiology* (5th ed.; pp. 220-284). Edinburgh, Scotland: Churchill Livingstone.

McIntosh, N., Van Veen, L., & Brameyer, H. (1994). Alleviation of the pain of heel prick in preterm infants. *Archives of Disease in Childhood, 70*, F177-F181.

Melzack, R., & Wall, P. (1965). Pain mechanisms: A new theory. *Science, 150*(699), 971-978.

Miller, H., & Anderson, G. (1993). Nonnutritive sucking: Effects on crying and heart rate in intubated infants requiring assisted mechanical ventilation. *Nursing Research, 42*(5), 305-307.

National Association of Neonatal Nurses (NANN) (Authored by Walden, M.). (1999). *Position paper on pain in neonates.* Glenview, IL: National Association of Neonatal Nurses.

National Association of Neonatal Nurses (NANN). (Authored by Walden, M.). (2001). *Pain assessment and management: Guideline for practice.* Glenview, IL: National Association of Neonatal Nurses.

Owens, M., & Todt, E. (1984). Pain in infancy: Neonatal reaction to a heel lance. *Pain, 20*(1), 77-86.

Porter, F., Miller, J., Cole, F., et al. (1991). A controlled clinical trial of local anesthesia for lumbar puncture in newborns. *Pediatrics, 88*(4), 663-669.

Porter, F., Wolf, C., & Miller, J. (1998). The effect of handling and immobilization on the response to acute pain in newborn infants. *Pediatrics, 102*(6), 1383-1389.

Porter, F., Wolf, C., & Miller, P. (1999). Procedural pain in newborn infants: The influence of intensity and development. *Pediatrics, 104*(1), e13-e16.

Ramenghi, L., Griffith, G., Wood, C., et al. (1996). Effect of non-sucrose sweet-tasting solution on neonatal heel prick responses. *Archives of Disease in Children, 74,* F129-F131.

Shah, V., & Ohlsson, A. (1999). Venipuncture versus heel lance for blood sampling in term neonates. *Neonatal Modules of the Cochrane Database of Systematic Reviews, 2,* 1-9.

Shah, V., Taddio, A., Bennett, S., & Speidel, B.D. (1997). Neonatal pain response to heel stick vs. venipuncture for routine blood sampling. *Archives of Disease in Childhood, 77*(2), 143-144.

Shapiro, C.R. (1993). Nurses' judgments of pain in term and preterm newborns. *Journal of Obstetric, Gynecologic, and Neonatal Nursing (JOGNN), 22*(1), 41-47.

Shiroiwa, Y., Kamiya, Y., & Uchibori, S. (1986). Activity, cardiac and respiratory responses of blindfold preterm infants in a neonatal intensive care unit. *Early Human Development, 14*(3-4), 259-265.

Skogsdal, Y., Eriksson, M., & Schollin, J. (1997). Analgesia in newborns given oral glucose. *Acta Paediatrica Scandinavia, 86*(2), 217-220.

Stevens, B., & Johnston, C. (1994). Physiological responses of premature infants to a painful stimulus. *Nursing Research, 43*(4), 226-231.

Stevens, B., Johnston, C., Franck, L., et. al. (1999). The efficacy of developmentally sensitive interventions and sucrose for relieving procedural pain in very low birth weight neonates. *Nursing Research, 48*(1), 35-43.

Stevens, B., Johnston, C., & Horton, L. (1993). Multidimensional pain assessment in premature neonates: A pilot study. *Journal of Obstetric, Gynecologic, and Neonatal Nursing (JOGNN), 22*(6), 531-541.

Stevens, B., Johnston, C., & Horton, L. (1994). Factors that influence the behavioral pain responses of premature infants. *Pain, 59*(1), 101-109.

Stevens, B., Johnston, C., Petryshen, P., et al. (1996). Premature infant pain profile: Development and initial validation. *Clinical Journal of Pain, 12*(1), 13-22.

Stevens, B., Johnston, C., Taddio, A., & Einarson, T. (1996). *The safety and efficacy of EMLA for heel lance in preterm neonates.* Vancouver, Canada: International Association for the Study of Pain, 8th World Congress on Pain, 181-182 (Abstract 239).

Stevens, B., & Ohlsson, A. (1998). Sucrose in neonates undergoing painful procedures. *Neonatal Modules of the Cochrane Database of Systematic Reviews* [Electronic database, 1-13].

Stevens, B., Taddio, A., Ohlsson, A., & Einarson, T. (1997). The efficacy of sucrose for relieving procedural pain in neonates: A systematic review and meta-analysis. *Acta Paediatrica, 86*(8), 837-842.

U.S. Department of Health and Human Services. (1992). *Acute pain management in infants, children, and adolescents: Operative and medical procedures* (AHCPR Publication. No. 92-0020). Rockville, Maryland: Author.

Walden, M., & Carrier, C.T. (2003). Sleeping beauties: The impact of sedation on neonatal development. *Journal of Obstretric, Gynecologic, & Neonatal Nursing (JOGNN), 32*(3), 393-401.

Walden, M., & Franck, L. (2003). Identification, management, and prevention of newborn/infant pain (pp. 843-856). In C. Kenner & J.W. Lott (Eds.), *Comprehensive neonatal nursing: A physiologic perspective* (3rd ed.). St. Louis: W.B. Saunders.

Walden, M., Penticuff, J.H., Stevens, B., et al. (2001). Maturational changes in physiological and behavioral responses of preterm neonates to pain. *Advances in Neonatal Care, 1*(2), 94-106.

# 13 Palliative Care

## Tanya Sudia-Robinson

Developmental care should benefit all infants, even those who are dying. The approach should be to provide individualized care based on the holistic needs, to foster positive growth and development or prevent complications. This approach is just as important to the child/family with a poor prognosis as it is to those for whom the outcome is bright. Palliative or end-of-life (EOL) care in many respects inherently incorporates the notion of developmental care—an individualized family-centered philosophy of care delivery.

Pediatric palliative care incorporates pain and symptom management for the child while attending to the psychological, social, and spiritual needs of the child and the family (American Academy of Pediatrics [AAP], 2000).

Palliative care can be incorporated into an existing developmental care program at any time, as the overall goals are congruent. Striving to deliver optimal care in a supportive family environment clearly reflects the desired outcomes of both philosophies.

Palliative care programs for newborns and infants and their families are still in the initial stages of integration into healthcare systems (Catlin & Carter, 2002) and are underutilized in many neonatal intensive care units (NICUs) in the United States and abroad (Hutton, 2002; Pierucci, Russell, & Leuthner, 2001; Sudia-Robinson, 2003). Comprehensive care cannot be provided if infants and parents do not have fully supportive intervention programs from the moment of birth to the moment of death. For the infant's parents and siblings, support and bereavement services should continue for as long as needed, to assist them as they progress through the grieving process.

In this chapter, palliative and EOL care in relationship to developmental care are discussed. The following section describes how aspects of developmental care can be continued or initiated for infants who are dying and their families.

## NORMALIZATION OF DYING

Dying occurs along a continuum. The time from diagnosis of a terminal condition to the moment of death can be as brief as minutes or hours. In other cases, the infant might live for a year or more. It is recommended that palliative care measures be incorporated into the existing plan of care at the time of diagnosis (AAP, 2000; Wolfe, Friebert, & Hilden, 2002; Wolfe, Klar, Grier, et al., 2000; Sahler, 2000). However, palliative care measures can be added at any point along this continuum and still provide benefit for the infant and family.

The newborn and infant care team can initiate the palliative care process by evaluating the infant's need for comfort and supportive measures. Just as parents should be involved in other aspects of the overall care plan for their infant, their parenting role should be affirmed by seeking their input. A comprehensive palliative care plan will reflect measures adapted to the infant's needs while simultaneously reflecting the parental preferences. This plan of care should not be static, but should change as the infant's condition warrants and as the family progresses through the anticipatory grieving phases.

## ALLEVIATING PAIN AND SUFFERING

Adequate pain management is an important component of optimal care throughout the time of dying. Continued, aggressive support until the moment of death often occurs for many infants (Pierucci, Russell, & Leuthner, 2001; Rebagliato, Cuttini, & Broggin, et al., 2000). This phenomenon raises questions about whether infants suffer needlessly during their last moments of life (Sudia-Robinson, 2003). Ensuring that adequate pain medication is provided is an initial step in promoting a more peaceful death for these infants (Abe, Catlin, & Mihara, 2001). Additionally, NICU care providers have an obligation to continue to explore additional supportive measures to further ease infant suffering. Such measures should include comfort positioning, alleviation of noxious stimuli, and elimination of noncurative tests and procedures.

## INCORPORATING SPECIFIC DEVELOPMENTAL CARE MEASURES

Although most aspects of developmental care can benefit infants in need of palliative care, the measures highlighted in this section include kangaroo care, music therapy, ambient lighting, aromatherapy, and infant massage.

### Kangaroo Care

Researchers have demonstrated the effectiveness of kangaroo care for preterm infants as well as the documented benefit to parents (Anderson, 1991; Gale Franck, & Lund, 1993). Among the most positive aspects of kangaroo care as a component of palliative care is that it provides parents precious moments, without interference, that they will treasure after their infant has died. Memories of how their infant felt when held skin-to-skin will linger forever in their minds.

It is important to note, however, that some parents upon initially seeing their infant in a NICU might not be ready to participate when first approached about kangaroo care. This hesitancy should be respected, and great care should be taken to avoid inadvertently causing any guilt for such a decision. Sometimes, parents need personal space and time to process the overwhelming feelings that accompany the birth of a baby that is not likely to survive (Lundqvist, Nilstun, & Dykes, 2002). They might be afraid that their holding their infant will cause his/her death to come more quickly. Usually, parents who initially distance themselves from their baby will eventually begin to touch and then hold their baby. Allowing parents to progress at their own pace respects their role as parents and as decision-makers for this new child. Acknowledging to parents that they can always make this decision later leaves the door open for this intervention when they are ready.

### Music Therapy

Music therapy is one of the easiest measures to incorporate in a NICU and can be continued if the infant is discharged to be cared for at home. In addition to the soothing aspects for infants and parents, adding music therapy provides the parents with another opportunity to enact their preferences for their infant's care.

The NICU team should provide initial guidance for families in the selection of music for their infant. Suggest a calming instrumental piece and place the volume indicator at the lowest setting. It is helpful if NICUs have a selection of appropriate CDs or audiotapes for parents to choose from. This is especially important when the active dying phase occurs shortly after birth. If the infant is hospitalized for a long time, the parents might wish to bring in their own music selections.

### Ambient Lighting

Adjustable ambient lighting at the infant's bedside has helped maintain day-night and sleep-wake cycles (Blackburn, 1996). There are various inexpensive ways to modify the bedside lighting, including individual adjustable lamps and shielding the light with blankets or cloth. When infants are in private rooms, the options for altered lighting are more varied. Lamps with soft, pastel blue light bulbs might help create a calming environment. Parents can be invited to share their preferences for adjustable lighting when possible in the NICU and encouraged to use this intervention if their infant is discharged home.

### Aromatherapy

There are no research studies to demonstrate the potential benefits of aromatherapy for critically ill infants and their families. However, there are indicators to suggest that such measures could prove beneficial (Kassity, Jones, Kenner, et al., 2003). Scents such as lavender and vanilla are usually perceived as calming. Eradicating the typical hospital smells and replacing them with a soothing, mild vanilla scent might help parents relax and would certainly leave a more pleasant memory of the environment. This intervention is an inexpensive measure to implement and can help with other measures to make the NICU a more calming environment.

### Infant Massage

In most cases, infant massage can be soothing to the infant. As with any additional care measures, the infant's reaction must be evaluated, and further plans for incorporation should be modified accordingly. Infant massage also provides an opportunity for parents to become involved in their infant's care if they feel comfortable doing so. The neonatal care team can use this parent/infant interaction to praise parents on their caregiving skills. Comments such as "He relaxes when you gently massage his back like that" and "She recognizes your gentle touch" provide powerful positive feedback to parents. Parents of critically ill infants need to feel that they can do something that all parents want to do—provide love and comfort to their child.

## PROVIDING OPPORTUNITIES FOR PARENTING

One of the most endearing gifts that the NICU team can give to parents is the opportunity to engage in parenting activities for their infant. For some parents, the interaction with their infant might be extremely limited by quantitative measurement—hours or days. However, their experience can be very memorable if planned from a qualitative perspective. It only takes a few moments to create memories that parents will hold onto forever.

NICU staff can provide parents with the opportunity to assist with most of their infant's personal care activities—cutting a lock of hair (instead of nurse cutting it, ask parents if one or both of them would like to). For parents who prefer not to engage in such activities, offer to do these things in their presence. Regardless of the activity, try to focus on something that the parents feel comfortable doing and something that will create a pleasant memory for the family, whether it is holding, touching, singing, or journaling.

Keep in mind that just because parents choose not to participate in one care measure, does not mean they will not want to participate in other caregiving activities. For example, a parent might find it difficult to cut a lock of hair, yet might desire to help dress the child. Another parent might consider the child too fragile to put clothing on, yet might welcome the opportunity to gently brush the child's hair. With sensitivity to their preferences, continue to extend opportunities for involvement. Respect, too, that some parents might not desire to touch or

photograph a dying child. Pictures that are taken can be placed in a file until parents are ready and request them.

## Timing of Opportunities for Involvement

Parents will be on an emotional roller coaster. Some days they will cope better than others and their level of energy for even the smallest of tasks will vary. They might be involved in their infant's care one day but return the next day preferring to stand at the bedside and watch. Again, an increased sensitivity to this is key in promoting further parenting opportunities.

## Differences between First-Time Parents and Parents with Other Children

Parents have different personal experiences that they draw upon as well as different parenting skills if they are already parents. Initial interventions to involve the parents should consider these differences.

First-time parents will not have any direct parenting experience to draw upon. Their thoughts about what they can do and what others might expect them to do might be in conflict. They might desire to be more involved in their infant's care, but feel uncomfortable verbalizing this to the staff. Their uncertainty might be more pronounced if they are very young parents or if they need additional support services.

Parents with other children bring a wide range of experiences and have varying degrees of expectations about their role. To assist staff in assessing potential parental expectations, it might be helpful to broadly categorize parents by the ages of their other children. Generally, the parenting experiences for parents with children under age 2 years will have focused on direct caretaking activities. These parents might feel very comfortable participating in care such as grooming.

Parents of preschool-age children might be primarily concerned about how to help their other children understand what is happening to their new baby brother or sister. Parents of young, school-age children might also need help explaining the sibling's pending death, and could benefit from help exploring the guilt feelings and fears that these siblings have. Parents of older children might need assistance with deciding how to involve these children in the visitation and care of their critically ill sibling. When available, age-appropriate sibling support groups should be offered to these families (Pearson, 1997).

Parents with children from previous marriages for whom the dying infant is a stepbrother or stepsister can have unique concerns. A stepsibling might be experiencing guilt, particularly if they were not happy about the pending birth of this child or about their parent's divorce/remarriage. They might be afraid that their thoughts about not wanting a new baby brother or sister actually caused the infant's illness. Appropriate support services for these children should also be explored.

## OPENNESS TO INNOVATIVE PRACTICES

Parents might suggest measures to the NICU staff that are unique to their cultural background or that they have read about. It is important that incorporation of these practices are evaluated in the same manner that they would be for any other infant. The most important question to consider is whether the proposed practice would cause any direct harm to the infant. Parents should not have to provide any evidence beyond their belief that a therapy might be beneficial for the team to consider their request. The ensuing evaluation for potential harm should come from the neonatal team directly caring for the infant. While remaining sensitive to the gravity of the infant's condition, it would be unethical to dismiss consideration of potential harmful effects. The NICU staff is obligated to continue to weigh the risks and benefits of their actions throughout the dying process.

When the infant's death is imminent, and the risk of harm seems unlikely, NICU staff should consider waving a formal review of their request to implement a culture-based practice. To meet their ethical obligation of weighing risks and benefits, the NICU staff directly involved in the infant's care and present at the bedside at that moment could briefly discuss the parents' request and allow them to proceed immediately. For example, the parents might request to rub an herbal ointment on their infant. Unless it is known that this substance will be painful once placed on the infant's skin, the NICU staff could allow the parents to apply it as they desire. However, if something is known to potentially cause the infant further pain or suffering, the practice should be avoided. Additional pain should never be inflicted or rationalized as acceptable simply because the infant will die anyway. The ethical obligation to avoid causing intentional harm to infants is just as important during the dying process as it is during the curative phase of care.

In cases in which the infant's death is not likely to occur in the next few days or weeks, NICU staff can take the time needed to evaluate the parents' request. However, proceeding with the evaluation as quickly as possible is in everyone's best interest, as the infant might, indeed, benefit, the parents will feel a sense of control and aiding their infant, and the parent/staff relationship will have an additional degree of mutual respect.

## CONCLUSION

Palliative care is a critical aspect of comprehensive newborn and infant and family-centered developmental care. A variety of measures can be instituted to help alleviate infant pain and suffering while simultaneously involving parents as valued primary caretakers for their infant. The neonatal care team, for possible incorporation, should explore existing and novel interventions that can assist in meeting these goals and incorporating them into the plan of care. Implementation of such practices can provide positive outcomes not only for the infant, but also for the parents and the neonatal care team. Parents feel less helpless and less like bystanders when they can suggest or participate in supplemental care practices. The neonatal care team benefits in that they might see an improvement in the comfort level of the infant, and they develop a more positive relationship with the parents. More research about ways to better support infants and families is needed in this area of caregiving.

Box 13-1 provides a list of additional resources for palliative care.

Box **13-1** Web and Other Resources for Palliative Care

American Academy of Pediatrics
141 Northwest Point Boulevard
Elk Grove Village, IL 60007
(847) 434-4000
*www.aap.org*
   The full text of the AAP guidelines for Pediatric Palliative Care can be viewed on this website.

Center to Advance Palliative Care
The Mount Sinai School of Medicine
1255 5th Avenue, Suite C-2
New York, New York 10029-6574
(212) 201-2670
*www.capc.org*
   This is a resource center for hospital and health systems interested in developing palliative care programs.

Children's International Project on Palliative and
   Hospice Services
National Hospice and Palliative Care
   Organization
1700 Diagonal Road, Suite 625
Alexandria, VA 22314
(877) 557-2847
*www.nhpco.org*
   Information about pediatric palliative care and hospice services can be obtained from this website.

The Initiative for Pediatric Palliative Care
Center for Applied Ethics and Professional
   Practice

Education Development Center, Inc.
55 Chapel Street
Newton, MA 02458-1060
(617) 618-2388
*www.ippcweb.org*
   This is the website of a consortium of eight children's hospitals currently working in collaboration with the National Association of Children's Hospitals and Related Institutions, The Society of Pediatric Nurses, and The New York Academy of Medicine to develop a curriculum for improving the quality of life for children with life-threatening illnesses.

National Academy of Sciences: Institute of
   Medicine
500 5th Street, NW
Washington, DC 20001
*www.IOM.org*
   The Institute of Medicine report *When Children Die: Improving Palliative and End-of-Life Care for Children and Families* (July 25, 2002) can be viewed in full at this website.

Promoting Excellence in End-of-Life Care
The Robert Wood Johnson Foundation
PO Box 2316
College Road East and Route 1
Princeton, NY 08543
(888) 631-9989
*www.promotingexcellence.org*
   This website provides links to pediatric palliative care projects and programs sponsored by the Robert Wood Johnson Foundation.

## REFERENCES

Abe, N., Catlin, A.J., & Mihara, D. (2001). End of life in the NICU: A study of ventilator withdrawal. *MCN: The American Journal of Maternal Child Care, 28*(3), 141-146.

American Academy of Pediatrics. (2000). Palliative care for children. *Pediatrics, 106*(2), 351-357.

Anderson, G.C. (1991). Current knowledge about skin-to-skin (kangaroo) care for preterm infants. *Journal of Perinatology, 11*(3), 216-226.

Blackburn, S.T. (1996). Research utilization: Modifying the NICU light environment. *Neonatal Network, 15*(4), 63-66.

Catlin, A., & Carter, B. (2002). Creation of a neonatal end-of-life palliative care protocol. *Journal of Perinatology, 22*(3), 184-185.

Gale, G., Franck, L., & Lund, C. (1993). Skin-to-skin (kangaroo) holding of the intubated premature infant. *Neonatal Network, 12*(6), 49-57.

Hutton, N. (2002). Pediatric palliative care: The time has come. *Archives of Pediatrics & Adolescent Medicine, 156*(1), 9-10.

Kassity, N.A., Jones, J, Kenner, C., et al. (2003). Complementary therapies. In C. Kenner & J.W. Lott (Eds.), *Comprehensive neonatal nursing: A physiologic perspective* (3rd ed., pp. 868-875). St Louis: W.B. Saunders.

Lundqvist, A., Nilstun, T., & Dykes, A.K. (2002) Experiencing neonatal death—Ambivalent transition to motherhood. *Pediatric Nursing, 28*(6), 610, 621-625.

Pearson, L. (1997). Family-centered care and the anticipated death of a newborn. *Pediatric Nursing, 23*, 178-182.

Pierucci, R.L., Russell, K., & Leuthner, S.R. (2001). End-of-life care for neonates and infants: The experience and effects of a palliative care consultation service. *Pediatrics, 108*(3), 653-660.

Rebagliato, M., Cuttini, M., Broggin, L., et al. (2000). Neonatal end-of-life decision making: Physicians' attitudes and relationship with self-reported practices in 10 European countries. *Journal of the American Medical Association, 284*(19), 2451-2459.

Sahler, O.J. (2000). Medical education about end-of-life care in the pediatric setting: Principles, challenges, and opportunities. *Pediatrics, 105*(3 Pt 1), 575-584.

Sudia-Robinson, T. (2003). Hospice and palliative care (pp. 127-131). In C. Kenner, & J.W. Lott (Eds.), *Comprehensive neonatal nursing: A physiologic perspective* (3rd ed.). St Louis: W.B. Saunders.

Wolfe, J., Friebert, S., & Hilden, J. (2002). Caring for children with advanced cancer integrating palliative care. *Pediatric Clinics North of America, 49*(5), 1043-1062.

Wolfe, J., Klar, N., Grier, H.E., et al. (2000). Understanding of prognosis among parents of children who died of cancer: Impact on treatment goals and integration of palliative care. *Journal of the American Medical Association, 284*(19), 2469-2475.

# 14 *Environmental Issues*

Lynda Law Harrison, Marilyn J. Lotas, and
Katherine M. Jorgensen

The neonatal intensive care unit (NICU) environment includes sources of both animate and inanimate stimulation that can affect infants, NICU staff, and visitors. This chapter includes a review of recent research related to effects of the environment, and interventions designed to reduce negative aspects of the environment and promote positive environmental influences. Aspects of the animate environment that are reviewed include tactile stimulation, activity levels, and parental involvement. Aspects of the inanimate environment that are reviewed include light, sound, and NICU design.

## ANIMATE ENVIRONMENT
### Tactile Stimulation

This section includes a review of research describing the types of tactile stimulation routinely received by infants in the NICU, as well as evaluations of supplemental tactile (with or without kinesthetic and vestibular) stimulation. For other reviews of this body of research, see recent papers by Harrison (Harrison, in press; Harrison, 2001b) and Vickers, Ohlsson, and Horsley (2001).

### Studies Describing Tactile Stimulation Routinely Received by Infants in the NICU

Most of the research describing the tactile stimulation routinely received by infants in the NICU was conducted between 1977 and 1995. There is a need for additional research to determine whether there have been changes in the types or amounts of tactile stimulation received by infants in the NICU, following the increased incorporation of developmental care principles in NICUs. Findings from research to date, suggest that most of the tactile stimulation received by infants in the NICU is associated with medical or nursing procedures, and this type of stimulation often has adverse effects, including sleep disruptions, hypoxia,

increased levels of intracranial pressure, heart rate (HR), respiratory rate, and blood pressure, and increased signs of behavioral distress (e.g., facial grimace, clenched fist, or gaze aversion) (Blackburn & Barnard, 1985; Catlett & Holditch-Davis, 1990; Danford, Miske, Headley, et al., 1983; Evans, 1991; Gottfried, Hodgman, & Brown, 1984; Lawson, Daum, & Turkewitz, 1977; Long, Philip, & Lucey, 1980; Miller & Holditch-Davis, 1992; Murdoch & Darlow, 1984; Norris, Campbell, & Brenkerd, 1982; Peters, 1992; Werner & Conway, 1990). Symon and Cunningham (1995) reported that preterm infants in the NICU might be handled as much as 28 to 71 times, for a total of 3.5 hours per day, and that infants on ventilators receive the most handling. The findings from two studies indicated that infants received little comforting or contingent touch in the NICU (Blackburn & Barnard, 1985; Werner & Conway, 1990). Miller and Holditch-Davis (1992) reported that parents provide more social touching than do nurses. Harrison and Woods (1991) found wide variability in the types and amounts of touch provided by parents and grandparents during NICU visits, and noted that parents provided less touch to infants who were younger than 28 weeks' gestational age (GA). These findings all suggest the need to exercise caution when handling infants in the NICU and the need for research to identify forms of tactile stimulation that might reduce stress and provide comfort to these fragile infants.

### Studies Evaluating Interventions Providing Supplemental Tactile, Kinesthetic, and/or Vestibular Stimulation

During the past 30 years, researchers have evaluated different types of tactile stimulation interventions designed to reduce stress and enhance health and developmental outcomes of infants hospitalized in the NICU. Some of these interventions have included only tactile stimulation, and others have also included kinesthetic (passive movement) or vestibular (rocking) stimulation. These interventions have included still, gentle touch, swaddling, massage/stroking, and kangaroo care (KC). Because KC research is addressed elsewhere in this book, it will not be reviewed in this chapter.

## Studies of Still, Gentle Touch

Still, gentle touch involves placing hands on the infant and leaving them for varying periods of time without providing any stroking or massage movements. The earliest study of this type of touch that was identified was based on a dissertation conducted by Jay (1982). In this study, 13 preterm infants (gestational ages 27 to 32 weeks), who were mechanically ventilated and had no congenital defects, received gentle touch for 12 minutes, four times a day for 10 days, beginning when they were younger than 96 hours old. The infants were in a supine position, and the investigator placed her warmed hands on the infants' heads and abdomens. The outcomes of the experimental group infants were compared with those of a matched control group of infants who had been hospitalized in the same NICU the previous year (1980-1981). There were no significant differences in the two groups on weight gain, temperature stability, length of hospital stay, or frequency of apnea and bradycardia episodes. However, infants in the experiment had higher hematocrits, received fewer blood transfusions, and required less oxygen from day 6 to 10 of the intervention (or a comparable period for control group infants). A major limitation of this study was the use of a matched control group of infants who had been hospitalized a year prior to providing the intervention to experimental group infants. Other changes in NICU care over this period might have contributed the study results.

Tribotti (1990) studied the responses of four stable preterm infants to gentle touch provided for 15 minutes once a day for 3 days. The infants were 27, 30, 31, and 34 weeks' gestational age (GA) at birth, and 33 to 35 weeks' GA at the time of the study. Although there were differences in the responses of the individual infants, the group data suggested a trend of decreased transcutaneous oxygen tension ($TcPO_2$) levels, increased respiratory regularity, and a slight decrease in motor activity from baseline to touch

during the first gentle touch session. During the second session, there was no change in the $TcPO_2$ level, an increase in regularity of respirations, and a decrease in activity level from the baseline to touch phase. By the third session, there were increases in $TcPO_2$ and respiratory regularity, and a continued decrease in motor activity from baseline to touch phases.

Harrison et al., conducted four studies evaluating gentle human touch (GHT) (Harrison, Olivet, Cunningham, et al., 1996; Harrison, Groer, Modrcin-McCarthy, & Wilkinson, 1992; Harrison, Williams, Berbaum, et al., 2000a, 2000b; Modrcin-McCarthy, 1992; Modrcin-Talbott, Harrison, Groer, et al., 2003). The touch consisted of the investigator placing one hand on the infant's head and the other on the infant's lower back and buttocks for 10 to 20 minutes.

In a small, pilot study, Harrison, Groer, Modrcin-McCarthy, and Wilkinson (1992) randomly assigned three infants to an E (experimental) group and three to a C (control) group. E-group infants received GHT for 15 minutes, three times a day for 10 days beginning when they were 7 to 9 days old. There were minimal changes in heart rate (HR), or oxygen saturation ($O_2$ sat) levels comparing baseline, touch, and posttouch periods, but there were fewer signs of behavioral distress and motor activity during periods of GHT. Infants in the experiment had fewer total days on supplemental oxygen, greater mean daily weight gain, decreased serum cortisol levels, fewer blood transfusions, and a shorter length of hospital stay. However, despite the randomization procedures, infants in the experimental group had higher birthweights and an older GA at birth than did control group infants.

In a second study that included 30 infants from 26 to 32 weeks' GA at birth, infants received 15 minutes of GHT each day for 5 days, beginning when they were 6 to 9 days old (Harrison, Olivet, Cunningham, et al., 1996). There was less active sleep, motor activity, and behavioral distress during periods of GHT. There were no differences in HR or $O_2$ sat levels comparing baseline, GHT, and posttouch phases. The only difference in outcomes noted between experimental and control group infants was that infants in the experimental group required more phototherapy.

Modrcin-Talbott, Harrison, Groer, et al. (2003) provided 20 minutes of GHT each day for 10 days to a group of Modrcin 10 preterm infants. Infants demonstrated lower levels of motor activity and behavioral distress cues during periods of GHT compared with baseline or posttouch phases, but there were no differences between the E and randomly assigned C group infants on weight gain in the NICU.

In the fourth study, 84 preterm infants between 27 and 33 weeks' GA at birth were assigned randomly to either an E or C group (Harrison, Williams, Berbaum, et al., 2000a, 2000b). E-group infants received three periods of GHT each day for 10 days, beginning when they were between 6 to 9 days of age. There were no differences between E- and C-group infants on any measures of morbidity, weight gain, or behavioral organization at the time of NICU discharge. There were no significant differences comparing baseline (B), touch (T), and posttouch (PT) phases in mean HR across the three phases. There was a significant decrease in $O_2$ sat from B to PT and from T to PT, although the difference in the means during these phases was very small and not clinically significant. There were also no differences in the percent of abnormally low HR or $O_2$ sat levels comparing B, T, and PT phases when using standard criteria (e.g., HR less than 100 beats per minute [bpm], more than 200 bpm, or $O_2$ sat less than 90 mg%). However there were more abnormally low levels of HR and $O_2$ sat and abnormally high HR levels comparing B and T phases using individualized criteria (HR or $O_2$ sat less than 1, 2, or 3 standard deviations [SD] from mean baseline value, or HR more than 1, 2, or 3 SDs from baseline value). This finding suggests that even the GHT intervention had physiologic effects on the infants, although the effects might not have been clinically significant (Harrison, Berbaum, Stem, et al., 2001). There were significantly lower levels of active sleep, motor activity, behavioral distress, and modified behavioral distress during periods of GHT compared with B and PT periods.

Findings from the studies of GHT suggest that this type of touch has no adverse effects on mean HR or $O_2$ sat levels, or on the percent of abnormal HR or $O_2$ sat levels using standard criteria. Study findings also suggest that still, gentle touch is associated with increased regularity; decreased levels of active sleep, motor activity, and behavioral distress respiratory; and increased levels of quiet sleep during periods of

gentle touch compared with baseline and posttouch periods (Harrison et al., 1992, 1996, 2000, 2000a, 2000b, Modrcin-McCarthy, 1992; Modricin-Talbott, Harrison, Groer, et al., 2003; Tribotti, 1990). There were no consistent longer-term benefits to the gentle touch interventions on outcome variables such as morbidity status, weight gain, or behavioral organization. These findings suggest that nurses could encourage parents and other caregivers to use gentle touch to reduce stress among infants in the NICU who might not be able to tolerate more vigorous forms of tactile stimulation, such as stroking or massage. However, the finding that there were more abnormally high levels of HR and abnormally low levels of $O_2$ sat and HR using individualized criteria suggests that nurses and caregivers should use caution when providing any type of tactile stimulation, and discontinue touch if the infant demonstrates adverse physiologic or behavioral responses.

## Studies Examining Preterm Infants' Responses to Stroking or Massage without Kinesthetic Stimulation

The studies of stroking and massage have included infants of varying GAs and morbidity levels, and have included different types and amounts of tactile stimulation. Because of these differences, findings across studies have been inconsistent. Adamson-Macedo and Attree (1994) suggested that the term *stroking* implies caressing the skin softly in one direction; *massage* implies kneading; and *rubbing* implies applying friction. These authors recommended clarifying the type of tactile stimulation provided to better compare findings across studies. Studies have evaluated both immediate and longer-term physiologic and behavioral outcomes of the stroking or massage interventions.

### Positive, Immediate Physiologic Effects of Stroking/Massage

Positive, immediate physiologic effects of stroking/massage interventions that have been identified include: decreased apnea, decreased salivary cortisol, and increased oxygenation. In an early study, Kattwinkel, Nearman, Fanaroff, et al. (1975) found decreased apnea in response to rubbing the extremities of preterm infants for 5 minutes out of every 15 minutes for 3 hours. The sample included only six infants who were 26 to 31 weeks' GA at birth and 2 to 35 days old at the time of the study. Acolet, Modi, Giannakoulpoulos, et al. (1993) studied the effects of a 20-minute massage provided to 11 preterm infants (23 to 34 weeks' GA and 4 to 132 days old). Serum cortisol levels were consistently decreased after the massage, suggesting that the massage intervention reduced stress levels. Daga, Ahuja, and Lunkad (1998) studied the effects of maternal stroking of the infant's back during a feeding. The sample included only seven preterm infants who were younger than 32 weeks' gestation and weighed less than 1600 g. Oxygen saturation levels were significantly higher in infants who received the stroking at 20 and 30 minutes after the feeding compared with a control group. De Róiste and Bushnell (2000) found no harmful effects of a stroking intervention on the heart rates, respiratory rates, or $TcPO_2$ levels of a group of 13 high-risk ventilated preterm infants.

## Positive, Immediate Behavioral Effects of Stroking/Massage

Harrison (2001a) studied the responses of six preterm infants (27 to 30 weeks' GA at birth) to a 10-minute massage intervention provided twice each day for 10 days in the NICU. Infants demonstrated more quiet sleep and slightly reduced levels of motor activity during the massage interventions compared with baseline, although the data were not analyzed statistically due to the small sample size.

## Negative, Immediate Physiologic Effects of Stroking/Massage

Findings from several studies have suggested that stroking/massage might result in decreased oxygenation. Oehler (1985) reported that the transcutaneous oxygen levels of preterm infants (26 to 30 weeks' gestation) tended to decrease during periods of stroking or stroking/talking, but that the levels stayed the same or increased during periods of auditory stimulation only. Adamson-Macedo, De Róiste, et al., (1997) studied 11 ventilated preterm infants and found that there were decreased $TcPO_2$ levels during and after 3- to 4-minute periods of

maternal intuitive touch. Harrison, Leeper, & Yoon (1991) evaluated responses of 36 preterm infants to touch provided by parents during visits to the NICU. The infants were 25 to 33 weeks' GA at birth. Although the types and amounts of touch provided by the parents varied considerably, there were more episodes of abnormally low $O_2$ sat levels during periods of parent touch compared with baseline periods.

Findings from other studies, however, have suggested that stroking/massage had no adverse effects on oxygenation. Adamson-Macedo et al. (1994, 1997) found that there were no significant decreases in $TcPO_2$ levels during or after the 3 to 4 minutes of a systematic light stroking intervention provided to 11 ventilated preterm infants. Scafidi, Field, Schanberg, et al. (1986) evaluated changes in $TcPO_2$ across four 15-minute stroking/kinesthetic stimulation sessions in a larger study reported by Scafidi, Field, Schanberg, et al. (1990). During the first of the four sessions, mean $TcPO_2$ levels decreased significantly from the baseline to the first tactile period and from baseline to the kinesthetic period, but increased from the stimulation periods to the posttouch period. There were no significant effects of the tactile or kinesthetic interventions on $TcPO_2$ during the fourth session. Most of the instances of decreased $TcPO_2$ levels occurred during the kinesthetic portion of the intervention, rather than during the stroking phase. Harrison (2001a) studied responses of six preterm infants (27 to 30 weeks' GA at birth) to a 10-minute massage intervention that was provided by a neonatal nurse twice each day for 10 days. There were no significant changes in $O_2$ sat during the massage, but infants demonstrated slight elevations in HR (averaging 6 bpm) during the massage compared with baseline periods.

## Negative, Immediate Behavioral Effects of Stroking/Massage

McGehee and Eckerman (1983) examined responses of preterm infants (27 to 32.5 weeks' GA) to three, 80-second periods of stimulation: talking, stroking, or a combination of talking and stroking. The infants exhibited more gasping, grunting, movement, and state transitions during periods of stroking and stroking/talking compared with parents of talking only. Oehler, Eckerman, and Wilson (1988) studied responses to the same type of intervention among 15 very low birthweight (VLBW) preterm infants who were 30 to 34 weeks' postconceptional age (PCA) at the time of the intervention. When the infants were in a sleep state at the beginning of the intervention, talking led to more time with eyes open, although stroking and talking together resulted in increased movement, particularly for the higher risk infants. Higher risk infants also showed more avoidance behaviors in response to stroking, such as facial grimace, tongue protrusion, yawn, and fussing/crying. Similarly, during the few times when infants were in a quiet, visually attentive state at the beginning of the intervention, higher risk infants showed more movement and avoidance cues in response to stroking or stroking/talking. A different pattern of response was noted when infants were in an active state at the beginning of the intervention. In this state, both higher- and lower-risk infants responded to talking with decreased body movement and more eye opening. When infants were in the active state at the beginning of the intervention, they continued to demonstrate movement and avoidance cues during the stroking or stroking/talking intervention, with no significant change in behavior.

Adamson-Macedo and Hayes (1998) compared the physiologic and behavioral responses of an extremely low birthweight (ELBW) ventilated infant (740 g) to stroking using both moderate and deep pressure. The infant exhibited more distress behaviors following the deep-pressure stroking compared with periods with moderate pressure stroking or no stroking, suggesting that deep pressure was distressing to the infant.

### Longer-Term Outcomes of Stroking/Massage Interventions

Positive longer-term outcomes of stroking or massage interventions that have been identified include increased weight gain, improved behavioral organization, and improved developmental outcomes. As with studies examining immediate effects of such interventions, the studies have included infants of differing GAs and with different levels of morbidity, and the types and amounts of tactile stimulation

have varied. As a result, findings across studies have not been consistent.

Solkoff, Yaffe, Weintraub, et al. (1969) studied the effects of a 5-minute stroking intervention provided each hour during the first 10 days after birth. The sample included 10 preterm infants whose birth weights ranged from 1190 to 1590 g. Compared with a control group, infants who received the stroking were more active during the hospitalization period, regained their birth weights faster, and had fewer developmental anomalies at 7 to 8 months after discharge. Solkoff and Matuszak (1975) evaluated a 7.5-minute stroking intervention that was provided once an hour for 16 hours per day, for 10 days. The sample included six infants who had a mean GA of 31.2 weeks at birth. Compared with infants in a control group, experimental group infants demonstrated more rapid habituation to light and sound, improved body tone, increased alertness, more consolability, more state changes, and more rapid avoidance of noxious stimuli.

Kramer, Chamorro, Green, et al. (1975) evaluated an intervention that consisted of 2 to 3 minutes of stroking before and after feedings (for a total of 48 minutes of extra touch each day) for a minimum of 2 weeks. The sample included eight preterm infants who had a mean GA of 33 weeks. Compared with infants in a control group, experimental group infants had increased rates of social development at 6 weeks and 3 months after transfer to a crib.

Adamson-Macedo (1985-1986) evaluated the effects of supplemental stroking for 10 minutes twice a day during the first week of life. The sample included 31 preterm infants who had a mean GA of 32 weeks. For 15 infants, the tactile intervention began within the first 48 hours after birth, and for the remaining infants the touch began 49 to 120 hours postbirth. Compared with infants in a control group, experimental group infants lost less weight during the week after the intervention. Infants in the early stimulation group lost the least amount of weight, suggesting that it might be beneficial to begin supplemental tactile stimulation programs soon after birth. Adamson-Macedo, Dattani, Wilson, et al. (1993) reported on a follow-up study of eight preterm infants who had received a supplemental stroking intervention in the NICU. At age 7 years, these eight children were compared with six matched controls. Children who had received the stroking intervention had higher scores on tests of mental, sequential, and simultaneous processing, and general intelligence.

De Róiste and Bushnell (1996) evaluated the effects of a similar stroking intervention that was provided for 20 minutes a day beginning the second or third day after birth. The intervention continued until the day before discharge from the NICU (for a mean of 17 days). The sample included 13 infants in the E and 13 in a matched C group. E-group infants progressed to total nipple feeding earlier, were discharged sooner, and had higher Bayley Mental Development Index scores at age 15 months.

Harrison (2001a) evaluated a 2-week gentle human touch (GHT) plus 2-week massage intervention. Infants in the E group received 10 days of GHT intervention for 10 minutes, twice each day beginning when they were 6 to 9 days old. They then received 10 days of massage intervention for 10 minutes, twice each day (beginning at age 20 to 23 days). The sample included 12 infants who were randomly assigned to the E group (n = 6) or to a control group, although the mean weight of E-group infants was 129 g more than C-group infants. E-group infants had lower total and average daily morbidity scores, fewer days in the hospital and on supplemental oxygen, lower neurobiologic risk scores, and higher average daily weight gain, although the small sample size precluded use of statistics to analyze these differences.

No studies were found that identified negative long-term outcomes of supplemental stroking/massage interventions provided in the NICU. Although the sample sizes in most studies have been small, and the types and amounts of touch provided have differed, the findings suggest that such interventions might have benefits including improved weight gain, reduced levels of morbidity, reduced lengths of hospital stay, improved behavioral organization, improved mental development, and increased activity levels.

## Studies of Massage Combined with Kinesthetic or Vestibular Stimulation

A number of studies have evaluated the effects of supplemental stimulation programs that have included stroking and massage combined with passive range of motion of the limbs or rocking. As with studies of gentle touch and stroking, there have been differences in the types and amounts of tactile stimulation, and in the characteristics of the samples, making it difficult to compare findings across studies. Researchers have examined both immediate and longer-term effects of the stimulation interventions.

## Immediate Effects of Interventions Combining Tactile with Kinesthetic and/or Vestibular Stimulation

Field et al. have conducted several studies evaluating the effects of a 15-minute tactile/kinesthetic stimulation protocol on stable preterm infants (Field, Schanberg, Scafidi, et al., 1986; Kuhn, Schanberg, Field, et al., 1991; Scafidi, Field, Schanberg, et al., 1990). The intervention consisted of 5 minutes of stroking, 5 minutes of kinesthetic stimulation (passive flexion/extension movements), and then 5 minutes of stroking. The infants were in a prone position during the stroking and in a supine position during the kinesthetic stimulation. In one of these studies, Morrow, Field, Scafidi, et al. (1991) described responses of a sample of the E infants to periods of stimulation and no stimulation, and differences in responses to the tactile and kinesthetic components of the intervention. During the periods of stimulation, the E-group infants spent more time in active sleep, less time in drowsy wakefulness, and more time with active limb movements. The infants were more active and more likely to be in active sleep during tactile compared with kinesthetic stimulation phases of the intervention.

White-Traut et al., have conducted a series of studies evaluating an intervention that includes auditory, tactile, visual, and vestibular (ATVV) stimulation, based on a procedure developed by Rice (1977) called the Rice Infant Sensorimotor Stimulation (RISS) massage technique. Early studies by this group evaluated the RISS technique (White-Traut & Tubeszewski, 1986; White-Traut & Pate, 1987; White-Traut & Goldman, 1988; White-Traut & Nelson, 1988). Subsequent studies described the intervention as the ATVV intervention (White-Traut, Nelson, Silvestri, et al., 1993, 1997, 1999, 2002). The intervention included continuous efforts to maintain eye contact with the infant throughout

10 minutes of stroking combined with infant-directed talk, followed by 5 minutes of rocking.

White-Traut and Pate (1987) evaluated changes in behavioral states among 16 preterm infants in response to the ATVV stimulation. Infants who received the ATVV intervention demonstrated more time in a quiet alert state during and following the intervention compared with infants in a control group. White-Traut and Goldman (1988) evaluated responses of 16 preterm infants to the ATVV stimulation and found that they responded with slight decreases in body temperature and slight increases in heart and respiratory rates, but that these responses stabilized by the end of the intervention. In a subsequent study with 20 infants assigned to an E and 20 to a C group, White-Traut, Nelson, Silvestri, et al. (1993) found that E infants demonstrated a statistically significant but minimal decrease in $O_2$ sat and an increase in behavioral state toward more alertness during the intervention. During the minute immediately following the intervention, E infants demonstrated more alert behavioral states compared with C-group infants, but there was no difference between the groups in HR or $O_2$ sat levels. In another study, White-Traut, Nelson, Silvestri, et al. (1997) compared responses of 54 clinically stable preterm infants to the different components of the ATVV intervention: auditory, tactile, auditory/tactile/visual, and auditory/tactile/visual/vestibular. Infants receiving any of the interventions with a tactile component demonstrated an increase in behavioral state, HR, and RR during stimulation. Infants receiving only tactile stimulation had a greater percentage of HR greater than 180 bpm, whereas the ATVV group had a greater percentage of HR less than 140 bpm. The authors suggested that the addition of vestibular stimulation might modulate the arousal that is stimulated by tactile stimulation alone.

## Longer-Term Effects of Interventions Combining Tactile with Kinesthetic and/or Vestibular Stimulation

Field, Schanberg, Scafidi, et al. (1986) provided the 15-minute tactile/kinesthetic intervention described earlier to 20 preterm infants who had a mean GA of 31 weeks and mean birth weight 1280 g. The intervention was provided three times daily for 10 days,

beginning when the infants were medically stable. Compared with 20 infants randomly assigned to a C group, E-group infants averaged a 47% higher daily weight gain, were more active and alert, and had more mature habituation, orientation, motor, and range of state behavior on the Brazelton Neonatal Behavioral Assessment Scale (BNBAS). In addition, they were discharged an average of 6 days earlier than C-group infants, resulting in a hospital cost savings of nearly $3000 per infant. Similar findings were obtained from a second study using similar methods with a different sample of 40 stable preterm infants (Kuhn, Schanberg, Field, et al., 1991; Scafidi, Field, Schanberg, et al., 1990). In this study, E-group infants averaged a 21% greater daily weight gain, were discharged 5 days earlier, and had more mature performance on the habituation cluster of the BNBAS scale.

White-Traut et al., have conducted several studies evaluating the long-term outcomes of the RISS and ATVV interventions. White-Traut and Tubeszewski (1986) evaluated the RISS intervention provided for 5 to 10 days for 17 infants. Although there were no significant differences between the E and 16 preterm C-group infants in terms of weight gain or length of hospital stay, results suggested a trend for greater weight gain and shorter hospitalizations among E-group infants. In a subsequent study, White-Traut and Nelson (1988) taught mothers to administer the ATVV intervention four times over the first 3 days after birth. The sample included a total of 33 preterm infants who were 28 to 35 weeks' GA. Mothers in the ATVV group ($n = 11$) had more positive interactions with their infants as measured by the Nursing Child Assessment and Feeding Scale (NCAFS) at the time of NICU discharge, compared with mothers in a control group ($n = 11$) or with mothers who were instructed only to talk or sing to their infants at comparable times to the intervention protocol ($n = 11$).

In two studies that included infants with periventricular leukomalacia (PVL), infants who received the ATVV stimulation program in the NICU were discharged an average of 9 days earlier than infants in a randomly assigned control group (White-Traut, Nelson, Silvestri, et al., 1999, 2002). In one of these studies, E-group infants received the ATVV stimulation from a researcher in the hospital and at home from their mothers until 2 months corrected age

(Nelson, White-Trout, Vasan, et al., 2001). Compared with infants in a randomly assigned control group, E-group infants had better mental and motor development scores and a lower incidence of cerebral palsy at age 1 year. These differences were not statistically significant, perhaps because the 1-year follow up data were available for only 26 of the original 37 infants who enrolled in the study.

## Summary of Studies of Tactile Stimulation

Vickers, Ohlsson, and Horsley (2001) recently published a meta-analysis of 14 controlled clinical trials evaluating the effects of gentle touch and massage interventions on preterm infants. Most of the subjects in the studies reviewed were 30 to 33 weeks' gestation and were medically stable before the start of the intervention. The authors noted that many of the massage interventions also included kinesthetic stimulation, and that although most interventions were provided for 5 to 10 days, one study (Rice, 1977) included massage provided by mothers for 30 days after hospital discharge. The authors concluded that massage and kinesthetic stimulation enhanced weight gain by 15% to 20%, or about 5.1 g per day. The length of hospital stays for infants receiving massage was 6 days fewer than that for infants in control groups. This finding has significant implications for healthcare costs, given the average daily charges for an infant in a NICU. Further research is needed to determine whether such reduced lengths of stay can be replicated with larger and more diverse samples. Infants receiving massage had more optimal scores on BNBAS scales for habituation, motor maturity, and range of state. There was not sufficient evidence to indicate the effects of massage on other developmental outcomes such as Bayley Developmental Index examination scores. Massage reduced postnatal complications, although 95% of the weighting for this analysis came from a study with a sample of only 30 infants. Massage, kinesthetic stimulation, and gentle touch did not have any adverse effects on the infants studied. Vickers, Ohlsson, and Horsley (2001) noted that there were methodologic problems in the reviewed studies including a failure to blind observers who assessed outcomes, and a failure to ensure that infants in experimental and control groups were treated similarly in all aspects other than the experi-

these methodologic [Oh]rsley, et al. (2001) [su]fficient evidence to [til] massage should be [NICU]. The authors advocate [studying t]he effects of massage [on outc]omes, controlling for methodologic problems by: (1) concealment of treatment allocation until the subject was entered into the trial; (2) ensuring the infants were treated similarly in all respects other than the experimental intervention; (3) blinding of observers assessing outcomes to the treatment assignment; (4) assessing whether there are differences in withdrawals from the study based on treatment group assignment; and (5) assessing longer term developmental outcomes.

## Parental Involvement

A key component of developmental care is providing support to parents to promote their involvement and competence as the primary nurturers of their infants (Als & Gilkerson, 1997). A key strategy for promoting parental involvement is incorporating principles of family-centered care (FCC). In this section, we review studies describing experiences and responses of parents to the birth of a high-risk infant, discuss principles of FCC, and review studies evaluating interventions for parents of high-risk infants in the NICU.

### Responses of Parents to the Birth of a High-Risk Infant

Findings from several studies suggest that the birth of a preterm or high-risk infant represents a crisis for parents, and that they often respond to this crisis with feelings of guilt, anxiety, anger, helplessness, depression, and chronic sorrow. Promoting parental involvement in caring for their high-risk infants might help parents cope with their negative emotional reactions.

Caplan, Mason, and Kaplan (2000), in a classic report originally published in 1965 and reprinted in 2000, presented findings from four related studies describing parental responses to the crisis associated with the birth of a premature infant. Data for the four studies were collected primarily during a series of home visits to a total of 86 families of preterm infants. In one of the studies, Kaplan and Mason

(1960) identified four major psychological tasks that appeared essential for parents to deal with the crisis of a preterm birth: (1) anticipatory grief; (2) acknowledging feelings of failure due to not delivering a normal, full-term baby; (3) resumption of the process of relating to the baby; and (4) understanding how a premature baby differs from a normal baby in terms of special needs and growth patterns. In another study, Caplan (1960) differentiated characteristics of parents who subsequently had healthy and unhealthy mental health outcomes. Parents who had healthy outcomes were characterized by efforts to gather as much information as possible about the infant, had realistic understandings of their infants' situations, were aware of and expressed their negative feelings, and actively sought help from within the family or community in relation to the tasks associated with caring for their baby. Parents rated as having unhealthy outcomes demonstrated little effort to seek information about their infants, and tended to suppress or avoid thoughts about the infant's situation. These parents rarely admitted or expressed negative feelings other than blaming others, and seemed unable to seek or accept help. Findings also suggested that it was possible to predict parents' mental health outcomes based on parents' patterns of reactions to their infants and the high-risk birth (Mason, 1963).

Findings from a number of studies have indicated that parents often experience anxiety and depression following a high-risk birth (Gennaro, 1986, 1988). Gennaro (1986) described high levels of anxiety in mothers of 40 preterm infants. There was no difference in the levels of anxiety of mothers based on the level of risk of their infants, suggesting that mothers of moderately ill preterm infants might be just as anxious as mothers of more critically ill infants.

Blackburn and Lowen (1986) conducted an exploratory survey to compare reactions of 59 parents and 83 grandparents to a preterm birth. Both parents and grandparents reported emotional reactions, such as anxiety, disappointment, grief, shock, and fear, but mothers reported more intense experiences with these feelings. Parents experienced higher levels of frustration than did grandparents. Only 11% of the grandmothers, and no grandfathers, participated in caregiving activities in the NICU. Although most grandparents were satisfied with their level of participation in the infant's care, 66% of the parents identified activities that they wanted grandparents to be able to participate in, such as touching, caressing, and holding the infant, or relieving parents at the infant's bedside.

Raines (1998) conducted qualitative interviews with 14 mothers of infants hospitalized in a NICU to explore the mothers' values and their preferences for involvement in the care of their infants. Mothers consistently identified their desire to be involved in their infants' care. There was consensus that they were told what would be or had been done to their infants, but mothers indicated that their participation was not usually solicited by the NICU staff. Many mothers identified a lack of knowledge related to the infant's needs, and although some wanted additional information, many did not want to ask for such information for fear of distracting staff from the infant's care.

Fenwick, Barclay, and Schmied (2001) conducted a grounded theory study of women's experiences of mothering in the NICU in Australia. Data were gathered from interviews with 28 mothers and 20 nurses, as well as observations of nurse-parent interactions and observations in the NICU. Women indicated that they gained access to their infants through nurses, and, thus, they saw the nurse-mother relationship as significantly influencing their mothering experience. Nursing interactions that facilitated the mothering role were consistent with principles of FCC, and included nurturing actions that helped mothers learn about their infants and participate in their care. Inhibitive nursing interactions, on the other hand, led to behaviors that the researchers categorized as "struggling to mother." Inhibitive nursing interactions incorporated an authoritarian style in which the nurse maintained a position as expert in control of the infant. Women who experienced such interactions described feeling disaffected, guarding, and disenfranchised. These findings reinforce the importance of incorporating principles of FCC in promoting positive parenting and minimizing stress for parents of hospitalized infants.

A number of studies have explored parents' perceptions of sources of support during their infant's NICU stay, based on the recognition that social support can be critical in helping to cope with any crisis or stressful situation. Prudhoe and Peters (1995) interviewed parents and grandparents of 14 preterm infants to identify sources of support and coping strategies. Informal support from family and friends was the most frequently identified type of support used by parents. Miles, Carlson, and Funk (1996) interviewed 158 parents 1 week after their infant's admission to the NICU (T1) to identify parents' perceptions of social support they had received. A week later (T2), they conducted a second interview with 89 of these parents. Parents reported receiving high levels of support from the NICU nurses. At T1 and T2, mothers reported the highest source of support as the baby's father, and identified nurses as the second highest source of support. Fathers reported similar perceptions at T2, but at T1 they reported that the nurses were the highest source of support, followed by the baby's mother. These findings suggest that nurses have an important role in providing support to help parents cope with the crisis of a high-risk birth.

Parents might experience increased stress at the time of the infant's discharge from the NICU, or transfer to another hospital before discharge home. Slattery, Flanagan, Cronenwett, et al. (1998) evaluated factors associated with the quality of parents' experiences associated with the "back transfer" of their infants from a regional level III NICU to a level I or II community NICU (CNICU) prior to hospital discharge. Experiences that are more positive were associated with fewer perceived differences in nursing and medical practices between the settings, fewer infant problems after transfer, and more pretransfer preparation. These findings suggest that communication between healthcare providers and preparation of parents can help reduce stressors associated with back transfer.

Fraley (1986) suggested that parents of premature infants often do not fully resolve their feelings about the loss of the expected normal pregnancy, and, as a result, might experience prolonged grief, which she labeled as "chronic sorrow." Hummel and Eastman (1991) administered questionnaires to 103 parents whose children attended a high-risk infant follow-up clinic to determine whether parents continued to experience grief and sorrow following their infants' discharge from the NICU. Mothers reported more distressing feelings and emotions than did fathers, including frustration, shock, emptiness, depression, hurt, irritability, anger, and feeling cut off and isolated. Different factors were associated with feelings of grief, loss, and fear in response to different potentially stressful experiences (e.g., during the initial hospitalization, a later illness of the child, the child's surgery, when first taking the baby home, visits to the follow-up clinic, or when parents perceived that the child might have a developmental delay).

## Factors Associated with Stress for Parents of High-Risk Infants

There are many factors that contribute to parental anxiety and distress following the birth of a high-risk infant, including the unexpected pregnancy outcome, parent-infant separation, hospitalization-related stresses, and the physical and behavioral characteristics of the infant (Harrison, 1997). The unexpected pregnancy outcome might be associated with uncertainty about the infant's condition and prognosis (Bennett & Slade, 1991; Gennaro, Brooten, Roncoli, et al., 1993). Separation from their infants can result in parents feeling a loss of control and can disrupt the attachment process (Bennett & Slade, 1991; Niven, Wiszniewski, & AlRoomi, 1993). Miles (1989) found that many aspects of the hospitalization were stressful to parents, including malfunctioning equipment; the sounds of alarms; seeing the infant turn blue or pale or stop breathing; observing the infant in pain, not knowing how to help the infant; and feeling that the staff were not communicating openly about the infant's condition. Aspects of the infant's physical and behavioral characteristics that can be stressful to parents include preterm infants' large and elongated heads, thin extremities, transparent skin, congenital defects, and immature reflexes, social behaviors, and cries (Frodi, Lamb, Leavitt, et al., 1978; Kaplan & Mason, 1960; Johnson & Grubbs, 1975; Miles, 1989).

Shields-Poe and Pinelli (1997) examined variables associated with stress in neonatal intensive care units (NICU) among a sample of 212 parents.

Parental trait anxiety and their perception of the infant's morbidity were the most significant predictors of their overall stress scores. Seeing the baby at birth or at transfer was associated with lower levels of stress than first seeing the baby in the NICU. One factor that was associated with increased stress for fathers was a discrepancy between the father's perception of the infant's morbidity status, and the actual morbidity of the infant. This finding suggests that clear explanations of the infant's health status might help to reduce stress for parents, particularly for fathers.

Miles, Funk, and Kasper (1991, 1992) developed a model to explain sources of stress and support experienced by parents of preterm infants. The model has been tested in numerous studies and refined as new data accumulate (Miles & Holditch-Davis, 1997). The model posits that sources of stress for parents include personal and family factors; prenatal and perinatal experiences; infant illness, treatments, and appearance; concerns about infant outcome; and loss of the parental role. Healthcare providers can provide much needed support to parents, or they might hinder parents' ability to cope with the NICU experience. Holditch-Davis and Miles (2000) reported the results of a qualitative study in which 31 mothers were asked to tell stories of their NICU experiences, when their preterm infants were 6 months corrected age. The analysis of the interview data confirmed the six major concepts of the Preterm Parent Distress Model.

Miles and Holditch-Davis (1997) summarized two decades of research related to parenting preterm infants, and presented a framework that expanded the parental stress model and identified pathways of influence in parenting prematurely born children. In this model, three factors were identified as interacting together prior to the infant's admission to the NICU: preexisting and current personal and family factors; prenatal, labor, and delivery experiences; and the birth of the preterm infant. In the NICU the three major factors identified were loss of the normal parental role; infant severity of illness, treatment, and appearance; and parental concerns about the infant's outcome. These various factors contribute to parental emotional distress, which subsequently influences the

parent's perception of the child and can lead to compensatory parenting and an altered parent-child relationship that influences child health and development outcomes.

## Summary of Research Related to Parental Reactions to a High-Risk Birth

Findings from studies conducted during the past 40 years suggest that parents experience a variety of stressors and emotional reactions following the birth of a high-risk infant, including anxiety, depression, guilt, and grief. Factors that influence parental reactions include personal and family factors; prenatal and perinatal experiences; infant illness, treatments, and appearance; concerns about infant outcome; and loss of the parental role (Miles, Funk, & Kasper, 1991, 1992; Holditch-Davis & Miles, 2000). Parents want to be involved in their infant's care, and have identified nurses as important sources of support in the NICU (Miles, Carlson, & Funk, 1996). However, some nursing interactions can inhibit the development of positive-parent interaction patterns (Fenwick, Barclay, & Schmied, 2001). The next section describes principles of FCC that have been identified as critical for helping parents adjust to the stressors associated with having a high-risk infant in the NICU.

## Principles of Family-Centered Care

Although the research suggests that there are common emotional reactions to the birth of a high-risk infant, it must be recognized that individual reactions vary, and that each parent develops different and unique coping strategies and styles (Sydnor-Greenberg & Dokken, 2000). Hurst (1993) stressed the need for assessing and documenting parental perceptions and reactions to their infants and to the NICU experience, to develop individualized and comprehensive care and promote parental involvement. During the past 20 years there has been increasing recognition of the importance of implementing principles of FCC in neonatal and pediatric settings—to promote optimal coping among families, and to empower parents as their child's optimal and most important caregivers. Although the specific definitions of FCC vary, most definitions encompass the four basic components outlined by the Institute for Family Centered Care (1998). In family-centered health care:

1. People are treated with dignity and respect
2. Health care providers communicate and share complete and unbiased information with patients and families in ways that are affirming and useful
3. Individuals and family members build on their strengths by participating in experiences that enhance control and independence
4. Collaboration among patients, families, and providers occurs in policy and program development and professional education, as well as in the delivery of care

Similar, but more specific, principles of FCC were developed during a 1992 meeting of physicians and parents of prematurely born infants that was planned to discuss problems experienced by parents and to explore possible solutions (Harrison, 1993) (Box 14-1). Johnson (1995) noted that FCC "empowers families and fosters independence; supports family caregiving and decision making; respects family choices; builds on family strengths; and involves families in all aspects of the planning, delivery, and evaluation of health services" (pp. 11-12).

Caregiving practices that reflect these principles include developing family resource rooms and parent-support groups, NICU designs that include family-friendly signage and spaces for families, including spaces for rest, child-care, and meal preparation. When FCC is implemented, parents are not seen as "visitors," but rather as members of the health team, and each family has a consistent team of healthcare providers who communicate with them openly, honestly, and frequently. They have access to the infant's chart and are encouraged to participate actively in rounds; their opinions are solicited and valued; and they work with other members of the team to develop policy and plan programs for the NICU (Harrison, 1993; Johnson, 1995). Developing a positive rapport with families and communicating with them in supportive ways are key to FCC. McGrath and Conliffe-Torres (1996) noted that "how information is said is often more important than what is said" (p. 379).

Gale and Franck (1998) incorporated FCC principles into a set of proposed standards for the care of parents of NICU infants (Box 14-2). Gretebeck, Shaffer, and Bishop-Kurylo (1998) developed clinical pathways for family-oriented developmental care in the NICU. The pathways included specific interventions designed to promote family involvement (Box 14-3). Staff on each shift could record whether the interventions were achieved, partially achieved, not addressed because of lack of opportunity, or still needed to be done. Krebs (1998) also developed a clinical pathway that focused on promoting parent-preterm infant interaction through education.

The expansion of technology in neonatal care has resulted in significant improvements in morbidity and mortality rates of the infants, but also has presented challenges to implementing FCC principles by increasing fragmentation of care, and demanding increased staff attention to the complex technology that they are required to master (Gordin & Johnson, 1999). Many developing countries that lack resources to support the use of new technologic innovations have incorporated creative strategies for involving parents in the care of their preterm and high-risk infants. For example, KC was first described and promoted in Colombia in a unit where preterm infants were dying from infections resulting from the practice of sharing beds and equipment due to limited resources. Consequently, mothers were encouraged to hold their infants skin-to-skin, until the infants could be discharged home. This practice decreased infant mortality and abandonment, decreased the incidence of apnea and bradycardia, and enhanced maternal lactation (Gale & VandenBerg, 1998). In Tallin, Estonia, neonatologist Adik Levin has pioneered the Humane Neonatal Care Initiative to promote minimum aggressive therapy and contact between sick newborns and medical staff, and maximum contact between mothers and infants. Mothers of preterm infants room in with their infants and assume primary responsibility for their infants' care, with nurses serving primarily as resources (Levin, 1994, 1999; Harrison & Klaus, 1994).

There are many barriers to fully implementing FCC in the NICU. Staff might have concerns about confidentiality issues if parents are involved in rounds and have access to the infant's health record (Grunwald, 1997), or it might be perceived that implementing FCC will take more time from their already overloaded work schedules (Griffin, 1998a,

Box **14-1** PRINCIPLES FOR FAMILY-CENTERED CARE DRAFTED BY PARENTS

Family-centered neonatal care should be based on open and honest communication between parents and professionals on medical and ethical issues.

1. To work with professionals in making informed treatment choices, parents must have available to them the same facts and interpretation of those facts as the professionals, including medical information presented in meaningful formats, information about uncertainties surrounding treatments, information from parents whose children have been in similar medical situations, and access to the chart and rounds discussions.
2. In medical situations involving very high mortality and morbidity, great suffering, and/or significant medical controversy, fully informed parents should have the right to make decisions regarding aggressive treatment for their infants.
3. Expectant parents should be offered information about adverse pregnancy outcomes and be given the opportunity to state in advance their treatment preferences if their baby is born extremely prematurely and/or critically ill.
4. Parents and professionals must work together to acknowledge and alleviate the pain of infants in intensive care.
5. Parents and professionals must work together to ensure an appropriate environment for babies in the NICU.
6. Parents and professionals should work together to ensure the safety and efficacy of neonatal treatments.
7. Parents and professionals should work together to develop nursery policies and programs that promote parenting skills and encourage maximum involvement of families with their hospitalized infant.
8. Parents and professionals must work together to promote meaningful long-term follow-up for all high-risk NICU survivors.
9. Parents and professionals must acknowledge that critically ill newborns can be harmed by overtreatment as well as by undertreatment, and we must insist that our laws and treatment policies be based on compassion. We must work together to promote awareness of the needs of NICU survivors with disabilities to ensure adequate support for them and their families. We must work together to decrease disability through universal prenatal care.

Adapted from Harrison, H. (1993). The principles for family-centered care. *Pediatrics, 92,* 643-650.
*NICU,* Neonatal intensive care unit.

1998b). Johnson (1995), however, suggests that implementing FCC ultimately lightens staff loads. NICU caregivers can also be limited by their own values and experiences, and might judge families based on their own conceptions rather than accepting and respecting differences in coping styles and patterns (Sydnor-Greenberg & Dokken, 2000). Some neonatal nurses are reluctant to give up control over the infant's care, and have a protective attitude toward the infant, fearing that sharing responsibility for the infant's care with parents might jeopardize the infant's welfare (Fenwick, Barclay, & Schmied, 2001).

There are many excellent resources that can be used to educate staff about FCC principles, evaluate the extent to which FCC principles are incorporated into the care provided in a given NICU, and implement change to promote FCC. The Institute for Family-Centered Care (IFCC) is a nonprofit organization that serves as an excellent resource for families, clinicians, educators, and policy-makers (see their website at www.familycenteredcare.org). Other resources for NICU staff and parents are listed in Boxes 14-4 and 14-5.

### Research Evaluating Programs to Promote Involvement of Parents of NICU Infants

The concept of FCC incorporates many specific strategies and different elements, as does the concept of developmental care. During the past 20 years,

## Box **14-2**   Proposed Standards for Care of Parents of NICU Infants*

Each NICU should develop formal policies, guidelines, and resources to ensure that the following activities and supports are available and offered to all NICU parents:

- Parental holding of NICU infants*
- Encouragement and support for parents to perform skin-to skin holding of their infant (Kangaroo care)*
- Support and guidance for parents to provide handling and physical care to their infant
- A policy of unrestricted parental participation in care and regular opportunities for inclusion of siblings
- Free child care provided by the hospital for siblings of NICU infants offered at least once per week
- Support group and networking opportunities for parents, including access to Internet support
- Parent-friendly signage (bulletin board, message board, orientation booklet)
- Information and resource materials for parents, including care of the newborn in the NICU and after discharge, and emotional and physical support for parents; provided in different reading levels, depths, and media formats
- Individualized education and support for parents, focused on helping parents understand their infant's behaviors[†]
- Teaching parents methods to reduce stress in their infant and promote appropriate development[†]
- Collaboration between NICU staff and parents to alleviate pain in the infant
- Affirmation of the parents' role as the ultimate decision makers about their infant's care
- Facilitation of parent's access to the infant's medical record, discussion of their infant's care during daily medical rounds, and medical ethics consultation
- Personalized environment for each infant's parents (e.g., individualized bedside, use of infant's first name, personal clothing)
- Recognition that the infant belongs to the parents and not to the NICU staff (i.e., nurses avoid referring to the infant as "my baby")
- Primary nursing care
- Breastfeeding support (i.e., lactation consultation, breast-feeding room, supplies, equipment, and storage)
- Designated "parent-only" space in (or close to) the NICU
- Chaplain services for families
- Early contact with parents (i.e., within 24 hours) by NICU nurses to assess attachment and how parents are doing (physically and emotionally) and to offer support
- Care provided by all members of the healthcare team, who are knowledgeable and sensitive to cultural, ethnic, and spiritual values of parents
- Preparation of parents for the transition to home, beginning well before discharge, and including contact with community follow-up services, practicing of infant care skills, and rooming-in before discharge
- Provision of maximal privacy for parents at the infant's bedside (e.g., curtains, screens) and private consultation rooms close to the NICU where staff can discuss the infant's care with the family in private

From Gale, G., & Franck, L.S. (1998). Toward a standard of care for parents of infants in the neonatal intensive care unit. *Critical Care Nurse, 18,* 62-74.

*NICU,* Neonatal intensive care unit

*Policies should be based on the infant's physiologic stability (not on weight or age alone).

[†]This service should be provided by nurses trained in neonatal developmental assessment, with ongoing support and consultation from a specialist in infant development.

Box 1**4**-3 Interventions to Promote Family Involvement

| Outcome | Intervention |
|---|---|
| Family receives social support and practical information | Give parents suggestions for nonstressful interaction with infant. |
| | Establish a plan for regular communication. |
| | Discuss ICN handbook with parents. |
| | Orient parents to resource library. |
| Family becomes educated about and involved with infant's developmental progress | Show parents their infants' stress signals and calming techniques. |
| | Offer kangaroo care or holding. |
| | Encourage parents to help during feeds and diaper changes. |
| | Encourage parents to use resource library or discuss books read or videotapes viewed. |
| Family is prepared for discharge | Facilitate participation of parents in all routine infant care activities. |
| | Initiate discharge teaching plans. |

Adapted from Gretebeck, R.J., Shaffer, D., &Bishop-Kurylo, D. (1998). Clinical pathways for family-oriented developmental care in the intensive care nursery. *Journal of Perinatal and Neonatal Nursing, 12,* 70-80.

researchers have begun to evaluate specific interventions that reflect FCC principles and that are designed to promote parental involvement and help reduce the stressors associated with the birth of a high-risk infant. Patteson and Barnard (1990) reviewed 19 studies evaluating programs designed to enhance parenting of preterm infants, and noted that 16 of the programs had positive outcomes. Successful programs involved active parent-infant interaction and focused on promoting parental satisfaction with caregiving by helping them learn to understand infants' cues and developmental needs. Griffin, Wishba, and Kavanaugh (1998) suggested that interventions to reduce stress and promote parental involvement in the NICU should include anticipatory guidance, to help parents process feelings surrounding their infant's birth and NICU experiences, and to help parents understand their infants' appearance, behavior, and conditions, promoting parent-infant interaction, and providing support. This section includes a review of studies evaluating interventions for families of NICU infants. Although many studies have evaluated long-term, home-based interventions provided after the infant's NICU discharge, the studies reviewed in this section focused only on interventions provided in the NICU.

## Studies Evaluating Educational or Support Programs Provided by Professionals

Interventions for parents that have been provided in the NICU have included single teaching sessions as well as more comprehensive, long-term programs. Griffin, Kavanaugh, Soto, et al. (1997) noted that although many hospitals offer tours of the NICU to parents with high-risk pregnancies, the effectiveness of these tours has not been systematically evaluated. These researchers questioned whether such tours might actually increase rather than decrease parental anxiety, noting that nurses have observed mothers crying following the NICU tour. They conducted naturalistic, qualitative interviews with 13 parents who had toured a NICU during their high-risk pregnancies, and subsequently coded the interviews to identify common themes. In general, the parents perceived the tour as having many benefits, including decreasing their fears, inspiring hope for their baby's prognosis, providing reassurance about NICU care, and preparing them for their infant's hospitalization. Although many parents acknowledged that the tour had been frightening or overwhelming, they acknowledged that it prepared them for the baby's admission, and all recommended that parents of high-risk infants should be offered tours prior to the infant's birth.

Box **14-4**   Resources and Training Organizations for NICU Staff

**GENERAL ORGANIZATIONS**

Association for the Care of Children's Health (ACCH)
7910 Woodmont Avenue, Suite 300
Bethesda, MD 20814
The ACCH is an educational and advocacy organization with a multidisciplinary membership of professionals and families in pursuit of excellence in caring for children and families. Parent Care Inc., an organization dedicated to support for parents in the NICU, became part of the ACCH in 1996.

Institute for Family Centered Care (IFCC)
7900 Wisconsin Avenue, Suite 405
Bethesda, MD 20814
(301) 652-0281
Website: *www.familycenteredcare.org*
The IFCC is a nonprofit organization that promotes the understanding and practice of family-centered care. It provides consultation, training, and technical assistance to hospitals, clinical practices, educational institutions, community organizations, and state and federal agencies. It facilitates collaboration among staff, patients, families, and others in bringing about change in newborn intensive care, pediatrics, maternity care, and programs serving other adults and their families.

**TRAINING IN NEONATAL DEVELOPMENTAL INTERVENTIONS**

Neonatal Individualized Developmental Care and Assessment Program (NIDCAP®; includes seven U.S. training centers and international sites).
Heidelise Als, PhD, Director
Enders Pediatric Research Laboratories, M 29
The Children's Hospital
Boston, MA 02115

NICU Training Project
Virginia Wyly, PhD and Jack Allen, MA
State College, State University of New York
Buffalo, NY 14222

Wee Care® Neonatal Systems Developmental Care Training Programs
Children's Medical Ventures
541 Main Street, Suite 220
South Weymouth, MA 02190

**RESOURCES FOR NICU ARCHITECTURE AND DESIGN FOR NICU SETTINGS**

Design Planning for Newborn Intensive Care
Planning tools and slides on innovative approaches to the architecture and design for newborn intensive care units. Cost: $55. Available from Institute for Family-Centered Care, 7900 Wisconsin Avenue, Suite 405, Bethesda, MD 20814; (301) 652-0281

Newborn Intensive Care: Resources for Family-Centered Practice
Assessment tools, guides for family-centered practice, participatory exercises, and bibliography. Cost: $40. Available from Institute for Family-Centered Care, 7900 Wisconsin Ave, Suite 405, Bethesda, MD 20814; (301) 652-0281.

Box **14-4**   Resources and Training Organizations for NICU Staff—cont'd

**BOOKS FOR NICU STAFF**

Kenner, C.K., & Lott, J.W. (Eds.) (2003). *Comprehensive neonatal nursing: A physiologic perspective.* (3rd ed.). St. Louis: W.B. Saunders.

Merenstein, G.B., & Gardner, S. (Eds.) (2002). *Handbook of neonatal intensive care* (5th ed.). St. Louis: Mosby.

Hinker, P., & Moreno, L.A. (1994). *Developmentally supportive care: Theory and application* (self-study module). South Weymouth, MA: Children's Medical Ventures Inc. Telephone: (800) 377-3449.

A great tool for learning the basics of the behavioral signals of infants.

*Infant and family-centered developmental care guidelines.* (1993). Petaluma, CA: National Association of Neonatal Nurses. Telephone: (800) 451-3795.

A helpful resource for writing protocols.

Wyly, M.V. (1995). *Premature infants and their families: Developmental interventions.* San Diego, CA: Singular Publishing Group Inc.

An excellent resource on interventions with infants and families in the NICU.

Klaus, M.H., Kennell, J.H., & Klaus, P.H. (1996). *Bonding: Building the foundations of secure attachment and independence.* London: Cedar.

One of the foundational works in the field, recently updated and expanded.

**CATALOGS FOR DEVELOPMENTAL CARE PRODUCTS AND PARENTING RESOURCES**

Centering Corporation
1531 North Saddle Creek Road
Omaha, NE 68104

Child Development Media Inc.
5632 Van Nuys Boulevard, Suite 286
Van Nuys, CA 94104

Children's Medical Ventures (developmental care products)
541 Main Street
South Weymouth, MA 02190
(800) 377-3449

Childbirth Graphics
PO Box 21207
Waco, TX 76702-1207

Communication Skill Builders
555 Academic Court
San Antonio, TX 78204-2498
(800) 228-0572

A Place to Remember (NICU bereavement resources)
1885 University Avenue, Suite 110
St. Paul, MN 55104
(800) 631-0973

Therapy Skill Builders
3830 East Bellevue/PO Box 42050-TS4
Tucson, AZ 85573
(602) 323-7500

VORT Corporation
PO Box 60880
Palo Alto, CA 94306
(415) 322-8282

**VIDEOS**

*Newborn intensive care: Changing practice, changing attitudes.* (1997). Bethesda, MD: Institute for Family-Centered Care. Telephone: (301) 652-0281. Cost: $100.

This nine-segment training video and user's guide describes the changes in family-centered and developmental care in the NICU at Phoenix Children's Hospital. Highly recommended.

Adapted from Gale, G., & Franck, L.S. (1998). Toward a standard of care for parents of infants in the neonatal intensive care unit. *Critical Care Nurse, 18,* 62-74.

*NICU,* Neonatal intensive care unit.

## Box **14-5**   RESOURCES FOR PARENTS

### BOOKS AND BOOKLETS

Zaichkin, J. (1996). *Newborn intensive care: What every parent needs to know.* Petaluma, CA: NICU Ink. Telephone: (888) NIC-Ulnk. Cost: $25.00.

This book is an excellent comprehensive resource for parents and covers most aspects of high-risk neonatal care (not just preemies). Some parents might find the amount of information overwhelming. The cost can be reduced by buying in quantity.

*Parenting your baby in the NICU: Suggestions for active parenting during your baby's stay.* (1995). Omaha, NE: Meyer Rehabilitation Institute Media Center. Telephone: (402) 559-7467. Cost: Approximately $2.50.

This beautifully designed pamphlet has removable cards inside that describe caregiving activities for parents at different stages of their baby's hospitalization. Developed at the University of Nebraska Medical Center, it can be used in almost all NICUs.

Fern, D., & Graves, C. (1996). *Developmental care guide for families with infants in the NICU.* South Weymouth, MA: Children's Medical Ventures. Telephone: (800) 377-3449. Cost: $1.00.

This booklet was written by two occupational therapists with many years of experience working with parents in the NICU. The language and pictures are reassuring. It can be purchased individually or by the case.

Flushman, B., Gale, G., Lackey, S., et al. (1991). *My special start: A guide for parents in the neonatal intensive care unit.* Palo Alto, CA: VORT Corp. Telephone: (415) 322-8282. Cost: About $6.00.

This pictorial booklet is written at a simple level. It discusses the ups and downs of parenting the NICU baby, how to read cues, and ways to protect the baby from stress. The second book in the series, *A Special Start*, is an excellent training tool for volunteers holding babies in the NICU.

Hussey-Gardner, B. (1988). *Understanding my signals.* Palo Alto, CA: VORT Corp. Telephone: (415) 322-8282. Cost: about $2.00.

This easy-to-read booklet is written from the infant's point of view and has pictures showing approach and advance signals. It is available in English and Spanish.

Centerwall, S., Boom, K., & Centerwall, W. (1987). *Low birth weight.* Redmond, WA: Medic Publishing. Telephone (206) 881-2883. Cost: About $1.35, but less if purchased by the case. Available from Medic Publishing, PO Box 89, Redmond, WA 98073-0089.

This booklet answers parents' questions about getting ready for their baby's discharge from the NICU. Although it is somewhat wordy, its tone is quite supportive. Helpful illustrations and photos illustrate developmental issues. It is a good source for parents who like to read.

*Your healing touch: For families and infants during hospitalization.* (1997). Albuquerque, NM: The Developmental Care Program, Children's Hospital of New Mexico. Telephone: (505) 272-3946. Cost: Free.

This pamphlet for parents is about infant massage they can do in the NICU. All the techniques shown are gentle and are appropriate for most infants in stable condition. The publication was produced by infant development specialists at the University of New Mexico.

Manginello, F., & DiGeronimo, T. (1993). *Your premature baby.* Omaha, NE: Centering Corp. Telephone: (402) 553-1200. Cost: $15.95.

This book is the classic resource for parents of preemies. Although much of the medical information is now out of date, the information about parenting and coping strategies remains extremely reassuring. It has wonderful photographs.

### VIDEOS

*Interview with Rochelle.* (1989). Oakland, CA: Children's Hospital Oakland. Time: 9 minutes. Available from Gay Gale at (510) 527-8999. Cost: $20.00.

This videotape is an edited 9-minute interview with an articulate low-income black woman for whom kangaroo care had an important impact on her relationship with her premature daughter. She is shown holding her daughter skin to skin.

*Kangaroo care: A parent's touch.* (1996). Chicago, IL: Northwestern Memorial Hospital. Time: Approximately 20 minutes. Telephone: (312) 908-7654. Cost: $60.00.

**B̲ox **14-5** R̲ESOURCES FOR P̲ARENTS—CONT'D**

This videotape covers physiologic benefits, developmental benefits, twins, and paternal Kangaroo care. It is also a good resource for teaching staff.

*Special beginning.* (1996). Omaha, NE: Centering Corp. Time: 30 minutes. Telephone: (402) 553-1200. Cost: $50.00.

NICU parents share their experiences and encouragement with new NICU parents.

*Getting to know your NICU.* (1996). Columbus, Ohio: Ross Products Division. Cost: Free.

*Special delivery: Understanding your premature infant.* (1982). Van Nuys, CA: Child Development Media. Time: 20 minutes. Telephone: (818) 994-0933.

This videotape was made at Children's Hospital, Oakland, California. The format is a letter of encouragement written from one parent to another that describes experiences of having a preemie. Supportive ways to participate in care and protect the baby from environmental stress are discussed. The emotions expressed are timeless. This tape is especially good for parents of newly admitted infants.

Als, H., et al. (1982). *Prematurely yours.* Boston, MA: Polymorph Films. Time: 20 minutes. Available in English and Spanish. Telephone: (800) 370-3456. Cost: $295.

Made by Heidelise Als and her team at Brigham and Women's Hospital in Boston, this video discusses signals and cues of the infant ready for interaction with parents. An excellent resource for parents, this tape might have more relevance for the parents when their infant is extubated.

Als, H., et al. (1985). *To have and not to hold.* Als H, et al. Boston, Mass: Polymorph Films. Time: 20 minutes. Telephone: (800) 370-3456. Cost: $295.00.

Made by Heidelise Als and her team at Brigham and Women's Hospital in Boston, this powerful video emphatically describes coping strategies for parents with babies in the NICU. A multicultural parent group is interviewed.

*A joyful tear: Parents of preemies remember.* (1988). Columbus, OH: Ross Products Division. Cost: Free. This wonderful video has timeless and moving content.

*Your baby and you.* (1992). Tucson, AR: Therapy Skill Builders. Time: 30 minutes. Telephone: (602) 323-7500. Cost: $110; includes 6 booklets in English and Spanish.

This video describes behavior of infants, behavioral cues, communication, and ways for parents to promote organization in their infant. It might be too much information for most parents to digest in a single sitting. English Spanish versions are included on the same tape. Accompanying booklets are excellent, and the material in them is easier to digest than that on the videotape. The booklets can be purchased separately.

**INTERNET RESOURCES FOR PARENTS**

The Internet abounds with resources for parents of NICU infants. Here are a few that come highly recommended. For a list of Web links to NICU parents' resources:

*www.medsch.wisc.edu/childrenshosp/parents_of_preemies/references.html*

*members.aol.com/MarAim/preemie.htm* (scroll to the Internet Resources section)

Parents of Preemies

*www.medsch.wisc.edu/childrenshosp/parents_of_preemies/overview.html*

This site provides NICU information and education, references, books, on-line/Internet resources, and support organizations. Much information is relevant for all NICU parents. The material is well written and nicely organized.

Preemie-L

To subscribe, send an e-mail message to majordomo@yarra.vicnet.net.au. In the body of your message type: SUBSCRIBE PREEMIE-L. (your name) but without the parentheses.

This is a discussion and support group for parents of infants born 6 weeks or more before the infants' due date. Other people who have an interest in premature children and neonatology, including doctors, nurses, and relatives, are also welcome to subscribe.

*Continued*

Box **14-5**   Resources for Parents—cont'd

Lactnet
To subscribe, send an e-mail message to listserv@library.unmed.edu. In the body of the message type: SUBSCRIBE LACTNET (your name and title) but without the parentheses.
LACTNET is a discussion group for those interested in issues associated with breastfeeding and lactation.

From Gale, G., & Franck, L.S. (1998). Toward a standard of care for parents of infants in the neonatal intensive care unit. *Critical Care Nurse, 18*, 62-74.
*NICU*, Neonatal intensive care unit.

An essential component of FCC is providing parents with information and education about their infant's condition and care, and about the NICU environment. Although most NICUs provide parents with written information, parents can become overwhelmed with such information if it is not presented at times when they are most ready to receive it, or they can misplace it and then be unable to find the information when they subsequently need it. Costello, Bracht, Van Camp, et al. (1996) described the use of parent information binders (PIB) to individualize education for parents of preterm infants. The PIB is a three-ring binder that is divided into five color-coded sections that include information about admission, feeding, parenting, clinical issues, and discharge planning. NICU staff provides parents with information as they need it. The binder was kept at the infant's bedside and was accessible to all of the infant's healthcare providers to provide a record of information previously shared with the family and to help ensure the provision of consistent information to the families. The authors noted that parents rated the binders positively.

Short-term interventions for parents in the NICU have included educational programs focused on preterm infant behaviors and characteristics and on common parental responses to the birth of a high-risk infant. Harrison and Twardosz (1986) provided mothers with a 1-hour instructional program that included watching a videotape and reviewing information in a pamphlet about physical and behavioral characteristics of preterm infants and common parental emotional reactions to a preterm birth. There were no differences in subsequent measures of maternal perceptions or behaviors comparing mothers who received the special instruction with mothers in one of two control groups.

Several studies have evaluated the effects of demonstrating behavioral assessment examinations to parents on subsequent parent-infant interaction patterns. Harrison et al. (1991) expanded the educational intervention tested by Harrison and Twardosz (1986). In addition to viewing the videotape and discussing a pamphlet describing preterm infant behaviors, 10 mothers in the first experimental group also observed the researcher assess their infants using the Brazelton Neonatal Behavioral Assessment Scale (BNBAS), and then assessed their infants using a modified version of the BNBAS, the Mother's Assessment of the Behavior of her Infant (MABI) scale. Ten mothers in a second experimental group received brief information about the MABI scale and then were asked to use it to assess their infants. A third group of 10 mothers (the control group) received routine NICU support but did not participate in a structured teaching program related to preterm infant behaviors. Mothers in the first experimental group had higher scores on a measure of mother-infant interaction, although the differences in scores among the three groups were not statistically significant. The researchers concluded that a larger sample might have resulted in significant group differences, and that greater effects might have resulted if they had provided more than one educational session for the mothers.

Culp, Culp, and Harmon (1989) evaluated the effects of demonstrating the Assessment of Preterm Infant Behavior (APIB) examination to parents and then providing them with feedback about their infants. Fourteen parents were alternately assigned to the intervention or control groups. Following the 40-minute intervention, fathers in the intervention group reported significantly lower anxiety than did fathers in the control group. Mothers and fathers in the intervention group had more realistic perceptions of their newborns, and mothers in this group had more accurate awareness of their newborns' abilities, compared with parents in the control group.

Pearson and Anderson (2001) evaluated a 90-minute "Parent's Circle" program that focused on supporting and validating the parenting experiences, teaching parents about preterm infant development, monitoring and tailoring interactions to support infant development, identifying ways they could participate in their infant's care and advocate for themselves and their infants, and providing information about hospital and community resources. A total of 104 parents were asked to evaluate the Parent's Circle program by identifying something new and helpful that they had learned, indicating whether they would recommend the program to others, and offering suggestions for improvement. Content analysis indicated that parents perceived the program as helpful and supportive, and that they valued learning about infant cues, ways to interact with their infants, and community resources. NICU staff perceived the program as helping to promote parental confidence.

Several studies evaluated more comprehensive and extensive educational interventions for parents in the NICU. Meyer, Garcia-Coll, Lester, et al. (1994) evaluated a family-based intervention that addressed four domains: infant behavior and characteristics; family organization and functioning; caregiving environment; and discharge planning. The interventions were individualized, based on an initial clinical interview by a care manager. The interventions ranged from 3 to 17 sessions (each lasting 1 to 1.5 hours) over 2 to 8 weeks. Parents were assigned randomly to the intervention ($n = 18$) or control ($n = 16$) group. Mothers in the intervention group reported less stress and less depression compared with mothers in the control group and had more positive interactions with their infants compared with control group mothers. Infants in the intervention group had fewer feeding problems compared with control group infants.

Lawhon (2002) used a multiple-case descriptive design to explore the effectiveness of an individualized parent-education program implemented in the NICU on parents' ability to appraise their infant's behaviors and integrate the appraisal into a supportive approach to handling their infants; and on parent and infant competence. The sample included 10 preterm infants and their 18 parents, and the intervention began within the first 10 days of the infant's life. The intervention included promoting critical appraisal of the infant's behavior through discussions of videotapes of parent-infant interactions at least once per week, through the infant's hospital stay. In addition, the nurse modeled and supported the parents in the critical appraisal process. The total number of sessions held with each parent ranged from 4 to 14. Although there was no comparison group, data indicated that the parents had higher scores on a measure of parent-infant interaction (the Nursing Child Assessment Feeding Scale, University of Washington, Seattle, WA) compared with scores of other groups of parents of preterm infants in previous studies. Similarly, infants had higher scores on measures of clarity of cues and responsiveness compared with samples of preterm infants in other studies. The researcher concluded that helping parents appreciate their infant's emerging competence supports their ability to promote their infant's development.

Another strategy that has been used to promote parental confidence in caring for their infants and prepare them for the infant's hospital discharge is to encourage parents to room-in with their infants and assume primary responsibility for the baby's care for at least a 24-hour period. Costello and Chapman (1998) conducted qualitative interviews with six mothers who had participated in such a care-by-parent program in a Toronto NICU. Mothers perceived the experience positively, and noted that it helped to reassure them that they were ready to care for their infant and that the infant was ready for discharge. They also reported that the experience helped them learn about responding to their baby's unique behaviors and cues, and that it allowed them to test the reality of caregiving in a safe environment.

In addition to providing parents with education about their infants' behaviors and interaction strategies, studies of parental reactions to high-risk birth suggest that parents also need help in coping with their emotional reactions to the birth. Macnab, Beckett, Park, et al. (1998) evaluated the use of journal writing as a social support strategy for parents of preterm infants. A total of 73 parents were enrolled in the study, received information about journal writing, and agreed to participate in follow-up telephone interviews 6 weeks after they entered the study. Although only 32% of the parents kept a journal, 68% of those who kept journals used their journals as a means to cope with the most stressful aspects of their NICU experiences. All parents who kept journals recommended the practice to other parents. Parents noted that the journals helped them to organize their thoughts and keep records of their experiences, and promoted their willingness to be involved in their infant's care.

## Studies of Parent-to-Parent Support Programs

Another strategy to promote parental involvement and to help parents cope with the stressors associated with the birth of a high-risk infant is parent-to-parent support provided through parent support groups or through volunteer parent mentor programs.

Findings from an early evaluation of a parent support group suggested that parent support groups can have positive benefits, including enhanced parent visiting in the NICU, enhanced interaction during visits, and enhanced involvement with their infants 3 months after NICU discharge (Minde, Shosenberg, Marton, et al., 1980). However, others have noted that support groups might not be appropriate for all parents, particularly if they are not accustomed to group participation (Lindsay, Roman, DeWys, et al., 1993). Alternately, others have noted that it is sometimes difficult to maintain attendance and commitment to parent support group programs (Stauber & Mahan, 1987; Del Bianco & Shankaran, 1987). Bracht, Ardal, Bot, et al. (1998) described the development and evaluation of a parent support group at a hospital in Ontario, Canada. A neonatal follow-up clinic nurse and social worker coordinated the group, and attendance ranges from 15 to 25 parents per session. The group meets for $1^1/_2$ hours each week, and features 11 different topics presented by an interdisciplinary team

of speakers. Questionnaires were sent to 100 parents who had participated in at least one group meeting to evaluate the group. All of the 41 parents who responded indicated a decrease in negative emotional states (e.g., hopelessness, despair, emptiness, pessimism) following group participation. Anecdotal observations from NICU staff suggested that parents who attended the group meetings were more self confident and interactive with their infants in the NICU.

Several researchers have evaluated parent-to-parent mentoring programs designed to provide emotional, informational, and role-modeling support to parents in the NICU. Lindsay, Roman, DeWys et al. (1993) described one such program established at Butterworth Hospital in Michigan. The program is coordinated by a paid hospital staff member who oversees recruitment, training, and continuing education of volunteer parents; matches volunteers with new parents; and oversees the volunteers' activities. Volunteers provide emotional as well as informational support to new parents through telephone and personal contacts, and maintain contact with the families following NICU discharge. Roman, Lindsay, Buger, et al. (1995) presented data evaluating the Butterworth Hospital parent-to-parent support program in which 27 mothers who had participated in the program were compared with a comparison group of 31 mothers. Mothers who participated in the program had less anxiety and higher self-esteem during the first 4 months after NICU discharge, and more positive interactions with their infants 1 year after discharge.

## Summary of Research Evaluating Interventions for Parents in the NICU

In summary, studies evaluating NICU-based parent interventions suggest that short-term educational programs have limited effectiveness, although they might enhance parental self confidence and understanding of preterm infant behaviors. More comprehensive programs that are continued throughout the NICU stay can help promote more positive parent-infant interactions, and can reduce levels of parental stress and depression. Parent support groups can help parents who are comfortable with group participation, and might promote increased parental confidence and interactions with their infants. Volunteer parent-to-parent mentoring programs provide parents with emotional and informational support and can help to reduce depression and anxiety and promote parental self-confidence and interactions.

Holditch-Davis and Miles (2000) reviewed the research related to parenting the prematurely born child, and noted that most studies were limited by not having a clear theoretic base, by failing to include longitudinal follow-up, and by using measures that were not sensitive to change. These researchers suggested that one particularly promising area for future research is the study of interventions in which the mother is given a specific and ongoing role in caring for her preterm infant, such as providing KC, massage therapy, or developmental care. There is a need for ongoing research to evaluate specific components of FCC and to continue to identify strategies to promote parental involvement and reduce the stressors associated with the birth of a high-risk infant.

## INANIMATE ENVIRONMENT
### Light: Research and Interventions

Consideration of ambient NICU light levels and lighting patterns (light/dark cycles vs continuous lighting) is a major component of most developmental care protocols. Existing protocols prescribe various interventions to reduce light levels experienced by hospitalized infants. These include consistently dimming overhead light and/or maintaining structured light/dark cycles throughout the 24-hour period. These protocols often include use of eye shields or incubator covers to reduce light reaching the baby. Each of these interventions is designed to respond to both concerns that excessively high light levels can negatively impact the developing preterm infant, and existing research describing excessively high NICU light levels. In the following section, we discuss: studies describing current NICU practice related to light; research on the effects of light on the preterm infant; the research base for interventions designed to modify infant light exposure; the existing standards of practice related to light; and recommendations for practice based on the best available evidence.

### Research on NICU Light Levels and Patterns

Studies describing light levels in NICUs were first reported in the mid-1980s through 1990. Four classic studies from this period clearly describe common light levels found in the NICUs at that time, the source of the highest light levels, and the presence or lack of any systematic variation in light levels over a 24-hour period (Hamer, Dobson, & Mayer 1984; Glass, Avery, Subramanian, et al., 1985; Landry, Scheidt, & Hammond, 1985). These studies, conducted in NICUs in the United Kingdom and the United States, consistently reported four findings: (1) light levels in the studied NICUs commonly ranged from 240 to 1500 lux (approximately 24 to 150 footcandles [ftc]) with reported means from 47 to 90 ftc; (2) peak light levels were associated with auxiliary light sources, including bedside treatment lamps (200 to 300 ftc), phototherapy lamps (300 to 400 ftc), and natural daylight from NICU windows (up to 1024 ftc); (3) light levels within NICUs demonstrated little structured diurnal variation; and (4) light levels were highest in the areas of highest infant acuity, usually associated with the youngest and, developmentally, most vulnerable infants. One study, (Landry, Scheidt, & Hammond, 1985) noted some seasonal variability in unit light levels based on proximity to direct window exposure.

In the mid-1990s through the present, a limited number of studies have reported on NICU light levels (Bullough & Rea, 1996; Fielder & Moseley, 2000; Gaddy, Rollag, & Brainard, 1993; Glozbach, Rowlett, Edgar, et al., 1993; Gray, Dostal, Ternullo-Retta, & Armstrong, 1998; Slevin, Farrington, Duffy, et al., 2000; Walsh-Sukys, Reitenbach, Hudson-Barr, et al., 2001). These studies document NICU light levels that are, on average, lower than those reported in the 1980s. However, the reported light levels vary widely, ranging from low levels of less than 1 to 25 ftc (Slevin, Farrington, Duffy, et al., 2000; Walsh-Sukys, Reitenbach, Hudson-Barr, et al., 2001), to excessively high levels of up to 235 ftc (Gray, Dostal, Ternullo-Retta, & Armstrong, 1998). Additionally, they continue to report little systematic diurnal variability in most units. These studies are limited in that each reports data collected from only one or two units, and by differences in instrumentation and data collection procedures.

In a recent study of current practice related to NICU lighting, Lotas, Seal, Ambrose, et al. (2003, under review) surveyed 56 randomly selected NICUs in the Southeastern region of the United States, asking staff to describe their unit's lighting practices. Descriptions were based on staff estimations, or actual measurements where available, and comparisons to light levels in other areas of each hospital. Most surveyed hospitals had level two or three neonatal units, eleven or more beds, and cared for infants born from 23 weeks PCA through term. Survey respondents were asked to describe their units in three ways: (1) Are there written policies or rules related to NICU lighting? (2) How would you rate your NICU light levels (low, moderate, or high)? and (3) How does the NICU lighting compare with the lighting in other areas of the hospital, such as the cafeteria, administrative offices, and other clinical units? An analysis of data from the survey indicated that most units (69%) have no rules or policies related to lighting levels or patterns; most units were described as having moderate to low lighting (75%) and being dimmer than the cafeteria (63%), other patient units (61%), and the administrative offices (70%).

In a follow-up study, Lotas and Seal (2003, under review) completed on-site light measurements in 18 units selected from the original survey sample through a stratified randomization procedure. In each of the units, lighting levels were measured at three times (8:00 to 10:00 AM; 6:00 to 8:00 PM; 12:00 to 2:00 AM) over the 24-hour period. At each data-collection time, measurements were taken at multiple sites within the units to ensure that the light levels reported were representative of the unit. Light measurements were recorded in footcandles using an Ex-Tech model 407026 (Ex-Tech Instrument Corp., Waltham, *MA*) light meter, and were taken with the light meter positioned at the approximate height of an infant's eyes when lying on an incubator mattress surface to approximate the actual light exposure experienced by an infant in the incubator. Overall, measured light levels ranged from 0.25 to 68.05 ftcs throughout the three different time points, but were not significantly correlated to the units' reported light levels in the earlier survey. The mean (28 ftc) and range of measured light levels are less than the early reports of NICU light levels. Although few units had formal policies related to maintaining light/dark cycles, an overall drop in light levels was noted during the nighttime hours.

Therefore, the literature at this time documents changes in practice in many NICUs, resulting in an overall lowering of NICU light levels. However, the literature also documents that a pattern of excessively high light levels continues to exist in many NICUs; that few units have formalized policies related to light reduction or light/dark cycling; and that few responders could accurately describe their unit light levels.

## Effects of Light on the Developing Preterm Infant

A substantive body of research exists exploring the effects of excessive light levels and lighting patterns on the developing premature infant. These studies can be considered in three groups: effects of light on the developing visual system, including the incidence of retinopathy of prematurity (ROP); light levels on nonvisual development and behavioral responses in preterm infants; and cycled light (structured light/dark cycles) versus noncycled light.

***Light Levels and Incidence of Retinopathy of Prematurity.*** Studies of the effects of excessive light on the visual system have focused predominantly on the influence of light levels on the development of ROP in the preterm infant. Concern regarding the relationship of light and the incidence of ROP evolved from four related premises (Glass, 1988, 1990; Moseley & Fielder, 1988; Robinson & Fielder, 1992):

- The NICU environment differs dramatically in light intensity from the intrauterine environment for which the preterm infant is physiologically adapted.
- The visual system of the preterm neonate is undergoing a period of intense development during the period from 23 to 32 weeks' PCA when most incidences of ROP occur.
- The preterm infant characteristically has few defensive mechanisms available to moderate the effect of bright light on the eye—that is, the infant's eyelids are thin and admit more light than a term baby; they have large pupils and a decreased ability to constrict their pupils in response to light stimuli;

they may spend more time with their eyes open; and, with the new recommendations for maintaining them in a supine position, they may spend time looking directly into ceiling lights.

• There is a plethora of early studies of the development of the visual system describing retinal damage in animals maintained in continuous, high levels of light (Sisson, Glauser, Glauser, et al., 1970; Messner, Maisels, & Leure-duPree, 1978; Lawwill, 1982; Noell, 1980).

Despite these concerns, however, the data have not demonstrated a consistent relationship between NICU light levels and the incidence of ROP. Studies by Glass, Avery, Subramanian, et al. (1985) described a significant reduction in the incidence of ROP in infants with birthweights less than 1000 g who were shielded from ambient light by covering the incubator with a sheet of transparent acetate. The Glass study using a historical control group is limited owing to significant changes in the way ROP was classified and staged over the time between the recruitment of the control group and the recruitment of the experimental group. Other studies attempting to replicate Glass's findings (Ackerman, Sherwonit, & Williams, 1989; Seiberth, Linderkamp, Knorz, et al., 1994; Reynolds, Hardy, Kennedy, et al., 1998) have found no significant differences between groups. In addition, a meta-analysis completed by Phelps and Watts (2001) also demonstrated no significant reduction in the incidence of ROP secondary to ambient light reduction. A recent study by Brandon, Holditch-Davis, and Belyea (2002) compared preterm infants maintained in near-darkness in the NICU with a group maintained in cycled light. One of the outcome variables measured by the investigators was incidence and severity of ROP. Although the groups did not differ in overall severity of ROP, the investigators reported an unexpected trend that the infants maintained in near darkness developed severe ROP earlier in gestation.

At this time, no studies have documented a clear relationship between the occurrence of ROP and NICU light levels; however, concern continues to focus on the effects of light levels and patterns on the developing visual system. The interaction of the infant's conceptional age, the developmental stage of the visual system, and optimal light levels have not yet been fully explored. Questions remain regarding the possible negative effects of near darkness on the developing retina as well as the possible adverse effects of excessive light on the visual system apart from ROP.

***Light Levels and Nonvision Effects on the Infant.*** In addition to the effects of light on the developing preterm visual system, nonvisual effects of NICU light levels and patterns have been extensively studied. Reported short-term effects from excessive, continuous lighting include a reversal of normal diurnal variability of amino acids (Mantagos, Moustogianni, Varvarigou, et al., 1989); reduction of oxygen saturation levels in infants born at younger than 28 weeks' gestational age (light levels of approximately 100 ftcs) (Shogan & Schumann, 1993); and higher respiratory rates, heart rates, and activity levels than infants maintained in lower light levels (Shiroiwa, Kamiya, Uchibori, et al., 1986). Other studies have focused on the effects of light on the development of biological rhythms, including sleep patterns, and the endocrine system, impact on growth and development, and the effects of light on infant state.

**Effects on the Development of Biological Rhythms.** Researchers and clinicians have been concerned about the effects of NICU lighting on the development of biological rhythms in the preterm infant because: (1) of the erratic patterns of light over the 24-hour period in many nurseries; (2) infants are often fed continuously, thus eliminating feeding cycles as a second organizing factor; and (3) the prematurely born infant has lost the natural organization imposed by the mother's own biological rhythms while the infant is in the uterine environment.

Circadian rhythms are thought to occur in most living beings, including man through the effects of structured 24-hour light cycles on the hypothalamic suprachiasmatic nuclei (SCN) via the retinohypothalamic tract projecting from the retina to the hypothalamus (Moore-Ede, Czeisler, & Richardson, 1983; Morin, 1994). Ultradian rhythms are those biological rhythms that occur in less than 24-hour cycles and, in infants, might be influenced by feeding cycles (Arendt, Minors, & Waterhouse, 1989). These rhythms serve the purpose of synchronizing and coordinating compatible physiologic functions and separating incompatible ones (Reppert, 1992; Moore-Ede, Sulzman, & Fuller, 1982). Physiologic functions considered to possess a circadian pattern include heart rate, body temperature, sleep/wake cycles, and the secretion of several hormones including cortisol, ACTH, and melatonin (Arendt, Minors, & Waterhouse, 1989; Moore-Ede, Sulzman, & Fuller, 1982; Rivkees, 2001).

In the human infant, early development of biological rhythms occurs in the fetus and is thought to be determined predominantly by maternal biological rhythms (Reppert, 1992). After birth, the development of circadian functions continues under the influence of the infant's environmental cues with light/dark cycles and feeding cycles. Recent work by Hao and Rivkees (1999), using a sample of preterm infant baboons, demonstrated that the SCN was responsive to light stimulation at ages equivalent to 24 weeks' PCA. This study's findings suggest that the period of hospitalization for most prematurely born infants is a time when they might be responsive to environment light levels and patterns in the development of circadian rhythms. Indeed, circadian patterns in heart rate, body temperature, and sleep have been shown to begin to emerge after the third week of life (Hellbrugge, 1974; Tenreiro, Dowse, D'Souza, et al., 1991; Glozbach, Edgar, & Ariagno, 1995). It is this development that can be disrupted if the preterm infant in the NICU environment receives inadequate or inappropriate environmental cues to develop normal circadian function.

## Research Describing the Effects of Interventions

*Light Reduction.* The reduction of NICU light levels is a component of virtually all of the existing developmental care protocols. Studies have described excessive NICU light levels associated with alterations in infant state organization, rest and sleep patterns (Moseley Thompson, Levene, et al., 1988; Robinson, Moseley, Thompson, et al., 1989; Shiroiwa, Kamiya, Uchibori, et al., 1986; Mann, Haddow, Stokes, et al., 1986). Reduced light levels have also been reported to increase the preterm infant's respiratory stability and to reduce heart rate, blood pressure, and motor activity (Als, Lawhon, Brown, et al., 1986; Blackburn &

Patteson, 1991; Shiroiwa, Kamiya, Uchibori et al., 1986). However, despite the fact that dimmed lighting or near-darkness has become a widespread intervention in nurseries implementing developmental care, an examination of existing studies reveals surprisingly little support for the benefits of dimmed light levels for the preterm infant. Dim lighting has been studied systematically in combination with other interventions but not as an individual strategy (Lotas & Walden, 1996). Intuitively, dimmed light levels seem more congruent with the intrauterine environment in which the preterm infant would normally be developing. However, the developing preterm infant is not the same as the developing fetus of the same PCA. To date, no studies have examined the issue of optimal environmental lighting in relation to the PCA of the infant—that is, does the optimal light level vary by PCA or determine the range of light levels that could be considered "dim"? In spite of these limitations, dimmed NICU light levels have not been shown to have negative effects and might contribute to improved rest, sleep, and physiologic stability. Additionally, the developing retina appears to need periods of very reduced light for retinal regeneration (Graven, 2002).

*Light/Dark Cycling.* A few studies have described the physiologic functioning of the preterm infants comparing the effects of light/dark cycled light in the NICU with the effects of continuous bright lighting (Mann, Haddow, Stokes, et al., 1986; Blackburn, & Patteson, 1991; Lotas & Medoff-Cooper, 2001 [under review]; Miller, White, Whitman, et al., 1995; Shiroiwa, Kamiya, Uchibori, et al., 1986; Tenreiro, Dowse, D'Souza, et al., 1991). Outcomes reported include:

- Decreased heart and respiratory rates during the dark cycle, in infants maintained in a light/dark cycled environment (Blackburn & Patteson, 1991; Lotas & Medoff-Cooper, 2001 [under review]; Shiroiwa, Kamiya, Uchibori, et al., 1986; Tenreiro, Dowse, D'Souza, et al., 1991).
- Increased weight gain for infants maintained in a light/dark cycled environment (Mann, Haddow, Stokes, et al., 1986; Miller, White, Whitman, et al., 1995; Brandon, Holditch-Davis, & Belyea, 2002)
- Increased sleep time for infants maintained in a light/dark cycled environment (Mann, Haddow, Stokes, et al., 1986).

- Decreased infant activity for infants maintained in a light/dark cycled environment (Blackburn & Patteson, 1991).

These studies provide findings that are suggestive but not conclusive in support of the benefits of a cycled light environment, at least for the infants of 29 weeks' gestation or older. The generalizability of the findings of these studies is limited owing to differences in lighting conditions used, in the timing and pattern of data collection in relation to the PCA of the infant, and the extremely small sample size in many of the studies. In addition, changes in lighting levels can also have influenced other aspects of the environment, such as noise levels and staff activity, which were not documented. These studies are further limited by lack of randomization in some, and serendipitous variations in light levels within the units during the study period. It should be noted that only one study (Brandon, Holditch-Davis, & Belyea, 2002) contrasted moderate to low light levels (20 to 23 ftc) with near-darkness in the light/dark cycled treatment. Additionally, few data are available for the ELBW infant.

*Use of Incubator Covers.* The use of incubator covers (IC) to reduce the light experienced by the preterm infant is one of the most widely used light-related nursing interventions. The implementation of this strategy varies substantively from unit to unit and within units in terms of when the covers are used, the kinds of covers used, and the consistency of use. In addition, a review of the literature produced no systematic evaluation of the effectiveness of this intervention in achieving improved infant rest and sleep. In a recent, small study of incubator use in one NICU, investigators identified 22 different kinds of covers used (Lee, Malakooti, & Lotas, 2003 [under review]). These covers varied in size, color, thickness, and porosity. Findings of this study included:

- Reduction of incubator light levels measured at the level of the infant's upper eye varied from more than 90% to less than 25%, depending on the cover used.
- Darker-colored covers produced greater reduction of light levels than did lighter-colored covers.
- Covers varied widely in the percent of the incubator surface covered (<20% to >85%), and the amount of incubator surface covered affected the level of light reduction achieved.

- Many of the popular hand-crocheted incubator covers produced relatively limited light reduction for the baby owing to the porosity of the fabric.

The inconsistency in light reduction achieved by different commonly used incubator covers, combined with the variability in the actual implementation of this strategy and the lack of studies evaluating the effects of the intervention limit the recommendations that can be made. However, this does not mean that there is no value in this intervention. However, it highlights the need for interventions such as the covering of incubators to be implemented consistently and systematically, and the need for well-controlled studies to be undertaken to evaluate this and other nursing interventions.

### Standards of Practice: Light

In the past, continuous lighting levels of 60 to 100 ftcs (approximately the light level of an office or classroom) were thought to be necessary to allow adequate evaluation of the infant's skin color and perfusion from any area of the NICU. Ambient light levels in excess of 60 ftcs are now thought to be excessive, except when necessary for caregiving or treatments. Although standards of practice related to light levels in the NICU have not been decisively established at this time, general recommendations for NICU design and practice related to light have been proposed by the Fifth Consensus Conference on Newborn ICU Design (White, 2002). These standards recommend that NICU light levels be adjustable over a range of 1 to 60 ftcs; that both natural and artificial light have controls that allow for sufficient darkening for trans-illumination; that electric light sources limit unnecessary ultraviolet or infrared radiation by the use of appropriate lamps, lens, or filters; and that no infant care space should have a source of direct ambient lighting, other than for necessary use during procedures (White, 2002). In addition, although the recommendations of the Fifth Consensus Conference (White, 2002) include the suggestion that NICU light levels should be "very dim for at least some part of the day for some babies" (p. 14), at this time data do not definitively support the importance of implementing light/dark cycles in the nursery; identify the optimal timing of such cycles; define the necessary degree of contrast between light levels in the "dark" period versus the "light" period; or distinguish optimal practices by gestational age. However, existing studies have not identified any negative consequences of maintaining light/dark cycling and have suggested possible benefits, particularly in relation to the development of circadian rhythms (Mirmiran & Ariagno, 2000). In addition, despite the lack of established standards for routine light levels in the NICU, within the concept of developmental care, lower light levels (± 20 ftcs to near darkness) have been recommended. Therefore, the following strategies for NICU light management are suggested:

- If no actual measurement of NICU light levels has been made, a survey of the unit using a light meter would be useful.
- Maintain ambient light levels at 20 ftcs or less unless more light is required for caregiving or treatments.
- Provide periods of dimmer than usual light levels for some part of the 24-hour cycle.
- Avoid the use of overhead lights and use individual lighting at the infant's bedside for caregiving and procedures.
- Use incubator covers during times when the infant is at rest to create a period of dimmer light for the infant.
- When using incubator covers, nurses should be aware that covers that are porous, light in color, and small, will provide significantly less light reduction than covers that are of tightly woven material, darker colored, and adequate to cover the entire top and most of the sides of the incubator.
- Outside windows represent the source of the highest light levels in the NICU. Outside windows should be glazed or have opaque shades of some type available to allow modifications of light levels.
- Infants, particularly those at less than 32 weeks PCA, should be placed away from direct sunlight.
- Place a screen between incubators where treatment lights or phototherapy lights are in use and adjacent incubators to protect those infants from random light excursions.
- Ensure that the infant is not looking directly into any light source. Particularly if the infant is placed in a supine position or a sidelying position, it is important to determine that no light source, including natural window lighting or procedural lighting

from adjacent incubators, is focused directly on the baby's face.

- Education of the family about the infant's development and caregiving needs should include explanations of the concerns about light levels and the precautions taken to protect the baby from excessive light.
- If an infant has received eye drops in preparation for an ophthalmic examination, consider that the pupil might be affected for up to 4 hours. The infant will be light-sensitive during this period and must be protected from direct light. Be mindful of the sensitivity during the examination itself.

## Sound in the NICU

Sound levels in the NICU environment have been a source of concern for clinicians and the focus for a substantive body of research. The concern has focused both on the conviction that NICU environment provides an acoustic environment that is inappropriate or toxic for the developing preterm infant, and the possibility that the ototoxic effects associated with some commonly used drugs might be exacerbated by NICU noise levels. Routine NICU sound levels have been described as frequently exceeding recommended levels, with sound excursions reaching levels associated with negative physical infant reactions and the potential for long-term alterations in infant behavioral responses and hearing. Researchers have measured sound levels within the incubator and in the surrounding room, described the components of NICU sound, and examined potential long-term effects of continuous excessive sound levels and the short term effects of brief sound excursions. In addition, a small number of studies have described the effect of sound reduction strategies in the NICU. In this section, we review studies describing the levels of NICU sound and the components of that sound; studies examining the long-term and short-term effects of excessive sound on the developing preterm infant; existing standards of practice for NICU sound and sound reduction; and recommendations for nurses in practice.

### NICU Sound Levels and Sources

During the past three decades, researchers have repeatedly documented consistent sound levels of 50 to 90 decibels (dBs) in the NICU with mean levels of 58 to 66 dBs and excursions to as high as 120 dBs (Anagnostakis, Petmezakis, Messaritakis, & Matsaniotis, 1980; Chang, Lin, & Lin, 2001; DePaul & Chambers, 1995; Long, Lucey, & Philip, 1980; Robertson & Philbin, 1996; Robertson, Cooper-Peel, & Vos, 1998; Thomas, 1989). For the purpose of comparison, 50 dBs approximates the sound level of light traffic, and 90 dBs approximates the sound level generated by light machinery. According to Occupational Safety and Health Administration (OSHA) standards, 80 dB is the highest sound level that does not produce measurable damage, regardless of the duration of the sound, and 90 dB is the limit imposed in industrial standards as the highest safe level for an 8-hour period for adults.

In addition, although no study reported systematic patterns of increased or decreased sound in the nurseries, higher levels of noise were identified with periods of "busyness" in the unit. Philbin and Gray (2002) noted that although sound excursions far exceed the average sound levels of a unit, "quiet periods" demonstrate only slight reductions from usual unit levels. In addition, the NICU noise level has been found to demonstrate little diurnal variation, and when fluctuations in sound occur, they do so in an unpredictable manner (Thomas, 1989). Investigations into the impact of incubators on the sound levels experienced by the infant have produced mixed findings. Noise levels within an incubator have been found to vary by manufacturer (Berens & Weigle, 1997; Robinson, Moseley, Thompson, et al., 1989) to be somewhat reduced in comparison to the outside environmental noise if no respiratory equipment is in use; and to be somewhat increased compared with the outside environment if respiratory equipment is in use (Robertson, Cooper-Peel, & Vos, 1999). In addition, incubators exacerbated the sound levels to the infant if the source of the sound was an object hitting the incubator wall or the opening and closing of the incubator latches. There are many sources of sounds found within the confines of the NICU. See Figure 14-1 for NICU sound levels and how they relate to common noises found in our everyday ambient environment.

In studies exploring the sources of sound in the NICU environment, researchers have identified both anticipated and unanticipated components of nursery sound. As expected, much of the sound present in the NICU is related to the hospital building itself, generated by heating, cooling, and ventilation systems; plumbing and communications; or the equipment used in the care of the infants, including incubators, oxygen-monitoring devices, ventilators, and infusion pumps (Robertson, Cooper-Peel, & Vos, 1999; Thomas, 1989; White, 2002). Furthermore, monitor alarms and telephones, as expected, contributed significantly to the high amplitude sound excursions. Less expected, however, were findings that demonstrated that many of the high amplitude sound excursions, 70 dBs or above, were related to staff activities, including closing doors, trash-can lids, incubator ports or drawers, laughter, and conversation (Long, Lucey, & Philip, 1980; Robertson, Cooper-Peel, & Vos, 1999; Chang, Lin, & Lin, 2001).

### Effects of Nursery Sound on the Preterm Infant

Three categories of effects of noise on the infant have been studied: the effects of excessive or inappropriate sound on sensorineural hearing; the effects of excessive or inappropriate sound on the infant's cognitive processing of sound; and the short-term effects on infant physiologic responses, including sleep and rest.

Estimates of the incidence of mild to moderate hearing loss in VLBW infants vary from 1.46% to 25% (Hack, Klein, & Taylor, 1995; Pettigrew, Edwards, & Henderson-Smart, 1988; Schendel, Stockbauer, Hoffman, et al., 1997). The increased risk for hearing loss in VLBW infants has been attributed to several factors, including significant intraventricular hemorrhage, prolonged oxygen therapy, hyponatremia, and the incidence of asphyxia, infection, and elevated serum bilirubin levels. The toxic effect of excessive nursery noise levels has also been proposed as a risk factor. Although common NICU noise levels are not higher than those levels found to be tolerated by adults (see OSHA recommendations earlier), the levels might be excessive for the immature auditory system of the preterm infant. In addition, the continuous nature of sound/noise in the NICU allows few periods of quiet for the infant's auditory system to recover. Studies of the effects of NICU sound levels on hearing loss, to date, have reported inconsistent

**NICU SOUND LEVELS (IN dB) RELATIVE
TO OTHER COMMON ENVIRONMENTS**

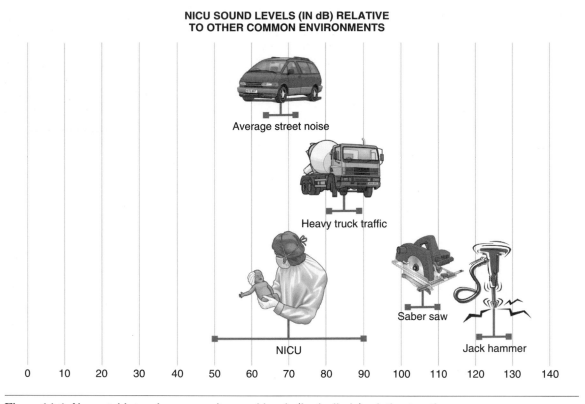

Figure **14-1** Neonatal intensive care unit sound levels (in decibels) relative to other common environments. (*From Littleton, L.Y., & Engebretson, J. [2002].* Maternal, neonatal, and women's health nursing. *Delmar Learning, a division of Thomson Learning.* www.thomsonrights.com.)

findings. Small samples, the lack of consistency in the timing and process of the hearing screening performed, and the difficulty in controlling for confounding variables in the clinical setting have limited studies. Also, because many of the existing studies were done in the 1970s and 1980s, changes in NICU care protocols limit generalizability to today's NICU population. However, it should be noted that in the early research, the hearing loss found in these infants has been described as most marked in the high frequency range (Pettigrew, Edwards, & Henderson- Smart, 1988) and that much of the equipment-related sound in the infant's environment, such as ventilators, incubators, and alarms is also often in the high-frequency range (Thomas, 1989). It is also worth noting that infants with the largest number of risk factors associated with sensorineural hearing loss are also likely to have the longest exposure to the ambient noise of the NICU.

Concerns related to the effects of nursery sound on infant hearing have also focused on the possible interaction of excessive ambient sound levels with ototoxic drugs the infant might receive while hospitalized. These drugs include, but are not limited to, the aminoglycosides such as gentamicin, kanamycin, vancomycin, streptomycin, and tobramycin, when used for more than 5 days. Again, studies exploring the synergism between ototoxic drugs and NICU sound levels have reported conflicting findings and have been limited by small samples, differences in the evaluation of hearing, and the existence of multiple confounding variables in the clinical setting.

A second area of concern related to the long-term effects of NICU noise on the LBW infant is whether, even in the absence of impairment of functional hearing, there might be some alteration in the infant's processing of auditory stimuli. The high level of continuous sound or "white noise" experienced by the infant in the incubator, the lack of predictability or rhythmicity of NICU sound, and the limited ability of the infant to associate a source, face, or event with sounds heard, all might permanently influence the way in which auditory stimuli are processed and understood by the infant. Certainly, the animal data describing developmental changes in the sensory and motor cortex secondary to altered sensory input (Philbin, Ballweg, & Gray, 1994; Spinelli, 1990) supports such a speculation, although the relationship has not been examined in human infants.

The final group of studies examining the issue of sound in the NICU has focused on what the long- and short-term outcomes of such sound might be on behavioral responses in hospitalized preterm infants. Researchers have examined the immediate responses of infants to noise in the nursery. Long et al. (1980) documented a repeated pattern of decreased transcutaneous oxygen tension, increased intracranial pressure, and increased heart and respiratory rates in two infants in response to sudden loud noise in the nursery. Gorski, Hole, Leonard, and Martin (1983) described mottling, apnea, and bradycardia in preterm infants exposed to sharp excursions in sound, such as telephones and monitor alarms and conversation during medical rounds. Both studies provide support for the notion that nursery noise levels are a disorganizing influence on the neurologically immature LBW infant and raise speculation regarding the energy cost to the infant these episodes represent.

In related work, Gadeke, Doring, Keller, et al. (1969), in a study of the effects of noise on the sleep patterns of term infants, reported that sound levels higher than 70 dBs were incompatible with infant sleep, and sound levels of 55 dBs aroused an infant from light sleep. Although this study has not been replicated with LBW infants, the reported sound levels are similar to those present in the NICU, suggesting that NICU noise might interfere with the development of sleep and rest patterns in these infants. Alternatively, the LBW infant in the NICU might be able to adapt to some degree to the continuous noise levels of her/his environment and, therefore, develop and maintain a pattern of sleep and rest. Again, this has not been studied in human infants.

Finally, a limited amount of research suggests a relationship among ambient noise levels, infant stress, and endocrine responses. Early research using a rat model demonstrated measurable increases in adrenocorticotropic hormone (ACTH) secretion with increased stress, including sound levels as low as 68 dBs (AAP, 1974; AAP Committee on Environmental Health, 1997). Recent research by Schanberg and Field (1987), using growth hormone (GH) secretion as a physiologic index of stress, reported that LBW infants stressed by handling manifested decreased growth hormone levels. Taken together these studies suggest that excessive noise levels might produce a stress response in infants, including alterations in endocrine function, and that one stress-related endocrine change in infants is a likely decrease in serum growth hormone levels. Certainly, each of these relationships is complex, measurement in human infants is difficult, and great caution must be used in extrapolating findings from animal studies to human infants. However, the premise that excessive noise in the NICU might contribute to poorer growth outcomes in infants is worthy of further exploration.

### Standards of Practice: Sound

In January 2002, the Fifth Consensus Conference on Newborn ICU Design, Robert D. White, Chairperson, published the monograph, *Recommended Standards for Newborn ICU Design*. Standard 23 of this document establishes specific recommendations for sound levels in NICU areas. These recommendations are summarized in the following.

- The combination of continuous background noise and transient sound in an infant care area shall not exceed an hourly Leq50 decibels (dB) A-weighted slow response. The term "hourly Leq" is a measurement representing the sound intensity that, if kept constant, would equal the variable sound levels during a 1-hour period. The term A-weighted slow response refers to a sound measurement scale or format that simulates human hearing. Therefore, 50 dBs, using an A-weighted scale is the maximum hourly "average" sound level that is acceptable in the NICU.

The hourly $L_{10}$ in the NICU should not exceed 55 dB A-weighted slow response. The term "$L_{10}$" refers to the level of sound that exceeds the $L_{eq}$ for 10% or more of the measurement period. Therefore, if a unit had an average sound level of 45 dB ($L_{eq}$), but 10% of the time the sound level was at 55 dB, then the $L_{10}$ would be 55 dB.

## Recommendations for Practice: Sound

A review of the research related to the effect of nursery sound on the developing LBW infant demonstrates substantive short-term physiologic changes, particularly in the cardiovasucular and respiratory systems. Although the literature does not provide definitive evidence of any long-term effects of excessive sound, it provides support for a realistic concern and justification for the modification of sound levels where possible. It should be noted that sound reduction in the NICU requires a combination of behavioral modifications on the part of the NICU staff and visitors, and significant modification of the physical environment itself. Neither approach is sufficient without the other. Several suggestions for sound reduction can be made:

- Units concerned about reducing the ambient sound level of their area should have equipment available to periodically measure the existing sound levels. Such measurements can be made with readily available, relatively inexpensive equipment.
  - If a unit is beginning the process of reducing sound levels, educational sessions for staff and visitors might be needed to raise awareness of the need to modify behaviors such as:
    - Conversations should be held away from the infants beside or out of the caregiving area completely.
    - Conversations should not be held by calling to another person across the room.
    - Opening and closing doors and drawers and manipulating equipment should be done in such a way that noise is kept to a minimum.
    - Minimized noise levels within incubators can be maintained by depressing the latch on the incubator ports prior to closing them or applying some felt stripping around the incubator doors.
    - Never use the incubator top to sit things on because the sound of anything impacting the incubator is intensified to the infant within.

- Modifications of the physical environment should include:
  - Replacement of metal equipment such as wastebaskets with plastic.
  - Removal of radios, intercoms, and other extraneous sources of sound from the NICU.
  - Modification of necessary equipment used in the nursery where possible to reduce the sound reaching the baby. Computer printers could be equipped with soundproofed covers. Telephones could be placed away from the caregiving area or equipped with flashers rather than ringers. Monitor alarms could be replaced with quieter audible alarms and/or with flashing alarms.
  - Carpeting, acoustical ceilings and other sound-absorbing materials should be used where possible.
  - When considering new or replacement equipment or other items for the nursery, the noise level generated by those items or equipment should be a primary consideration. Sound levels inside the incubator are determined in large part by the noise of the machinery itself, and such noise levels should become part of the selection criteria.
  - Specific guidelines for acceptable noise levels should be established for the NICU. These could be used as a standard when selecting nursery equipment and would serve to encourage manufacturers to design and develop quieter equipment for use in the NICU. Such guidelines could also be used to evaluate caregiving procedures.

A final caveat for staff seeking to enhance their NICU as a developmentally supportive environment is to limit the addition of auditory stimuli for infants. At this time, no definitive evidence exists documenting the value of interventions such as adding music, voices, or heartbeats to the infant's environment. Unanswered questions include how long such stimulation should be provided; what sound levels are appropriate for continuous auditory stimulation; and does the amount, kind, and level of auditory stimulation differ by PCA.

## NICU Design

The previous sections of this chapter concern environmental issues that must be considered when promoting individualized, family-centered developmental care (IFDC). These issues require careful consideration of the overall NICU design. The structural design of the NICU has changed and continues to change in response to the research that abounds regarding light and sound. Much of this research describes the noxious effects, both short- and long-term, that the traditional NICU provides (Benini, Magnavita, Lago, et al., 1996; Blackburn, 1996, 1998; Long, Lucey, & Philip, 1980; Lotas, 1992; Magnavita, Arslan, & Benini, 1994; Morris, Philbin, & Bose, 2000; Philbin, 2000; Shogan & Schumann, 1993; Zahr & Balian, 1995). In addition, research as well as consumer pressure has identified and supported the need to incorporate families in a more inclusive manner into the care and environment of their infant (Bialoskurski, Cox, & Hayes, 1999; Harrison, 1993; Levy-Shiff, Sharir, & Mogilner, 1989; Meyer, Garcia-Coll, Lester, et al., 1994; Sullivan, 1999).

Many of the necessary changes can be incorporated within current unit settings with the comprehensive integration of developmentally supportive care and family-centered care concepts. However, alterations within the NICU will enhance staff efforts and more readily promote success. In the early 1990s, Dr. Stanley Graven at University of South Florida, Tampa, FL, convened a group of experts to examine the literature and develop recommendations for NICU design (Graven, Bowen, Brooten, et al., 1992). Over the years, these recommendations have been updated to incorporate the ongoing research and provide evidence-based standards. These recommendations address the needs of the infant and the family, as well as the staff working within this area. The Recommended Standards for Newborn ICU Design are available at *www.nd.edu/~kkolberg/DesignStandards.htm.*

Lighting requires a multilayered approach that combines both direct and indirect lighting options. The use of natural lighting, when available, must be integrated into the overall design. The windows require shielding to prevent too much light from entering the clinical area; however, this shielding should allow the adults in the setting the opportunity to see the outside environment. Direct or task lighting is necessary for procedures being performed upon the infant as well as for staff tasks requiring such lighting. Care must be observed to protect the infant's eyes at such times of increased luminance. The NICU Design recommendations suggest this lighting be available at 100 ftc or 1000 lux (White, Nelson, Silvestri, et al., 2002). This should be provided on an individualized basis to limit the disruption to other infants in the area. Indirect lighting for ambient lighting and non–task related activities should be flexible and not interfere with the infant's ability to sleep. The recommendation for this lighting is less than 60 ftc or 600 lux (White, 2002). Even at this level, the infant will require protection within the microenvironment to prevent direct light onto their eyes and to optimize sleep time between periods of care. In addition, research now clearly indicates the need for day-night cycling or support of the circadian rhythm (Blackburn & Patteson, 1991; Glozbach, Rowlett, Edgar, et al., 1993; Mann, Haddow, Stokes, et al., 1986; Miller, White, Whitman, et al., 1995; Mirmiran & Ariagno, 2000). This requires only small fluctuations in the lighting from dim to about 20 ftc or 200 lux (Rivkees, 2003) while still protecting the infant's eyes from direct exposure. This must be incorporated into any lighting strategy being planned to provide consistency and identification of the appropriate infants.

NICU design must also address the amount of noise the infant is exposed to. The AAP recommendation is to maintain the noise below 50 dB (AAP Committee on Environmental Health, 1997). Materials which will decrease the transmission of noise should be used on the floor and within the ceiling (Evans & Philbin, 2000). The selection of such materials must be made with cleaning consideration kept in mind. For example, carpet might be quieter; however, it is more difficult to maintain. Equipment must be placed at an appropriate level and in a location that permits the staff easy and quick access to alarms and other noise-producing events. Designated functional areas for staff activities away from the clinical area will also contribute to a quieter unit. These areas would include a medication area, a feeding preparation area, a charting area, and an area designated for communications.

The current recommendations for increased space at each bed further assists with the individualization of light and the reduction of noise. The recommended bed space has grown to 120 square feet to accommodate the increased amount of equipment being used and to provide privacy for the infant and family (White, 2002). Many units are using a private or semiprivate room design versus the multibed ward configuration. The single-patient room configuration offers the family increased privacy and access to their infant, with many designs incorporating a sleep space for the parents. The multibed unit can provide privacy with a variety of structural configurations that limit visual access into all bedspaces or, with the use of bedside curtains, individualize environments as desired.

Additional space to support the parents includes a sitting area outside or nearby the clinical area, space for confidential meetings with care providers, lactation support rooms, a sibling area, and a resource room with educational opportunities, including Internet access. Sleeping space adjacent to the unit prevents separation during acute periods of illness and rooming-in before discharge for teaching and parent comfort in providing independent care.

Staff working in the area also needs appropriate space to provide patient care as well as other associated professional and personal activities. These spaces include a medication preparation area, space for nutrition preparation, charting, and a communication area, as mentioned previously. In addition, a conference area for education, and a lounge area for relaxation and self-care provide staff support.

## Activity

The topic of activity must be examined on two levels; the activity occurring around the infant, and the activity involving the infant. Increased activity in the environment around the infant carries with it the additional consequence of increased light and increased noise. The unit should be a designated space with controlled access and devoid of traffic going to other clinical areas (White, 2002). Nonessential activity should be moved out to the clinical area, as discussed in the section on NICU design. Infants should be situated within the unit based on their environmental needs rather than the available bed space. Light and sound readings

obtained at each bedside will provide a 'map' of the unit so that infant needs and bedspace characteristics can be matched. The most fragile and sensitive infant requires the bedspace with the greatest protection. The bedspaces in high traffic areas and in environments that cannot be controlled should only be used if absolutely necessary.

The level of activity that is associated with his/her care also affects the infant. Research findings of physiologic changes as related to handling indicate the adverse effects on the ill neonate (Evans, 1991; Harrison, 1997; Lawrence-Black & Peters, 1996; Long, Philip, & Lucey, 1980). This activity should be minimized and consolidated to ensure uninterrupted periods of sleep to promote healing, growth, and neurodevelopment. Clustered care must occur across all disciplines to avoid numerous interruptions of sleep by numerous care providers with varied tasks and roles. This coordination of care must incorporate the assessment of behavioral cues and the use of supported 'time-outs' to minimize the degree of fatigue and stress the infant might experience.

Families are with their infants to provide support and positive tactile experiences. Integration of these needs is an essential component for the care provided to the infant. Encouraging the parents to be with their infant providing this important role is necessary for healing and attachment. Coordination of this interaction during scheduled care times is optimal; however, if that is not possible, the parent should not be denied access between the identified times.

## CONCLUSION

In this chapter, we reviewed the research in the areas of the animate environment, tactile-touch, parental influences, and inanimate environment of light and sound stimuli, and their effects on both the infant and family. These areas of research represent essential components of developmental care. Further research is needed to continue the growing body of evidence of the impact of the NICU environment on the growing neonate/infant and family. Recommendations for practice should be grounded in our interdisciplinary research as we strive to promote positive growth and development. Recommendations for NICU design should follow the recommended guidelines set forth by White (2002).

# REFERENCES

Ackerman, B., Sherwonit, E., & Williams, J. (1989). Reduced incidental light exposure: Effect on the development of retinopathy of prematurity in low birth weight infants. *Pediatrics, 83*, 958-962.

Acolet, D., Modi, N., Giannakoulpoulos, X., et al. (1993). Changes in plasma cortisol and catecholamine concentrations in response to massage in preterm infants. *Archives of Disease in Childhood, 68*, 29-31.

Adamson-Macedo, E.N. (1985-1986, Winter). Effects of tactile stimulation on low and very low birthweight infants during the first week of life. *Current Physiological Research and Reviews, 6*, 305-308.

Adamson-Macedo, E.N., & Attree, J.L.A. (1994). TAC-TIC therapy: The importance of systematic stroking. *British Journal of Midwifery, 2*, 264-269.

Adamson-Macedo, E.N., Dattani, I., Wilson, A., et al. (1993). A small sample follow-up study of children who received tactile stimulation after pre-term birth: Intelligence and achievements. *Journal of Reproductive and Infant Psychology, 11*, 165-168.

Adamson-Macedo, E.N., De Róiste, A., et al. (1994). TAC-TIC therapy with high-risk, distressed, ventilated preterms. *Journal of Reproductive and Infant Psychology, 12*, 249-252.

Adamson-Macedo, E.N., De Róiste, A., et al., (1997). Systematic gentle/light stroking and maternal random touching of ventilated preterms: A preliminary study. *International Journal of Prenatal and Perinatal Psychology and Medicine, 9*, 17-31.

Adamson-Macedo, E.N., & Hayes, J.A. (1998). Sensitivity and susceptibility to deep or light touch? *Infant Behavior and Development, 21*, 4.

Als, H., & Gilkerson, L. (1997). The role of relationship-based developmentally supportive newborn intensive care in strengthening outcomes of preterm infants. *Seminars in Perinatology, 21*, 178-189.

Als, H., Lawhon, G., Brown, E., Gibes, R., Duffy, F.H., McAnulty, G., et al. (1986). Individualized behavioral and environmental care for the very low birth weight preterm infant at high risk for bronchopulmonary dysplasia: Neonatal intensive care unit and developmental outcome. *Pediatrics, 78*, 1123-1132.

American Academy of Pediatrics (AAP). (1974; updated 1997, October). Policy statement. Noise: A hazard for the fetus and newborn (RE9728). Committee on Environmental Health, *Pediatrics, 100*(4), 724-727.

American Academy of Pediatrics (AAP) Committee on Environmental Health. (1997). Noise: A hazard for the fetus and newborn. *Pediatrics, 100*(4), 724-727.

Anagnostakis, D., Petmezakis, J., Messaritakis, J., & Matsaniotis, N. (1980, November). Noise pollution in neonatal units: A potential health hazard. *Acta Paediatrica Scandinavica, 69*, 771-773.

Arendt, J., Minors, D., & Waterhouse, J. M. (Eds.). (1989). *Biological rhythms in clinical practice.* London: John Wright.

Benini, F., Magnavita, V., Lago, P., et al. (1996). Evaluation of noise in the neonatal intensive care unit. *American Journal of Perinatology, 13*(1), 37-41.

Bennett, D.E., & Slade, P. (1991). Infants born at risk: Consequences for maternal post-partum adjustment. *British Journal of Medical Psychology, 64*, 159-172.

Berens, R.J., & Weigle, C.G. (1997). Noise analysis of three newborn infant isolettes. *Journal of Perinatology, 17*, 351-354.

Bialoskurski, M., Cox, C.L., & Hayes, J.A. (1999). The nature of attachment in a Neonatal Intensive Care Unit. *Journal of Perinatal Neonatal Nursing, 13*(1), 66-77.

Blackburn, S. (1996). Research utilization: Modifying the NICU light environment. *Neonatal Network, 15*(4), 63-66.

Blackburn, S. (1998). Enviromental impact of the NICU on developmental outcomes. *Journal of Pediatric Nursing, 13*(5), 279-289.

Blackburn, S., & Barnard, K. (1985). Analysis of caregiving events relating to preterm infants in the special care unit (pp. 113-130). In A.W. Gottfried & J.L. Gaiter (Eds.). *Infants under stress: Environmental neonatology.* Baltimore: University Park Press.

Blackburn, S., & Lowen, L. (1986). Impact of an infant's premature birth on the grandparents and parents. *Journal of Obstetric, Gynecologic, and Neonatal Nursing (JOGNN), 15*, 173-178.

Blackburn, S., & Patteson, D. (1991). Effects of cycled light on activity state and cardiorespiratory function in preterm infants. *Journal of Perinatal and Neonatal Nursing, 4*, 47-54.

Bracht, M., Ardal, F., Bot, A., et al. (1998). Initiation and maintenance of a hospital-based parent group for parents of premature infants: Key factors for success. *Neonatal Network, 17*, 33-37.

Brandon, D.H., Holditch-Davis, D., & Belyea, M. (2002, February). Preterm infants born at less than 31 weeks' gestation have improved growth in cycled light compared with continuous near darkness. *Journal of Pediatrics, 140*, 192-199.

Bullough, J., & Rea, M. (1996). Lighting for neonatal intensive care units: Some critical information for design. *Lighting Research and Technology, 28*(4), 189-198.

Caplan, G. (1960). Patterns of parental response to the crisis of premature birth. *Psychiatry, 23*, 365-374.

Caplan, G., Mason, E.A., & Kaplan, D.M. (2000; reprinted from 1965). Four studies of crisis in parents of prematures. *Community Mental Health Journal, 36*, 25-45.

Catlett, A.T., & Holditch-Davis, D. (1990). Environmental stimulation of the acutely ill premature infant: Physiological effects and nursing implications. *Neonatal Network, 8*, 19-26.

Chang, Y.J., Lin, C.H., & Lin, L.H. (2001). Noise and related events in a neonatal intensive care unit. *Acta Paediatrica Taiwanica, 42*, 212-217.

Costello, A., Bracht, M., Van Camp, K., et al. (1996). Parent information binder: Individualizing education for parents of preterm infants. *Neonatal Network, 15,* 43-46.

Costello, A., & Chapman, J. (1998). Mothers' perceptions of care-by-parent program prior to hospital discharge of their preterm infants. *Neonatal Network, 17,* 37-42.

Culp, R.E., Culp, A.M., & Harmon, R.J. (1989). A tool for educating parents about their premature infants. *Birth, 16,* 23-26.

Daga, S.R., Ahuja, V.K., & Lunkad, N.G. (1998): A warm touch improves oxygenation in newborn babies. *Journal of Tropical Pediatrics, 44,* 170-172.

Danford, D., Miske, S., Headley, J., et al. (1983): Effects of routine care procedures on transcutaneous oxygen of neonates: A quantitative approach. *Archives of Disease in Childhood, 58,* 20-23.

Del Bianco, L.A., & Shankaran, S. (1987). The design, organization and evaluation of a support group for parents of critically ill neonates. *Canadian Critical Care Nursing, 4,* 13-15.

DePaul, D, & Chambers, S. (1995). Environmental noise in the neonatal intensive care unit: Implications for nursing practice. *The Journal of Perinatal and Neonatal Nursing, 8*(4), 71-76.

De Róiste, A., & Bushnell, I. (1996). Tactile stimulation: Short and long-term benefits for premature infants. *British Journal of Developmental Psychology, 14,* 41-53.

De Róiste, A., & Bushnell, I. (2000). Cardiorespiratory and transcutaneous oxygen monitoring of high-risk preterms receiving systematic stroking. *International Journal of Prenatal and Perinatal Psychology and Medicine, 12*(8), 89-95.

Evans, J.B., & Philbin M.K. (2000). The acoustic environment of hospital nurseries. *Journal of Perinatology, 20*(8)(Pt 2), S105-S112.

Evans, J.C. (1991). Incidence of hypoxemia associated with caregiving in premature infants. *Neonatal Network, 10,* 17-24.

Fenwick, J., Barclay, L., & Schmied, V. (2001). Struggling to mother: A consequence of inhibitive nursing interactions in the neonatal nursery. *Journal of Perinatal and Neonatal Nursing, 15,* 49-64.

Field, T.M., Schanberg, S.M., Scafidi, F., et al. (1986): Tactile/kinesthetic stimulation effects on preterm neonates. *Pediatrics, 77,* 654-658.

Fielder, A.R., & Moseley, M.J. (2000). Environmental light and the preterm infant. *Seminars in Perinatology, 24,* 291-298.

Fraley, A.H. (1986). Chronic sorrow in parents of premature children. *Children's Health Care, 15,* 114-118.

Frodi, A.M., Lamb, M.E., Leavitt, L.A., et al. (1978). Fathers' and mothers' responses to the faces and cries of normal and premature infants. *Developmental Psychology, 14,* 490-498.

Gaddy, J.R., Rollag, M.D., & Brainard, G.C. (1993). Pupil size regulation of threshold of light-induced melatonin suppression. *Journal of Clinical Endocrinology and Metabolism, 77,* 1398-1401.

Gadeke, R., Doring, B., Keller, F., et al. (1969). The noise level in a childrens hospital and the wake-up threshold in infants. *Acta Paediatrica Scandinavica, 58,* 164-170.

Gale, G., & Franck, L.S. (1998). Toward a standard of care for parents of infants in the neonatal intensive care unit. *Critical Care Nurse, 18,* 62-74.

Gale, G., & VandenBerg, K.A. (1998). Kangaroo care. *Neonatal Network, 17,* 69-71.

Gennaro, S. (1986). Anxiety and problem-solving ability in mothers of premature infants. *Journal of Obstetric, Gynecologic, and Neonatal Nursing (JOGNN), 15,* 160-164.

Gennaro, S. (1988). Postpartal anxiety and depression in mothers of term and premature infants. *Nursing Research, 37,* 82-85.

Gennaro, S., Brooten, D., Roncoli, M., et al. (1993). Stress and health outcomes among mothers of low-birth-weight infants. *Western Journal of Nursing Research, 15,* 97-113.

Glass, P. (1988). Role of light toxicity in the developing retinal vasculature. *Birth Defects Original Article Series, 24,* 103-117.

Glass, P. (1990). Light and the developing retina. *Documenta Ophthalmologica Advances in Ophthalmology, 74,* 195-203.

Glass, P., Avery, G.B., Subramanian, K.N., et al. (1985). Effect of bright light in the hospital nursery on the incidence of retinopathy of prematurity. *New England Journal of Medicine, 313,* 401-404.

Glozbach, S.F., Edgar, D.M., & Ariagno, R.L. (1995). Biological rhythmicity in preterm infants prior to discharge from neonatal intensive care. *Pediatrics, 95,* 231-237.

Glozbach, S.F., Rowlett, E.A., Edgar, D.M., et al. (1993). Light variability in the modern neonatal nursery: Chronobiologic issues. *Medical Hypotheses, 41,* 217-224.

Gordin, P., & Johnson, B.H. (1999). Technology and family-centered perinatal care: Conflict or synergy? *Journal of Obstetric, Gynecologic, and Neonatal Nursing (JOGNN), 28,* 401-408.

Gorski, P.A., Hole, W.T., Leonard, C.H., & Martin, J.A. (1983). Direct computer recording of premature infants and nursery care: Distress following two interventions. *Pediatrics, 72,* 198-202.

Gottfried, A., Hodgman, J., & Brown, K. (1984): How intensive is newborn intensive care? An environmental analysis. *Pediatrics, 74,* 292-294.

Graven, S.N. (2002, January 13-16). The Physical and Developmental Environment of the High Risk Infant Conference, Sheraton Sand Key, Clearwater Beach, FL.

Graven, S.N., Bowen, F.W.J., Brooten, D., et al. (1992). The high-risk infant environment. Part 1. The role of the neonatal intensive care unit in the outcome of high-risk infants. *Journal of Perinatology, 12,* 164-172.

Gray, K., Dostal, S., Ternullo-Retta, C., & Armstrong, M.A. (1998). Developmentally supportive care in a neonatal intensive care unit: A research utilization project. *Neonatal Network, 17*(2), 33-38.

Gretebeck, R.J., Shaffer, D., & Bishop-Kurylo, D. (1998). Clinical pathways for family-oriented developmental care in the intensive care nursery. *Journal of Perinatal and Neonatal Nursing, 12*, 70-80.

Griffin, T. (1998a). The visitation policy. *Neonatal Network, 17*, 75-76.

Griffin, T. (1998b). Visitation patterns: The parents who visit "too much." *Neonatal Network, 17*, 67-68.

Griffin, T., Kavanaugh, K., Soto, C.F., et al. (1997). Parental evaluation of a tour of the neonatal intensive care unit during a high-risk pregnancy. *Journal of Obstetric, Gynecologic, and Neonatal Nursing (JOGNN), 26*, 59-65.

Griffin, T., Wishba, C., & Kavanaugh, K. (1998). Nursing interventions to reduce stress in parents of hospitalized preterm infants. *Journal of Pediatric Nursing, 13*, 290-295.

Grunwald, P. (1997). Family-centered care in the NICU. *Exceptional Parent, 27*(5), 58.

Hack, M., Klein, N.K., & Taylor, H.G. (1995). Long-term developmental outcomes of low birth weight infants. *The Future of Children/Center for the Future of Children the David and Lucile Packard Foundation, 5*, 176-196.

Hamer, R.D., Dobson, V., & Mayer, M.J. (1984). Absolute thresholds in human infants exposed to continuous illumination. *Investigative Ophthalmology and Visual Science, 25*, 381-388.

Hao, H., & Rivkees, S.A. (1999). The biological clock of very premature primate infants is responsive to light. *Proceedings of the National Academy of Sciences of the United States of America, 96*, 2426-2429.

Harrison, H. (1993). The principles for family-centered neonatal care. *Pediatrics, 92*, 643-650.

Harrison, L. (1997). Research utilization: Handling preterm infants in the NICU. *Neonatal Network, 16*(3), 65-69.

Harrison, L.L. (1997). Parenting the high-risk neonate (pp. 1409-1431). In F.H. Nichols & E. Zwelling (Eds.). *Maternal-newborn nursing: Theory and practice.* Philadelphia: W.B. Saunders.

Harrison, L.L. (2001a). *Effects of massage on preterm infants and mothers* (unpublished manuscript). Birmingham, AL: The University of Alabama School of Nursing, The University of Alabama at Birmingham.

Harrison, L.L. (2001b). The use of comforting touch and massage to reduce stress for preterm infants in the neonatal intensive care unit. *Newborn and Infant Nursing Reviews, 1*, 235-241.

Harrison, L.L. (In press). Tactile stimulation of NICU preterm infants. In T.M. Field. (Ed.), *Touch research book.* Skillman, NJ: Johnson & Johnson.

Harrison, L.L., Berbaum, M., Stem, J.T., et al. (2001). Use of individualized versus standard criteria to identify abnor-

mal levels of heart rate or oxygen saturation in preterm infants. *Journal of Nursing Measurement, 9*, 181-200.

Harrison, L.L., Groer, M., Modrcin-McCarthy, M., & Wilkinson, J. (1992). Effects of gentle human touch on preterm infants: Results from a pilot study. *Infant Behavior and Development, 15*, 12.

Harrison, L., & Klaus, M.H. (1994). Commentary: A lesson from Eastern Europe. *Birth, 21*, 45-46.

Harrison, L.L., Leeper, J., & Yoon, M. (1991). Preterm infants' physiologic responses to early parent touch. *Western Journal of Nursing Research, 13*, 698-713.

Harrison, L.L., Olivet, L., Cunningham, K., et al. (1996). Effects of gentle human touch on preterm infants: Report from a pilot study. *Neonatal Network, 15*, 35-42.

Harrison, L.L., Sherrod, R.A., Dunn, L., et al. (1991). Effects of hospital-based instructions on interactions between parents and preterm infants. *Neonatal Network, 9*, 27-33.

Harrison, L.L., & Twardosz, S. (1986). Teaching mothers about their preterm infants. *Journal of Obstetric, Gynecologic, and Neonatal Nursing (JOGNN), 15*(2), 165-172

Harrison, L., Williams, A., Berbaum, M., et al. (2000a). Effects of developmental, health status, behavioral and environmental variables on preterm infants' responses to a gentle human touch intervention. *International Journal of Prenatal and Perinatal Psychology and Medicine, 12*, 109-122.

Harrison, L., Williams, A., Berbaum, M., et al. (2000b). Physiologic and behavioral effects of gentle human touch on preterm infants. *Research in Nursing and Health, 23*, 435-446.

Harrison, L.L., & Woods, S. (1991). Early parental touch and preterm infants. *Journal of Obstetric, Gynecologic, and Neonatal Nursing (JOGNN), 20*, 299-306.

Hellbrugge, T. (1974). The development of circadian and ultradian rhythms of premature and full-term infants (pp. 339-341). In L. Sheving, F. Halberg, & J. Pauly (Eds.), *Chronobiology.* Tokyo: Igaku Shoin.

Holditch-Davis, D., & Miles, M.S. (2000). Mothers' stories about their experiences in the neonatal intensive care unit. *Neonatal Network, 19*, 13-21.

Hummel, P.A., & Eastman, D.L. (1991). Do parents of preterm infants suffer chronic sorrow? *Neonatal Network, 10*, 59-65.

Hurst, I. (1993). Facilitating parental involvement through documentation. *Journal of Perinatal and Neonatal Nursing, 7*, 80-90.

Institute for Family Centered Care. (1998). Core principles of family-centered health care. *Advances in Family-Centered Care, 4*, 2-4.

Jay, S.S. (1982). The effects of gentle human touch on mechanically ventilated very-short-gestation infants. *Maternal Child Nursing Journal, 11*, 199-256.

Johnson, B.H. (1995). Newborn intensive care units pioneer family-centered change in hospitals across the country. *Zero to Three, 15*, 11-17.

Johnson, S.H., & Grubbs, J.B. (1975). The premature infant's reflex behaviors: Effect on the maternal-child relationship. *Journal of Obstetric, Gynecologic, and Neonatal Nursing (JOGNN), 4*, 15-21.

Kaplan, D., & Mason, E.A. (1960). Maternal reactions to premature birth viewed as an acute emotional disorder. *American Journal of Orthopsychiatry, 30*, 539-547.

Kattwinkel, J., Nearman, H.S., Fanaroff, A.A., et al. (1975). Apnea of prematurity: Comparative therapeutic effects of cutaneous stimulation and nasal continuous positive airway pressure. *The Journal of Pediatrics, 86*, 588-592.

Kramer, M., Chamorro, I., Green, D., et al. (1975). Extra tactile stimulation of the premature infant. *Nursing Research, 24*, 324-334.

Krebs, T.L. (1998). Clinical pathway for enhanced parent and preterm infant interaction through parent education. *Journal of Perinatal and Neonatal Nursing, 12*, 38-49.

Kuhn, C.M., Schanberg, S.M., Field, T., et al. (1991). Tactile-kinesthetic stimulation effects on sympathetic and adrenocortical function in preterm infants. *Journal of Pediatrics, 119*, 434-440.

Landry, R.J., Scheidt, P.C., & Hammond, R.W. (1985). Ambient light and phototherapy conditions of eight neonatal care units: A summary report. *Pediatrics, 75*(2)(Pt 2), 434-436.

Lawhon, G. (2002). Facilitation of parenting the premature infant within the newborn intensive care unit. *Journal of Perinatal and Neonatal Nursing, 16*, 71-82.

Lawrence-Black, T, & Peters, K. (1996). Physiological responses to caregiving maneuvers in preterm infants. *Tenth Ross Conference in Pediatrics*, 45-50.

Lawson, K., Daum, C., & Turkewitz, G. (1977). Environmental characteristics of a neonatal intensive care unit. *Child Development, 48*, 1633-1639.

Lawwill, T. (1982). Three major pathologic processes caused by light in the primate retina: A search for mechanisms. *Transactions of the American Ophthalmological Society, 80*, 517-579.

Lee, Y.H., & Malakooti, N., & Lotas, M. (2003, under review).

Levin, A. (1994). The mother-infant unit at Tallinn Children's Hospital, Estonia: A truly baby-friendly unit. *Birth, 21*, 39-44.

Levin, A. (1999). Humane neonatal care initiative. *Acta Paediatrica, 88*, 353-355.

Levy-Shiff, R.M., Sharir, H., & Mogilner, M.B. (1989). Mother- and father-preterm infant relationship in the hospital preterm nursery. *Child Development, 60*(1), 93-102.

Lindsay, J.K., Roman, L., DeWys, M., et al. (1993). Creative caring in the NICU: Parent-to-parent support. *Neonatal Network, 12*, 37-43.

Long, J.G., Lucey, J.F., & Philip, A.G. (1980). Noise and hypoxemia in the intensive care nursery. *Pediatrics, 65* (Jan), 143-145.

Long, J.G., Philip, A. & Lucey, J.F. (1980). Excessive handling as a cause of hypoxemia. *Pediatrics, 65*, 203-207.

Lotas, M.J. (1992). The effects of light and sound in the neonatal intensive care unit environment on the low birth weight infant. NAACOG's (Nursing Association of the College of Obstetrics and Gynecology). *Clinical Issues in Perinatal & Women's Health Nursing, 3*(1), 34-44.

Lotas, M.J., & Medoff-Cooper, B. (2001, under review). Effects of light-dark cycles in the NICU environment on heart rate in the preterm infant.

Lotas, M.J., Seal, L., Ambrose, B., et al. (2003, under review). NICU lighting levels and patterns revisited: A study in research utilization.

Lotas, M.J., & Walden, M. (1996). Individualized developmental care for very low-birth-weight infants: A critical review. *Journal of Obstetric, Gynecologic, and Neonatal Nursing (JOGNN), 25* (8), 681-687.

Macnab, A.J., Beckett, L.Y., Park, C.C., & Sheckter, L. (1998). Journal writing as a social support strategy for parents of premature infants: A pilot study. *Patient Education and Counseling, 33*, 149-159.

Magnavita, V., Arslan, E., & Benini, F. (1994). Noise exposure in the neonatal intensive care units. *Acta Otorhinolaryngology, Italy, 14*(9), 489-501.

Mann, N.P., Haddow, R., Stokes, L., et al. (1986). Effect of night and day on preterm infants in a newborn nursery: Randomised trial. *British Medical Journal (Clinical Research Ed), 293*, 1265-1267.

Mantagos, S., Moustogianni, A., Varvarigou, A., et al. (1989). Effect of light on diurnal variation of blood amino acids in neonates. *Biology of the Neonate, 55*, 97-103.

Mason, E.A. (1963). A method of predicting crisis outcome for mothers of premature babies. *Public Health Reports, 78*, 1031-1035.

McGehee, I.J., & Eckerman, C.O. (1983): The preterm infant as social partner: Responsive but unreadable. *Infant Behavior and Development, 6*, 461-470.

McGrath, J.M., & Conliffe-Torres, S. (1996). Integrating family-centered developmental assessment and intervention into routine care in the neonatal intensive care unit. *Nursing Clinics of North America, 31*, 367-385.

Messner, K., Maisels, M., & Leure-duPree, A. (1978). Phototoxicity in the newborn primate retina. *Investigative Ophthalmology and Visual Science, 17*, 178-182.

Meyer, E.C., Garcia-Coll, C.T., Lester, B.M., et al. (1994). Family-based intervention improves maternal psychological well-being and feeding interaction of preterm infants. *Pediatrics, 93*(2), 241-246.

Miles, M.S. (1989). Parents of critically ill premature infants: Sources of stress. *Critical Care Nursing Quarterly, 12*, 69-74.

Miles, M.S., Carlson, J., & Funk, S.G. (1996). Sources of support reported by mothers and fathers of infants hospitalized in a neonatal intensive care unit. *Neonatal Network, 15*, 45-52.

Miles, M.S., Funk, S., & Kasper, M.A. (1991). The neonatal intensive care unit environment: *American Association of Critical Care Nursing (AACN) Clinical Issues in Critical Care Nursing, 2*, 346-352.

Miles, M.S., Funk, S., & Kasper, M.A. (1992). The stress response of mothers and fathers of preterm infants. *Research in Nursing and Health, 15*, 261-269.

Miles, M.S., & Holditch-Davis, D. (1997). Parenting the prematurely born child: Pathways of influence. *Seminars in Perinatology, 21*, 254-266.

Miller, C., White, R., Whitman, T., et al. (1995). The effects of cycled versus noncycled lighting on growth and development in preterm infants. *Infant Behavior and Development, 18*, 87-95.

Miller, D.B., & Holditch-Davis, D. (1992). Interactions of parents and nurses with high-risk preterm infants. *Research in Nursing and Health, 15*, 187-197.

Minde, K., Shosenberg, N., Marton, P., et al. (1980). Self-help groups in a premature nursery: A controlled evaluation. *Journal of Pediatrics, 96*, 933-940.

Mirmiran, M., & Ariagno, R.L. (2000). Influence of light in the NICU on the development of circadian rhythms in preterm infants (review). *Seminars in Perinatology, 24* (4), 247-257.

Modrcin-McCarthy, M.A. (1992). The physiological and behavioral effects of a gentle human touch nursing intervention on preterm infants, Doctoral Dissertation. Knoxville, TN: University of Tennessee *Dissertation Abstracts International, 54B*, 1336.

Modrcin-Talbott, M.A., Harrison, L.L., Groer, M.W., et al. (2003). The biobehavioral effects of gentle human touch on preterm infants. *Nursing Science Quarterly, 16*, 60-67.

Moore-Ede, M.C., Czeisler, C.A., & Richardson, G.S. (1983). Circadian timekeeping in health and disease. Part 1. Basic properties of circadian pacemakers. *New England Journal of Medicine, 309*(9), 469-476.

Moore-Ede, M., Sulzman, F., & Fuller, C. (1982). *The clocks that time us*. Cambridge: Harvard University Press.

Morin, L.P. (1994). The circadian visual system. *Brain Research Reviews, 19*, 102-127.

Morris, B.H, Philbin, M.K, & Bose, C. (2000). Physiological effects of sound on the newborn. *Journal of Perinatology, 20*(8)(Pt 2) S55-S60.

Morrow, C.J., Field, T.M., Scafidi, F.A., et al. (1991). Differential effects of massage and heelstick procedures on transcutaneous oxygen tension in preterm neonates. *Infant Behavior and Development, 14*, 397-414.

Moseley, M.J., & Fielder, A.R. (1988). Phototherapy: An ocular hazard revisited. *Archives of Disease in Childhood, 63*, 886-887.

Moseley, M.J., Thompson, J.R., Levene, M.I., et al. (1988). Effects of nursery illumination on frequency of eyelid opening and state in preterm neonates. *Early Human Development, 18*, 13-26.

Murdoch, D.R. & Darlow, B.A. (1984). Handling during neonatal intensive care. *Archives of Disease in Childhood, 59*(1), 957-961.

Nelson, M.N., White-Traut, R.C., Vasan, U., et al. (2001). One-year outcome of auditory-tactile-visual-vestibular intervention in the neonatal intensive care unit: Effects of severe prematurity and central nervous system injury. *Journal of Child Neurology, 16*, 493-498.

Niven, C.A., Wiszniewski, C., & AlRoomi, L. (1993). Attachment in mothers of pre-term babies. *Journal of Reproductive and Infant Psychology, 11*, 175-185.

Noell, W. (1980). Possible mechanism of photoreceptor damage by light in mammalian eyes. *Vision Research, 20*, 1163-1171.

Norris, S., Campbell, L., & Brenkerd, S. (1982). Nursing procedures and alterations in transcutaneous oxygen tension in premature infants. *Nursing Research, 31*, 330-336.

Oehler, J.M. (1985). Examining the issue of tactile stimulation for preterm infants. *Neonatal Network, 4*, 25-33.

Oehler, J.M., Eckerman, C.O., & Wilson, W.H. (1988). Social stimulation and the regulation of premature infants' state prior to term age. *Infant Behavior and Development, 11*, 333-351.

Patteson, D., & Barnard, K.E. (1990). Parenting of low birthweight infants: A review of issues and interventions. *Infant Mental Health Journal, 11*, 37-56.

Pearson, J., & Anderson, K. (2001). Evaluation of a program to promote positive parenting in the neonatal intensive care unit. *Neonatal Network, 20*, 43-48.

Peters, K. (1992). Does routine nursing care complicate the physiologic status of the premature neonate with respiratory distress syndrome? *Journal of Perinatal & Neonatal Nursing, 6*, 67-84.

Pettigrew, A.G., Edwards, D.A., & Henderson-Smart, D.J. (1988). Perinatal risk factors in preterm infants with moderate-to-profound hearing deficits. *Medical Journal of Australia, 148*, 174-177.

Phelps, D.L., & Watts, J.L. (2001). Early light reduction for preventing retinopathy of prematurity in very low birth weight infants. *Cochrane Database of Systematic Reviews*, CD000122. Available online at *www.cochrane.org/cochrane/revabstr/AB000122.htm*.

Philbin, M.K. (2000). The influence of auditory experience on the behavior of preterm newborns. *Journal of Perinatology, 20*(8)(Pt 2), S77-S87.

Philbin, M.K., Ballweg, D.D., & Gray, L. (1994). The effect of an intensive care unit sound environment on the development of habituation in healthy avian neonates. *Developmental Psychobiology, 27*, 11-21.

Philbin, M.K., & Gray, L. (2002). Changing levels of quiet in an intensive care nursery. *Journal of Perinatology, 22*, 455-460.

Prudhoe, C.M., & Peters, D.L. (1995). Social support of parents and grandparents in the neonatal intensive care unit. *Pediatric Nursing, 21*, 140-146.

Raines, D.A. (1998). Values of mothers of low birth weight infants in the NICU. *Neonatal Network, 17,* 41-46.

Reppert, S.M. (1992). Pre-natal development of a hypothalamic biological clock. *Progress in Brain Research, 93,* 119-131; discussion 132.

Reynolds, J.D., Hardy, R.J., Kennedy, K.A., et al. (1998). Lack of efficacy of light reduction in preventing retinopathy of prematurity. Light Reduction in Retinopathy of Prematurity (LIGHT-ROP) Cooperative Group. *New England Journal of Medicine, 338,* 1572-1576.

Rice, R.D. (1977). Neurophysiological development in premature infants following stimulation. *Developmental Psychology, 13,* 69-76.

Rivkees, S.A. (2001). Mechanisms and clinical significance of circadian rhythms in children. *Current Opinion in Pediatrics, 13,* 352-357.

Rivkees, S. (2003). *The development of circadian rhythms.* Presented at The Physical and Developmental Environment of the High-Risk Infant Conference, Clearwater Beach, FL, January 29, 2003.

Robertson, A., Cooper-Peel, C., & Vos, P. (1998). Peak noise distribution in the neonatal intensive care nursery. *Journal of Perinatology, 18,* 361-364.

Robertson, A., Cooper-Peel, C., & Vos, P. (1999). Contribution of heating, ventilation, and air conditioning airflow and conversation to the ambient sound in a neonatal intensive care unit. *Journal of Perinatology, 19,* 362-366.

Robertson, A., & Philbin, M.K. (1996). *Studies of sound and auditory development.* Paper presented at the Physical and Developmental Environment of the High Risk Neonate, Clearwater Beach, FL: University of South Florida College of Medicine.

Robinson, J., & Fielder, A.R. (1992). Light and the immature visual system. *Eye (London England), 6*(Pt 2), 166-172.

Robinson, J., Moseley, M.J., Thompson, J.R., et al. (1989). Eyelid opening in preterm neonates. *Archives of Disease in Childhood, 64,* 943-948.

Roman, L.A., Lindsay, J.K., Buger, R.P., et al. (1995). Parent-to-parent support initiated in the neonatal intensive care unit. *Research in Nursing and Health, 18,* 385-394.

Scafidi, F.A., Field, T.M., Schanberg, S.M., et al. (1990). Massage stimulates growth in preterm infants: A replication. *Infant Behavior and Development, 13,* 176-188.

Scafidi, F.A., Field, T.M., Schanberg, S.M., et al. (1986). Effects of tactile/kinesthetic stimulation on the clinical course and sleep/wake behavior of preterm neonates. *Infant Behavior and Development, 9,* 91-105.

Schanberg, S.M., & Field, T.M. (1987). Sensory deprivation stress and supplemental stimulation in the rat pup and preterm human neonate. *Child Development, 58,* 1431-1447.

Schendel, D.E., Stockbauer, J.W., Hoffman, H.J., et al. (1997). Relation between very low birth weight and developmental delay among preschool children without disabilities. *American Journal of Epidemiology, 146*(9),740-749.

Seiberth, V., Linderkamp, O., Knorz, M.C., et al. (1994). A controlled clinical trial of light and retinopathy of prematurity. *American Journal of Ophthalmology, 118,* 492-495.

Shields-Poe, D., & Pinelli, J. (1997). Variables associated with parental stress in neonatal intensive care units. *Neonatal Network, 16,* 29-37.

Shiroiwa, Y., Kamiya, Y., Uchibori, S., et al. (1986). Activity, cardiac and respiratory responses of blindfold preterm infants in a neonatal intensive care unit. *Early Human Development, 14,* 259-265.

Shogan, M.G., & Schumann, L.L. (1993). The effect of environmental lighting on the oxygen saturation of preterm infants in the NICU. *Neonatal Network, 12*(5), 7-13.

Sisson, T.R., Glauser, S.C., Glauser, E.M., et al. (1970). Retinal changes produced by phototherapy. *Journal of Pediatrics, 77,* 221-227.

Slattery, M.J., Flanagan, V., Cronenwett, L.R., et al. (1998). Mothers' perceptions of the quality of their infants' back transfer. *Journal of Obstetric, Gynecologic, and Neonatal Nursing (JOGNN), 27,* 394-401.

Slevin, M., Farrington, N., Duffy, G., et al. (2000). Altering the NICU and measuring infants' responses. *Acta Paediatrica, 89,* 577-581.

Solkoff, N., & Matuszak, D. (1975). Tactile stimulation and behavioral development among low–birthweight infants. *Child Psychiatry and Human Development, 61,* 33-37.

Solkoff, N., Yaffe, S., Weintraub, D., et al. (1969). Effects of handling and the subsequent development of premature infants. *Development Psychology, 1,* 864-866.

Spinelli, D.N. (1990). Plasticity triggering experiences, nature, and the dual genesis of brain structure and function. *Clinics in Perinatology, 17*(1), 77-82.

Stauber, S.R., & Mahan, C.K. (1987). Successes and struggles of parent support groups in neonatal intensive care units. *Journal of Perinatology, 7,* 140-144.

Sydnor-Greenberg, N., & Dokken, D. (2000). Coping and caring in different ways: Understanding and meaningful involvement. *Pediatric Nursing, 26,* 185-190.

Sullivan, J.R. (1999). Development of father–infant attachment in fathers of preterm infants. *Neonatal Network, 18*(7), 33-39.

Symon, A., & Cunningham, S. (1995). Handling premature neonates: A study using time-lapse video. *Nursing Times, 91*(17), 35-37.

Tenreiro, S., Dowse, H.B., D'Souza, S., et al. (1991, November). The development of ultradian and circadian rhythms in premature babies maintained in constant conditions. *Early Human Development, 27,* 33-52.

Thomas, K.A. (1989). How the NICU environment sounds to a preterm infant. *MCN: The American Journal of Maternal Child Nursing, 14,* 249-251.

Tribotti, S.J. (1990). Effects of gentle touch on the premature infant (pp. 80-89). In N. Gunzenhauser (Ed.), *Advances in touch: New implications in human development.* Skillman, NJ: Johnson & Johnson.

Vickers, A., Ohlsson, A.J., & Horsley, A. (2001). *Massage therapy for preterm and/or low birthweight infants* (pp. 1-30). Available online at *silk.nih.gov/silk/cochrane/vickers/vickers.htm.*

Walsh-Sukys, M., Reitenbach, A., Hudson-Barr, D., et al. (2001). Reducing light and sound in the neonatal intensive care unit: An evaluation of patient safety, staff satisfaction and costs. *Journal of Perinatology, 21,* 230-235.

Werner, N.P., & Conway, A.E. (1990). Caregiver contacts experienced by premature infants in the neonatal intensive care unit. *Maternal Child Nursing Journal, 19,* 21-43.

White, R.D. (2002). *Recommended standards for newborn ICU design.* Report of the Fifth Consensus Conference on Newborn ICU Design, January 2002, Clearwater Beach, Florida, Committee to Establish Recommended Standards for Newborn ICU. Available online at *design://www.nd.edu/~kkolberg/DesignStandards.htm.*

White-Traut, R.C., & Goldman, M.B.C. (1988). Premature infant massage: Is it safe? *Pediatric Nursing, 14,* 285-289.

White-Traut, R.C., & Nelson, M.N. (1988). Maternally administered tactile, auditory, visual, and vestibular stimulation: Relationship to later interactions between mothers and premature infants. *Research in Nursing and Health, 11,* 31-39.

White-Traut, R.C., Nelson, M.N., Silvestri, J.M., et al. (1993). Patterns of physiologic and behavioral response of intermediate care preterm infants to intervention. *Pediatric Nursing, 19,* 625-629.

White-Traut, R.C., Nelson, M.N., Silvestri, J.M., et al. (1997). Responses of preterm infants to unimodal and multimodal sensory intervention. *Pediatric Nursing, 23,* 169-175, 193.

White-Traut, R.C., Nelson, M.N., Silvestri, J.M., et al. (1999). Developmental intervention for preterm infants diagnosed with periventricular leukomalacia. *Research in Nursing and Health, 22,* 131-143.

White-Traut, R.C., Nelson, M.N., Silvestri, J.M., et al. (2002). Effect of auditory, tactile, visual, and vestibular intervention on length of stay, alertness, and feeding progression in preterm infants. *Developmental Medicine and Child Neurology, 44,* 91-97.

White-Traut, R.C., & Pate, C.M.H. (1987). Modulating infants state in premature infants. *Journal of Pediatric Nursing, 2,* 96-101.

White-Traut, R.C., & Tubeszewski, K.A. (1986). Multimodal stimulation of the premature infant. *Journal of Pediatric Nursing, 1,* 90-95.

Zahr, L.K., & Balian, S. (1995). Responses of premature infants to routine nursing interventions and noise in the NICU. *Nursing Research, 44,* 179-183.

# 15 *Caregiving and the Environment*

## Carol Spruill Turnage-Carrier

Prematurity comes with the potential for later learning disabilities or behavioral problems even when surviving without serious medical complications. Long-term outcomes include motor delays, mild to severe cognitive disability, visual-motor deficits, language impairment, behavioral and social problems, and increased need for special education services (Bhutta, Cleves, Casey, et al, 2002; Cherkes-Julkowski, 1998; Cloonan, Maxwell, & Miller, 2001; Hack & Fanaroff, 2000; Hack, Taylor, Klein, et al., 1994; Lewis, Singer, Fulton, et al., 2002; McGrath & Sullivan, 2002; McGrath, Sullivan, Lester, & Oh, 2000; Msall & Tremont, 2002; Taylor, Klein, Minich, & Hack, 2000; Taylor, Klein, & Hack, 2000; Vohr, Wright, Dusick, et al., 2000). In a study comparing very low birthweight infants (VLBW) to normal birthweight infants, the VLBW group demonstrated lower mathematical skills, higher incidence of grade retention, and a need for special academic assistance 2.8 times greater in the academic setting (Schraeder, Heverly, O'Brien, et al., 1997).

Early intervention (EI) to minimize the stress and negative developmental impact of the neonatal intensive care unit (NICU) on preterm infants presents a challenge to NICU care teams (Hernandez-Reif & Field, 2000). Designing appropriate interventions is only one aspect of the challenge. Understanding when to implement interventions and better methods to evaluate both short- and long-term outcomes is an ongoing goal of developmental research. For now, careful evaluation as to quality of the research is required to determine what evidence supports the use of a particular developmental intervention in the clinical setting. Some researchers are concerned that atypical sensory stimulation might adversely affect later developing senses, resulting in perceptual and behavioral difficulties (Foushee & Lickliter, 2002; Lickliter, 2000a, 2000b; Lickliter & Bahrick, 2000; Lickliter & Stoumbos, 1992; McBride & Lickliter, 1994; Sleigh & Lickliter, 1995, 1998). Other researchers argue that supplemental stimulation is beneficial for optimizing preterm growth and neurobehavioral development (Als, Lawhon, Duffy, et al., 1994; Buehler, Als, Duffy, et al., 1995; Feldman, Eidelman, Sirota, & Weller, 2002; Gale & VandenBerg, 1998; Pinelli & Symington, 2000a, 2000b). A common-sense approach is recommended by Glass (1999) that considers the hierarchical organization and integration of sensory development and function as the framework for intervention. Guiding principles for these interventions can be found in Box 15-1 (Glass, 1999). In this chapter, the research related to individualized, family-centered, developmental care (IFDC) interventions in the caregiving environment of the NICU is discussed. IFDC interventions are discussed within the sensory system most affected: vestibular; taste and smell; auditory; and visual. Tactile interventions are addressed in Chapter 14. Caregiving interventions, in general, are examined. However, discussion of more programmatic forms of IFDC interventions, such as Newborn Individualized Developmental Care Assessment Program (NIDCAP®) (Boston, MA) and Wee Care® (Norwell, MA), are not to be discussed, as they are examined in several other sections of this book, and their outlines are available in the Appendixes. The IFDC intervention of skin-to-skin holding is addressed. Recommendations for caregiving practice based on the supporting evidence are made.

## VESTIBULAR SYSTEM

The fetus' early experience with vestibular stimulation is contingent upon his/her own actions and on the noncontingent activities of the mother. Periodic oscillations and movements generated by the fetus or mother, or both, occur in the fluid-filled environment of the womb. As the environment becomes more restrictive, through less amniotic

## Box 15-1   Guiding Principles for Developmental Intervention

Individualize intervention based on assessment, knowledge of preterm infant development, and each infants current and past medical status; physiologic stability; autonomic, motor, and behavioral state responses to the environment and caregiving, thresholds, vulnerabilities, strengths; and social and physical needs.

Organize intervention to follow the normal maturational course of development so that the most mature sensory system is supported first without attempts to accelerate the developmental process (i.e., type, timing, amount).

Consider the most natural occurring opportunities as optimal for normal development (i.e., mother, breast, skin-to-skin, nonnutritive sucking).

Protect infants from environmental stressors.

Support behavioral state development (i.e., undisturbed rest, gentle arousal).

Use positioning and containment to promote autonomic, state, and motor stability.

Consider using natural smells and tastes that have biological significance as early as possible (i.e., breast milk, parent smell).

Introduce graded tactile-vestibular intervention based on infant's tolerance before auditory input saving visual stimulation for last and only when stable alerting and interest in the environment is demonstrated.

Remove any sensory stimulation when stress behaviors manifest.

Maintain ongoing responsive interaction based on individual infant communication.

Ensure opportunities for parents to participate in nurturing and caring for their infant beginning at admission.

Data from Glass, P. (1999). The vulnerable neonate and the neonatal intensive care environment. In G.B. Avery, M.A. Fletcher, & M.G. MacDonald (Eds.), *Neonatology: Pathophysiology and management of the newborn* (5th ed.). Philadelphia: Lippincott, Williams & Wilkins.

fluid and space, the vestibular experience is more a result of mother's activities, which are slower as the time of birth approaches. Behavioral state is affected by vestibular stimulation as moving to upright increases arousal and slow side-to-side rocking, walking, or pacing is often followed by drowsiness or sleep (Glass, 1999). This early functional system might explain the calming of term infants to gentle, rhythmic rocking movements and the increase in activity that accompanies fast, arrhythmic movements. Research using vestibular stimulation is often conducted along with other sensory modalities, making it difficult to understand the benefits of added stimulation to this sensory system alone.

Infants must be able to balance their bodies and adjust their movements to remain steady and attend to other stimuli in their world. It is important for these postural adjustments during movement to take place unconsciously, so that infants are free to explore and develop motor, auditory, and visual skills. The vestibular system functions through an interplay with other sources of information. Three intact sources of sensory information, necessary for balance and self-movement, include:

1. Proprioceptive input from the skin, joints, and muscle
2. Vestibular stimulation from the semicircular canals of the inner ear
3. Optical flow stimulation from movements in the visual field (Berk, 2000)

Optical flow is defined as movements within the visual field that indicate the body is in motion, resulting in postural adaptation, so that the body remains upright. Although the vestibular system is anatomically complete, this system and other sources of information, such as the visual system, are not functionally mature. This might explain why repositioning and transferring from bed to mother might be particularly stressful for preterm infants.

The typical newborn already has a sense of balance and control that is further refined by experience and motor development (Berk, 2000). All other sensory systems appear to rely on appropriate input that influences specification of neuronal connections for normal development (Peusner, 2001). The infant in the NICU, especially the premature infant, experiences a reduction in the usual vestibular stimulation. Is there opportunity to support this sensory system in the clinical setting?

Six randomized, controlled experimental studies have demonstrated safety and efficacy in reduction of apnea of prematurity using a specialized, oscillating waterbed for premature infants with uncomplicated apnea (Korner, 1999). The device was set to move in the rhythm of maternal breathing (12 to 14 breaths/min) at an amplitude of less than 2.5 mm over the surface, in a head to toe motion. Infants who were placed on the oscillating waterbed demonstrated more organized sleep; more mature motor patterns; fewer jittery or jerky movements; decreased irritability; more time spent in a visually alert, quiet state; and significantly better attention and pursuit of inanimate and animate visual and auditory stimuli. Korner and others (Korner, 1999; Symington & Pinelli, 2002) found no effect of vestibular stimulation (oscillating waterbed) on physiologic parameters (heart rate, respiratory rate, or body temperature). In a meta-analysis of developmental intervention research (Symington & Pinelli, 2002), vestibular stimulation showed no effects on feeding, growth as in weight gain, or length of stay. Three trials included in the analysis found no evidence that vestibular stimulation is beneficial for improving neurodevelopmental outcomes (each study used different neurobehavioral assessment instruments).

Cordero, Clark, and Schott (1986) randomized 17 preterm infants who weighed less than 1.5 kg to either a rocking or traditional incubator and found a significant increase in quiet sleep in the treatment group. Thoman, Ingersoll, and Acebo (1991) studied the effects of a breathing bear versus a nonbreathing bear on 45 premature infants (29 to 33 weeks' gestation) in incubators during a 3-week period. Infants were able to move toward and away from the breathing bear. Breathing-bear infants demonstrated significantly more quiet sleep and spent longer time in quiet sleep at postterm. Preterm infants with the breathing bear spent more time in physical contact with the bear than control infants receiving the nonbreathing bear. This intervention might provide a self-regulating experience that is controlled by the infant's own efforts of moving toward or away from the stimulus.

Other modes of vestibular stimulation, such as rocking chairs, swings, and hammocks have not undergone similar investigation (Glass, 1999). Rhythm and motion provided by rocking is controlled by the adult and can be adjusted or stopped based on an infant's response. Swings are not justified by research or consideration of the preterm infant's vulnerabilities, especially airway, due to the extreme upright position and the fast rate of oscillation, which is generally not adjustable. Infants should not be left in any device for prolonged periods, and, if quietly alert, it is an opportunity to support that behavioral state through face-to-face interaction with a parent or caregiver.

Theoretically it makes sense to provide interventions for an early developing sensory system. From the evidence, it appears that vestibular stimulation enhances behavioral state, in particular, quiet sleep, and, possibly, maturation of sleep. The role of vestibular stimulation remains unclear; however, careful use of gentle vestibular stimulation might be considered within the boundaries of infant tolerance and based on current evidence. There is no literature that provides information on the optimal way to support this sensory system, particularly for the smallest, most fragile low birthweight infants.

## TASTE AND SMELL

The chemical senses are often forgotten in the NICU, at least the pleasurable ones. NICU smells generally include alcohol, povidone-iodine, and other clinical odors. As infants improve, they begin to receive more exposure to the smell of their parents and breast milk or formula. Taste is most often not stimulated during parenteral nutrition, unless the infant's mouth is cleaned with a flavored swab. Once an infant can take fluid by mouth, noxious oral medications can be administered, as well as breastmilk or formulas.

Taste buds have formed by the 8th or 9th week of gestation. At 16 weeks, taste receptors are present and by term are at adult levels (Glass, 1999). Term neonates show different facial expressions for different tastes, such as a relaxed expression in response to sweetness, pursed lips to sour, and the unique open arch-like mouth when exposed to bitter (Berk, 2000). Swallowing behavior of amniotic fluid in 34- to 39-week-old fetuses was shown to increase when the fluid was injected with sweet flavor and decreased with bitter (Glass, 1999). Preterm infants respond to sour taste by puckering their mouths.

Onset of function for olfaction (smell) has been demonstrated prenatally in rat fetuses (Glass, 1999). Infants at 1 week of age turn their heads from noxious odors, such as ammonia (Reiser, Yonas, & Wilkner, 1976). Infants only 3 days old orient more to their mother's amniotic fluid than the fluid of another mother (Marlier, Schaal, & Soussignan, 1998a, 1998b). Breastfed newborn infants within 2 weeks postbirth have shown preference for their own mother's axillary odor over that of another lactating mother (Cernoch & Porter, 1985). No preference was observed in bottle-fed infants nor was the preference extended to fathers.

Olfactory cortical activity in 23 healthy, full-term infants has been observed (Bartocci, Winberg, Ruggiero, et al., 2000) using near-infrared spectroscopy (NIRS) to detect changes in oxygenated hemoglobin (Hb $O_2$) and deoxygenated Hb during an olfactory stimulus (colostrums, vanilla, and distilled water control). Results showed a statistical difference between groups in post hoc comparison as follows: (1) control versus colostrum, $P < 0.0004$; (2) control versus vanilla, $P < 0.0001$; and (3) colostrums versus vanilla, $P < 0.0001$. The significant rise in oxygenated hemoglobin (Hb) was viewed as a positive response. Bartocci, Winberg, Papendieck, et al. (2001) conducted a similar study on preterm infants (mean postconceptional age—postconceptual age [PCA] of 35.5 weeks + 2.75 standard deviations [SD]) using the odors of disinfectant or a detergent. Both oxygenated Hb and total Hb decreased with exposure to these odors. Although the significance of this response is not known, these findings suggest that a cortical hemodynamic response might occur when infants are exposed to the odors commonly used in the NICU. Studies such as these have potential application in the clinical setting as caregivers try to minimize exposure to

noxious odors and provide biologically meaningful olfactory experiences to NICU patients.

Olfactory learning has been demonstrated in term newborns within the first 48 hours after birth (Sullivan, Taborsky-Barba, Mendoza, et al., 1991). Infants in the experimental group were videotaped receiving 10 30-second paired stimuli consisting of both a citrus odor and a tactile stimulus (stroking) as the reinforcing stimulus. Results analyzed by observers unaware of infant training status showed that only the treatment infants exhibited the conditioned response of turning their heads toward the odor.

A study of 44 healthy newborns presented with either their own mother's odor, another mother's odor, a clean hospital gown, and no gown was conducted by investigators who held the hospital gowns or nothing close to the infants out of their visual field (Sullivan & Toubas, 1998). Both breast- and bottle-fed infants stopped crying when exposed to their own mother's and another mother's maternal odor ($P < 0.01$). Crying infants exposed to their own mother's smell significantly increased their mouthing behaviors ($P < 0.05$). Awake infants responded specifically to their own mother's smell and showed significantly increased mouthing ($P < 0.05$). These findings suggest that maternal odor is soothing to the crying infant and might be beneficial in fostering the preparatory response to feeding and nipple acceptance.

Two studies now suggest that the fetus can learn odors from their pregnant mother's diet. Treatment groups exposed to anise flavor from their pregnant mother in the third trimester demonstrated a stable preference for anise odor over the study period (Schaal, Marlier, & Soussignan, 2000). Infants given carrot juice in their cereal consumed significantly more cereal and spent a longer time eating the carrot-flavored cereal than infants eating plain cereal (Mennella, Jagnow, & Beauchamp, 2001).

A pilot study (Bingham, Abassi, & Sivieri, 2003) of the effect of milk odor on nonnutritive sucking (NNS) by premature infants was conducted in a blinded, crossover design using breast or formula milk versus placebo (water) in a specially modified pacifier held by the nose. Digital recordings were performed during tube feedings for total number of sucks and sucking bursts. Subjects treated to breast milk odor showed more sucks and sucking bursts compared with either of the other groups, but results did not reach significance.

Use of routine interventions involving chemoreceptors has not been well studied, with one exception. Sucrose for modulating the pain response in term and preterm infants older than 26 weeks' gestation has undergone extensive investigation (Abad, Diaz, Domenech, et al., 1996; Blass & Watt, 1999; Franck & Gilbert, 2002; Gibbins & Stevens, 2001; Gibbins, Stevens, Hodnett, et al., 2002; Johnston, Stremler, Horton, & Friedman, 1999; Noerr, 2001; Renqvist & Fellman, 2000; Stevens & Ohlsson, 2000; Stevens, Taddio, Ohlsson, & Einarson, 1997; Stevens, Yamada, & Ohlsson, 2001). The sweet taste appears to be the mechanism of action, implying positive stimulation of taste receptors. Although not discussed in this chapter, a more thorough presentation on the value of sucrose is detailed in Chapter 12.

Research is still needed in this area to understand how best to use the olfactory and gustatory senses as positive stimuli in the NICU. A balanced exposure to pleasant smells/tastes, as well as the more aversive ones, in the NICU might have benefits for premature and high-risk infants. There can be positive gains for the feeding of preterm infants who have been exposed to the smell of breastmilk or formula during gavage feeding and/or given small amounts of milk in the mouth to stimulate taste sensations prior to oral feeds. Further study is needed in this area to identify interventions that have positive value for infants in the NICU. The NICU nurse can minimize an infant's exposure to the typical clinical smells that are malodorous and encourage skin-to-skin or holding to familiarize them with their parents' scents (Figure 15-1). Providing the smell of breastmilk during tube feeding might be another harmless means of enriching the feeding experience through the olfactory sense. Providing a small taste of breast milk or formula on the tongue might enhance preparation for oral feeding.

Biologically meaningful odors and tastes are the ones devised by nature to include mother's smell, colostrums, and breastmilk aroma and taste. The premature infant might benefit from exposure to these smells, whereas the older infant might begin to

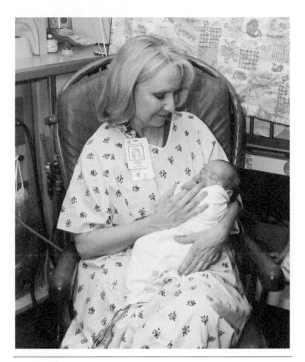

Figure **15-1** Traditional holding (*Courtesy Texas Children's Hospital, Dallas, TX; photographer Jim DeLeon.*)

appreciate a wider variety of experiences. Research remains sparse concerning the best interventions for the chemical senses for infants in the NICU. The literature suggests the chemical senses are important in recognition of parents and in appreciation of taste/odors for pleasure. As such, interventions that use smell/taste might offer pleasurable experiences to offset disturbing events common to the NICU.

## AUDITORY SYSTEM

In recent years there has been a growing concern about the effects of noise exposure in the NICU on the developing preterm and term infant (Abrams & Gerhardt, 2000; Evans & Philbin, 2000; Graven, 2000; Jennische & Sedin, 1998; Philbin, 1996, 2000a; Philbin & Gray, 2002; Robertson, Cooper-Peel, & Vos, 1998, 1999; Walsh-Sukys, Reitenbach, Hudson-Barr, & DePompei, 2001). Studies suggest that exposure to typical patterns of sound levels in the NICU might result in disruption of sleep patterns and physiologic/ behavioral responses of premature and term infants requiring such treatment

(Anderssen, Nicolaisen, & Gabrielsen, 1993; Gadeke, Doring, Keller, & Vogel, 1969; Graven, 2000; Long, Lucey, & Philip, 1980; Morris, Philbin, & Bose, 2000; Philbin, 1996, 2000b; Wharrad & Davis, 1997; Zahr & Balian, 1995). An understanding of the NICU sound environment (see Chapter 14) is necessary in making the acoustic and personnel behavior changes that support sleep, normal development, and optimal parent-infant interaction.

The research available on auditory stimulation in isolation and within a multimodal context for healthy and high-risk infants is scant and full of methodologic limitations. There is much to learn concerning the type, timing, harmonic range, intensity, duration, and frequency of sound stimuli appropriate for recovering high-risk and developing preterm infants. Much larger sample sizes from diverse populations are necessary to generalize findings. The range and frequency of sounds administered for experimental infants must be measured before interventions can be extrapolated and used in the clinical setting. Intensity and frequency of sound and the resulting effects on the infants' physical, motor, and state response needs better definition and should be included in any research investigating auditory stimulation. Patterns of stimulation required for early auditory pathway and speech are needed to design programs that foster speech and language development.

## THE FETUS AND SOUND

Physiologic responses to acoustic stimulation are seen in the fetus as early as 23 to 25 weeks' gestation (Abrams & Gerhardt, 2000; Crade, 1988; Gerhardt & Abrams, 2000; Hall, 2000). External stimulation from vibroacoustic devices placed on the abdomen over the uterus (e.g., electronic artificial larynx, vibroacoustic stimulators) has been associated with prolonged tachycardia, excessive fetal movements, and disorganization of fetal behavioral state (Gagnon, 1989; Viser et al., 1993).

### Infant Responses to Noise

Long, Lucey, and Philip (1980) reported hypoxemia, crying, agitation, and increased anterior fontanelle pressure in infants exposed to sudden loud sounds of approximately 80 decibels (dB) intensity. This research has been further supported by more recent research that demonstrated autonomic instability associated with auditory stimulation in both term and preterm infants (Anderssen, Nicolaisen, & Gabrielsen, 1993; Long, Lucey, & Philip, 1980; Zahr & Balian, 1995). Zahr and Balian (1995) studied 55 infants weighing between 480 and 1930 g, with gestational ages ranging from 23 to 27 weeks. Acute drops in oxygen saturation and acute increases in heart and respiratory rate were associated with sudden noise occurrences. Fussing or crying was noted in 43% of the infants in response to a noise stimulus.

Wharrad and Davis (1997) compared the patterns of motor activity, heart rate, and respirations in 20 preterm and 22 full-term neonates. The preterm group demonstrated significantly increased motor activity and heart rate, with decreased respiratory rate during sound stimuli, compared with full-term infants. This increase in arousal could result in energy expenditure and oxygen consumption in preterm infants, who have little reserve.

### Waking Thresholds

Gadeke, Doring, Keller, et al. (1969) studied the effects of sound level on sleep in a controlled laboratory environment using 126 healthy, term infants ranging in age from 3 to 63 weeks. A broadband noise stimulus with frequencies between 100 and 7000 Hertz (Hz) and intensities ranging from 50 to 80 dB (in 5-dB increments) during 6 time periods was used in the study. Each infant was presented with one randomly assigned stimulus during the night while in a deep sleep state. Noise levels between 70 and 75 dB caused sleep disturbance or awakening of 33% to 50% of the infants after only 3 minutes, and in all the infants by 12 minutes. About 33% of the infants awakened or changed sleep state after 3 minutes of sound intensities at 65 dB. Sound levels of 75 dB consistently disrupted sleep or resulted in waking the infants. Wedenberg (1963) observed similar results with audiograms of 20 newborns. These infants were roused from deep sleep at around 70 to 75 dB and from light or shallow sleep at about 55 dB. Extrapolating these findings to the preterm population provides a rationale for why these infants seldom reach or maintain a deep sleep in the NICU.

## Hearing and Speech

Premature infants are thought to be particularly susceptible to loud noise because of sensitive cochlea and an immature organ of Corti (Beckham & Mishoe, 1982). The developmental and psychosocial impact of hearing loss can be overwhelming, especially if other developmental disorders are present. The prevalence of hearing loss in very and/or extremely low birthweight infants treated in NICUs ranges from 0.5% to 12.3%. (Hearing loss in very preterm and VLBWs, when tested at the age of 5 years, was the population down from a nationwide cohort [Veen, Sassen, Schreuder, et al., 1993].) Former LBW infants have demonstrated low-to-moderate rates of language delay, even when no serious sensory impairment is present (Byrne, Ellsworth, Bowering, & Vincer, 1993). In one study of 151 former LBW infants (<1000 g), language delays were found in 31% of the children (Monset-Couchard, de Bethmann, & Kastler, 2002). Others have also reported increased rates of speech delay, including problems with auditory memory and processing, articulation, comprehension, receptive and expressive language, auditory discrimination, and word fluency (Byrne, Ellsworth, Bowering, & Vincer, 1993; Davis, Doyle, Ford, et al., 2001; Jennische & Sedin, 1999, 2001; Monset-Couchard, de Bethmann, & Kastler, 2002; Whitfield, Grunau, & Holsti, 1997). Whether the NICU sound environment is a contributing factor remains to be seen.

## The NICU Sound Environment

Currently there is no substantial evidence of the long-term effects of noise exposure in a traditional NICU environment on the high-risk or preterm newborn. There is concern that NICU noise might interfere with developing auditory pathways necessary for communication and language skills by masking or distortion of socially relevant sounds of the human voice needed for language development (Byrne, Ellsworth, Bowering, & Vincer, 1993; Davis, Doyle, Ford, et al., 2001; Jennische & Sedin, 1999, 2001; Whitfield, Grunau, & Holsti, 1997). Reducing the impact of the sound environment through noise abatement can be achieved through structural renovation or construction emphasizing acoustic improvements and staff participation to minimize the human contribution to NICU noise levels.

## Modifying the Sound Environment

Acoustic and personnel behavior changes that support sleep, normal development, and optimal parent-infant interaction are the most natural ways to create an environment responsive to the needs of preterm and high-risk infants. Supplemental auditory stimulation for preterm infants has not been supported through extensive, rigorous investigation that includes both short- and long-term effects of stimuli such as tape recordings, radio, or music therapy.

## Scheduled Quiet Times

The effects of one "quiet hour" protocol that included specific times, noise control, and no infant disruption unless medically necessary, were evaluated (Strauch, Brandt, & Edwards-Beckett, 1993). Mean noise levels decreased significantly ($P < 0.005$) during "quiet hours" versus control periods. Infant states were significantly improved ($P < 0.0005$) during "quiet hour" as demonstrated by 85% of infants in light or deep sleep compared with 34% of controls. Fourteen percent of infants were crying during the control periods compared with 2% during "quiet hour." Both nurses and parents reported decreased stress levels during the "quiet hour," an unforeseen effect.

Premature infants wearing earmuffs that decreased the sound level by 7 dB (Natus Corp., San Carlos, CA) demonstrated significant clinical and behavioral benefits such as higher mean oxygen saturation levels, less fluctuation in oxygen saturation, less frequent behavioral state changes, more time in quiet sleep, and longer bouts in the sleep state (Zahr & de Traversay, 1995). This study demonstrates a benefit to a quieter environment, but does not support the routine use of earmuffs that could adversely affect development of hearing and auditory processing pathways.

Quiet time for longer bouts of protected sleep might require that administration and staff evaluate the daily routines and redefine care delivery schedules. Overall efforts at decreasing ambient noise, lights, and attention to behavioral state prior to care will also be effective ways to support sleep in the NICU.

## Structural Modification to Abate Sound

Structural modification in NICU design and staff education have been shown to improve sound levels

(Philbin & Gray, 2002; Robertson, Kohn, Vos, & Cooper-Peel, 1998; Strauch, Brandt, & Edwards-Beckett, 1993; Walsh-Sukys, Reitenbach, Hudson-Barr, & DePompei, 2001). Modifications (Walsh-Sukys, Reitenbach, Hudson-Barr, & DePompei, 2001) to an existing level III NICU led to lower sound levels compared with the control nursery in $L_{eq}$ (64.2 vs 71.8 dB; $P < 0.001$); $L_{max}$ (65.7 vs 72 dB; $P < 0.001$); and $L_{10}$ (64.5 vs 71.8 dB; $P < 0.01$). In a quasiexperimental, prospective, longitudinal study, Philbin and Gray (2002) compared sound levels from an open design NICU to a new NICU with eight smaller bedrooms that included removal of the central workstation to the outside, away from patient beds. Staff education on the effects of sound on the newborn and preterm infant was provided before the new unit was built. After the renovation, levels were decreased to $L_{min}$s (minimum levels) of 47 to 51 dB and $L_{max}$s of 68 to 84 dBA. These levels compare to the previous nursery when 80% of sound levels were between 62 and 70 dBA, similar to NICUs in the literature reports on sound (American Academy of Pediatrics [AAP] Committee on Environmental Health, 1997; Philbin & Gray, 2002; Robertson, Cooper-Peel, & Vos, 1998; Robertson, Kohn, Vos, & Cooper-Peel, 1998; Thomas & Martin, 2000; Zahr & Balian, 1995). Because sound levels or decibels are measured and perceived on a logarithmic rather than linear scale, an increase of 10 dB is heard as twice as loud, a decrease by 10 dB is perceived as half as loud, and a change of 5 dB is clearly detectable. Therefore, relatively small changes in the sound pressure level can be perceived as less noisy and improve the environment for sleep and parent-infant interaction.

## Unimodal and Multimodal Supplemental Sound Stimulation in the NICU

There is little evidence that infants need more supplemental sound stimulation than that provided by parents. Physiologic effects in response to a sound stimulus occur as early as 23 weeks' gestation (Graven, 2000). The most salient auditory experience for the fetus is the mother's voice. As such, it is no surprise that newborn infants demonstrate preference for their own mother's voice and specific language soon after birth. Audio recordings are not recommended for routine use

for infants left unattended during their use (Gerhardt & Abrams, 2000). How this early introduction to communication influences later speech and language development is not understood at this time. Cusson (2003) examined factors influencing language development in preterm infants. She found that maternal sensitivity to communication cues is very important to later language acquisition, especially in the preterm infant at risk for language delays. Socially relevant sounds that are distorted or obscured by the more chaotic NICU environment might actually interfere with the developing pathways necessary for speech and language acquisition. Few studies are available related to sound as a single stimulus; often studies include several sensory modalities simultaneously, making interpretation difficult and inspiring caution before applying the techniques in the clinical setting.

## Supplemental Intervention Using Sound Stimulation

Few well-controlled studies are available providing guidance in the use of supplementary auditory stimuli for preterm infants. Philbin and Klass (2000) and Symington and Pinelli (2002) provide reviews of research regarding planned supplemental stimulation for preterm infants.

Music therapy has been advocated for infants in the NICU, starting as early as 28 weeks (Burke, Walsh, Oehler, et al., 1995; Caine, 1991; Kaminski & Hall, 1996; Kurihara, Chiba, Shimizu, et al., 1996; Standley, 1998, 2002; Standley & Moore, 1995; Symington & Pinelli, 2002). In a meta-analysis of the efficacy of music therapy for preterm infants, an overall beneficial effect was observed (Standley, 2002). Recorded lullaby music inside the incubator starting at 28 weeks of age showed improved oxygen saturations, increased weight gain, and decreased length of stay (LOS). Live singing and multimodal stimulation including auditory, begun at 32 weeks of age, produced shortened LOS and increased tolerance for stimulation, with time. Recorded lullabies in concert with pacifier sucking were associated with more nonnutritive sucking at 30 weeks for infants reinforced with 10 seconds of music. The pacifier-activated-lullaby was shown to increase the feeding rate of poor feeders at 34 to 36 weeks of age. However, caution must be used in interpreting the results of research promoting the use of music therapy for preterm infants until more substantial studies that include additional short- and long-term outcomes from well-designed randomized, controlled trials with appropriate sample size have been completed. Of concern are the documented levels of sound stimulus used, with ranges usually between 65 to 80 dB, clearly exceeding recommended standards for sound levels. It is even more worrisome that these sound levels were often provided using earphones directing the sound into the ear canal or in the incubator where sound is reflected off plastic walls and resonates throughout the chamber.

Limitations of most of the multimodal stimulation studies include use of added stimuli over the constant NICU background, small samples, dissimilarity of measurement methods, contamination of NICU practices, pre-/post-test design with one or two groups, and lack of long-term neurodevelopmental follow-up. One improvement for such studies might be the use of a data acquisition device that captures continuous physiologic parameters, as well as, sound, light, and temperature fluctuations before, during, and after the stimulation. In addition, behavioral data should be collected in a time sampling fashion synchronized to the computer timed data acquisition software.

## Multimodal Stimulation
### Auditory and Tactile
Ingersoll and Thoman (1994) studied the effects of the breathing bear (BrBr) as a source of optional rhythmic stimulation that reflects the breathing pattern of the individual infant (Ingersoll & Thoman, 1994). A bear with rhythmic breathing sounds and chest wall movement was placed in the incubator where the infant could touch or cuddle with the bear or move away from it, minimizing the possibility of overstimulation and providing a source of rhythmic vestibular stimulation that can be escaped as needed. The bear's breathing is very quiet and set to reflect the baby's own respiration rate in quiet sleep (QS). At 33 weeks, 19 premature infants were randomized to receive a BrBr and 17 infants a non-

breathing bear (N-BrBr). At 35 weeks, the BrBr babies exhibited slower and more regular respirations during QS than N-BrBr babies. At 35 and 45 weeks, the BrBr babies' respiration regularity correlated with the amount of QS. The findings of this and previous studies suggest that this type of optional, rhythmic auditory and tactile stimulation might be beneficial for the neurodevelopment of premature infants. In 1991 (Thoman, Ingersoll, & Acebo, 1991), infants (33 weeks at enrollment) exposed to the BrBr for 22 to 24 days had significantly more quiet sleep periods and greater duration of quiet sleep than control infants during the 5 weeks after discharge. Many factors other than the BrBr stimulus might have impacted this outcome, however, including quality of care and interventions associated with inability to blind caregivers to group assignment.

### Auditory, Tactile, Vestibular, and Visual
White-Traut, Nelson, Silvestri, et al. (2002) studied 37 preterm infants with and without central nervous system (CNS) injury (periventricular leukomalcia [PVL] and/or intraventricular hemorrhage [IVH]) to determine the effects of auditory, tactile, vestibular, and visual (ATVV) attributes on length of stay, alertness, and feeding progression. The intervention was provided for 15 minutes twice daily, for 5 days each week, to the treatment infants from 33 weeks' PCA until discharge. The intervention (ATVV) group demonstrated increased alertness ($P < 0.05$), earlier discharge (mean of 1.6 weeks; $P < 0.05$), and more rapid progression to full oral feeding ($P < 0.0001$) than control infants.

Standley (1998) divided 40 infants into a control and treatment group of 20 each. The infants were more than 32 weeks' gestation, older than 10 days of age, weighed more than 1700 g, and all had been referred for developmental stimulation by medical staff (Standley, 1998). Experimental infants received reciprocal, multimodal stimulation consisting of ATVV in combination with line singing of *Brahms' Lullaby*. Infants received the stimulation for 15 to 30 minutes, one or two times a week from referral until discharge. Male and female infants gained significantly more weight each day than their control counterparts, and female infants left the hospital an average of 11.9 days earlier than control females. Both male and female infants' tolerance for stimulation increased across stimulation intervals, with females showing more rapid rates of tolerance than males.

Another study (White-Traut, Nelson, Silvestri, et al., 2002) of 37 preterm infants with and without CNS injury (PVL and/or IVH) was conducted to determine the effects of ATVV on LOS, alertness, and feeding progression. The intervention was provided for 15 minutes, twice daily, for 5 days each week to the treatment infants from 33 weeks PCA until discharge. The intervention (ATVV) group demonstrated increased alertness ($P < 0.05$), earlier discharge (mean of 1.6 weeks; $P < 0.05$), and more rapid progression to full oral feeding ($P < 0.0001$) than control infants.

White-Traut, Silvestri, Cunningham, et al. (1997) studied the responses of 54 clinically stable preterm infants to two forms of unimodal stimulation: (1) auditory only (A); (2) tactile (T) only; (3) auditory, tactile, and visual (ATV); and (4) auditory, tactile, visual and vestibular (ATVV). The convenience sample of preterm infants, 33 to 34 weeks' PCA, was randomly assigned to five groups: control (C); (A); (T); (ATV); and (ATVV). Infants received stimulation for 15 minutes once a day for 4 consecutive days. Stimulation was provided in the following manner: (1) auditory stimulation, by soothing female voice; (2) tactile, by massage; (3) visual, by attempting eye-to-eye contact; and (4) vestibular, by rocking.

Stimulation was provided contingent upon each infant's cues, and adapted accordingly. Infants in this study were more likely to have pulse rates of more than 180 bpm (beats per minute) and respiratory rates of more than 60 breaths per minute when receiving tactile-only stimulation. Infants receiving any intervention with a tactile component showed more arousal states and increased pulse rates and respiratory rates. Group ATVV had significantly more pulse rates higher than 140 and increased alertness following the stimulation that was sustained over the 30-minute, postintervention observation. Infants receiving the auditory-only intervention responded with an increase in quiet sleep (11.8% baseline vs 29% following stimula-

tion). It is unclear whether the sustained alertness was a hyperalert state or whether the QS was post-stimulus fatigue.

Simultaneous use of various forms of stimulation make it difficult to ascertain whether one type of stimulation is more beneficial or if some are potentially harmful. It is also difficult to determine if all types of the stimuli in ATVV are necessary to achieve the outcomes reported. Supplemental stimulation research treatments, when provided in the NICU environment, are most likely contaminated by the ambient background and intermittent bursts of noise, lighting, and general activity that are difficult to control. When these continuous environmental stimuli are not measured during the study, it is impossible to factor them out or adjust for them using statistical methods.

## Conclusions and Recommendations for the Sound Environment

Auditory experiences in the NICU might alter CNS organization as auditory pathways develop during hospitalization. Research is still needed to establish safe limits, and to guide principles for adding auditory stimulation over the NICU sounds already in place. It seems prudent and reasonable to be cautious when introducing auditory stimulation, especially to developing preterm infants, whose auditory and cognitive pathways are being organized during their NICU stay. The general principles of developmental care seem appropriate until more evidence base is available.

As each individual infant matures and recovers, the amount and type of auditory input will change. Any additional sound input over and above the NICU environmental sound must be carefully evaluated. If added sound is provided, then efforts to minimize the NICU background noise should take place before the intervention. It is critical that infant's be monitored after any stimulus is started to determine whether a delayed response will occur. Sound that is soothing, simple, repetitive, low intensity, and harmonic within a limited dynamic range might work best until more is known about added sound stimulation for preterm infants.

Speech and nonspeech sounds stimulate different parts of the cerebral hemispheres. Exposure to speech sounds might be critical to the development of speech and language. Parents might need encouragement, environmental modification, comfortable furniture, and support from staff to provide the singing and soft speech that occurs in the home setting. They can learn to provide the appropriate sound input using sensitivity to their individual infant's responses so they can titrate the amount and intensity of the interaction. Parents need support and encouragement to feel comfortable enough to talk to their infant in the primary language used in the home. This would be normal for that infant's early auditory experience and include cultural variations important to the infant and family.

Sound measurements inside the incubator can be as intense as the sound levels in open NICU beds. Robertson, Stuart, & Walker (2001) suggest that only midfrequency speech requiring an increased vocal effort can be heard due to signal transmission loss in the incubator (in $L_{eq}$). The loss of transmitted speech results from motor noise, position of the person speaking, incubator port (open or closed), and frequency (Hz) of the sound (Robertson, Stuart, & Walker, 2001). Continuous background noise coupled with equipment, conversation, alarms, and other NICU-related conditions create an atypical sound environment that interferes with normal interactions between parent and child.

Therefore, extreme caution must be used when adding any supplemental auditory stimulation while the infant is nursed in the clinical setting. Acoustical foam padding has been shown to decrease noise levels inside the incubator by an average 3.27 dB (Johnson, 2001) and might prove useful in managing the resonance problems in incubators.

Finally, NICU staff must consider that the effects of the sound environment might not be limited to one stimulated sensory system. Staff can combine their knowledge of infant organization and sensory system integration to provide the conceptual framework for developmental assessment and intervention. It seems prudent to begin intervention with the most mature system (i.e., touch) and support the normal maturational process without trying to accelerate it (Glass, 1999). The natural resource for intervening with the infant is the mother, then the family.

By working together with families, administrators, staff, medical/nursing management, individual bedside caregivers, and architects, and considering each infant's individual characteristics, a more normalizing sound environment might be achieved that supports optimal opportunity for auditory development while minimizing the impact of the NICU environment. Box 15-2 lists some recommendations for the sound environment of term and preterm infants that were developed by the expert review panel from the Study Group on NICU sound based

---

**Box 15-2** CONCLUSIONS AND RECOMMENDATIONS ON SOUND AND THE DEVELOPING INFANT

1. Mother's voice during daily activities, body sounds, and those of a normalized environment are sufficient for fetal auditory development.
2. Supplemental stimulation is not required by the fetus, and such programs to enhance the auditory experience or advance maturity is not recommended.
3. Noise levels should be regularly assessed and kept within recommended levels.
4. NICUs need ongoing programs for noise control.
5. Ample opportunity should be provided for infants to be with parents and hear their voices naturally, not through artificial means (e.g., recorded tapes).
6. Earphones and other sound transmission devices should not be used.
7. Little evidence is available to support the addition of recorded music or speech to the environment of premature and high-risk infants.

Audio recordings are not recommended for routine use nor should infants be left unattended during their use.

From Graven, S.N. (2000). Sound and the developing infant in the NICU: Conclusions and recommendations for care. *Journal of Perinatology, 20*(8)(Pt 2), S88-S93; and Philbin, M.K., Robertson, A., & Hall, J.W. 3rd. (1999). Recommended permissible noise criteria for occupied, newly constructed or renovated hospital nurseries (The Sound Study Group of the National Resource Center). *Journal of Perinatology, 19*(8)(Pt 1), 559-563.

out of the Physical and Developmental Environment of the High-Risk Infant Center (Graven, 2000). Desired outcomes of a more stable and natural environment include: (1) stable physiology; (2) improved growth; (3) consistent neurosensory progression and maturation; (4) natural parent-infant interaction; (5) parent-infant attachment; (6) normal maturation of sleep/wake organization; and (7) fewer speech and language difficulties.

## VISUAL STIMULATION

As reviewed in earlier chapters, the visual system is not stimulated in utero as are other developing systems; therefore, this system does not have a history of experience preparing for the intense visual milieu of the NICU. Significant maturation and differentiation of the retinal connections to the visual cortex that typically occur in utero during the last trimester might have to develop in the atypical intensive care environment. Psychobiologic research with animal models have shown that early stimulation to the immature visual system can result in behavioral and perceptual consequences that alter the developmental course of the visual and other sensory systems (Banker & Lickliter, 1993; Casey & Lickliter, 1998; Foushee & Lickliter, 2002; Honeycutt & Lickliter, 2001; Lickliter, 2000a, 2000b; Sleigh, Columbus, & Lickliter, 1996; Sleigh & Lickliter, 1995, 1998).

### Visual System Characteristics

The visual system is the least mature for the term infant and much more so for the preterm (Glass, 1999; Graven, 2000). Although term infants are limited in the ability to focus (accommodate visually to near and far distances) and discriminate (visual acuity), they will actively explore their environment. Responsiveness to visual stimulation and acuity or accommodation is not as developed in the preterm infant. In general, preterm infants exposed to light, reduced lighting, and early visual stimulation in the NICU have not shown accelerated visual acuity development in visual evoked potential (VEP) and preferential looking (PL) studies (Birch & O'Connor, 2001). VEPs are electrical signals from the occipital cortex made in response to visual stimulation, and PL measures an infant's consistent gaze preference. PL is dependent on visual attention and oculomotor

fixation ability and develops slower than VEP acuity that reveals maturity of both the retina and striate cortex.

Although preterm infants might attend to a visual stimulus by 30 or 32 weeks, they can become disorganized or stressed by the effort. The need for patterned stimulation (high-contrast black and white patterns) is questionable and can be damaging because the intensity of such stimuli might evoke an obligatory, staring response by the immature infant who is unable to regulate incoming information and break away from it (Glass, 1999). This behavior is not appropriate or desired from preterm or term infants. An expert panel who has extensively reviewed the literature (Blackburn, 1996; Glass, 1999; Holditch-Davis, Blackburn, & VandenBerg, 2003) and the current published NICU Design Standards (White, 2002) can make recommendations for the visual environment (see Chapter 14), including the precautionary statement that visual stimulation programs have not been substantiated by clinical trials demonstrating their value or the lack of harmful effects both short- and long-term. Practical considerations (Glass, 1999; Hunter, 2001; Mirmiran & Ariagno, 2000; White, 2002) for support of the visual system are listed in Box 15-3.

## Research: Illumination and Visual Stimulation

### Light Reduction

Kennedy, Fielder, Hardy, et al. (2001) used goggles to reduce visible light by 97% in a study of 359 premature infants (mean gestational age 27 weeks, range 23 to 30 weeks) and found no difference in the medical outcomes (weight gain, duration of oxygen therapy, mechanical ventilation, length of stay, IVH, or retinopathy of prematurity [ROP]) between infants experiencing light reduction in the first 4 to 6 weeks of life and control infants. Medical outcomes in this study could have been influenced by the tactile irritation of wearing goggles; however, no difference in outcomes also suggests that reduced lighting is neither harmful nor beneficial. These investigators (Kennedy, Ipson, Birch, et al., 1997) also examined the effects of light reduction on

## Box 15-3   Guidelines for Research Evaluation

1. Is the purpose of the study clearly identified?
2. Are the research questions or hypothesis specific and logically linked to the outcome variables and treatments or tests? Do the research questions/hypotheses flow from the study purpose?
3. Does a thorough critical review of relevant literature describe previous work or useful theory that supports the need for this study?
4. Is the research design well-described with thorough description and definition of each variable?
5. Was the manner of collecting data planned before subjects received any treatment?
6. Is the subject population appropriate to the type of research being conducted?
7. Are the inclusion/exclusion criteria appropriate and complete? Are the reasons that some subjects withdrew or refused to participate provided?
8. Is it clear how the sample size was determined? Was a power analysis used to determine sample size to detect an appropriate magnitude of effects of a treatment?
9. Is randomization or stratification used and, if so, well-described?
10. Is the procedure for when and how data will be collected thoroughly described?
11. Are all instruments used to collect data described along with a discussion of validity and reliability? Are scoring procedures described? Is the process for obtaining data presented for qualitative research?
12. Are all data collectors reliable in using tests or instruments such as behavioral state observations and scoring?
13. Is the method of group assignment clear? Are the groups homogenous? Is there a strong rationale used when matching subjects? Is there a control group? Is one high-risk group being compared with another high-risk group? Is an additional well-infant control used to compare with both high-risk control and high-risk intervention groups?
14. If subjects serve as their own controls, is the order of treatment and control condition randomized and not just alternated? Are the least well-controlled assignment methods avoided (such as assignment because of availability of subjects or convenience)?
15. Is informed consent with due privacy obtained?
16. Are the treatment, test, or procedures clearly explained, including potential contaminating environmental factors such as sound, light, and activity levels?
17. Are the activity, sleep, care disruptions, painful experiences collected as needed to identify possible extraneous contributing factors?
18. What level of blinding or masking to treatments or subjects was performed? Was a placebo condition used?
19. Are lost or withdrawn subjects described and potential effects analyzed?
20. Are both negative and undesired results reported along with the positive and beneficial responses? Are long-term consequences evaluated and reported? Is the cost of the treatment evaluated and reported?
21. Are the presentation and analysis of the data clear and concise? Were appropriate statistical tests used for the data collected? Is the analysis complete with appropriate statistics reported (i.e., mean, median, range, standard deviation, proportion)? Were the statistical or analytic techniques used to answer each research hypothesis or question appropriate and fully reported?
22. Are the results interpreted cautiously with reasonable considerations and limitations addressed?
23. Are recommendations consistent with the results from the study? Are recommendations for practice overstated and without full support from the study's findings?
24. Are there reservations about using the treatment, procedures, and tests in the clinical setting at this time?

Cited from Philbin, M.K., & Klaas, P. (2000). Evaluating studies of the behavioral effects of sound on newborns. *Journal of Perinatology, 20,* S61-S67.

retinal development and function by electroretino-gram (ERG). Sixty-one preterm infants weighing less than 1251 g and aged younger than 31 weeks' gestation were randomly assigned to a control group and treatment group who wore light-filtering goggles for 4 weeks or until 31 weeks' gestational age. At 36 weeks' PCA, no difference between the two groups was found in ERG, visual acuity, ROP, feeding tolerance, rate of weight gain, and LOS.

One level III NICU significantly reduced sound levels ($P < 0.01$) and modified nursery lighting from continuous, fixed lighting with high output of 193 lux to individualized, variable lighting capable of reduction to 12 lux (Walsh-Sukys, Reitenbach, Hudson-Barr, et al., 2001). Patient safety outcomes, such as medication errors, intravenous infiltrates, accidental extubations, nosocomial infection rate, mortality, and number of patient days were not impacted by the environmental changes when evaluated at 6 months postmodification.

A small sample of premature infants from younger than 29 weeks' to 32 weeks' PCA received either complete visual occlusion or traditional care. No difference was found in the pattern visual-evoked responses at 41 and 51 weeks' PCA and at 3 years (Roy, Caramelli, Orquin, et al., 1999). Reduced lighting, as an intervention for immature infants, has not been found to negatively impact visual development, medical outcomes, or safety by these investigators. These findings suggest that light reduction for younger preterm infants is a safe alternative to continuous bright light or day/night cycling. Incubator covers are another method of light reduction (Figures 15-2 and 15-3). But some units are using a combination of covers and cycled lighting.

### Cycled Lighting

Brandon, Holditch-Davis, & Belyea (2002) reported significantly faster weight gain for preterm infants cared for with cycled lighting starting at birth and at 32 weeks PCA than infants not receiving cycled lighting until 36 weeks PCA. Near darkness for the study was measured at 5 to 10 lux, while cycled light was increased to 200 to 225 lux; which is considerably below the amount of lighting recommended by the AAP for observation in the NICU (Warren,

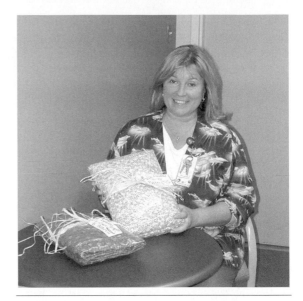

Figure **15-2** Crib cover material ready to sew by parents.(*Courtesy Texas Children's Hospital, Dallas, TX.*)

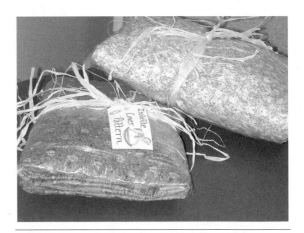

Figure **15-3** Crib cover patterns for parents. (*Courtesy Texas Children's Hospital, Dallas, TX.*)

2002). No differences in medical outcomes, including ROP, were reported. Measures of a functional visual system other than the presence/absence of ROP were not collected. Other studies of day/night cycled lighting for healthy preterm infants have shown lower heart rate and activity during the reduced light cycle (Blackburn & Patterson,

1991); increased sleep time, improved feeding efficiency, and faster weight gain at 6 and 12 weeks after discharge (Mann, Haddow, Stokes, et al., 1986); and better weight gain, less time to oral feeding, and fewer ventilator days (Miller, White, Whitman, et al., 1995). Most of the studies were done with healthy, preterm infants and with variation between continuous light and cycled lighting conditions.

More studies that include ophthalmic follow-up and visual-motor performance must be conducted to determine long-term significance of lighting conditions during prematurity. Until more is known about light and the development of vision in the premature infant in the extrauterine environment, the most conservative and intuitive guide for intervention is that of the intrauterine experience of dim lighting. During the critical period of visual development after term birth, it is essential that enough light is present for infants to see patterns and forms clearly. Medical benefits might not be observed in preterm infants cared for in reduced light; however, early light exposure greater than expected by the developing visual system might result in the pathogenesis of other ophthalmic sequelae or disturbances in visual-motor processing (Fielder & Moseley, 2000; O'Connor, Stephenson, Johnson, et al., 2002; Sullivan & Margaret, 2003). The impact of early light stimulation on other sensory systems should also be considered. The value of day/night cycled lighting for preterm infants is not clear due to a lack of appropriate follow-up information, and until the long term effects of this intervention are known, a conservative approach to illumination in the NICU is most prudent.

### Circadian Rhythm

Daily organization of sleep, melatonin and cortisol levels, body temperature, and neurobehavioral performance are influenced by a biologic clock (circadian pacemaker) that is sensitive to light. Fetal diurnal rhythms (Mirmiran & Ariagno, 2000; Shanahan & Czeisler, 2000) of heart rate are entrained during the third trimester of pregnancy by maternal rest-activity cycles, heart rate, cortisol, melatonin, and body temperature.

Human infants show no sign of circadian rhythm at birth. Circadian body temperature has been seen in infants at 1 month of age (Mirmiran & Ariagno, 2000). Melatonin and cortisol rhythmicity in term infants have been demonstrated between 10 and 12 weeks. Circadian rhythms might be influenced by the fetal prenatal experience and postnatal environment. Preterm infants are deprived of the maternal influence during pregnancy, and both term and preterm infants are exposed to the NICU postnatal environment. Currently, there are insufficient data showing that day/night cycled lighting support earlier development of circadian rhythms in preterm infants. Individual differences also exist and are not well understood. Neither do preterm infants seem to show a difference in the timing of maturation of circadian rhythms compared with term infants.

Maturation, day/night cycled light, plus decreasing nighttime caregiver interruption/intervention after discharge might be more important determinants of circadian rhythm development for both preterm and term infants. It is unclear what the role of the NICU environment or caregiving practices might be in facilitating normal maturation of the biological clock. Providing parents with information about circadian rhythms and how illumination can affect the setting of this biological clock can help parents intervene in the home setting by varying the lighting conditions appropriately.

### Phototherapy

Phototherapy (Fielder & Moseley, 2000) is a known hazard for the visual system, with light exposure ranging from 200 to 280 footcandles (ftc) (2400 to 3000 lux) and small amounts of ultraviolet radiation (UV) from 330 to 400 nanometers (nm). Eye patches reduce approximately 90% of the phototherapy light when securely attached. One study found that more than 50% of the eye shields observed had slipped and were not in place to protect the eyes from the potential photokeratitis from UV exposure and retinal injury associated with the use of blue light. Careful monitoring of eye shields is required for continuous protection of infants' eyes during phototherapy.

### Procedures

Pupillary dilatation for eye examinations can leave infants sensitive to light for as long as 18 hours

(Fielder & Moseley, 2000). Protective eye shielding is not routinely provided for infants after pupil dilation and eye examinations (Glass, 1999). Medication-induced dilation can last 2 to 4 hours, and protection from light sources during this time might be warranted. It has been estimated that exposure for approximately 2 minutes to indirect ophthalmoscope at maximum power as routine for eye examinations is equal to 2000 ftc or 20,000 lux for 3 hours.

### Abrupt Lighting Variations

Sudden illumination is stressful for preterm infants. Significantly lower oxygen saturations at 1 and 5 minutes were observed in preterm infants when lighting was increased from 5 to 100 ftc (about 50 to 1000 lux). Saturations were changed significantly when lights were lowered after 30 minutes (Shogan & Schumann, 1993). Having a quick method for shielding eyes is important if light levels must be suddenly increased to avoid potential hypoxemia in particularly sensitive infants.

### Supplemental Visual Stimulation

There are no randomized, well-controlled trials for supplemental visual stimulation alone for the preterm infant. Multimodal sensory stimulation studies have included visual stimulation but do not provide information on the effects of visual stimulation separate from additional modalities. In fact, studies of any additional stimulation, regardless of the type, is influenced by the general environmental conditions of light, noise, activity, and routines of a busy intensive care unit. Caution and careful consideration of the quality of the research must be used when deciding to implement any intervention that will affect the growth and development of a human being.

Staff must cautiously consider the impact of the complex visual milieu in the NICU on the developing premature infant. For both preterm and unstable term infants, care should be taken to minimize the influence of overwhelming, chaotic visual surroundings. Brief emerging alert states in preterm infants do not mean they are ready for intense visual stimulation. Early stimulation to the visual system might interfere with the normal maturational processes for both vision and other developing sensory systems and have serious perceptual and behavioral consequences that could explain later school difficulties and visual-motor problems in former preterm infants.

## CARE DELIVERY

NICU nurses have more control over the care routines by virtue of being at the bedside all day, every day. The art of collaborating effectively with other disciplines is necessary to negotiate timing, intensity, and appropriateness of interventions, tests, and procedures. The moment-by-moment observation and responsiveness to infant cues requires nurses to alter care routines and techniques according to developmentally supportive principles. In a society that has evolved to a fast-paced, get tasks done quickly and efficiently attitude, the developmental paradigm means that nurses have to be "in the moment" during each episode of care without looking ahead to "what has to be done next." It is a slower-paced, more thoughtful way of going about delivering care to infants and their families in the NICU. Until staffs have fully integrated these principles, developmental care will probably take more time, as nurses assimilate the knowledge, skills, and attitudes (KSAs) into practice.

### Modifying Care Procedures/Techniques

Routine care such as diaper changes, bathing, and repositioning can be stressful for preterm infants. "Routine" care implies the same approach is provided to all infant care. Developmental principles emphasize an individual approach that must be operationalized to caregiving practices. Individualizing care might require modification of procedure/techniques to minimize the disruption resulting from necessary care. Modifications such as changing diapers with infants in the sidelying position and carefully removing and applying diapers without raising the extremities, is one suggested developmentally supported technique. No research has been done to validate this practice.

Another modification to routine practice that has been recommended is swaddled bathing. No formal research is available to validate this practice, although it has been used in research of the effects of overall individualized developmental care for low-risk preterm infants (Buehler, Als, Duffy, et al., 1995). Research has shown that traditional bathing is extremely stressful with marked physical and behavioral consequences. This is another form of handling that appears to be linked to stress (Peters, 1999). Anecdotal evidence suggests benefits to swaddled bathing for some preterm infants, including: decreased physiologic and motor signs of stress; decreased flailing of limbs and startle movements; better state control during the procedure (i.e., decreased crying and agitation); successful self-regulatory behaviors, and improved ability to breastfeed or bottle-feed immediately after bathing.

Currently, nurses often use innovative means to minimize the stress of care based on individual observation of infants. Research efforts toward identifying some useful interventions that have demonstrated benefits would add to the repertoire of available options to meet the needs of individual infants.

## State Responsive Timing of Care

Care routines that respect individual infants state behaviors have been suggested. There is little research evidence showing what state is best for care and what to do for the preterm infant with brief alert periods. In one study, infants who received care (excluding emergencies) when beginning to awaken spontaneously had better growth, physiologic parameters, and decreased hospital stay compared with traditional care irrespective of behavioral state. It was recommended that the quiet, alert state is a time when aversive procedures should be avoided.

It is also important to consider the impact of uncomfortable, invasive procedures on stress or maturation if started while an infant is waking or in a light sleep. Older infants can become hyperalert or vigilant if continually experiencing stressful procedures in their beds. The bed can become a place that is not safe and an added source of stress. It is important to remember that trust versus mistrust is the developmental task of infancy, and infants in the NICU need to achieve this task as a building block to later development. It is unclear how these activities influence the development of restful, mature sleep states. It makes sense to avoid starting a proce-

dure when an infant is sleeping and to gently arouse before any care event, aversive or otherwise.

The balance between impersonal or intrusive care and nurturing experiences during awake periods might be beneficial. Until more is known concerning the effects of care and behavioral state maturation, consideration of sleep states, gentle arousal for care or procedures, providing comfort and recovery time after procedures, and including nurturing, loving opportunities aside from routine nursing care makes intuitive sense.

## Clustered Care

"Clustered" care has been recommended as a means to provide NICU infants the opportunity for more rest and to protect from overwhelming, stressful care events. There is no published research on the impact of clustered care on preterm infants. Care epochs need to be individualized using infant cues to determine when to stop a "cluster" or whether a "time out" for recovery is needed before continuing care. The type of care in the cluster might include care that is routine (diapering) or aversive and even painful (suctioning, blood sampling, heelstick). How and whether to mix certain types of care with others is not known. Some infants can tolerate longer episodes or combined types of care while others cannot. An infant might tolerate a particular cluster during one care event and later that same "cluster" might be too overwhelming. Containment has been shown to help preterm infants tolerate and recover more quickly from some necessary interventions, such as heelstick, eye examination, and suctioning (Corff, Seideman, Venkataraman, et al., 1995; Fearon, Kisilevsky, Hains, et al., 1997; Schraeder, Heverly, O'Brien, et al., 1997; Slevin, Murphy, Daly, et al., 1999).

Careful thought by nursing staff is essential in deciding how much care is included in a "cluster" followed by continuous observation for signs of stress or fatigue during each care event. A care cluster does not mean getting all the care done if it results in sensory overload, significant energy and oxygen consumption, and a disorganized, stressed infant. Many times care can be delayed to support optimal infant functioning. Nurses have the most opportunity to impact care routines in the NICU to support optimal timing, type, and amount of stimulation to reduce stress and provide appropriate opportunity for growth, rest, and development.

## SKIN-TO-SKIN HOLDING OR KANGAROO CARE

A recent survey of 90 U.S. hospitals showed 98% of the NICUs used skin-to-skin holding or kangaroo care (KC) as an intervention for premature infants (Field, 2003), confirming the wide acceptance of this practice. In some countries KC has been used as a practical means of providing warmth in hospitals with limited nursing resources and lacking facilities such as incubators (Kirsten, Bergman, & Hann, 2001). In Bogota, Colombia, KC led to lower morbidity and mortality rates. In the United States, KC has been recommended for fostering neurobehavioral development, parent-infant intimacy, and attachment, and to encourage breastfeeding.

The term "kangaroo care" was coined because of the similarity to the marsupial's way of carrying their young protected in their pouch. NICU parents maintain skin-to-skin contact with their diaper-clad infant resting prone and semi-upright on a bared chest and covered by a blanket. Stimulation to the infant includes warmth, rise and fall of the chest (vestibular), tactile sensation of skin to skin, smell of parents (olfactory) and maternal breast, and the parent's tender, quiet, vocalizations, breathing sounds, and heartbeat (auditory). All the earlier developing senses receive appropriate input through this intervention modality.

The efficacy and safety of KC has been researched since the 1980s, revealing many positive benefits of this intervention. Few studies are available supporting KC for sicker, more premature infants and only one study reports use in intubated infants. Currently, no quality randomized, controlled trial provides enough evidence that KC is beneficial with no risk of harm in that subcategory of NICU infants (McGrath & Brock, 2002).

### Research Evidence: Physiologic and Behavioral Parameters

Kangaroo care for stable, nonventilated, premature infants is reported to reduce incidence and severity of illness, decrease nosocomial infection rates,

improve duration of breastfeeding, improve state organization, increase infant weight gain, shorten length of stay, and even provide analgesia during heel lancing (Acolet, Sleath, & Whitelaw, 1989; Anderson, 1991; Bier, Ferguson, Morales, et al., 1996; Charpak, de Calume, & Ruiz, 2000; Charpak, Figueroa, & Ruiz, 1998; Charpak, Ruiz-Pelaez, & Figueroa de Calume, 1996; Cleary, Spinner, Gibson, & Greenspan, 1997; Conde-Agudelo, Diaz-Rossello, & Belizan, 2000; Feldman, Eidelman, Sirota, et al., 2002; Gray, Watt, & Blass, 2000; Hurst, Valentine, Renfro, et al., 1997; Kirsten, Bergmann, & Hann, 2001; Ludington-Hoe, Anderson, et al., 1999; Ludington-Hoe, Nguyen, Swinth, & Satyshur, 2000; McGrath & Brock, 2002; Messmer, Rodriguez, Adams, et al., 1997; Roberts, Paynter, & McEwan, 2000; Tornhage, Stuge, Lindberg, et al., 1999; Whitelaw, Histerkamp, Sleath, et al., 1988).

Hurst, Valentine, Renfro, et al. (1997) reported significantly increased milk volume in mothers who provided KC to their stable, preterm infants on nasal continuous positive airway pressure (NCPAP). No adverse effects of KC were reported in these infants (mean 27.7 weeks' gestation) compared with a non-KC control group. A major limitation for this study was the retrospective review of control group data. In 138 KC events, two infants experienced brief desaturation during the first session and both times the saturations returned to normal limits without need for intervention. Cardiorespiratory, body temperature, and oxygenation monitoring before, during, and after KC should be maintained as with any intervention in the NICU.

Other reported advantages to KC include maintenance of skin temperature; reduction of apnea and bradycardia; less variability of heart rate and transcutaneous oxygen levels; increased frequency/duration of quiet sleep; less time crying; lower activity levels; and no increase in energy expenditure in preterm infants compared with control non-KC infants (Anderson, 1991; Bauer, Sontheimer, Fischer, et al., 1996; Bauer, Uhrig, Sperling, et al., 1997; Bohnhorst, Heyne, Peter, et al., 2001; Charpak, Figueroa, & Ruiz, 1998; Charpak, Ruiz-Pelaez, & Figueroa de Calume, 1996; Conde-Agudelo, Diaz-Rossello, & Belizan, 2000; Feldman, Eidelman, Sirota, et al., 2002; Fohe, Kropf, & Avenarius, 2000;

Hurst, Valentine, Renfro, et al., 1997; Ludington-Hoe, Anderson, et al., 1999; Ludington-Hoe, Nguyen, et al., 2000; Ludington-Hoe, Thompson, Swinth, et al, 1994; McGrath & Brock, 2002; Messmer, Rodriguez, Adams, et al., 1997; Roberts, Paynter, & McEwan, 2000). A goal of care is to reduce energy expenditure and oxygen consumption to support optimal functioning of preterm infants. KC appears effective at reducing thermal instability and motor activity that can impede recovery.

The most vulnerable phase of KC occurs during the transfer of the infant from bed to parent and back to bed. The effects of two transfer techniques (parent transfer or nurse to parent transfer) were evaluated on 15 ventilated preterm infants (mean weight of 1094 g) assigned to receive each transfer method alternated randomly on 2 consecutive days (Neu, Browne, & Vojir, 2000). Oxygen saturation decreased and heart rate increased regardless of transfer method, returning to baseline during and after KC. During transfer by either method, infants showed decreased muscle tone, less self-regulatory efforts, more physiologic and motor disorganization as scored continuously on the Assessment of Behavioral Systems Observation (ABSO). These physiologic and behavioral parameters stabilized during and after KC. More caregiver facilitation was required during transfer than active KC periods. More research is needed to identify better transfer methods for fragile infants to minimize the physiologic and behavioral costs of moving infants for KC. Transferring fragile infants to their parents might require more than one nurse or therapist and uninterrupted ventilation for infants requiring ventilator support even when stable.

## Preterm Infant Development and Kangaroo Care

Feldman et al. (Feldman & Eidelman, 2003; Feldman, Eidelman, Sirota, et al., 2002; Feldman, Weller, Sirota, et al., 2002) have examined both short and longer-term outcomes of KC on parenting and preterm infant development. In one study (Feldman, Eidelman, Sirota, & Weller, 2002), 73 infants who received KC were compared with 73 matched controls. No differences were found between groups before KC. At term, KC infants demonstrated more mature state distribution and better organized sleep/wake

cycles than controls. By 3 months, the KC group exhibited improved arousal modulation during increasingly complex stimuli. At 6 months, KC infants manifested better mother-infant shared attention and sustained exploring behaviors during a toy session. They (Feldman & Eidelman, 2003) also studied a group of 70 infants, 50% receiving KC, and found improved autonomic functioning, state regulation, and neurobehavioral development in the KC-treated infants. Vagal tone matured more rapidly in the KC group between 32 and 37 weeks PCA ($P < 0.029$). State organization was improved in KC infants as evidenced by longer duration of quiet sleep ($P < 0.016$) and quiet alerting ($P < 0.013$) and decreased amounts of active sleep ($P < 0.023$). Habituation and orientation was better for KC infants than non-KC controls. These results emphasize the potential of KC intervention for supporting the autonomic, self-regulatory, and state development of preterm infants (Figure 15-4).

## Parenting Outcomes with Kangaroo Care

Kangaroo care is often hypothesized to promote bonding and attachment. Feldman, Eidelman, Sirota, and Weller (2002) examined the effects of KC on parent-infant interaction using 73 KC infants matched (birthweight, gestational age, medical severity, and demographics) with 73 control infants who received

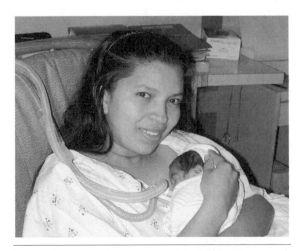

Figure **15-4** Kangaroo care. (*Courtesy Texas Children's Hospital, Dallas, TX; photographer Paul Kuntz.*)

traditional incubator care. Mothers and infants were observed at 37 weeks prior to discharge, and after discharge at 3 and 6 months' corrected age. At 37 weeks, KC mothers demonstrated more positive affect, touch, and responsiveness to infant cues, and their infants showed significantly more alerting and less gaze aversion than controls. KC mothers reported less depression and perceived their infants as more normal than non-KC control mothers. Home environments at 3 months were better as scored on the Home Observation for Measurement of the Environment (HOME) variables. Maternal and paternal sensitivity to their infants needs, organization of the environment, and variety of experiences were more optimal for KC infants than controls. At 6 months, KC infants were more socially alert and scored significantly higher on the mental (Motor Developmental Index [MDI] mean: 96.39) and psychomotor index (Psychomotor Developmental Index [PDI] mean: 85.47) scores on the Bayley Scales of Infant Development II than control subjects (MDI mean: 91.81; PDI mean: 80.53). Mothers were scored as more sensitive, adaptive to their infants, and affectionate during social interaction at 6 months. These findings need further research validations but provide impressive evidence that KC is beneficial in promoting parenting and parent-infant interaction both in the hospital and after discharge.

Finally, it is important to remember that fathers can also provide KC. A small study of 11 infants (median age 29 weeks and 22 days old) showed no differences in the effects of maternal and paternal Kangaroo care on oxygen consumption, carbon dioxide production, calculated energy expenditure, heart and respiratory rates, arterial oxygen saturation, and behavioral states (Bauer, Uhrig, Sperling, et al., 1997). Similar increases in skin temperature occurred during both maternal and paternal KC. These findings suggest that fathers can safely provide KC for their infants. More research is needed to discover the benefits of KC for both father and infant.

In summary, Kangaroo or skin-to-skin care appears to be a positive intervention for preterm infants and their parents. As with all interventions, it is necessary to individualize the approach and techniques as needed to accommodate individual differences between parents and preterm infant pairs. Parents (both mothers and fathers) who choose to provide KC need to be supported in their decision, and those who do not should be encouraged, without judgment to hold their infants according to their own beliefs and values.

## INDIVIDUALIZED DEVELOPMENTAL CARE AS AN INTERVENTION

Individualized developmental care programs such as NIDCAP® (Boston, MA) and others developed by Ohmeda Medical (Columbia, MD) and Children's Medical Ventures (Norwell, MA) have been widely implemented on an international scale. The positive effects of individualized care on medical, neurodevelopmental, and cost outcomes have been reported in randomized, controlled trials (Als, Lawhon, Duffy, et al., 1994; Buehler, Als, Duffy, et al., 1995; Fleisher, VandenBerg, Constantinou, et al., 1995; Heller, Constantinou, VandenBerg, et al., 1997; Kleberg, Westrup, & Stjernqvist, 2000; Kleberg, Westrup, Stjernqvist, et al., 2002; Westrup, Kleberg, von Eichwald, et al., 2000). More such trials need to be done with any developmental care program.

Consistency of care by caregivers familiar with each infant is necessary for subtle behavior changes to be appraised and care modified at that moment in time. This is very difficult given the staff shortages and rotation of staff from outside the NICU. Developmental care philosophy requires NICU staff to assess their KSAs, reflect on their own practice, and expand their horizons beyond the traditional medical and nursing models of care. It also requires integration of the family into the developmental care team (Figure 15-5).

## CONCLUSION

Philbin and Klaas (2000) suggest a checklist for evaluating research for use in the clinical setting (see Box 15-3). The checklist questions help the practitioner evaluate a study's validity (findings are true) and reliability (repeated trials produce same results). Not all interventions have an accumulated evidence-base and must be considered using infant characteristics, including current thresholds, vulnerabilities, and capabilities, medical status, corrected age, and developmental principles along with risk of harm or potential benefit.

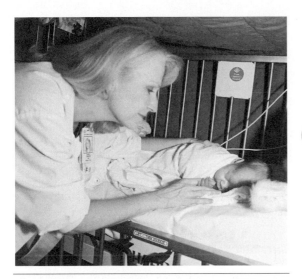

Figure **15-5** Soft touch.(*Courtesy Texas Children's Hospital, Dallas, TX; photographer Jim DeLeon.*)

Developmental literature should be reviewed for quality and strength of the evidence base (Carteaux, Cohen, Check, et al., 2003; Saunders, Abraham, Crosby, et al., 2003) using criteria similar to the following, with level 1 as the highest quality evidence base: (1) evidence strongly recommended by at least one systematic review of multiple quality, randomized controlled studies; (2) strong evidence from one or more well-designed randomized, controlled trials with adequate sample size; (3) well-designed studies lacking randomization but including single-group pre- and posttest, cohort, time-series or matched case control; (4) nonexperimental, well-designed, multicenter trials; (5) authoritative opinion based on solid clinical evidence, qualitative or descriptive studies, or expert panel review; (6) supported by neuropsychobiology and/or developmental theory; or (7) intuitive or anecdotal experience.

Developmental research is increasing substantially. Developmental teams must continually update themselves on current literature and make decisions concerning appropriate application of interventions in the NICU. Nurses, practitioners, therapists, and physicians should systematically review the developmental literature before applying any practice that has the potential for significant short- and long-term

effects on the developing preterm infant. Research on many of the IFDC interventions described inconclusive. There is just not enough evidence to support many of these interventions. What must be remembered is that developmental intervention with the preterm infant in the NICU must be individualized. What works with one infant might not work with another. Even if the evidence for a particular intervention appears positive, results might not be positive with the infant in question. Vigilant assessment of infant response both during and after initiation of any new stimuli must be a part of the intervention process. There is still much research that needs to be done in the area of IFDC intervention in the NICU. This chapter is focused on what is known and what is yet to be discovered between caregiving and the use of developmental care.

## REFERENCES

Abad, F., Diaz, N.M., Domenech, E., Robayna, M., et al. (1996). Oral sweet solution reduces pain-related behaviour in preterm infants. *Acta Paediatrica, 85*(7), 854-858.

Abrams, R.M.G., Gerhardt, K.J. (2000). The acoustic environment and physiological responses of the fetus. *Journal of Perinatology, 20*(8), S31-S37.

Acolet, D., Sleath, K., & Whitelaw, A. (1989). Oxygenation, heart rate and temperature in very low birthweight infants during skin-to-skin contact with their mothers. *Acta Paediatrica Scandinavia, 78*(2), 189-193.

Als, H., Lawhon, G., Duffy, F.H., et al. (1994). Individualized developmental care for the very low-birth-weight preterm infant: Medical and neurofunctional effects. *Journal of the American Medical Association (JAMA), 272*(11), 853-858.

American Academy of Pediatrics (AAP) Committee on Environmental Health. (1997). Noise: A hazard for the fetus and newborn. *Pediatrics, 100*(4), 724-727.

Anderson, G.C. (1991). Current knowledge about skin-to-skin (kangaroo) care for preterm infants. *Journal of Perinatology, 11*(3), 216-226.

Anderssen, S.H., Nicolaisen, R.B., & Gabrielsen, G.W. (1993). Autonomic response to auditory stimulation. *Acta Paediatrica, 82,* 913-918.

Banker, H., & Lickliter, R. (1993). Effects of early and delayed visual experience on intersensory development in bobwhite quail chicks. *Developmental Psychobiology, 26*(3), 155-170.

Bartocci, M., Winberg, J., Papendieck, G., et al. (2001). Cerebral hemodynamic response to unpleasant odors in the preterm newborn measured by near-infrared spectroscopy. *Pediatric Research, 50*(3), 324-330.

Bartocci, M., Winberg, J., Ruggiero, C., et al. (2000). Activation of olfactory cortex in newborn infants after odor stimulation: A functional near-infrared spectroscopy study. *Pediatric Research*, *48*(1), 18-23.

Bauer, J., Sontheimer, D., Fischer, C., et al. (1996). Metabolic rate and energy balance in very low birth weight infants during kangaroo holding by their mothers and fathers. *Journal of Pediatrics*, *129*(4), 608-611.

Bauer, K., Uhrig, C., Sperling, P., et al. (1997). Body temperatures and oxygen consumption during skin-to-skin (kangaroo) care in stable preterm infants weighing less than 1500 grams. *Journal of Pediatrics*, *130*(2), 240-244.

Beckham, R.W., & Mishoe, S.C. (1982). Sound levels inside incubators and oxygen hoods used with nebulizers and humidifiers. *Respiratory Care*, *27*(1), 33-40.

Berk, L.E. (2000). *Child development* (5th ed.). Needham Heights: Allyn and Bacon.

Bhutta, A.T., Cleves, M.A., Casey, P.H., et al. (2002). Cognitive and behavioral outcomes of school-aged children who were born preterm: A meta-analysis. *Journal of the American Medical Association (JAMA)*, *288*(6), 728-737.

Bier, J.A., Ferguson, A.E., Morales, Y., et al. (1996). Comparison of skin-to-skin contact with standard contact in low-birth-weight infants who are breast-fed. *Archives of Pediatric and Adolescent Medicine*, *150*(12), 1265-1269.

Bingham, P.M., Abassi, S., & Sivieri, E. (2003). A pilot study of milk odor effect on nonnutritive sucking by premature newborns. *Archives of Pediatric and Adolescent Medicine*, *157*(1), 72-75.

Birch, E.E., & O'Connor, A.R. (2001). Preterm birth and visual development. *Seminars in Neonatology*, *6*(6), 487-497.

Blackburn, S.T. (1996). Research utilization: Modifying the NICU light environment. *Neonatal Network*, *15*(4), 63-66.

Blackburn, S., & Patterson, D. (1991). Effects of cycled light on activity, state, and cardiorespiratory function in preterm infants. *Journal of Perinatal and Neonatal Nursing*, *4*(4), 47-54.

Blass, E.M., & Watt, L.B. (1999). Suckling- and sucrose-induced analgesia in human newborns. *Pain*, *83*(3), 611-623.

Bohnhorst, B., Heyne, T., Peter, C.S., et al. (2001). Skin-to-skin (kangaroo) care, respiratory control, and thermoregulation. *Journal of Pediatrics*, *138*(2), 193-197.

Brandon, D.H., Holditch-Davis, D., & Belyea, M. (2002). Preterm infants born at less than 31 weeks' gestation have improved growth in cycled light compared with continuous near darkness. *Journal of Pediatrics*, *140*(2), 192-199.

Buehler, D.M., Als, H., Duffy, F.H., et al. (1995). Effectiveness of individualized developmental care for low-risk preterm infants: Behavioral and electrophysiologic evidence. *Pediatrics*, *96*(5 Pt 1), 923-932.

Burke, M., Walsh, J., Oehler, J., et al. (1995). Music therapy following suctioning: Four case studies. *Neonatal Network*, *14*(7), 41-49.

Byrne, J., Ellsworth, C., Bowering, E., & Vincer, M. (1993). Language development in low birth weight infants: The first two years of life. *Journal of Developmental & Behavorial Pediatrics*, *14*(1), 21-27.

Caine, J. (1991). The effects of music on the selected stress behaviors, weight, caloric and formula intake, and length of hospital stay of premature and low birth weight neonates in a newborn intensive care unit. *Journal of Music Therapy*, *28*(4), 180-192.

Carteaux, P., Cohen, H., Check, J., et al. (2003). Evaluation and development of potentially better practices for the prevention of brain hemorrhage and ischemic brain injury in very low birth weight infants. *Pediatrics*, *111*(4)(Pt 2), e489-e496.

Casey, M.B., & Lickliter, R. (1998). Prenatal visual experience influences the development of turning bias in bobwhite quail chicks (*Colinus virginianus*). *Developmental and Psychobiology*, *32*(4), 327-338.

Cernoch, J.M., & Porter, R.H. (1985). Recognition of maternal axillary odors by infants. *Child Development*, *56*(6), 1593-1598.

Charpak, N., de Calume, Z.F., & Ruiz, J.G. (2000). The Bogota Declaration on kangaroo mother care: Conclusions at the second international workshop on the method. Second International Workshop of Kangaroo Mother Care. *Acta Paediatrics*, *89*(9), 1137-1140.

Charpak, N., Figueroa, Z., & Ruiz, J.G. (1998). Kangaroo mother care. *Lancet*, *351*(9106), 914.

Charpak, N., Ruiz-Pelaez, J.G., & Figueroa de Calume, Z. (1996). Current knowledge of kangaroo mother intervention. *Current Opinions in Pediatrics*, *8*(2), 108-112.

Cherkes-Julkowski, M. (1998). Learning disability, attention-deficit disorder, and language impairment as outcomes of prematurity: A longitudinal descriptive study. *Journal of Learning Disabilities*, *31*(3), 294-306.

Cleary, G.M., Spinner, S.S., Gibson, E., et al. (1997). Skin-to-skin parental contact with fragile preterm infants. *Journal of American Osteopathic Association*, *97*(8), 457-460.

Cloonan, H.A., Maxwell, S.R., & Miller, S.D. (2001). Developmental outcomes in very low birth weight infants: a six-year study. *West Virginia Medical Journal*, *97*(5), 250-252.

Conde-Agudelo, A., Diaz-Rossello, J.L., & Belizan, J.M. (2000). Kangaroo mother care to reduce morbidity and mortality in low birthweight infants. *Cochrane Database System Reviews*, 4, CD002771.

Cordero, L., Clark, D.L., & Schott, L. (1986). Effects of vestibular stimulation on sleep states in premature infants. *American Journal of Perinatology*, *3*(4), 319-324.

Corff, K.E., Seideman, R., Venkataraman, P.S., et al. (1995). Facilitated tucking: A nonpharmacological comfort measure for pain in preterm neonates. *Journal of*

*Obstetric, Gynecology, and Neonatal Nursing (JOGNN)*, 24(2), 143-147.

Crade, M.L.S. (1988). Fetal response to sound stimulation: Preliminary report exploring use of sound stimulation in routine obstetrical ultrasound examination. *Journal of Ultrasound Medicine*, 7(9), 499-503.

Cusson, R.M. (2003). Factors influencing language development in preterm infants. *Journal of Obstetric, Gynecologic, and Neonatal Nursing (JOGNN)*, 32(3), 402-409.

Davis, N.M., Doyle, L.W., Ford, G.W., et al. (2001). Auditory function at 14 years of age of very-low-birth-weight. *Developmental Medicine and Child Neurology*, 43(3), 191-196.

Evans, J.B., & Philbin, M.K. (2000). Facility and operations planning for quiet hospital nurseries. *Journal of Perinatology*, 20(8)(Pt 2), S105-S112.

Fearon, I., Kisilevsky, B.S., Hains, S., et al. (1997). Swaddling after heel lance: Age-specific effects on behavioral recovery in preterm infants. *Journal of Developmental and Behavioral Pediatrics*, 18, 222-232.

Feldman, R., & Eidelman, A.I. (2003). Skin-to-skin contact (kangaroo care) accelerates autonomic and neurobehavioural maturation in preterm infants. *Developmental Medicine and Child Nuerology*, 45(4), 274-281.

Feldman, R., Eidelman, A.I., Sirota, L., & Weller, A. (2002). Comparison of skin-to-skin (kangaroo) and traditional care: Parenting outcomes and preterm infant development. *Pediatrics*, 110(1 Pt 1), 16-26.

Feldman, R., Weller, A., Sirota, L., et al. (2002). Skin-to-skin contact (kangaroo care) promotes self-regulation in premature infants: Sleep-wake cyclicity, arousal modulation, and sustained exploration. *Developmental Psychology*, 38(2), 194-207.

Field, T.M. (2003). Stimulation of preterm infants. *Pediatric Reviews*, 24(1), 4-11.

Fielder, A.R., & Moseley, M.J. (2000). Environmental light and the preterm infant. *Seminars in Neonatology*, 24(4), 291-292.

Fleisher, B.E., VandenBerg, K., Constantinou, J., et al. (1995). Individualized developmental care for very-low-birth-weight premature infants. *Clinics in Pediatrics (Philadelphia)*, 34(10), 523-529.

Fohe, K., Kropf, S., & Avenarius, S. (2000). Skin-to-skin contact improves gas exchange in premature infants. *Journal of Perinatology*, 20(5), 311-315.

Foushee, R.D., & Lickliter, R. (2002). Early visual experience affects postnatal auditory responsiveness in bobwhite quail (*Colinus virginianus*). *Journal of Complementary Psychology*, 116(4), 369-380.

Franck, L., & Gilbert, R. (2002). Reducing pain during blood sampling in infants. *Clinical Evidence*, 7, 352-366.

Gadeke, R., Doring, B., Keller, F., et al. (1969). The noise level in a children's hospital and the wake-up threshold in infants. *Acta Paediatrica Scandinavia*, 58, 164-170.

Gagnon, R. (1989). Stimulation of human fetuses with sound and vibration. *Seminars in Perinatology*, 13, 393-402.

Gale, G., & VandenBerg, K.A. (1998). Kangaroo care. *Neonatal Network*, 17(5), 69-71.

Gerhardt, K.J.A., & Abrams, R.M. (2000). Fetal exposures to sound and vibroacoustic stimulation. *Journal of Perinatology*, 20(8), S21-S30.

Gibbins, S., & Stevens, B. (2001). Mechanisms of sucrose and non-nutritive sucking in procedural pain management in infants. *Pain Research Management*, 6(1), 21-28.

Gibbins, S., Stevens, B., Hodnett, E., et al. (2002). Efficacy and safety of sucrose for procedural pain relief in preterm and term neonates. *Nursing Research*, 51(6), 375-382.

Glass, P. (1999). The vulnerable neonate and the neonatal intensive care environment. In G.B. Avery, M.A. Fletcher, & M.G. MacDonald (Eds.), *Neonatology: Pathophysiology and management of the newborn* (5th ed.). Philadelphia: Lippincott, Williams & Wilkins.

Graven, S.N. (2000). Sound and the developing infant in the NICU: Conclusions and recommendations for care. *Journal of Perinatology*, 20(8)(Pt 2), S88-S93.

Gray, L., Watt, L., & Blass, E.M. (2000). Skin-to-skin contact is analgesic in healthy newborns. *Pediatrics*, 105(1), e14.

Hack, M., & Fanaroff, A.A. (2000). Outcomes of children of extremely low birthweight and gestational age in the 1990s. *Seminars in Neonatology*, 5(2), 89-106.

Hack, M., Taylor, H.G., Klein, N., et al. (1994). School-age outcomes in children with birth weights under 750 g. *New England Journal of Medicine*, 331(12), 753-759.

Hall, J.I. (2000). Development of the ear and hearing. *Journal of Perinatology*, 20(8), S12-S20.

Heller, C., Constantinou, J.C., VandenBerg, K., et al. (1997). Sedation administered to very low birth weight premature infants. *Journal of Perinatology*, 17(2), 107-112.

Hernandez-Reif, M., & Field, T. (2000). Preterm Infants benefit from early interventions (pp. 298-319). In J.D. Osofsky & H.E. Fitzgerald (Eds.), *Infant mental health in groups at high risk* (vol. 4). New York: John Wiley & Sons.

Holditch-Davis, D., Blackburn, S.T., & VandenBerg, K.A. (2003). Newborn and infant neurobehavioral development (pp. 236-284). In C. Kenner & J.W. Lott (Eds.), *Comprehensive neonatal nursing: A physiologic perspective* (3rd ed.). St. Louis: W.B. Saunders.

Honeycutt, H., & Lickliter, R. (2001). Order-dependent timing of unimodal and multimodal stimulation affects prenatal auditory learning in bobwhite quail embryos. *Developmental Psychobiology*, 38(1), 1-10.

Hunter, J. (2001). The neonatal intensive care unit. In J. Case-Smith (Ed.), *Occupational therapy for children* (4th ed.). St. Louis: Mosby.

Hurst, N.M., Valentine, C.J., Renfro, L., et al. (1997). Skin-to-skin holding in the neonatal intensive care unit influences maternal milk volume. *Journal of Perinatology*, 17(3), 213-217.

Ingersoll, E.W., & Thoman, E.B. (1994). The breathing bear: Effects on respiration in premature infants. *Physiology and Behavior, 56*(5), 855-859.

Jennische, M., & Sedin, G. (1998). Speech and language skills in children who required neonatal intensive care. I. Spontaneous speech at 6.5 years of age. *Acta Paediatrica, 87*(6), 654-666.

Jennische, M., & Sedin, G. (1999). Speech and language skills in children who required neonatal intensive care: Evaluation at 6.5 y of age based on interviews with parents. *Acta Paediatrica, 88*(9), 975-982.

Jennische, M., & Sedin, G. (2001). Linguistic skills at 6 1/2 years of age in children who required neonatal intensive care in 1986–1989. *Acta Paediatrica, 90*(2), 199-212.

Johnson, A.N. (2001). Neonatal response to control of noise inside the incubator. *Pediatric Nursing, 27*(6), 600-605.

Johnston, C.C., Stremler, R., Horton, L., & Friedman, A. (1999). Effect of repeated doses of sucrose during heel stick procedure in preterm neonates. *Biology of the Neonate, 75*(3), 160-166.

Kaminski, J., & Hall, W. (1996). The effect of soothing music on neonatal behavioral states in the hospital newborn nursery. *Neonatal Network, 15*(1), 45-54.

Kennedy, K.A., Fielder, A.R., Hardy, R.J., et al. (2001). Reduced lighting does not improve medical outcomes in very low birth weight infants. *Journal of Pediatrics, 139*(4), 527-531.

Kennedy, K.A., Ipson, M.A., Birch, D.G., et al. (1997). Light reduction and the electroretinogram of preterm infants. *Archives of Disease in Child Fetal Neonatal Education, 76*(3), F168-F173.

Kirsten, G.F., Bergman, N.J., & Hann, F.M. (2001). Kangaroo mother care in the nursery. *Pediatric Clinics North America, 48*(2), 443-452.

Kleberg, A., Westrup, B., & Stjernqvist, K. (2000). Developmental outcome, child behaviour and mother-child interaction at 3 years of age following Newborn Individualized Developmental Care and Intervention Program (NIDCAP®) intervention. *Early Human Development, 60*(2), 123-135.

Kleberg, A., Westrup, B., Stjernqvist, K., et al. (2002). Indications of improved cognitive development at one year of age among infants born very prematurely who received care based on the Newborn Individualized Developmental Care and Assessment Program (NIDCAP®). *Early Human Development, 68*(2), 83-91.

Korner, A.F. (1999). Vestibular stimulation as a neurodevelopmental intervention with preterm infants: Findings and new methods of reevaluating intervention effects. In E. Goldson (Ed.), *Nurturing the premature infant: Developmental interventions in the neonatal intensive care nursery.* New York: Oxford University Press.

Kurihara, H., Chiba, H., Shimizu, Y., et al. (1996). Behavioral and adrenocortical responses to stress in neonates and the stabilizing effects of maternal heartbeat on them. *Early Human Development, 46*, 117-127.

Lewis, B.A., Singer, L.T., Fulton, S., et al. (2002). Speech and language outcomes of children with bronchopulmonary dysplasia. *Journal of Communication and Disorders, 35*(5), 393-406.

Lickliter, R. (2000a). Atypical perinatal sensory stimulation and early perceptual development: Insights from developmental psychobiology. *Journal of Perinatology, 20*(8 Pt 2), S45-S54.

Lickliter, R. (2000b). The role of sensory stimulation in perinatal development: Insights from comparative research for care of the high-risk infant. *Journal of Developmental & Behavorial Pediatrics, 21*(6), 437-447.

Lickliter, R., & Bahrick, L.E. (2000). The development of infant intersensory perception: Advantages of a comparative convergent-operations approach. *Psychology Bulletin, 126*(2), 260-280.

Lickliter, R., & Stoumbos, J. (1992). Modification of prenatal auditory experience alters postnatal auditory preferences of bobwhite quail chicks. *Quality Journal Experimental Psychology, B, 44*(3-4), 199-214.

Long, J., Lucey, J., & Philip, A. (1980). Noise and hypoxemia in the intensive care nursery unit. *Pediatrics, 65*, 143-145.

Ludington-Hoe, S.M., Anderson, G.C., et al. (1999). Birth-related fatigue in 34-36-week preterm neonates: Rapid recovery with very early kangaroo (skin-to-skin) care. *Journal of Obstetric, Gynecologic, and Neonatal Nursing (JOGNN), 28*(1), 94-103.

Ludington-Hoe, S.M., Nguyen, N., Swinth, J.Y., & Satyshur, R.D. (2000). Kangaroo care compared to incubators in maintaining body warmth in preterm infants. *Biology Research Nursing, 2*(1), 60-73.

Ludington-Hoe, S.M., Thompson, C., Swinth, J., et al. (1994). Kangaroo care: Research results, and practice implications and guidelines. *Neonatal Network, 13*(1), 19-27.

Mann, N.P., Haddow, R., Stokes, L., et al. (1986). Effect of night and day on preterm infants in a newborn nursery: Randomised trial. *British Medical Journal (Clinical Research Education), 293*(6557), 1265-1267.

Marlier, L., Schaal, B., & Soussignan, R. (1998a). Bottle-fed neonates prefer an odor experienced in utero to an odor experienced postnatally in the feeding context. *Developmental Psychobiology, 33*(2), 133-145.

Marlier, L., Schaal, B., & Soussignan, R. (1998b). Neonatal responsiveness to the odor of amniotic and lacteal fluids: A test of perinatal chemosensory continuity. *Child Development, 69*(3), 611-623.

McBride, T., & Lickliter, R. (1994). Specific postnatal auditory stimulation interferes with species-typical visual responsiveness in bobwhite quail chicks. *Developmental Psychobiology, 27*(3), 169-183.

McGrath, J.M., & Brock, N. (2002). Efficacy and utilization of skin-to-skin care in the NICU. *Newborn and Infant Nursing Reviews, 2*(1), 17-26.

McGrath, M., & Sullivan, M. (2002). Birth weight, neonatal morbidities, and school age outcomes in full-term and preterm infants. *Issues Comprehensive Pediatric Nursing, 25*(4), 231-254.

McGrath, M.M., Sullivan, M.C., Lester, B.M., & Oh, W. (2000). Longitudinal neurologic follow-up in neonatal intensive care unit survivors with various neonatal morbidities. *Pediatrics, 106*(6), 1397-1405.

Mennella, J.A., Jagnow, C.P., & Beauchamp, G.K. (2001). Prenatal and postnatal flavor learning by human infants. *Pediatrics, 107*(6), E88

Messmer, P.R., Rodriguez, S., Adams, J., et al. (1997). Effect of kangaroo care on sleep time for neonates. *Pediatric Nursing, 23*(4), 408-414.

Miller, C., White, R., Whitman, T., et al. (1995). The effects of cycled versus noncycled lighting on growth and development in preterm infants. *Infant Behavioral Development, 18*, 87-95.

Mirmiran, M., & Ariagno, R.L. (2000). Influence of light in the NICU on the development of circadian rhythms in preterm infants. *Seminars in Perinatology, 24*(4), 247-257.

Monset-Couchard, M., de Bethmann, O., & Kastler, B. (2002). Mid- and long-term outcome of 166 premature infants weighing less than 1,000 g at birth, all small for gestational age. *Biology of Neonate, 81*(4), 244-254.

Morris, B.H., Philbin, M.K., & Bose, C. (2000). Physiological effects of sound on the Newborn. *Journal of Perinatology, 20*(8), S55-S60.

Msall, M.E., & Tremont, M.R. (2002). Measuring functional outcomes after prematurity: Developmental impact of very low birth weight and extremely low birth weight status on childhood disability. *Mental Retardation & Development Disability Research Reviews, 8*(4), 258-272.

Neu, M., Browne, J.V., & Vojir, C. (2000). The impact of two transfer techniques used during skin-to-skin care on the physiologic and behavioral responses of preterm infants. *Nursing Research, 49*(4), 215-223.

Noerr, B. (2001). Sucrose for neonatal procedural pain. *Neonatal Network, 20*(7), 63-67.

O'Connor, A.R., Stephenson, T., Johnson, A., et al. (2002). Long-term ophthalmic outcome of low birth weight children with and without retinopathy of prematurity. *Pediatrics, 109*(1), 12-18.

Peters, K.L. (1999). Infant handling in the NICU: Does developmental care make a difference? An evaluative review of the literature. *Journal Perinatal Neonatal Nursing, 13*(30), 83-100.

Peusner, K.D. (2001). Development of the gravity sensing system. *Journal of Neuroscience and Research, 63*(2), 103-108.

Philbin, M.K. (2000a). The influence of auditory experience on the behavior of preterm newborns. *Journal of Perinatology, 20*(8)(Pt 2), S77-S87.

Philbin, M.K. (2000b). The influence of auditory experience on the behavior of preterm newborns. *Journal of Perinatology, 20*(8), S77-S87.

Philbin, M.K. (1996). Some implications of early auditory development for the environment of hospitalized preterm infants. *Neonatal Network, 15*(8), 71-73.

Philbin, M.K., & Gray, L. (2002). Changing levels of quiet in an intensive care nursery. *Journal of Perinatology, 22*(6), 455-460.

Philbin, M.K., & Klass, P. (2000). Evaluating studies of the behavioral effects of sound on newborns. *Journal of Perinatology, 20*(8 Pt 2), S61-S67.

Pinelli, J., & Symington, A. (2000a). How rewarding can a pacifier be? A systematic review of nonnutritive sucking in preterm infants. *Neonatal Network, 19*(8), 41-48.

Pinelli, J., & Symington, A. (2000b). Non-nutritive sucking for promoting physiologic stability and nutrition in preterm infants. *Cochrane Database System Review, 2*, CD001071.

Reiser, J., Yonas, A., & Wilkner, K. (1976). Radial localization of odors by human neonates. *Child Development, 47*, 856-859.

Renqvist, H., & Fellman, V. (2000). [Sucrose reduces pain reaction to heel lancing in newborn infant]. *Duodecim, 116*(18), 1977-1981.

Roberts, K.L., Paynter, C., & McEwan, B. (2000). A comparison of kangaroo mother care and conventional cuddling care. *Neonatal Network, 19*(4), 31-35.

Robertson, A., Cooper-Peel, C., & Vos, P. (1998). Peak noise distribution in the neonatal intensive care nursery. *Journal of Perinatology, 18*(5), 361-364.

Robertson, A., Cooper-Peel, C., & Vos, P. (1999). Contribution of heating, ventilation, and air conditioning airflow and conversation to the ambient sound in a neonatal intensive care unit. *Journal of Perinatology, 19*(5), 362-366.

Robertson, A., Kohn, J., Vos, P., & Cooper-Peel, C. (1998). Establishing a noise measurement protocol for neonatal intensive care units. *Journal of Perinatology, 18*(2), 126-130.

Robertson, A., Stuart, A., & Walker, L. (2001). Transmission loss of sound into incubators: Implications for voice perception by infants. *Journal of Perinatology, 21*(4), 236-241.

Roy, M.S., Caramelli, C., Orquin, J., et al. (1999). Effects of early reduced light exposure on central visual development in preterm infants. *Acta Paediatrica, 88*(4), 459-461.

Saunders, R.P., Abraham, M.R., Crosby, M.J., et al. (2003). Evaluation and development of potentially better practices for improving family-centered care in neonatal intensive care units. *Pediatrics, 111*(4 Pt 2), e437-e449.

Schaal, B., Marlier, L., & Soussignan, R. (2000). Human foetuses learn odours from their pregnant mother's diet. *Chemical Senses, 25*(6), 729-737.

Schraeder, B.D., Heverly, M.A., O'Brien, C., et al. (1997). Academic achievement and educational resource use of very low birth weight (VLBW) survivors. *Pediatric Nursing, 23*(1), 21-25, 44.

Shanahan, T.L., & Czeisler, C.A. (2000). Physiological effects of light on the human circadian pacemaker. *Seminars Neonatology, 24*(4), 299-320.

Shogan, M.G., & Schumann, L.L. (1993). The effect of environmental lighting on the oxygen saturation of preterm infants in the NICU. *Neonatal Network, 12*(5), 7-13.

Sleigh, M.J., Columbus, R.F., & Lickliter, R. (1996). Type of prenatal sensory experience affects prenatal auditory learning in bobwhite quail (*Colinus virginianus*). *Journal of Comprehensive Psychology, 110*(3), 233-242.

Sleigh, M.J., & Lickliter, R. (1995). Augmented prenatal visual stimulation alters postnatal auditory and visual responsiveness in bobwhite quail chicks. *Developmental Psychobiology, 28*(7), 353-366.

Sleigh, M.J., & Lickliter, R. (1998). Timing of presentation of prenatal auditory stimulation alters auditory and visual responsiveness in bobwhite quail chicks *(Colinus virginianus). Journal of Comprehensive Psychology, 112*(2), 153-160.

Slevin, M., Murphy, J.F.A., Daly, L., et al. (1999). Retinopathy of prematurity screening, stress related responses, the role of nesting. *British Journal of Ophthamology, 81*, 762-764.

Standley, J.M. (1998). The effect of music and multimodal stimulation on responses of premature infants in neonatal intensive care. *Pediatric Nursing, 24*(6), 532-538.

Standley, J.M. (2002). A meta-analysis of the efficacy of music therapy for premature infants. *Journal Pediatric Nursing, 17*(2), 107-113.

Standley, J.M., & Moore, R.S. (1995). Therapeutic effects of music and mother's voice on premature infants. *Pediatric Nursing, 21*(6), 509-512, 574.

Stevens, B., & Ohlsson, A. (2000). Sucrose for analgesia in newborn infants undergoing painful procedures. *Cochrane Database System Reviews, 2*, CD001069.

Stevens, B., Taddio, A., Ohlsson, A., & Einarson, T. (1997). The efficacy of sucrose for relieving procedural pain in neonates: A systematic review and meta-analysis. *Acta Paediatrica, 86*(8), 837-842.

Stevens, B., Yamada, J., & Ohlsson, A. (2001). Sucrose for analgesia in newborn infants undergoing painful procedures. *Cochrane Database System Review, 4*, CD001069.

Strauch, C., Brandt, S., & Edwards-Beckett, J. (1993). Implementation of a quiet hour: Effect on noise levels and infant sleep states. *Neonatal Network, 12*(2), 31-35.

Sullivan, M.C., & Margaret, M.M. (2003). Perinatal morbidity, mild motor delay, and later school outcomes. *Developmental Medicine Child Neurology, 45*(2), 104-112.

Sullivan, R.M., Taborsky-Barba, S., Mendoza, R., et al. (1991). Olfactory classical conditioning in neonates. *Pediatrics, 87*(4), 511-518.

Sullivan, R.M., & Toubas, P. (1998). Clinical usefulness of maternal odor in newborns: Soothing and feeding preparatory responses. *Biology of Neonate, 74*(6), 402-408.

Symington, A., & Pinelli, J. (2002). Distilling the evidence on developmental care: A systematic review. *Advances in Neonatal Care, 2*(4), 198-221.

Taylor, G.H., Klein, N., & Hack, M. (2000). School-age consequences of birth weight less than 750 g: A review and update. *Developmental Neuropsychology, 17*(3), 289-321.

Taylor, G.H., Klein, N.M., Minich, N.M., & Hack, M. (2000). Verbal memory deficits in children with less than 750 g birth weight. *Neuropsychology Development Cognitive Section C Child Neuropsychology, 6*(1), 49-63.

Thoman, E.B., Ingersoll, E.W., & Acebo, C. (1991). Premature infants seek rhythmic stimulation, and the experience facilitates neurobehavioral development. *Journal of Developmental & Behavioral Pediatrics, 12*(1), 11-18.

Thomas, K.A., & Martin, P.A. (2000). NICU sound environment and the potential problems for caregivers. *Journal of Perinatology, 20*(8)(Pt 2), S94-S99.

Tornhage, C.J., Stuge, E., Lindberg, T., et al. (1999). First week kangaroo care in sick very preterm infants. *Acta Paediatrica, 88*(12), 1402-1404.

Veen, S., Sassen, M.L., Schreuder, A.M., et al. (1993). Hearing loss in very preterm and very low birthweight infants at the age of 5 years in a nationwide cohort. *International Journal of Pediatric Otorhinolaryngology, 26*, 11-28.

Viser, G.H.M., et al. (1993). The effect of vibroacoustic stimulation on fetal behavioral state organization. *American Journal of Indian Medicine, 23*, 531-539.

Vohr, B.R., Wright, L.L., Dusick, A.M., et al. (2000). Neurodevelopmental and functional outcomes of extremely low birth weight infants in the National Institute of Child Health and Human Development Neonatal Research Network, 1993–1994. *Pediatrics, 105*(6), 1216-1226.

Walsh-Sukys, M., Reitenbach, A., Hudson-Barr, D., & DePompei, P. (2001). Reducing light and sound in the neonatal intensive care unit: An evaluation of patient safety, staff satisfaction and costs. *Journal of Perinatology, 21*(4), 230-235.

Warren, I. (2002). Facilitating infant adaptation: The nursery environment. *Seminars in Neonatology, 7*, 459-467.

Wedenberg, E. (1963). Objective auditory tests on noncooperative children: A follow-up examination of 50 newborn infants and pre-school children with suspected hearing loss. *Acta Otolaryngology, 175*(Suppl), 1-32.

Westrup, B., Kleberg, A., von Eichwald, K., et al. (2000). A randomized, controlled trial to evaluate the effects of the newborn individualized developmental care and assessment program in a Swedish setting. *Pediatrics, 105*(1) (Pt 1), 66-72.

Wharrad, H.J., & Davis, A.C. (1997). Behavioural and autonomic responses to sound in pre-term and full-term babies. *British Journal of Audiology, 31*(5), 315-329.

White, R. (2002). *Recommended standards for newborn ICU design.* Committee to Establish Recommended Standards for Newborn ICU Design, 5th Consensus Conference, Clearwater Beach, FL. Available online at *www.nd.edu/~kkolberg/frmain.htm.*

Whitelaw, A., Histerkamp, G., Sleath, K., et al. (1988). Skin to skin contact for very low birthweight infants and their mothers. *Archives of Disease in Children, 63*(11), 1377-1381.

White-Traut, R.C., Nelson, M.N., Silvestri, J.M., et al. (2002). Effect of auditory, tactile, visual, and vestibular intervention on length of stay, alertness, and feeding progression in preterm infants. *Development Medicine and Child Neurology, 44*(2), 91-97.

White-Traut, R.C., Silvestri, J.M., Cunningham, N., et al. (1997). Responses of preterm infants to unimodal and multimodal sensory intervention. *Pediatric Nursing, 23*(2), 169-175.

Whitfield, M.F., Grunau, R.V., & Holsti, L. (1997). Extremely premature (<800 g) schoolchildren: Multiple areas of hidden disability. *Archives of Disease in Children, Fetal and Neonatal Education, 77*(2), F85-F90.

Zahr, L.K., & Balian, S. (1995). Responses of premature infants to routine nursing interventions and noise in the NICU. *Nursing Research, 44*(3), 179-185.

Zahr, L.K., & de Traversay, J. (1995). Premature infant responses to noise reduction by earmuffs: Effects on behavioral and physiologic measures. *Journal of Perinatology, 15*(6), 448-455.

# 16 *Positioning*

### Jan Hunter

Essential competencies for neonatal intensive care unit (NICU) caregivers encompass more than medical sophistication. Current standards for excellence in neonatal nursing require knowledgeable and technically superior clinicians to successfully address the nonmedical needs of the baby and family. This opportunity presents a challenge for committed neonatal nurses to advance their skills in areas of developmental support, such as therapeutic positioning, that have long-reaching implications for improved functional outcomes of NICU graduates.

Therapeutic positioning can promote the normal structural alignment and neuromotor control necessary for optimal development of an infant's posture and motor skills. Conversely, lack of caregiver attention to an infant's developing postures and movement patterns can inadvertently create short-term and long-term functional problems, even in the absence of overt brain pathology. This chapter is focused on the rationale and techniques of developmentally supportive positioning as a necessary caregiver intervention for immature and ill infants in the NICU.

## PREDISPOSITION OF NICU INFANTS TO POSTURAL AND MOVEMENT PROBLEMS

Factors that encourage a flexed posture after birth and promote early motor development in healthy term newborns do not necessarily occur with infants born very early; preterm infants at term age equivalency look motorically different than newborn term infants (Palmer, Dubowitz, Verghote, & Dubowitz, 1982). Birth that occurs significantly before optimal fetal musculoskeletal and neurologic maturation has been completed places the early-born infant at risk for atypical postures and movement patterns (Riegger-Krugh, 1993; Sweeney & Gutierrez, 2002).

## Implications of Preterm Birth on Musculoskeletal Maturation

Prenatally, a fetus in the womb has dynamic circumferential boundaries at all times. Active movements occur within consistent and predictable boundaries; resting posture is typically flexed and contained with midline orientation of the head and extremities. Limited intrauterine space in a full-term pregnancy creates a postural bias toward flexion (called *physiologic flexion*), and temporarily limits range of motion in knees, hips, elbows, and shoulders (Amiel-Tison, 1976; Hoffer, 1980).

Conversely, infants in the NICU tend to assume flattened postures with the trunk, pelvis, and extremities flat on the bed surface, owing to the effects of prematurity (i.e., incomplete musculoskeletal development, maturation-related hypotonia, immature neuromotor control, primitive reflexes), illness, and gravity (Hunter, 2001) (Figure 16-1). The forceful prenatal motor pattern of active extension, as the fetus kicked and stretched in the womb, is no longer counterbalanced for the NICU infant by consistent uterine boundaries that compelled the fetus to return to a flexed midline position. Arching with excessive neck and trunk hyperextension often evolves from strong active extension, from postural asymmetry as gravity and primitive reflexes pull the head out of midline, and from positional effects of endotracheal intubation and mechanical ventilation.

## Principle of Activity-Dependent Development

The principle of activity-dependent development refers to the influence of repetitive use in the formation of neural connections and pathways. In this "use it, or lose it" framework, neural connections that are frequently activated strengthen and become dominant; potential neural pathways that are rarely used weaken or disappear (van Heijst, Touwen & Vos, 1999; Penn & Schatz,

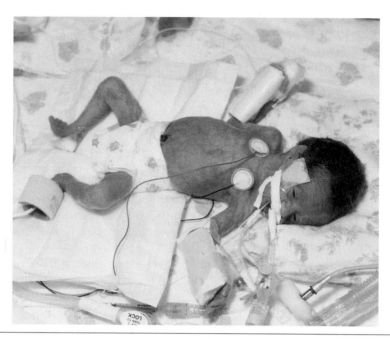

Figure **16-1**  Hypotonic preemie (hypotonic posture of preterm infant). Without therapeutic positioning, the "W" configuration of arms, "frogged" posture of legs, and asymmetric head position can promote positional deformities and developmental gaps or delays. (*From Hunter, J.G. [2001]. The neonatal intensive care unit. In J. Case-Smith [Ed.], Occupational therapy for children [4th ed.; pp. 636-707]. St. Louis: Mosby.*)

1999). In other words, "neurons that fire together, wire together; neurons that don't, won't" (Penn, 2001).

Important neural connections are being formed and reinforced during the last trimester of pregnancy that emphasize a return to flexion and midline as the normal baseline resting posture for the developing infant. The central nervous system of a third-trimester fetus is undergoing rapid development as cortical neurons layer, organize, specialize, and form vital connections and pathways; formation of synaptic connections at this stage is particularly vulnerable to circumstances and environment. The protection afforded by the consistency of the womb typically allows a much more controlled and predictable progression of this neuronal development than does the variable high-tech environment of the NICU.

Application of the principle of activity-dependent development to body posture and movement suggests that neuronal pathways supporting extremity flexion and symmetrical body alignment are constantly reinforced in the womb. Active stretching and kicking by the normal fetus is always followed by a return to midline and flexion, due to uterine constraints. In contrast, the resting posture of a NICU infant *without* therapeutic positioning is often flat, extended, asymmetrical with the head to one side (usually to the right), and with the extremities abducted and externally rotated. Active extension of the trunk and extremities still occurs as it did in utero; but, without boundaries, the baby does not spontaneously return to a flexed midline posture. With time, neuronal connections are reinforced that favor a flat, externally rotated and asymmetric resting posture as baseline for that infant; active extension and arching become dominant or unopposed motor patterns.

## IMPACT OF POSITIONING ON INFANTS IN THE NICU

Both correct and incorrect positioning affects the neurobehavioral organization, musculoskeletal development, and neuromotor functioning of

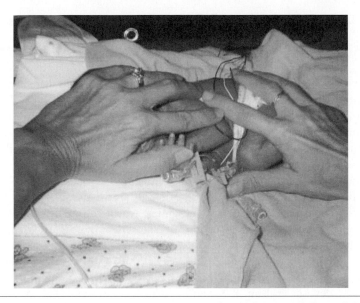

Figure **16-2** Facilitative tuck. A facilitative tuck, which is gentle but firm swaddling of the baby in the caregiver's hands, can calm a stressed or disorganized preterm infant and has been recommended as a nonpharmacologic option to assist with pain management in the NICU. (*From Hunter, J.G. [2001]. The neonatal intensive care unit. In J. Case-Smith [Ed.], Occupational therapy for children [4th ed.; pp. 636-707]. St. Louis: Mosby.*)

infants in the NICU. Some adverse consequences of inadequate positioning, such as arching or lateral skull flattening, might be apparent during hospitalization. Other unfavorable outcomes are not evident until after hospital discharge. The term *new morbidity* has been applied to neurodevelopmental delays or dysfunction of the NICU graduate in the absence of known brain pathology; inappropriate positioning can be a contributing factor (Johnson, 2000).

### Neurobehavioral Organization

Preterm infants left in unsupported extended positions frequently exhibit increased stress and agitation with decreased physiologic stability. Persistent and extreme extensor posturing can increasingly interfere with caregiving and with the infant's ability to attend and interact appropriately within his environment. Appropriate therapeutic positioning promotes improved rest and neurobehavioral organization; the baby is calmer and easier to care for (Petryshen, Stevens, Hawkins, & Stewart, 1998). Less crying and reduced restless or frenetic activity conserves calories needed for growth, physiologic recovery, and functional activities such as oral feeding. Swaddling and facilitated tucking ("hand swaddle") are calming to the infant and have been recommended as nonpharmacologic options to assist with pain management in the NICU (Campos, 1989; Corff, Seideman, Venkataraman, et al., 1995; Fearon, Kisilevsky, Hains, et al., 1997; Short, Brooks-Brunn, Reeves, et al., 1996) (Figure 16-2).

### Iatrogenic Positional Deformities and Developmental Consequences

Undesirable muscular and skeletal changes in the NICU infant are promoted when inattention to correct positioning allows abnormal body alignment to persist. These changes can initiate a cascade of atypical resting postures, acquired positional deformities, and atypical movement patterns that can adversely affect the NICU graduate's future motor development, play skills, attractiveness, and social attachment.

### Head Position

Both preterm and full-term infants demonstrate spontaneous preferential head-turning to the right, maintaining this position up to 70% to 80% of the time when supine (Konishi, Mikawa, & Suziki, 1986). Preferential head-turning has been linked to asymmetrical skull deformation (flattened occiput on preferred side, with or without a corresponding bulging of the forehead), torticollis, lateral trunk curvature that does not disappear on ventral suspension, a visual and functional preference for the right hand that occurs too early (because that hand is constantly in the visual field), and asymmetric gait patterns with increased external rotation of the left lower extremity (Boere-Boonekamp, van der Linden-Kuiper, & van Es, 1997; Chadduck, Kast, & Donahue, 1997; Dias, Klein, & Backstrom, 1996; Geerdink, Hopkins, & Hoeksma, 1994; Hamanishi & Tanaka, 1994; Konishi, Mikawa, & Suziki, 1986). These outcomes, which occur more frequently and are more sustained in preterm infants than in full-term infants (Konishi, Mikawa, & Suziki, 1986), have been accentuated by sudden infant death syndrome (SIDS) recommendations to place infants supine for sleeping (American Academy of Pediatrics [AAP] Task Force on Infant Sleep Position and SIDS, 2000; Chadduck, Kast, & Donahue, 1997; Hunter and Malloy, 2002). Some infants with this preferential head turning and early right-hand preference have been mistakenly diagnosed with left hemiparetic cerebral palsy, causing the parents considerable anxiety and misusing scarce early-intervention resources in the process.

### Deformational Plagiocephaly

Deformational plagiocephaly refers to the development of an abnormal head shape in infants from prenatal or postnatal external molding forces. Plural birth infants have an increased risk of deformational plagiocephaly due to factors such as in utero constraints, prematurity, supine sleeping position, and torticollis (Littlefield, Beals, Manwaring, et al., 1998). Preterm infants are especially vulnerable to postural deformation, as their skulls are thinner and softer than the skulls of full-term infants (Baum &

Searls, 1971; Cartlidge & Rutter, 1988; Huang, Cheng, Lin, et al., 1995).

Dolichocephaly (also called scaphocephaly) refers to progressive lateral skull flattening that results in a narrow and elongated "preemie-shaped" head (Cartlidge & Rutter, 1988; Rutter, Hinchcliffe, & Cartlidge, 1993) (Figure 16-3). Persistent lateralization of the head in supine and prolonged motor asymmetries have been linked to this narrow head shape (Geerdink, Hopkins, & Hoeksma, 1994; Konishi, Mikawa, & Suziki, 1986). Lateral head flattening also has implications for infant attractiveness, which can affect social attachment and, as a result, might increase the risk of abuse (Alley, 1981; Budreau, 1987, 1989; Elmer & Gregg, 1979; Frodi, et al., 1978, Semmler, 1989). No effect on brain development has been reported (Elliman, Bryan, Elliman, & Starte, 1986).

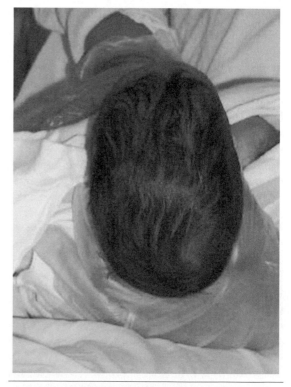

Figure **16-3** Dolichocephaly. Narrow and elongated head shape of preterm infant with lateral skull flattening. Also called scaphocephaly.

Brachycephaly is another type of deformational plagiocephaly that has increased in both preterm and full-term infants since the introduction of the "Back to Sleep" initiative to prevent SIDS (Argenta, David, Wilson, & Bell, 1996; Davis, Moon, Sachs, et al., 1998; Dewey, Fleming, & Golding, 1998; Jantz, Blosser, & Fruechting, 1997; Huang, Cheng, Lin, et al., 1995; Huang, Mouradian, Cohen, & Gruss, 1998; Kane, Mitchell, Craven, & Marsh, 1996; Pollack, Loskan, & Fasick, 1997). In addition to supine sleeping, overuse of infant carriers and neonatal medical problems resulting in relative immobility can contribute to posterior positional molding. Clinical features of brachycephaly include unilateral occipital flattening with alopecia (bald spot), and forward displacement of the ipsilateral ear, forehead, and maxilla. Torticollis, a condition in which the head is tilted with tightness of the ipsilateral sternocleidomastoid muscle, is common and usually right-sided; male infants are more frequently affected than females (Chadduck, Kast, & Donahue, 1997). Physical therapy and/or head-shaping helmets are the most widespread interventions; surgery is usually reserved for deformations involving craniosynostosis (Cavadas & Alvarez-Garijo, 1997; Kelly, Littlefield, Pomatto, et al., 1999; Littlefield, Kelly, Pomatto, & Beals, 1999; Persing, 1997; Taylor & Norton, 1997; VanderKolk & Carson, 1994). Although many infants with brachycephaly have associated developmental delays and mobility problems, there is no evidence of compressive brain pathology (Chadduck, Kast, & Donahue, 1997).

### Extensor Tone and Asymmetry

Compared with term babies, preterm infants with a low probability of neurologic impairment tend to demonstrate increased active extension of the trunk and neck with subsequent motor asymmetries well past term age equivalency; this is especially true of infants who were small for gestation and/or younger than 32 weeks' gestation at birth (de Groot, Hopkins, & Touwen, 1992, 1997). In one study of infants with asymmetry at 4 months corrected age, approximately 50% displayed asymmetrical oculomotor responses, and 33% remained asymmetrical in voluntary hand and gross motor

performance at 1 year of age (de Groot, Hopkins, & Touwen, 1997). It has been suggested that sensory feedback from early movement patterns is incorporated into developing neural networks, and that repetitive use of specific developing neural pathways strengthens those connections while less-used pathways weaken (principle of activity-dependent development) (Hadders-Algra, Brogren, & Forssberg, 1997; van Heijst, Touwen, & Vos, 1999; Penn & Schatz, 1999). Consequently, preventing early abnormal postures and movement patterns becomes even more significant with the preterm population.

### Upper Extremities

Shoulder external rotation and retraction with scapular adduction are common upper extremity positional deformities occurring in the NICU (Georgieff & Bernbaum, 1986; Monfort & Case-Smith, 1997). A persistent "W" arm position has a profound negative impact on an infant's early development. Hand-to-mouth activity used for self-calming and hand-to-hand midline play are more difficult and less frequent. Increased tone in the neck and trunk is facilitated, reinforcing a tendency toward arching; the resultant tone and posture might then contribute to persistent motor asymmetry (de Groot, Hopkins, & Touwen, 1997). When arms are held out to the side rather than underneath the body in prone, the infant is unable to successfully prop on forearms and quickly learns to dislike this uncomfortable and nonfunctional "tummy time" (Figure 16-4). The development of shoulder girdle contraction necessary for distal fine motor control (i.e., reaching against gravity in midline, or hand play in supine and sitting) is impaired without the proprioceptive input that occurs when the humerus presses into the shoulder socket during forearm propping. Lack of tummy time also inevitably delays subsequent gross motor skills (balanced head control, rolling, hands and knees crawling, transitional movements from the floor to upright positions) and can promote abnormal functional compensations, such as scooting along the floor in supine for floor mobility. By default, any delays in fine and gross motor skills interfere with the spontaneous play and exploration needed for optimal cognitive development during the first year (or more) of life.

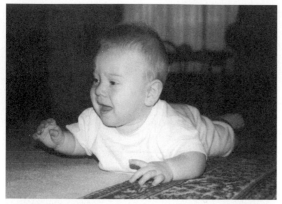

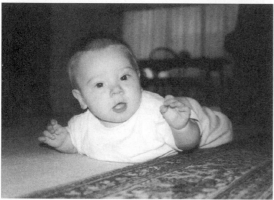

Figure **16-4** "W" arm position and belly time. Normal 6-month-old infant with "W" position of the arms and insufficient tummy play time. His arms are held to the side; they should be aligned under his chest to support body weight and to allow balanced head lifting/chin tucking. Head lifting for this infant is accomplished with increased extensor tone in the neck and trunk. Because this position is uncomfortable and nonfunctional, the baby soon cries and parents often become reluctant to encourage prone play. Developmental gaps and delays result. (*From Hunter, J.G. & Malloy, M.H. [2002]. Effect of sleep and play positions on infant development, reconciling developmental concerns with SIDS prevention. Newborn and Infant Nursing Reviews, 2, 9-16.*)

## Lower Extremities

Lower-extremity hip abduction, external rotation, knee flexion, external tibial torsion (rotation of the tibia), and ankle eversion frequently result when the infant's legs rest on the bed surface in a "frogged" or "M" shape (Davis, Robinson, Harris, & Cartlidge, 1993; Downs, Edwards, McCormick, et al., 1991; Katz, Krikler, Wielunsky, & Merlob, 1991; Lacey, Henderson-Smart, & Edwards, 1990; Sweeney & Gutierrez, 2002). These positional deformities can cause delays in motor skills such as crawling and walking during the first year of life (Fay, 1988; Monterosso, Coenen, Percival, & Evans, 1995). A possible association with toe walking for up to 18 months of age (Fay, 1988; Bottos & Stefani, 1982), and persistence of out-toeing that has not resolved by 3 to 4.5 years (Davis, Robinson, Harris, & Cartlidge, 1993) or up to 8 years (Katz, Krikler, Wielunsky, & Merlob, 1991), have also been reported.

Because independent walking is a momentous motor milestone to most parents, lower extremity positional deformities frequently promote significant parental concern and prompt referrals to early intervention programs, physical therapists, and/or to orthopedic surgeons. Parental anxiety is typically prolonged, as lower extremity positional deformities are apparent during the early months of life; however, the extent of residual sequelae often cannot be determined definitively until after the first birthday when the child is walking well independently.

### Decreased Rib-Cage Depth

Decreased depth of the rib cage has also been noted in NICU graduates, which can be detrimental to infants who already experience respiratory compromise from chronic lung disease (Semmler, 1989).

### Grooved Palate

The relationship between grooved palates and prolonged oral intubation continues to be investigated with, sometimes conflicting, conclusions (Ash & Moss, 1987; Behrstock, Ramos, & Kaufman, 1977; Budreau & Kleiber, 1987; Carillo, 1985; Duke, Coulson, Santos, & Johnson, 1976; Erenberg & Nowak, 1984; Hanson, Smith, & Cohen, 1976; Monteli & Bumstead, 1986; Procter, Lether, Oliver, & Cartlidge, 1998; Saunders, Easa, & Slaughter, 1976; Seow, 1997; vonGonten, Meyer, & Kim, 1995; Warwick-Brown, 1987; Watterberg & Munsick-Bruno, 1986). A persistently grooved palate can cause future problems with feeding, some speech

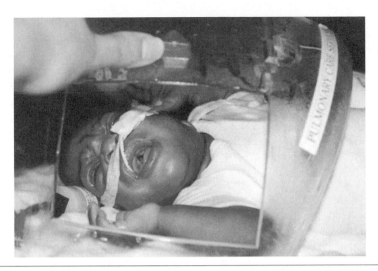

Figure **16-5** Grooved palate. Neonatal intensive care unit infant with a deep palatal groove from prolonged oral intubation.

sounds, and dental development requiring orthodontic intervention (Figure 16-5).

No research was found that compared the development of speech and language in infants who were orally, versus nasally intubated. Both practices are used and the tendency to use one over the other tends to be more practice based and related to success in a particular nursery. Most outcomes noted in the literature are short-term, such as need for re-intubation or decrease in number of self-extubations. Research that examines the long-term effects of intubation and mechanical ventilation has not been able to tease-out what truly causes what, and no interventions have been studied well enough to facilitate a change in practice thus far.

However, there seems to be more documented trauma with oral intubation. In preterm infants, the hard palate is soft and still growing. The presence of an endotracheal tube in the oral cavity can produce pressure on the developing palate, and a groove is the result. This depth of the groove is dependent on duration of intubation, movement of the tube, and maturation of the infant. Incidence of an oral groove in infants intubated 1 week or less has been reported as high as 39.5%, with an increase to 87.5% in infants intubated 15 days or more (Loochtan & Loochtan, 1989). It has been reported that preterm infants who suck vigorously on their endotracheal tube might

have even deeper grooves. This groove could later delay speech development and/or be related to speech impediments, but no direct cause/effect relationship has been found or investigated.

Bier, Ferguson, Cho, and Vohr (1993) found that preterm infants who were intubated for prolonged periods in the NICU experienced more difficulties with feeding than preterm infants who had not been intubated or who were intubated for less than 1 week. The numbers of days of oxygen therapy (most likely an indicator of severity of illness) and the postconceptional age (PCA) at first bottle-feeding were the most powerful predictors of later sucking abilities. In addition, an oral groove was noted in 45% of the infants who had endured prolonged intubation. These researchers suggest that prolonged intubation can be viewed as a marker for potential oral motor problems (Bier, Ferguson, Cho, & Vohr, 1993). Although there are suggestions in the literature for using palate protection during intubation, few nurseries use this type of equipment routinely.

## GENERAL PRINCIPLES AND CONCEPTS OF THERAPEUTIC POSITIONING

Alignment and shaping of the musculoskeletal system occur during each body position that infants experience while in the NICU; complacency in positioning can quickly lead to asymmetry and deformities (Sweeney & Gutierrez, 2002). Physiologic and developmental benefits to the infant mandate that appropriate positioning become a personal and unit-based standard of care in the NICU.

Therapeutic positioning in the NICU uses external supports to compensate for the infant's immature motor control in an environment where the womb is absent and the influence of gravity is relentless. Ideally, comfortable and secure boundaries contain the preterm or ill infant with gentle flexion and midline orientation of the extremities, and with the head and trunk supported in neutral alignment. Containment is not restraint; the infant must be able to move for the musculoskeletal system to develop normally.

A comfortable, soft, nest with secure and deep boundaries (commercial positioning products, high blanket rolls), or swaddling, can simulate the benefits of intrauterine positioning. An effective nest should have high boundaries closely surrounding the baby; boundaries are only effective if contact with the infant is sufficient to promote flexion and flexible containment. Concave nests formed from a blanket or sheepskin draped over blanket rolls are frequently too wide and shallow to provide adequate containment, flexion, and/or midline orientation (Figure 16-6).

Swaddling provides the easiest, most secure containment, and can be used with other positioning aids. Swaddling provides neutral warmth that helps relax the infant, reduces extraneous movement, promotes the development of flexor tone by containing the extremities in flexion, improves the neuromuscular development of preterm infants, and can be a useful adjunct in managing infant pain (Campos, 1989; Mouradian & Als, 1994; Short, Brooks-Brunn, Reeves, et al., 1996).

Uncontrolled or excessive motor activity expends significant calories (Thureen, Phillips, Baron, et al., 1998) needed by the preterm infant for growth, recovery, and basic physiologic processes such as breathing. Motor disorganization is often most pronounced in supine (Figure 16-7), and can be improved by prone positioning, supported sidelying, circumferential boundaries, or swaddling. Infants under phototherapy need boundaries; postural support that reduces excessive movements and agitation can be provided without undue compromise of body exposure (Figure 16-8).

Oversized diapers on a small preterm infant passively maintain the hips in an exaggerated externally rotated and abducted "frog-leg" position. Excessive diaper bulk between the legs can prevent achievement of more normal hip alignment even when boundaries

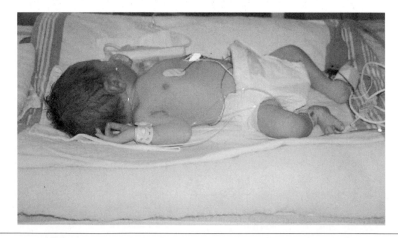

Figure **16-6** Concave nest. This sheepskin nest is too wide and shallow to provide adequate positioning. There is no containment to support the head and extremities toward midline, and no boundary available for foot bracing.

are provided around the infant. Conversely, consistent use of appropriately sized diapers combined with therapeutic positioning to maintain normal hip alignment can help reduce or prevent this typical positional deformity of the lower extremities.

Infants should be repositioned at least every 2 to 4 hours, or when behavioral cues suggest discomfort that might be relieved by a position change. Keep in mind that a fetus forcefully extends in utero, and is passively brought back into flexion by the uterine wall. After preterm birth, active extension is frequent and not yet balanced by purposeful flexion of the extremities. Avoid confusing this imbalanced motor control with infant preference (i.e., "He doesn't like

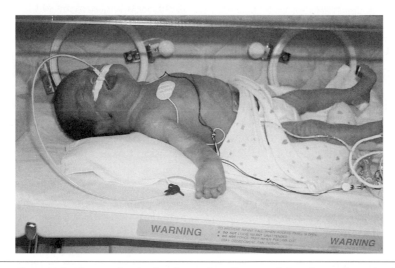

Figure **16-7** Motor disorganization and agitation in supine. Preterm infant in supine who has escaped his boundaries and is burning significant calories from excessive motor activity and agitation.

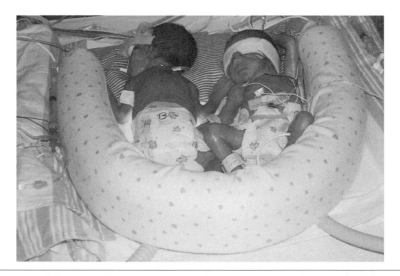

Figure **16-8** Co-bedded twins receiving phototherapy. Although positioning is affected by double-bank phototherapy (overhead and bili blanket), these twins have gel pillows to reduce lateral skull flattening, a soft flexible boundary for side support and foot bracing, and each other for co-regulation.

to be contained; he always pushes out of his nest"). Often this infant needs *more* boundaries, either more secure and/or circumferential (surrounding the whole body, including up around the head).

*Flexion. Midline. Containment. Comfort.* Remembering and implementing these four key concepts will provide the most consistent and supportive therapeutic positioning.

## POSITIONING TECHNIQUES

Assessment of positioning supports for their effectiveness in providing comfortable containment in midline and gentle flexion should be routine for NICU caregivers. Therapeutic positioning will only occur with ongoing caregiver attention; the presence of commercial positioning products or blanket rolls in the baby's bed does not guarantee appropriate positioning (Figure 16-9). Specific positioning suggestions follow.

### Supine

Supine positioning with head in midline has been recommended for micropreemies during the first few days of life to prevent functional obstruction of cerebral venous drainage and prevent elevation of cerebral blood flow (Pellicer, Gaya, Madero, et al., 2002).

Regardless of age, however, supporting the head in (or near) midline when a NICU baby is supine provides an opportunity to relieve weight-bearing pressure on the sides of the skull and might help minimize lateral skull flattening (dolichocephaly). Secure orotracheal ventilator tubing at the level of midoral cavity to minimize contact of the endotracheal tube on the baby's palate; secure nasotracheal ventilator tubing to avoid soft tissue pressure that distorts the nares. All ventilator tubing should be positioned to avoid pulling the infant's head to one side.

If a gel or water pillow is used to cushion the baby's head for reduction of head flattening, avoid conductive heat loss by pre-warming the pillow before placing it underneath the infant; heat from the radiant warmer or incubator will keep the pillow warm. Excessive neck flexion that can cause airway occlusion can be prevented by extending the pillow to nipple level; rather than placing it only under the baby's head; the pillow can be used as a mattress under the head and body of a micropreemie to maintain proper body alignment. If an infant's body weight or active movement flatten a gel pillow, gel can be displaced from the sides to the middle of a pillow while underneath an infant by pushing downward on both ends of the pillow simultaneously.

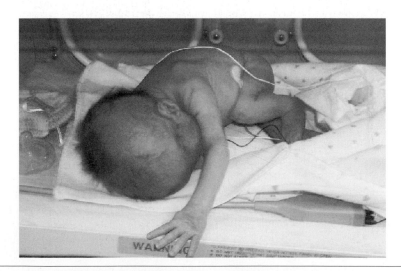

Figure **16-9** Escaping baby. Preterm infant in incubator who is escaping both her boundaries and her diaper. Babies do move, and neonatal intensive care unit caregivers must frequently assess whether positioning supports are still providing a flexed, midline, and contained posture.

Theoretically, neck rolls help maintain airway patency by preventing hyperflexion of the neck. In practice, neck rolls tend to be overused and oversized. Intubated infants rarely benefit from the addition of a neck roll. If an occasional nonintubated baby (usually one who is extremely hypotonic, sedated, and/or has lateral head flattening with a prominent occiput) seems to need the extra support of a neck roll in supine, it should be small enough to provide neutral alignment of the head and trunk without neck hyperextension. Proper use of a gel pillow to decrease the development of scaphocephaly and to maintain neutral alignment of the head, neck, and upper trunk is preferred.

Use surrounding boundaries to maintain the upper extremities tucked close to the body with shoulders gently rounded forward (not flat on surface) and elbows in flexion; elbow flexion more than 90 degrees can cause occlusion of some percutaneous catheters. Hips should be partially flexed and adducted toward midline (*not* medial to neutral alignment, as adduction with internal rotation places the neonate's hips in an unstable "dislocatable" position). Knees should be partially flexed with feet *inside* surrounding boundaries; a boundary under the baby's thighs with the lower part of the legs dangling over might compromise circulation and does not provide a support for the infant to use foot bracing as a self-regulatory strategy.

## Prone

Supporting the infant's head on a gel pillow and alternating head position between the right and left sides might help reduce lateral skull flattening. As with supine, neutral alignment of the head and trunk is important; placing the bottom edge of the gel pillow at the infant's nipple line will prevent excessive neck extension. Arms can be tucked around the sides of the pillow to avoid shoulder retraction and facilitate shoulder protraction (rounding). Using the gel pillow lengthwise as a mattress under a micropreemie, or folded in half lengthwise as a prone roll, is often successful; occasionally, the softer surface can compromise respiratory function.

Prone rolls elevate the infant's upper body to promote flexion of the extremities without placing excessive pressure on the fragile skin of knees and elbows. A small cloth folded to the width of an infant's torso (or a gel pillow folded and taped lengthwise) is placed lengthwise under the infant from the umbilicus to the top of the head; this allows the infant's shoulders to round forward over the sides of the roll, and the legs to gently flex and remain in midline over the bottom edge of the roll. Stable external boundaries (e.g., swaddling, bunting, Bendy-Bumper) are needed to help the infant maintain a secure balanced and flexed position on the prone roll; this is especially crucial if the infant is intubated, so that an accidental extubation is avoided (Figure 16-10). Provide secure lower boundaries for the baby to use in foot-bracing.

## Sidelying

When positioned correctly, sidelying decreases the extensor effects of gravity, facilitates midline orientation of the head and extremities, and encourages hand-to-hand, hand-to-mouth, or hand-to-face activity. Some neonatologists do not advocate prolonged sidelying for micropreemies (except in treatment of specific air leaks, such as pulmonary interstitial emphysema [PIE]), owing to concern that excessive time in this position might promote atelectasis of the dependent lung; thus, clinical practice regarding sidelying with very small infants varies among NICUs.

A single blanket roll behind the infant's back (or a blanket roll placed firmly behind the infant, flattened between the legs, and up along the baby's chest) does not provide adequate positioning support or containment. Sidelying is most secure with swaddling and/or commercial positioning products (Figure 16-11). To maintain sidelying (and to avoid extremity extension and retraction, as well as increased infant stress from positional instability), position the infant's top hip and shoulder slightly forward of the weight-bearing hip and shoulder. Be careful not to trap the bottom arm in an uncomfortable position underneath the baby's body, and avoid bundling so tightly that chest expansion is compromised by forceful upper extremity midline orientation. Having the infant hug a small roll, such as a folded cloth diaper or a Beanie Baby, will encourage forward tucking.

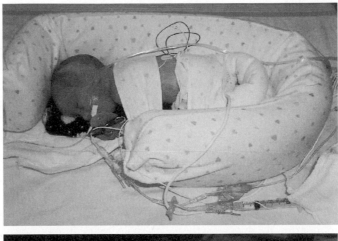

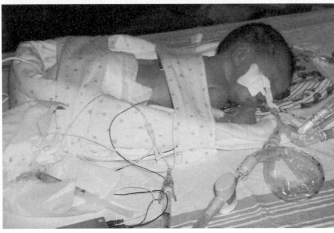

Figure **16-10** Infants on prone roll and surrounding boundaries. Preterm infants on gel pillows and prone roll with surrounding boundaries. The infant with both a Snuggle-Up and Bendy-Bumper (Children's Medical Ventures, Norwell, MA) has a tendency to arch and self-extubate (*top*). The other infant is acutely ill and inactive; his surrounding boundaries do not need to be quite as secure. (*Top photo from Hunter, J.G. [2001]. The neonatal intensive care unit. In J. Case-Smith [Ed.],* Occupational therapy for children *[4th ed.; pp. 636-707]. St. Louis: Mosby.*)

## POSITIONING TRANSITION FROM THE NICU TO HOME

It is important to transition the baby to positioning that will be used in the home before hospital discharge. There is not a current common standard among NICUs on how to transition infants out of positioning aids and into supine sleeping in preparation for discharge to home. The general sequence of events is to move from very secure boundaries, to looser positioning aid support, to swad-

dling without positioning aids, to just covering the clothed infant with a blanket. Timing varies, and this last step can occur after the infant is home. The reader is referred to Chapter 11 and to journal articles by Lockridge, Taquino, and Knight (1999) and Hunter & Malloy (2002) for additional information on SIDS and sleep positions. Discharge teaching should impress upon the parents the importance of frequent and consistent prone play during the early months at home to avoid preventable developmental gaps and delays (Hunter & Malloy, 2002).

## MEDICAL AND DEVELOPMENTAL CONSIDERATIONS IN POSITIONING

No position is totally benign in its effects on NICU infants. Although medical stability is top priority, developmental issues are also important. Awareness of both medical and developmental considerations in neonatal positioning options allows the NICU caregiver to improve physiologic stability, increase infant comfort, minimize positional deformities, and facilitate optimal muscle tone and movement patterns. Table 16-1 provides a referenced summary of the medical and developmental advantages and disadvantages of various positioning options.

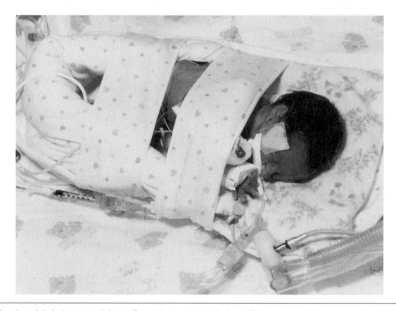

Figure **16-11** Baby in sidelying position. Small, preterm infant (the same baby as in Figure 16-1) supported in sidelying with flexion and midline orientation of the extremities. (*From Hunter, J.G. [2001]. The neonatal intensive care unit. In J. Case-Smith [Ed.],* Occupational therapy for children *[4th ed.; pp. 636-707]. St. Louis: Mosby.*)

Table **16-1** Medical and Developmental Considerations of Positioning in the NICU

**PRONE**

| Medical Advantages | Developmental Advantages |
| --- | --- |
| Improved oxygenation and ventilation (despite increased work of breathing) in infants with and without ventilatory support[1, 6, 9, 26, 38, 49, 52, 55, 66, 69] | Facilitates development of flexor tone[2] |
| | Facilitates hand-to-mouth activity for self-calming[2] |
| Better gastric emptying than in supine (unless feeds pool regardless)[23, 68, 71] | Facilitates active neck extension and head raising, forearm propping, and subsequent floor-based gross motor skills[39] |
| Reduced reflux, especially if head of bed is elevated 30 degrees[10, 53, 60] | Improved coping with extrauterine environment (i.e., if sleep more, cry less)[11] |

*Continued*

## Table 16-1   MEDICAL AND DEVELOPMENTAL CONSIDERATIONS OF POSITIONING IN THE NICU—CONT'D

Decreased episodes of bradycardia and hypoxemia with head of bed elevated 15 degrees vs. prone horizontal[21, 40]

Recommended sleep position for infants with complicated reflux unresponsive to medical and dietary measures[3, 24]

Decreased risk of aspiration[33]

Term and preterm infants sleep more and cry less when prone rather than supine[11, 14, 58]

Less energy expenditure in prone vs. supine[51]

Less sleep apnea in prone vs. supine in term infants[38] and preterm infants[32, 44]

Increased heart rate during sleep[62]

Can expose diaper rash to air or heat lamp

With early placement of head to alternating sides, might decrease persistent head turning to right, with subsequent skull asymmetry

Can be used to gently reduce occasional abnormal hip flexion contractures (i.e., as potentially with arthrogryposis or fetal compression syndrome) without extra handling for passive range of motion by combined effect of body weight and gravity when legs are extended in neutral alignment

| Medical Disadvantages | Developmental Disadvantages |
|---|---|
| Access for some acute medical procedures is more difficult | Flattened "frogged" posture develops because of downward force of gravity if on flat surface with no intervention[22, 56] |
| Agitated or active infant might self-extubate | Contributes to dolichocephaly, lateralized head position, and potential prolonged motor asymmetries[29, 42] |
| Prone sleep position is associated with increased risk of SIDS[3, 4, 24, 45, 61] | Visual exploration more difficult for baby |
|  | Face-to-face social contact more difficult between baby and caregiver |

**SUPINE**

| Medical Advantages | Developmental Advantages |
|---|---|
| Easier access to infant for medical care | Easier visual exploration by infant |
| Supine (in hammock) increases sleep time for preterm infants (vs. "flat" supine)[12] | Facilitates face-to-face social contact between baby and caregiver |
| Recommended position to reduce risk of SIDS (when near and after discharge)[3, 4, 24, 45, 61] | Supine (in hammock) might facilitate midline position[12] |
|  | Can keep head in midline to reduce lateral head flattening |

| Medical Advantages | Developmental Advantages |
|---|---|
| Decreased arterial oxygen tension, lung compliance and tidal volume compared with prone[1, 49, 50, 69] | Encourages extension rather than flexion (i.e., increased muscle tone with hyperextension of head, neck, and shoulders)[2] |

Table **16-1** MEDICAL AND DEVELOPMENTAL CONSIDERATIONS OF POSITIONING
IN THE NICU—CONT'D

More reflux than in prone at any time, or than in upright sitting if infant is awake[53, 60]

Greater risk for aspiration than in prone or right sidelying[33]

Term and preterm infants sleep less and cry more in supine than prone[11, 14, 58]

Supine in hammock might decrease respiration if infant has decreased lung compliance (i.e., respiratory distress syndrome)[12]

Greater energy expenditure in supine vs. prone[51]

Encourages external rotation positional deformities of arms and legs (with subsequent delay in hands-to-midline and reaching activities, plus out-toeing gait)

Supine sleep position (as per SIDS recommendations) has been correlated to posterior plagiocephaly and later developmental delays in motor skills[5, 17–19, 35–37, 39, 41, 42, 54, 57, 59]

**SIDELYING**

| Medical Advantages | Developmental Advantages |
|---|---|
| Left side: Better gastric emptying than supine or right sidelying (as effective as prone)[23, 68] <br><br> Right side: Better gastric emptying than supine or left sidelying (about same as prone)[71] <br><br> Infant with unilateral lung disease has better oxygenation with good lung positioned on top[13, 31] <br><br> Can be used to treat pulmonary interstitial emphysema by placing affected lung in dependent (bottom) position[20, 63] | Encourages midline orientation of head and extremities <br><br> Counteracts external rotation of limbs; promotes extremity flexion and adduction <br><br> Facilitates hand-to-mouth pattern for self-calming <br><br> Facilitates hand-to-hand activity |

| Medical Disadvantages | Developmental Disadvantages |
|---|---|
| Right side: Decreased gastric emptying compared to prone or left side[23, 68] <br><br> Left side: Decreased gastric emptying compared to prone or right side[71] <br><br> Might contribute to atelectasis of dependent (bottom) lung in micropreemie <br><br> Increased risk of SIDS compared to supine[4, 45, 61] | Might be difficult to maintain flexed sidelying position with active, irritable, and/or hypertonic extended infant |

**SEMI-RECLINED/SITTING**

| Medical Advantages | Developmental Advantages |
|---|---|
| Alternative position (i.e., for variety, skin integrity) <br><br> Increased lung compliance and decreased pulmonary resistance (possibly due to increased pulmonary functional residual capacity) in semi-sitting vs. supine[16] | Upright is an alerting posture <br><br> Encourages infant visual exploration <br><br> Encourages social interaction <br><br> Might allow use of swing for older NICU infants <br><br> Might help temporarily inhibit (relax) high tone (i.e., with hips flexed >90 degrees) |

*Continued*

Table **16-1**   MEDICAL AND DEVELOPMENTAL CONSIDERATIONS OF POSITIONING
IN THE NICU—CONT'D

| Medical Disadvantages | Developmental Disadvantages |
|---|---|
| Infant seat or car seat elevated 60 degrees increases the frequency and duration of reflux[60] | Might be difficult to maintain proper head, neck, and trunk alignment as baby is more upright[15] |
| More upright (95 degrees) increases heart rate and mean arterial pressure in preterm infants, as compared to more reclined car seat positions of 110 degrees and 140 degrees[65] | Neck flexion (if it occurs) increases airway resistance and predisposes infant to obstructive apnea[15, 16, 67] |
| Decreased oxygen saturation, apnea and bradycardia might occur in smaller premature infants and some healthy term infants in semi-reclined/car seat positioning[7 8, 15, 70] | Overuse of infant carriers might contribute to the development of posterior plagiocephaly[18] |
| | Unless infant's head is supported in midline, asymmetric head position will predominate |

**HEAD POSITION/HEAD IN MIDLINE**

| Medical Advantages | Developmental Advantages |
|---|---|
| Head in midline seems to decrease intracranial pressure and intraventricular hemorrhage[30] | Head in midline might reduce lateral head flattening and asymmetric plagiocephaly |
| Elevation of head of bed 30 degrees might reduce intracranial pressure[30] | Midline positioning reduces postural asymmetry and encourages development of antigravity flexion |
| | Waterbeds (and water pillows) might reduce head flattening (dolichocephaly, scaphocephaly)[25, 28, 43, 48, 64] |

| Medical Disadvantages | Developmental Disadvantages |
|---|---|
| Might create pressure sore on occiput if head remains in midline too long on firm surface without pressure relief | Head midline positioning is not possible in prone |

Adapted with permission from Hunter, J. (2001). The NICU. In J. Case-Smith, (Ed.), *Occupational therapy for children* (4th ed.; pp. 704-707). St. Louis: Mosby.

1. Hutchison, A.A., Ross, K.R., & Russell, G. (1979). The effect of posture on ventilation and lung mechanics in preterm and light-for-date infants. *Pediatrics, 64*(4), 429–432.
2. Anderson, J., & Auster-Liebhaber, J. (1984). Developmental therapy in the neonatal intensive care unit. *Physical and Occupational Therapy in Pediatrics, 4,* 89–106.
3. American Academy of Pediatrics. (1992). Policy statement: Positioning and SIDS (RE9254). *Pediatrics, 89,* 1120–1126.
4. American Academy of Pediatrics. (1996). Policy statement: Positioning and sudden infant death syndrome (SIDS) update (RE9254). *Pediatrics, 98,* 1216–1218.
5. Argenta, L., David, L., Wilson, J., & Bell, W. (1996). An increase in infant cranial deformity with supine sleeping position. *Journal of Craniofacial Surgery, 7*(1), 5–11.
6. Baird, T.M., Paton, J.B., & Fisher, D.E. (1992). Improved oxygenation with prone positioning in neonates: Stability of increased transcutaneous $PO_2$. *Neonatal Intensive Care, 5,* 43–44, 46.
7. Bass, J.L., Mehta, K.A., & Camara, J. (1993). Monitoring premature infants in car seats: Implementing the American Academy of Pediatrics policy in a community hospital. *Pediatrics, 91*(6), 1137–1141.
8. Bass, J.L., & Mehta, K.A. (1995). Oxygen desaturation of selected term infants in car seats. *Pediatrics, 96*(2)(Pt 1), 288–290.

9. Bjornson, K., Deitz, J., Blackburn, S., et al. (1992). The effect of body position on the oxygen saturation of ventilated preterm infants. *Pediatric Physical Therapy*, 109–115.

10. Blumenthal, I., & Lealman, G.T. (1982). Effect of posture on gastroesophageal reflux in the newborn, *Archives of Disease in Childhood*, *57*(7), 555–556.

11. Bottos, M., & Stafani, D. (1982). Postural and motor care of the premature baby (letter). *Developmental Medicine and Child Neurology*, *24*(5), 706–707.

12. Bottos, M., Pettenazzo, A., Giancola, G., et al. (1985). The effect of a containing position in a hammock versus the supine position on the cutaneous oxygen level in premature and term babies. *Early Human Development*, *11*(3–4), 265–273.

13. Bozynski, M., Naglie, R., Nicks, J., et al. (1988). Lateral positioning of the stable ventilated very low birthweight infant. *American Journal of Diseases in Children*, *142*(2), 200–202.

14. Brackbill, Y., Douthitt, T., & West, H. (1973). Psychophysiologic effects in the neonate of prone versus supine placement. *Journal of Pediatrics*, *82*(1), 82–83.

15. Callahan, C.W., & Sisler, C. (1997). Use of seating devices in infants too young to sit. *Archives of Pediatric and Adolescent Medicine*, *151*(3), 233–235.

16. Carlo, W.A., Beoglos, A., Siner, B.S., & Martin, R.J. (1989). Neck and body position effects on pulmonary mechanics in infants. *Pediatrics*, *84*(4), 670–674.

17. Cartlidge, P.H.T., & Rutter, N. (1988). Reduction of head flattening in preterm infants. *Archives of Disease in Childhood*, *63*(7 Spec No), 755–757.

18. Chadduck, W.M., Kast, J., & Donahue, D.J. (1997). The enigma of lamboid positional molding. *Pediatric Neurosurgery*, *26*(6), 304–311.

19. Chan, J.S.L., Kelley, M.L., & Khan, J. (1995). Predictors of postnatal head molding in very low birth weight infants. *Neonatal Network*, *14*(4), 47–52.

20. Cohen, R., Smith, D., Stevenson, D., et al. (1984). Lateral decubitus position as therapy for persistent focal pulmonary interstitial emphysema in premature infants. *Pediatrics*, *104*(3), 441–443.

21. Dellagrammaitics, H., Kapetanakes, J., Papadimitriou, M., & Kourakis, G. (1991). Effect of body tilting on physiological functions in stable very low birthweight neonates. *Archives of Disease in Childhood*, *66*(4 Spec No), 429–432.

22. Downs, J.A., Edwards, A.D., McCormick, D.C., et al. (1991). Effect of intervention on the development of hip posture in very preterm babies. *Archives of Disease in Childhood*, *66*(7 Spec No), 197–201.

23. Ewer, A.K., James, M.E., & Tobin, J.M. (1999). Prone and left lateral positioning reduce gastro-oesophageal reflux in preterm infants. *Archives of Disease in Childhood: Fetal and Neonatal Edition*, *81*, F201-F205.

24. Faure, C., Leluyer, B., Aujard, Y., et al. (1996). Sleeping position, prevention of sudden infant death syndrome and gastroesophageal reflux. *Archives de Pediatrica*, *3*(6), 598–601.

25. Fay, M.J. (1988). The positive effects of positioning. *Neonatal Network*, *8*(5), 23–28.

26. Fox, M., & Molesky, M. (1990). The effects of prone and supine positioning on arterial oxygen pressure. *Neonatal Network*, *8*(4), 25–29; erratum in *8*(5), 17

27. Fox, R., & Viscardi, R., Tackiak, V., et al. (1993). Effect of position on pulmonary mechanics in healthy preterm newborn infants. *Journal of Perinatology*, *13*(3), 205–211.

28. Fowler, K., Kum-Nji, P., Wells, P.J., & Mangrem, C.L. (1997). Water beds may be useful in preventing scaphocephaly in preterm very low birth weight neonates. *Journal of Perinatology*, *17*, 397.

29. Geerdink, J.J, Hopkins, B., & Hoeksma, J.B. (1994). The development of head position in preterm infants beyond term age. *Developmental Psychobiology*, *27*(3), 153–168.

30. Goldberg, R.N., Joshi, A., Moscoso, P., & Castillo, T. (1983). The effect of head position on intracranial pressure in the neonate. *Critical Care Medicine*, *11*(6), 428–430.

31. Heaf, D.P., Helms, P., Gordon, I., & Turner, H.M. (1983). Postural effects of gas exchange in infants. *New England Journal of Medicine*, *308*(25), 1505–1508.

32. Heimler, R., Langlois, J., Hodel, D., et al. (1992). Effect of positioning on the breathing pattern in premature infants. *Archives of Disease in Childhood*, *67*(3), 312–314.

33. Hewitt, V. (1976). Effect of posture on the presence of fat in tracheal aspirate in neonates. *Australian Pediatric Journal*, *12*, 267–271.

34. Hoshimoto, T., et al. (1983). Postural effects on behavioral states of newborn infants: A sleep polygraphic study. *Brain Development*, *5*, 286–291.

35. Huang, C-S, Cheng, H-S, Lin, W-Y, et al. (1995). Skull morphology affected by different sleep positions in infancy. *Cleft Palate–Craniofacial Journal*, *32*(5), 413–419.

36. Huang, M.H., Mouradian, W.E., Cohen, S.R., & Gruss, J.S. (1998). The differential diagnosis of abnormal head shapes: Separating craniosynostosis from positional deformities and normal variants. *Cleft Palate-Craniofacial Journal*, *35*(3), 204–211.

37. Hunt, C.E., & Puczynski, M.S. (1996). Does supine sleeping cause asymmetric heads? *Pediatrics*, *98*(1), 127–129.

38. Hutchison, A., Ross, K., & Russell, G. (1979). The effects of posture on ventilation and lung mechanics in preterm and light-for-date infants. *Pediatrics, 64*(4), 429–432.

39. Jantz, J.W., Blosser, C.D., & Fruechting, L.A. (1997). A motor milestone change noted with a change in sleep position. *Archives of Pediatric and Adolescent Medicine, 151*(6), 565–568.

40. Jenni, O.G., von Siebenthal, K., Wolf, M., et al. (1997). Effect of nursing in the head elevated tilt position (15°) on the incidence of bradycardic and hypoxemic episodes in preterm infants. *Pediatrics, 100*(4), 622–625.

41. Kane, A.A., Mitchell, L., Craven, K.P., & Marsh, J.L. (1996). Observations on a recent increase in plagiocephaly without synostosis. *Pediatrics, 97*(6)(Pt 1), 877–885.

42. Konishi, Y., Mikawa, H., & Suziki, J. (1986). Asymmetrical head-turning of preterm infants: Some effects on later postural and functional lateralities. *Developmental Medicine and Child Neurology, 28*(4), 450–457.

43. Kramer, L.I. & Pierpont, M.E. (1976). Rocking waterbeds and auditory stimuli to enhance growth of preterm infants. *Journal of Pediatrics, 88*(2), 297–299.

44. Kurlak, L.O., Ruggins, N.R., & Stephenson, T.J. (1994). Effect of nursing position on incidence, type, and duration of clinically significant apnea in preterm infants. *Archives of Disease in Childhood, 71*, F16-F19.

45. Lockridge, T. (1997). Now I lay me down to sleep: SIDS and infant sleep positions. *Neonatal Network, 16*(7), 25–31.

46. Long, T., & Soderstrom, E. (1995). A critical appraisal of positioning infants in the neonatal intensive care unit. *Physical and Occupational Therapy in Pediatrics, 15*, 17–31.

47. Mansell, A., Bryan, C., & Levison, H. (1972). Airway closure in children. *Journal of Applied Physiology, 33*(6), 711–714.

48. Marsden, D.J. (1980). Reduction of head flattening in preterm infants. *Developmental Medicine and Child Neurology, 22*(4), 507–509.

49. Martin, R.J, Herrell, N., Rubin, D., & Fanaroff, A. (1979). Effect of supine and prone positions on arterial oxygen tension in the preterm infant. *Pediatrics, 63*(4), 528–531.

50. Martin, R.J., DiFore, J.M., Korenke, C.B., et al. (1995). Vulnerability of respiratory control in healthy preterm infants placed supine. *Journal of Pediatrics, 127*(4), 609–614.

51. Masterson, J., Zucker, C., & Schulze, K. (1987). Prone and supine effects on energy expenditure and behavior of low birth weight neonates. *Pediatrics, 80*(5), 689–692.

52. Mendoza, J., Roberts, J., & Cook, L. (1991). Postural effects on pulmonary function and heart rate of preterm infants with lung disease. *Journal of Pediatrics, 118*(3), 445–448.

53. Meyers, W.F., & Herbst, J.J. (1982). Effectiveness of position therapy for gastroesophageal reflux. *Pediatrics, 69*(6), 768–772.

54. Mildred, J., Beard, K., Dallwitz, A., et al. (1995). Play position is influenced by knowledge of SIDS sleep position recommendations. *Journal of Pediatric Child Health, 31*(6), 499–502.

55. Mizuno, K., Itabashi, K., & Okuyama, K. (1995). Effect of body position on the blood gases and ventilation volume of infants with chronic lung disease before and after feeding. *American Journal of Perinatology, 12*, 275–277.

56. Monfort, K.P., & Case-Smith, J. (1997). The effects of a neonatal positioner on scapular rotation. *American Journal of Occupational Therapy, 51*(5), 378–384.

57. Mulliken, J.B., VanderWoude, D.L., Hansen, M., et al. (1999). Analysis of posterior plagiocephaly: Deformational versus synostotic. *Plastic & Reconstructive Surgery, 103*(2), 371–380.

58. Myers, M.M., Fifer, W.P., Schaeffer, L., et al. (1998). Effects of sleeping position and time after feeding on the organization of sleep/wake states in prematurely born infants. *Sleep, 21*(4), 343–349.

59. Najarian, S.P. (1999). Infant cranial molding deformation and sleep position: Implications for primary care. *Journal of Pediatric Health Care, 13*(4), 173–177.

60. Orenstein, S., Whitington, P., & Orenstein, D. (1983). The infant seat as treatment for gastroesophageal reflux. *New England Journal of Medicine, 309*(13), 760–763.

61. Oyen, N., Markestad, T., Skaerven, R., et al. (1997). Combined effects of sleeping position and prenatal risk factors in sudden infant death syndrome: The Nordic epidemiological SIDS study. *Pediatrics, 100*(4), 613–621.

62. Sahni, R., Schulze, K.F., Kashyap, S., et al. (1999). Body position, sleep states, and cardiorespiratory activity in developing low birth weight infants. *Early Human Development, 54*(3), 197–206.

63. Schwartz, A., & Graham, B. (1986). Neonatal tension pulmonary interstitial emphysema in bronchopulmonary dysplasia: Treatment with lateral decubitus positioning. *Radiology, 161*(2), 351–354.

64. Schwirian, P., Eesley, T., & Cuellar, L. (1986). Use of water pillows in reducing head shape distortion in preterm infants. *Research in Nursing and Health, 9*(3), 203–207.

65. Smith, P., & Turner, B. (1990). The physiologic effects of positioning premature infants in car seats. *Neonatal Network, 9*(4), 11–15.

66. Squire, S.J., & Kirchhoff, K.T. (1992). Positional oxygenation changes in air-transported neonates. *Heart & Lung: Journal of Critical Care, 21*(3), 255–259.

67. Thach, B.T., & Stark, A.R. (1979). Spontaneous neck flexion and airway obstruction during apneic spells in preterm infants. *Journal of Pediatrics, 94*(2), 275–281.

68. Tobin, J.M., McCloud, P., & Cameron, D.J. (1997). Posture and gastro-esophageal reflux: A case for left lateral positioning. *Archives of Disease in Childhood, 76*(3), 254–258.

69. Wagaman, M.J., Shutack, J.G., Moomjian, A.S., et al. (1979). Improved oxygenation and lung compliance with prone positioning of neonates. *Journal of Pediatrics, 94*(5), 787–791.

70. Willett, L., Leuschen, M.P., Nelson, L.S., & Nelson, R.M. (1986). Risk of hypoventilation in premature infants in car seats. *Journal of Pediatrics, 109*(2), 245–248.

71. Yu, V.Y.H. (1975). Effect of body position on gastric emptying in the neonate. *Archives of Disease in Childhood, 50,* 500–504.

## REFERENCES

Alley, T.R. (1981). Head shape and the perception of cuteness. *Developmental Psychology, 17,* 650-654.

American Academy of Pediatrics (AAP) Task Force on Infant Sleep Position and SIDS. (2000). Changing concepts of sudden infant death syndrome: Implications for infant sleeping environment and sleep position. *Pediatrics, 105,* 650-656.

Amiel-Tison, C. (1976). A method for neurological evaluation within the first year of life. In L. Gluck (Ed.), *Current problems in pediatrics* (pp. 1-50). Chicago: Year Book Medical Publishers.

Argenta, L., David, L., Wilson, J., & Bell, W. (1996). An increase in infant cranial deformity with supine sleeping position. *Journal of Craniofacial Surgery, 7*(1), 5-11.

Ash, S.P., & Moss, J.P. (1987). An investigation of the features of the preterm infant palate and the effect of prolonged oral intubation with and without protective appliances. *British Journal of Orthodontics, 14*(4), 253-261.

Baum, J.D., & Searls, D. (1971). Head shape and size of preterm low birth-weight infants. *Developmental Medicine and Child Neurology, 13*(5), 576-581.

Behrstock, B., Ramos, A., & Kaufman, N. (1977). Does prolonged oral intubation contribute to medial hypertrophy of the lateral palatine ridges and possibly to iatrogenic cleft palate? *Journal of Pediatrics, 91*(1), 171.

Bier, J.B., Ferguson, A., Cho, C., & Vohr, B.R. (1993). The oral motor development of low-birth-weight infants who underwent orotracheal intubation during the neonatal period. *American Journal of Developmental C, 147*(8), 858-862.

Boere-Boonekamp, M.M., van der Linden-Kuiper, A.T., & van Es, P. (1997). Preferential posture in infants: Serious demands on health care. *Nederlands Tijdschr voor Geneeskd, 141,* 769-772.

Bottos, M., & Stefani, D. (1982). Postural motor care of the premature baby. *Developmental Medicine and Child Neurology, 5,* 706-707.

Budreau, G. (1987). Postnatal cranial molding and infant attractiveness: Implications for nursing. *Neonatal Network, 5*(5), 13-19.

Budreau, G. (1989). The perceived attractiveness of preterm infants with cranial molding. *Journal of Obstetric, Gynecologic, & Neonatal Nursing (JOGNN), 18*(1), 38-44.

Budreau, G., & Kleiber, C. (1987). Nursing management of the infant with an intraoral appliance. *Journal of Obstetric, Gynecologic, and Neonatal Nursing (JOGNN), 16*(1), 23-25.

Campos, R.G. (1989). Soothing pain-elicited distress in infants with swaddling and pacifiers. *Child Development, 60*(4), 781-792.

Carillo, P.J. (1985). Palatal groove formation and oral endotracheal intubation. *American Journal of Diseases in Children, 139,* 859-860.

Cartlidge, P.H.T., & Rutter, N. (1988). Reduction of head flattening in preterm infants. *Archives of Disease in Childhood, 63*(7 Spec No), 755-757.

Cavadas, P.C., & Alvarez-Garijo, J.A. (1997). Surgical correction of posterior plagiocephaly, original technique (letter). *Plastic and Reconstructive Surgery, 99*(5), 1465-1466.

Chadduck, W.M., Kast, J., & Donahue, D.J. (1997). The enigma of lamboid positional molding. *Pediatric Neurosurgery, 26*(6), 304-311.

Corff, K.E., Seidman, R., Venkataraman, P.S., et al. (1995). Facilitated tucking, a nonpharmacologic comfort measure for pain in preterm neonates. *Journal of Obstetric, Gynecologic, & Neonatal Nursing (JOGNN), 24*(2), 143-147.

Davis, B.E., Moon, R.Y., Sachs, H.C., et al. (1998). Effects of sleep position on infant motor development. *Pediatrics, 102*(5), 1135-1140.

Davis, P.M., Robinson, R., Harris, L., & Cartlidge, P.H.T. (1993). Persistent mild hip deformation in preterm infants. *Archives of Disease in Childhood, 69*(5), 597-598.

de Groot, L., Hopkins, B., & Touwen, B. (1992). A method to assess the development of muscle power in preterm infants beyond term age. *Neuropediatrics, 23*(4), 172-179.

de Groot, L., Hopkins, B., & Touwen, B. (1997). Motor asymmetries in preterm infants at 18 weeks corrected age and outcomes at 1 year. *Early Human Development, 48*(1-2), 35-46.

Dewey, C., Fleming, P., & Golding, J. (1998). Does the supine sleeping position have any adverse effects on the child? Development in the first 18 months. *Pediatrics Electronic Pages, 101,* E5.

Dias, M.S., Klein, D.M., & Backstrom, J.W. (1996). Occipital plagiocephaly, deformation or lamboid synostosis, parts I and II. *Pediatric Neurosurgery, 24,* 61-68.

Downs, J.A., Edwards, A.D., McCormick, D.C., et al. (1991). Effect of intervention on development of hip posture in very preterm babies. *Archives of Disease in Childhood, 66*(7 Spec No), 797-801.

Duke, P.M., Coulson, J.D., Santos, J.L., & Johnson, J.D. (1976). Cleft palate associated with prolonged orotracheal intubation in infancy. *Journal of Pediatrics, 89*(6), 990-991.

Elliman, A.M., Bryan, E.M., Elliman, A.D. & Starte, D. (1986). Narrow heads of preterm infants: Do they matter? *Developmental Medicine and Child Neurology, 28*(6), 745-748.

Elmer, E., & Gregg, G. (1979). Developmental characteristics of abused children. *Pediatrics, 40*, 596-602.

Erenberg, A., & Nowak, A.J. (1984). Palatal groove formation in neonates and infants with orotracheal tubes. *American Journal of Diseases in Children, 138*(10), 974-975.

Fay, M.J. (1988). The positive effects of positioning. *Neonatal Network, 6*(5), 23-28.

Fearon, I., Kisilevsky, B.S., Hains, S.M., et al. (1997). Swaddling after heel lance: Age-specific effects on behavioral recovery in preterm infants. *Journal of Developmental and Behavioral Pediatrics, 18*(4), 222-232.

Frodi, A.M., et al. (1978). Fathers' and mothers' responses to the faces and cries of normal and premature infants. *Developmental Psychology, 14*, 490-498.

Geerdink, J.J, Hopkins, B., & Hoeksma, J.B. (1994). The development of head position in preterm infants beyond term age. *Developmental Psychobiology, 27*(3), 153-168.

Georgieff, M. & Bernbaum, J. (1986). Abnormal shoulder girdle muscle tone in premature infants during their first 18 months of life. *Pediatrics, 77*(5), 664-669.

Hadders-Algra, M., Brogren, E., & Forssberg, H. (1997). Nature and nurture in the development of postural control in human infants. *Acta Paediatrica Supplement, 422*, 48-53.

Hamanishi, C., & Tanaka, S. (1994). Turned head–adducted hip–truncal curvature syndrome. *Archives of Disease in Childhood, 70*(6), 515-519.

Hanson, J.W., Smith, D.W., & Cohen, M.M. (1976). Prominent lateral palatine ridges, development and clinical relevance. *Journal of Pediatrics, 89*(1), 54-58.

Hoffer, M. (1980). Joint motion limitations in newborns. *Clinical Orthopaedics and Related Research, 148*, 94-96.

Huang, C-S, Cheng, H-S, Lin, W-Y, et al. (1995). Skull morphology affected by different sleep positions in infancy. *Cleft Palate–Craniofacial Journal, 32*(5), 413-419.

Huang, M.H., Mouradian, W.E., Cohen, S.R., & Gruss, J.S. (1998). The differential diagnosis of abnormal head shapes, separating craniosynostosis from positional deformities and normal variants. *Cleft Palate-Craniofacial Journal, 35*(3), 204-211.

Hunter, J.G. (2001). The neonatal intensive care unit. In J. Case-Smith (Ed.), *Occupational therapy for children* (4th ed.; pp. 636-707). St. Louis: Mosby.

Hunter, J.G., & Malloy, M.H. (2002). Effect of sleep and play positions on infant development, reconciling developmental concerns with SIDS prevention. *Newborn and Infant Nursing Reviews, 2*(1), 9-16.

Jantz, J.W., Blosser, C.D., & Fruechting, L.A. (1997). A motor milestone change noted with change in sleep position. *Archives Pediatric and Adolescent Medicine, 151*(6), 565-568.

Johnson, T. (2000). Neonatal neurophysiology overview, neurodevelopment. Presented at *Preconference A, The National Conference of Neonatal Nursing*. Seattle, WA, April 11-12.

Kane, A., Mitchell, L., Craven, K., & Marsh, J. (1996). Observations on a recent increase in plagiocephaly without synostosis. *Pediatrics, 97*(6)(Pt 1), 877-885.

Katz, K., Krikler, R., Wielunsky, E., & Merlob, P. (1991). Effect of neonatal posture on later lower limb rotation and gait in premature infants. *Journal of Pediatric Orthopedics, 11*(4), 520-522.

Kelly, K.M., Littlefield, T.R., Pomatto, J.K., et al. (1999) Importance of early recognition and treatment of deformational plagiocephaly with orthotic cranioplasty. *Cleft Palate-Craniofacial Journal, 36*(2), 127-130.

Konishi, Y., Mikawa, H., & Suziki, J. (1986). Asymmetrical head-turning of preterm infants, some effects on later postural and functional lateralities. *Developmental Medicine and Child Neurology, 28*(4), 450-457.

Lacey, J.L., Henderson-Smart, D.J., & Edwards, D.A. (1990). A longitudinal study of early leg postures of preterm infants. *Developmental Medicine and Child Neurology, 32*(2), 151-163.

Littlefield, T.R., Beals, S.P., Manwaring, K.H., et al. (1998). Treatment of craniofacial asymmetry with dynamic orthotic cranioplasty. *Journal of Craniofacial Surgery, 9*(1), 11-19.

Littlefield, T.R., Kelly, K.M., Pomatto, J.K., & Beals, S.P. (1999). Multiple birth infants at higher risk for development of deformational plagiocephaly. *Pediatrics, 103*(3), 565-569.

Lockridge, T., Taquino, L.T., & Knight, A. (1999). Back to sleep: Is there room in that crib for both AAP recommendations and developmentally supportive care. *Neonatal Network, 18*(5), 29-33.

Loochtan, A.M., & Loochtan, R.M. (1989). Damage to neonatal oral structures: Effects of laryngoscopy and intubation. *Respiratory Care, 34*(10), 879-889.

Monfort, K.P., & Case-Smith, J. (1997). The effects of a neonatal positioner on scapular rotation. *American Journal of Occupational Therapy, 51*(5), 378-384.

Monteli, R.A., & Bumstead, D.H. (1986). Development and severity of palatal grooves in orally intubated newborns. *American Journal of Diseases in Children, 140*, 357-359.

Monterosso, L., Coenen, A., Percival, P., & Evans, S. (1995). Effect of a postural support nappy on 'flattened posture' of the lower extremities in very preterm infants. *Journal of Paediatric and Child Health, 31*(4), 350-354.

Mouradian, L.E., & Als, H. (1994). The influence of neonatal intensive care unit caregiving practices on motor functioning of preterm infants. *American Journal of Occupational Therapy, 48*(6), 527-533.

Palmer, P.G., Dubowitz, L.M.S., Verghote, M., & Dubowitz, V. (1982). Neurological and neurobehavioral differences between preterm infants at term and full term newborn infants. *Neuropediatrics, 13*(4), 183-189.

Pellicer, A., Gaya, F., Madero, R., et al. (2002). Noninvasive continuous monitoring of the effects of head position on brain hemodynamics in ventilated infants. *Pediatrics, 109*(3), 434-440.

Penn, A.A. (2001). *The role of endogenous and sensory-driven neural activity in development.* Presented at The Physical and Developmental Environment of the High Risk Infant, Clearwater Beach, FL, January 29-February 1.

Penn, A.A., & Schatz, C.J. (1999). Brain waves and brain wiring: The role of endogenous and sensory-driven neural activity in development. *Pediatric Research, 45*(4)(Pt 1), 447-458.

Persing, J. (1997). Controversies regarding the management of skull abnormalities. *Journal of Craniofacial Surgery, 8*(1), 4-5.

Petryshen, P., Stevens, B., Hawkins, J., & Stewart, M. (1998). Comparing nursing costs for preterm infants receiving conventional vs developmental care. *Neonatal Intensive Care, 11*, 18-24.

Pollack, I.F., Loskan, H.W., & Fasick, P. (1997). Diagnosis and management of posterior plagiocephaly. *Pediatrics, 99*(2), 180-185.

Procter, A.M., Lether, D., Oliver, R.G., & Cartlidge, P.H.T. (1998). Deformation of the palate in preterm infants. *Archives of Disease in Childhood, Fetal and Neonatal Edition, 78*, F29-F32.

Riegger-Krugh, C. (1993). Relationship of mechanical and movement factors to prenatal musculoskeletal development. *Physical and Occupational Therapy in Pediatrics, 12*, 19-37.

Rutter, N., Hinchcliffe, W., & Cartlidge, P.H.T. (1993). Do preterm infants always have flattened heads? *Archives of Disease in Childhood, 68*(5 Spec No), 606-607.

Saunders, B.S., Easa, D., & Slaughter, R.J. (1976). Acquired palatal groove in neonates. *Journal of Pediatrics, 89*(6), 988-989.

Semmler, C. (1989). Positioning and deformities. In C. Semmler (Ed.), *A guide to care and management of very low birth weight infants: A team approach.* Tuscon: Therapy Skill Builders.

Seow, W.K. (1997). Effects of preterm birth on oral growth and development. *Australian Dental Journal, 42*(2), 85-91.

Short, M.A., Brooks-Brunn, J.A., Reeves, D.S., et al. (1996). The effects of swaddling versus standard positioning on neuromuscular development of very low birth weight infants. *Neonatal Network, 15*(4), 25-31.

Sweeney, J.K., & Gutierrez, P. (2002). Musculoskeletal implications of preterm infant positioning in the NICU. *Journal of Perinatal and Neonatal Nursing, 16*(1), 58-70.

Taylor, J.L., & Norton, E.S. (1997). Developmental muscular torticollis, outcomes in young children treated by physical therapy. *Pediatric Physical Therapy, 9*, 173-178.

Thureen, P.J., Phillips, R.E., Baron, K.A., et al. (1998). Direct measurement of the energy expenditure of physical activity in preterm infants. *Journal of Applied Physiology, 85*(1), 223-230.

van Heijst, J.J., Touwen, B.C.L., & Vos, J.E. (1999). Implications of a neural network model of sensori-motor development for the field of developmental neurology. *Early Human Development, 55*(1), 77-95.

VanderKolk, C.A., & Carson, B.S. (1994). Lamboid synostosis. *Clinics in Plastic Surgery, 21*(4), 575-584.

vonGonten, A.S., Meyer, J.B. Jr., & Kim, A.K. (1995). Dental management of neonates requiring prolonged oral intubation. *Journal of Prosthodontics, 4*(4), 221-225.

Warwick-Brown, M.M. (1987). Neonatal palatal deformity following oral intubation. *British Dental Journal, 162*(7), 258-259.

Watterberg, K., & Munsick-Bruno, G. (1986). Incidence and persistence of acquired palatal groove in preterm neonates following prolonged oral intubatio. *Clinical Research, 34*, 113A.

# 17 Feeding

## Jacqueline M. McGrath

Many times the importance of feeding interventions and techniques are lost or forgotten in the high-tech environment of the NICU.

A. Conway (1994, pg. 71)

The environment of the neonatal intensive care unit (NICU) is, for the most part, noxious. As previous sections of this text have indicated, the environment plays a big role in the infant and family's development. Research in the area of "environmental neonatology" is mounting; however, evidence of the long-term consequences remains mostly unknown. Given this situation, avoidance of prolonged hospitalization in the NICU is an appropriate goal. Until recently, low birthweight (LBW), preterm infants were cared for in the NICU until 40 or more weeks' postconceptional age (PCA). However, because of healthcare reform, the managed care movement, and intensified utilization review, these infants are now routinely discharged at 35 to 37 weeks' PCA. The criteria used to determine the stability of the preterm infant before earlier discharge often includes cardiorespiratory stability, consistent weight gain, and successful bottle-feeding (even when the mother intends to breastfeed) (Kenner, Bagwell, & Torok, 2003; Merritt, Piller, & Prows, 2003) (Box 17-1). These criteria have become the "gold standard" for stability in the preterm infant before discharge. In addition, many nurseries are beginning to consider discharging a preterm infant who weighs 1800 g, regardless of PCA. Because of these changes, implementation of successful gastric and later, oral breastfeeding or bottle-feeding in the NICU is becoming a critical developmental milestone for infants leaving the NICU and a competency for families. In this chapter, feeding is reviewed: as a developmental milestone; with regard to interventions to successfully support this process; and through examination of the supporting research for these practices. Focus is on issues related to supporting the family during the transition to oral feeding and the transition to home. Oral feeding success is an important milestone for both the infant and the parent in the NICU.

## THE IMPORTANCE OF FEEDING

Nursing generally has not recognized bottle-feeding a preterm or high-risk infant as an intervention requiring the expertise of the professional nursing staff. Bottle-feeding an infant is commonly thought to be instinctual for both the infant and the caregiver; therefore, it is believed that *anyone* can feed a baby. The skills for both partners are believed to develop naturally with time and patience. When oral feeding is unsuccessful, the caregiver is just as likely to be found at fault as the infant.

Feeding success has implications for fostering parent-child bonding. The first task a new mother judges herself on is the ability to feed her infant; feeding her child often becomes a lifelong benchmark she uses to evaluate her parenting success (Bishop, 1995). For families, mealtime is a social event involving interaction and interchange as well as nourishment. It is usually a time of family bonding, sharing, and togetherness. Many cultural celebrations (e.g., holidays, birthdays, weddings, birth, and death ceremonies) involve meals. Thus, when a family has a child who is a difficult eater, the entire family is affected.

Feeding issues are even more significant for preterm infants because of the relative uncertainty of their growth and development. Once the preterm infant has attained cardiorespiratory stability, successful gastric and breast or bottle-feeding is usually the next major objective of care in the NICU (Conway, 1994). PCA and consistent weight gain are still often used to assess oral bottle-feeding readiness, but some practitioners are beginning to use behavioral competencies as useful criteria. However, nursing practices

Box **17-1**   SUGGESTED CRITERIA FOR EARLY DISCHARGE

- Cardiorespiratory stability
- No apnea or bradycardia for 5 to 7 days
- Consistent weight gain
- Thermal regulation
- Successful bottle-feeding (even if the mother intends to breastfeed)
- Parents actively participating in caregiving
- Parents confident in feeding skills
- Home environment calm and prepared for care of infant

Data from Merritt, T.A., Piller, D., & Prows, S.L. (2003). Early NICU discharge of very low birth weight infant: A critical review and analysis. *Seminars in Neonatalogy, 8,* 95-115.

and protocols in the NICU generally are based more on routines ("the way we've always done it") than on research findings. As Conway (1994; p. 71) stated, "Few other routine tasks of neonatal nursing require as much expertise and offer as few objective measurements of the outcome as bottle-feeding the premature infant."

Families of preterm infants might not be prepared to feed their high-risk infants. The NICU's emphasis on technology and numbers rather than on infant behaviors as well as the standardized way in which care is often delivered leads to what has been termed as the "medicalization" of families in the NICU (Pinch & Spielman, 1990). The importance of feeding can get lost amid the chaos and routines and, thus, families might not be as well prepared to feed their infants after discharge. Families of preterm infants are already at greater risk for difficulties with bonding, attachment, and parenting that can only be compounded by problems with breast or bottle-feeding (Miles, Funk, & Kasper, 1991). Therefore, oral feeding is an area of neonatal nursing care that cannot be overlooked. It might even need to be assigned a higher priority, given the managed care environment of the future, in which preterm infants might be discharged earlier with breastfeeding or bottle-feeding interventions occurring more and more in the home environment.

## GASTROINTESTINAL TRACT: ANATOMIC AND PHYSIOLOGIC LIMITATIONS

At birth, the neonate's gastrointestinal (GI) system must be able to provide a multitude of functions, including: nutrient digestion and absorption; fluid

and electrolyte maintenance; and immunologic protection against various toxins and bacteria. To support the neonate's energy requirements for basal metabolism and growth, the GI tract must have the functional capacity for efficient digestion and absorption of carbohydrates, fats, and proteins.

In utero, the placenta provides for the nutritional needs of the fetus and facilitates function of the fetal gastrointestinal tract while it is maturing. At approximately 4 weeks' gestation, the stomach develops from the ectoderm (Moore & Persaud, 2003). The endoderm becomes the lining of the intestinal tract, and is supported by the mesoderm. The mesoderm is believed to be responsible for expression of the first digestive enzymes. Functionality of the gastrointestinal tract begins with the development of these enzymes. Intestinal villi begin to develop at 7 weeks and develop throughout the entire intestine by 14 weeks (Blackburn, 2003). The GI track has a muscle structure that consists of two layers—an inner circular sheath overlaid by an outer longitudinal coating of muscle tissues. The circular layer begins to develop at 5 weeks' gestation while the outer layer is not appreciated until approximately 8 weeks' gestation. The layers thicken with increasing gestational age and are responsible for motility within the GI tract. At 25 weeks' gestation, gastric motility is approximately 60% of that of a term infant (Fletcher, 1998).

In the premature and critically ill child, the provision of adequate nutritional support for growth and development is an ongoing challenge (Pereira & Balmer, 1996). Limitations of gastrointestinal function cause the infants to be at risk for dehydration, reflux, malabsorption, electrolyte imbalance, and necrotizing enterocolitis (NEC). Because the development of motility and peristalsis occur during the third trimester, premature infants have higher risks. Infants who have cardiorespiratory disease require assisted ventilation, and those who are physiologically unstable will also have a delay in oral-motor coordination as well as GI function, as the gut might be compromised secondary to these other medical conditions.

Gastrointestinal function that is immature at birth increases the risk of malabsorption and malnutrition. Functional and anatomic maturation includes the suck-swallow reflexes, esophageal motility, function of the lower esophageal sphincter, gastric emptying, intestinal motility, and development of the absorptive surface area. Esophageal motility is decreased in the newborn during the first 12 hours. The lower esophageal sphincter (LES) is primarily above the diaphragm and subject to intrathoracic pressures, which results in esophageal reflux. Esophageal reflux is common and can be seen on a radiographic film in 38% of normal term infants in the first week of life; more than 70% of preterm infants have reflux; however, most are asymptomatic. The sphincter remains small and inadequate in these high-risk infants for the first 6 to 12 months. Gastric emptying takes a minimum of 2 to 6 hours.

Although the anatomic development of the fetal gut is essentially complete by 20 weeks' gestation, maturation of physiologic function does not occur until later in gestation, and extends throughout the early postnatal period (Slater-Myer, Saslow, & Stahl, 1996). Thus, at full-term birth, although structurally mature, the functional ability of the GI tract of the neonate is continuing to develop, and is somewhat inefficient in its capabilities for digestion, fluid and electrolyte maintenance, and immunologic protection. These concerns are even more apparent for the preterm infant.

When determining the preterm infant's physiologic capacity for safe and effective oral feeding, the infant's gestational age (GA) and PCA are important factors to consider. This means that the infant's ability to establish and maintain successful oral feeding by breast or bottle will primarily depend on the degree of structural and functional development of the preterm infant's GI tract and oral cavity (Table 17-1). In a discussion of the anatomic and physiologic limitations imposed by an immature GI tract, Mason-Wyckoff, McGrath, Griffin, et al. (2003) identified 7 develop-

mental handicaps that might disrupt or delay the successful transition to oral feeds:

- Immature suck-swallow-breathe coordination
- Absent or weak cough and gag reflexes
- Incompetent gastroesophageal (GE) sphincter
- Delayed gastric emptying
- Decreased intestinal motility
- Incompetent ileocecal valve
- Impaired rectosphincteric reflex

Intestinal motility has been described and identified by the PCA at which motility dramatically improves (Berseth, 1990; Morriss, Moore, Weisbrodt, et al., 1986). The investigators found that there was considerable improvement at 32 weeks' gestation, and infants whose mothers had received prenatal steroids demonstrated a more mature pattern than that of infants of comparable gestations. Motility appears to be a function of gestation, postnatal maturation, and disease state, with a link to central nervous system (CNS) maturation. There is a fourfold increase noted in gastric motility between 28 and 38 weeks' PCA. If intestinal motility is the limiting factor in the progression of enteral feedings, it should be identified as such before several formula changes are tried. It is essential to identify the specific source of the enteral feeding characteristics so that a plan can be devised to eliminate the causative factor. The gastric capacity of an infant is approximately 6 ml/kg of body weight (Blackburn, 2003). Increased gastric volumes might compromise respiratory function and interfere with delivery of adequate nutrients. In preterm infants, large residual gastric volumes might develop, leading to gastric distention and vomiting.

## ENTERAL FEEDING
### Minimal Enteral Nutrition Feedings

Many nurseries are introducing minimal enteral nutrition (MEN) feedings or trophic gavage feedings that are early subnutritional feedings to preterm within a few days of life rather than holding feeds in an effort to wait for greater physiologic stability. These feedings are usually small (a few ml), dilute (often 50%-strength formula or expressed breastmilk), and frequent (every 2 to 3 hours), and are most often provided by gravity via a gavage tube. Results from research are varied; however, there seems to be greater evidence from both retrospective analysis and

Table **17-1** ANATOMICAL DIFFERENCES BETWEEN THE FULL-TERM INFANT AND PRETERM INFANT MOUTH AND PHARYNX

| Structure | Full-Term Infant | Preterm Infant |
| --- | --- | --- |
| Oral cavity | "Potential space" | Large space |
| Buccal pads | Large | Small or absent |
| Lips | Large, inactive | Small, inactive |
| Tongue | Relative size | Small |
| Soft palate | Full closure | Weak, incomplete |
| Jaw | Stable | Hypermobile |
| Hyoid | Stable | Unstable |
| Larynx | Muscular closure | Weak closure |
| Arytenoids | Large | Smaller bulk |
| Nasal passage | Nose breathers | Often $O_2$ dependent |

controlled trials of increased feeding tolerance, fewer residuals, fewer numbers of days to full feeding with a decreased incidence of NEC (Berseth, 1990; Berseth, Bisquera, & Paje, 2003; Troche, Harvey-Wilkes, Engle et al., 1995). Ho, Yen, Hsieh, et al. (2003) did a retrospective study to evaluate two forms of nutrition given to 17 premature infants with respiratory distress syndrome (RDS). Their findings were that those infants who received early feedings had less time to full enteral feedings and regained any weight loss experienced and decreased days on the ventilator and on aminophylline than those infants who received later supplementation. de Pipaon, VanBeek, Quero, et al. (2003) studied the effect of MEN on leucine uptake by splanchnic tissues. This uptake is a physiologic indicator of maturation of these GI tissues. They found that there was an increase in maturation of splanchnic tissue and protein synthesis with MEN. The enhancement of protein synthesis could act as a protection for premature, sick infants, and increase their ability to wound heal. GI tract maturation in general might be fostered with MEN, especially if this is done with expressed breastmilk. Breastmilk contains fats that increase the immunologic function of this system and decrease infections. It also contains nutrients such as glutamate, threonine, peptide growth factors (e.g., glucagon-like peptide [GLP-2]), and hormones that stimulate GI growth, maturation, and ability to digest enteral nutrition (Burrin & Stoll, 2002). Nutritional support for premature infants is essential if we are to

decrease the incidence of extrauterine growth restriction (EUGR) (Clark, Wagner, Merritt, et al., 2003). MEN appears to be one way to do that. Although more evidence is needed to support various aspects of MEN, research findings are mounting to support its use in the NICU.

### Gavage Feedings

Gavage feedings are provided for premature infants before the maturation of suck, swallow, and breathing. Box 17-2 shows the progression of sucking and swallowing development. The gavage tube can be placed either orally or nasally and is usually a semi-soft catheter of 3.5 to 8 French, depending on the size of the infant.

### Tube Placement

For placement, the tube is first measured by extending it from the xiphoid process to the ear of the infant and then to mouth or nares and adding 1 cm. The tube can be inserted quickly and smoothly into the nares or mouth while the infant is offered a pacifier. Insertion orally can be slightly more difficult; however, the same technique can be utilized to decrease the stress of insertion. The tube is secured to the side of the mouth or nares with tape or other clear adhesive dressing. Many of the clear adhesive dressings are kinder and gentler to the delicate skin of the preterm infant. The tube can be removed after each feeding or left indwelling for 1 to 3 days. However, some of the softer

Box 17-2    Postconceptual Age and Associated Feeding Behaviors

| Postconceptional Age (PCA) | Behavior |
|---|---|
| 9.5 weeks | Perioral stimulation produces mouth opening and movement. |
| 12 to 17 weeks | Active swallowing and sucking routinely noted. |
| 14 weeks | Basic tastebud morphology and nerve supply develops. |
| 16 to 17 weeks | Swallowing regulates the amount of amniotic fluid. |
| 24 weeks | Ganglion cells have innervated the gastrointestinal system |
| 28 weeks | Rooting, swallowing, and sucking reflex are present but slow/imperfect. |
| 32 weeks | Gag reflex present. |
|  | Nonnutritive sucking present. |
| 34 weeks | Functional suck/swallow/breath pattern but poor endurance. |
| 36 weeks | Coordinated suck/swallow/breath pattern. |

Data from Moore, K.L., & Persaud, T.V.N. (2003). *The developing human: Clinically oriented embryology* (7th ed.). St Louis: W.B. Saunders.

Silastic tubes might be left in place for a month or more. In the past, checking for placement was done by inserting air into the tube and listening for a gastric bubble; recently this technique has been found to be somewhat inaccurate, and checking the aspirate from the tube for gastric pH might be a more reliable technique for assessing tube placement into the stomach of infants.

## Oral Gastric Versus Nasal Gastric Feedings

Enteral tube feedings minimize the premature infant's energy expenditure during feeding; however, which method is best nasal gastric (NG) or oral gastric (OG)? This issue has been debated throughout the literature and practice differs from nursery to nursery as well as from individual caregiver to caregiver. With proper tube placement into the stomach and not into the lower end of the esophagus, Symington, Ballantyne, Pinelli, et al. (1995) found no difference in weight gain, apnea, or bradycardia between matched groups of preterm infants who received either indwelling NG or intermittent OG feedings. However, it has been hypothesized that indwelling feeding with an NG might be less optimal because of the increased airway resistance in the nares and the continuous inhibition of the esophageal sphincter, increasing the risk of reflux. Even the placement of the tube can adversely affect breathing and, if left in place, sucking

as well (Shiao, Youngblut, Anderson, et al., 1995). Symington, Ballantyne, Pinelli, et al. (1995) suggest that indwelling tubes might be more economical (changed less often), and cited this as the only clinically significant difference in the two methods of enteral feedings. In spite of which method the caregiver chooses, insertion might be what causes the greatest distress for the infant and should be done skillfully with a pacifier in a fluid process. Once the tube is placed, the feeding should be administered by gravity for 15 to 30 minutes; if too large a feeding tube is used, the feeding could flow in too fast and increase the risk for reflux.

## CONTINUOUS VERSUS BOLUS FEEDINGS

More research is focusing on the use of continuous feedings versus intermittent gavage feedings rather than just the question of an indwelling catheter or not. Premji and Chessell (2001) conducted a systematic review of studies that had been done in this area. The infants across the studies were all premature and weighed less than 1500 g. They found that it was difficult to do comparisons across groups because consistent variables and outcomes were not examined, and most studies had very small sample sizes. Although no recommendation as to which feeding method to use could be made from this systematic review, they did find that continuous feedings resulted in a longer period of time to reach full enteral feedings. There were no differences in days to maximal growth or discharge or in the incidence of NEC. This is another area of infant feeding that requires more research.

## Nursing Interventions during Gavage Feedings

Routine nursing care during gavage feedings should include abdominal assessments consisting of palpation, auscultation, and abdominal girths at least every 4 hours, with more close assessment when any one parameter has changed in the previous 4 hours. It has been suggested that aspirates/residuals should be checked before feeding and should not exceed either the hourly rate (if continuous) or what would have been given if the bolus feedings were hourly. These parameters can be altered by the infant's intolerance for stress from the NICU environment, handling and/or procedures. Thus, the infant's behavioral cues also need to be a part of this routine assessment. Always consider what has been happening to and around the infant when examining the infant. Transition to bottle-feeding can be facilitated during gavage feeding in a number of ways. Some are listed in Box 17-3, with supporting rationale from the literature.

Pickler, Mauck, and Geldmaker (1997) examined the medical records of 40 preterm infants to study their bottle-feeding histories. Records were examined for physical characteristics related to and predictive of bottle-feeding initiation and progression. Infant morbidity ratings were closely correlated with PCA at first bottle-feeding, full bottle-feeding, and discharge. Therefore, prematurity and disease status as well as stability were related to initiation and transition time. Pridham, Kosorok, Greer, et al. (1999) also examined medical records for similar indications of feeding progression and found that individual infant characteristics as well as environmental and historical characteristics contributed significantly to shortening or lengthening transition time. However, Kliethermes, Cross, Lanese, et al. (1999) found that infants receiving gavage-feeding supplementation rather than bottlefeeding supplementation during the transition to breastfeeding were 4.5 times more likely to be breastfeeding at discharge and 9.4 times more likely to be fully breastfed than infants who received supplementation with bottles. These findings suggest that how an infant is transitioned from gavage feeding to breastfeeding might affect long-term ability to breastfeed, and that bottle-feeding should be avoided

## Box 17-3   INTERVENTIONS TO FACILITATE TRANSITION TO ORAL BOTTLE-FEEDING

| Nursing Intervention | Supportive Rationale |
| --- | --- |
| Nonnutritive sucking | Accelerates maturation of the sucking reflex |
| | Improves weight gain |
| | Decreases oxygen consumption |
| | Facilitates earlier advancement to full oral feeding and earlier discharge |
| Prone or sidelying position during and after feeding | Improves gastric emptying |
| | Decreases regurgitation and aspiration |
| Folded and flexed into a semi-upright position | Promotes flexed posture |
| | Encourages social interaction |
| | Decreases regurgitation and aspiration |
| Reduction of noxious environmental stimulation | Reduces hypoxia |
| | Decreases fluctuations in oxygenation that could affect the GI tract |
| | Promotes behavioral state that is conducive to social interaction (alertness) |
| Skin-to-skin holding | Increases social interaction |
| Kangaroo care | Decreases stress and increases sleep |

if full breastfeeding is the goal. This practice is contrary to most feeding practices in NICUs in the United States.

## BREASTFEEDING

Breastfeeding is an age-old practice that falls in and out of fashion. Ahluwalia, Morrow, Hsia, et al. (2003) examined breastfeeding initiation and continuation among women in 10 states in the United States. They used the Pregnancy Risk Assessment and Monitoring System surveillance data from the Centers for Disease Control and Prevention (CDC), Atlanta, GA, from 1993 to 1998. They found an 18% rise in the initiation of breastfeeding across all socioeconomic groups. However, those women at highest risk for having vulnerable infants did not continue breastfeeding whereas women less vulnerable and generally of higher socioeconomic status continued breastfeeding. This trend was supported by others who studied mothers of premature and sick infants and their incidence of breastfeeding (Griffin, Meier, Bradford, et al., 2000; Meier, 2001). With these trends in mind, this rise even in the initiation of breastfeeding might be related to the emphasis on "Breast is the Best Infant Feeding" campaigns. In the past two decades, more research has focused on the benefits of breastmilk on the premature infant's well-being. Immunologic enhancement, GI growth, and fewer morbidities are associated with breastfeeding. Physiologic stability, in the form of heart and respiratory rates and oxygen saturation, has been found to be linked with breastfeeding (Dowling, 1999; Meier & Anderson, 1987; Meier & Brown, 1996). The American Academy of Pediatrics (AAP) (1996-1997) developed a policy statement supporting breastfeeding for all infants. Breastfeeding, when initiated among this group, fails at a rate of approximately 50% (Mason-Wyckoff, McGrath, Griffin, et al., 2003). Failure is defined as cessation of breastfeeding before or immediately after discharge (Mason-Wyckoff, McGrath, Griffin, et al., 2003). To successfully breastfeed in an intensive care environment, there needs to be an interdisciplinary team approach and a commitment to its promotion (DiGirolamo, Brummer-Strawn, & Fein, 2003; Nascimento & Issler, 2003). Meier and Mangurten (1993) recommend a

five-phase temporal model for supporting lactation in the NICU. This model is based on their ongoing research in the area of breastfeeding support. The five phases are: (1) assisting the mother with milk collection and storage, (2) gavage feeding of expressed mother's milk, (3) managing in-hospital breastfeeding, (4) breastfeeding support following the infant's discharge, and (5) consultation with the family or NICU staff/lactation consultant or both. This model incorporates use of nonpharmacologic supports to increase milk volume and ease of breastfeeding. These supports include use of breast pumps at the infant's bedside, Kangaroo care (KC), and nonnutritive sucking (NNS) (Griffin, Meier, Bradford, et al., 2000; Mason-Wyckoff, McGrath, Griffin, et al., 2003; Meier, 2001).

There are many aspects of breastfeeding that are beyond the scope of this book; however, some guidelines are presented to assist those who wish to breastfeed. Protocols to support enteral feedings including breastfeeding can be found in Kenner and Lott (2004).

Vidyasagar, Theorell, and Peters (2003) offer the following guidelines for breastfeeding.

## UNIVERSITY OF ILLINOIS AT CHICAGO MEDICAL CENTER CLINICAL CARE GUIDELINE

### Subject: Breastfeeding for the Newborn Infant in the NICU/ICN

#### Objective

To establish the nurse's role for the promotion and support of breastfeeding mothers and their infants who require specialized care in the NICU or intermediate care nursery (ICN).

#### Position Statements

The University of Illinois and Chicago Medical Center supports breastfeeding/breastmilk as the feeding method of choice for newborns, but especially those who are compromised by acute illness or prematurity, as long as mother is not one of the very few for whom breastfeeding is contraindicated.

All mothers should have adequate information antenatally concerning breastfeeding to make an informed choice. Frequently the premature birth or illness of a term infant is unexpected, and breastfeeding should be discussed with the mother again in light of its benefits to an already compromised infant. Expressing milk for a limited time while the child is ill should be presented as a viable option and will be facilitated if mother chooses to.

The ideal is to have the baby feed directly from the breast. Due to varying situations in the NICU/ICN, that might not be possible. A mother might choose to only pump milk for the baby and never put the baby to breast. Ultimately, our goal is to provide the mother with as much information as possible concerning her different options, and facilitate and support whatever decision she makes.

## Standards

1. Every mother whose infant is admitted to the NICU/ICN will be assessed by a registered nurse or lactation consultant for willingness to pump milk during the infant's hospital stay, even if her long-term plan is to formula feed.
2. When maternal breastfeeding problems requiring medical consultation are noticed, the mother will be referred back to her obstetric (OB) care provider for consultation as needed. If the mother has no OB care provider and needs to be seen urgently, she can be seen by the attending OB physician on call in Labor and Delivery (L & D) in triage visit.
3. The mother should be assisted in getting baby to breast, when possible, if mother chooses to do so. Getting the baby to actually latch on at the breast might be a slow process requiring a number of attempts. In many cases, the mother will be encouraged to continue to pump milk with an electric pump, even though baby is doing some feedings at breast, so she does not loose her milk supply, as it reflects the amount of stimulation provided.

## Procedure

### Milk expression and collection:

1. Instruct mother to always wash hands thoroughly with soap and water before handling the breast, pump, and attachments.
2. Instruct the mother how to set up the pump equipment properly.

3. Instruct the mother to wash all breast pump equipment that has contact with the breast or breastmilk. They should be washed thoroughly with hot, soapy water, rinsed to ensure all soap is removed, and left to air dry on clean towel. Instruct her once a day to boil equipment (everything but the tubing) for 10 minutes and then let air dry (or use a dishwasher).
4. Instruct mother to begin milk expression as soon as possible after birth—ideally in the first few hours.
5. Instruct the mother to pump, with a hospital-grade electric pump, using a double collection kit, every $2^1/_2$ hours for 10 to 15 minutes, or until milk stops flowing, to initiate lactation. Encourage mother to keep a log of the time of day that she pumped and volume expressed.
6. Instruct mother to use lowest pump setting for pumping; the highest setting can injure breast tissue. It is possible that the mother will see no or very little breastmilk for the first four days of pumping, but she should continue to pump to initiate lactation. Without pumping she will be limiting milk production. It is possible that the mother will make more breastmilk than the baby needs initially; excess should be frozen. If the mother delays beginning pumping, it is possible that mother will go on to not develop a full milk supply.
7. Reassure the mother that uterine cramping during pumping is a normal physiologic response from the release of oxytocin and expected in the early days of milk expression. It is safe to take ibuprofen for pain relief without harming the infant, as long as the mother has not been prohibited from taking it.
8. Mothers receiving magnesium sulfate and most intravenous (IV) antibiotics while on postpartum unit are not prohibited from beginning pumping breastmilk.
   - For premature infants who are physiologically stable and at least 28 weeks' PCA, encourage NNS (after mother has pumped during kangaroo care).
   - Encourage nutritive sucking at the breast when infant is tolerating NNS well, shows some oral-motor coordination, and has physician approval/support.

- Instruct the mother on different positions that might assist the small preemie to latch on.

**Estimating intake:**

- Can use pre- and post-weights to estimate intake.
- Use the electronic infant scale and make sure that it is balanced and nothing is touching the edges.
- Weigh the baby before breastfeeding. It is best to disconnect baby from monitor, but have the monitor lead wires fully on the scale.
- After feeding, weigh baby again in exactly the same condition (i.e., same diaper, T-shirt, blanket).

**Documentation**

Reassessment of mother's willingness to pump milk and instructions on how to pump milk will be documented in Gemini (computer system) under patient education. Periodic assessment of mother's adequacy of pumping will also be documented in Gemini (computer system).

**On the NICU/ICN flowsheet:**

- When double-checking breastmilk, the RN checking will initial on the flow sheet on the page documenting intake volumes.
- The type of milk being given will be indicated on the intake page—colostrums (Co), fresh or previously frozen milk (FBRM), and fortified milk (fresh BRM).
- When the infant goes to the breast, document if the baby latched onto the breast, duration of breastfeeding one or both breasts, behavioral response of the infant.
- If pre- and post-weights are done, the estimate will be recorded in the "volume" space with an asterisk

GUIDELINES FOR STORING/THAWING MOTHER'S MILK FOR FEEDING PRETERM INFANTS

| Milk Type | To Be Fed within | Warming/Thawing | Special Considerations |
|---|---|---|---|
| Fresh, unrefrigerated | 1 hour | Not necessary | Extra milk can be refrigerated or frozen after 1 hour at room temperature. |
| Fresh, refrigerated | 48 hours | Warm slowly over 30 minutes to approximately body temperature. *Do not overheat. Do not microwave.* | Literature indicates milk is suitable for 48 hours with refrigeration less than or equal to 4 °C. "Cream" layer separates with refrigeration, so milk be shaken vigorously before use. Milk remaining after 48 hours should be discarded, not frozen. |
| Frozen | 24 hours after thawing | Thaw gradually (over 1 hour) to approximately body temperature. Do not overheat. Do not microwave. Take care not to contaminate milk if warm water bath is used. | Do not refreeze milk. Do not add fresh milk to bottles of frozen milk; use separate containers. The exception would be with colostrums. Discard unused milk after 24 hours of refrigeration. Frozen milk will keep 3 to 4 months in freezer compartment of refrigerator, and 6 months in deep freezer (0° For less). |

From University of Illinois Medical Center at Chicago Women's and Children's Nursing Services. Chicago, IL: University of Illinois Medical Center at permission by Dharmapuri Vidyasagar, MD; Catherine Theorell, RNC, MSN, NNP; and Beena Peters, RN, MS.

(*), which will be defined as meaning "estimated by scale".

**Unit equipment logs:**

- Temperature of the refrigerator and freezers used for breastmilk will be recorded daily on a log by the equipment technician.
- Equipment technician will be responsible for periodic cleansing of refrigerator and freezers, and cleaning the electric breast pumps daily with topical disinfectant.

**Breastmilk fortifier:** Should be added to fresh or thawed frozen milk in amounts that will be used in less than 24 hours. Milk that is already fortified should be discarded after 24 hours if not used.

**Labeling of milk:** Containers of milk should be labeled by mother or nurse: with infant's name, date/time expressed. Fresh milk should be labeled as such. Colostrum should have an additional label with "Colostrum" written on it. Date and time of thawing should be written on frozen milk.

## PHYSIOLOGY AND DEVELOPMENT OF SUCKING AND SWALLOWING

Reflexes required for oral intake mature in the fetus during the third trimester. Physiologic maturation appears to have a greater influence on the development of nutritive sucking (NS) abilities and swallowing than "experience" with bottle-feeding, although there is some evidence to support experience playing a complimentary role in the development of NS. Research in this area needs to be further explored. Coordination of suck, swallow, and breathing has been considered the most complex task of infancy. All components are present by 28 weeks but they are not at all mature. The swallowing reflex is well developed by 28 to 30 weeks, but is easily exhausted. The swallowing reflex is completely functional by 34 weeks' PCA. NS can be demonstrated in infants by 26 weeks, but a rhythmic pattern is not developed until 32 to 34 weeks. The gag reflex is complete at 34 weeks. Coordination of breath, suck, and swallow occurs beginning at 32 to 34 weeks for short periods; however, these mechanisms are not yet coordinated enough to sustain the infant's nutritional needs. True synchrony of suck, swallow, and breath in a 1:1:1 pattern does not occur until 36 to 38 weeks' PCA.

Infants with a physiologic disability in which the absence or the weakness of the gag and cough reflexes exist should be monitored for an increased risk of aspiration. The assessment for the presence of a gag reflex can be performed by direct observation during the passing of a feeding tube. However, the adequacy of the gag reflex can be more difficult to assess and the risk of aspiration should be a consideration in all infants receiving nasal or oral gastric tubefeeding.

The development of competent oral feeding skills is a requisite for physiologic adaptation and survival during infancy (Bu'Lock, Woolridge, & Baum, 1990; Medoff-Cooper & Ray, 1995). Oral feeding is a highly organized and intricate behavior that encompasses the activities of food seeking/obtaining, ingestion, and swallowing (Rudolph, 1994). Physiologically, oral feeding involves complex interaction of the brain and CNS, oral-motor reflexes, and multiple muscles of the mouth, pharynx, esophagus, and face (Tuchman & Walter, 1994). Infant oral feeding requires the rhythmic coordination of sucking and swallowing a bolus of fluid while at the same time balancing the demands for breathing (Timms, DiFiore, Martin, et al., 1993).

---

Box **17-4**   PHYSIOLOGIC INFLUENCES ON THE EFFICACY OF SUCKING IN THE PRETERM INFANT

- Immature sucking response
- Decreased muscle tone
- Poor state regulation
- Autonomic instability
- Disorganized sucking, swallowing, and breathing patterning
- Inability to effectively switch from nonnutritive to nutritive sucking.

Data from Case-Smith, J., Cooper, P., & Scala, V. (1989). Feeding efficiency of premature neonates. *American Journal of Occupational Therapy, 43*(4), 245-250.

Oral feeding has been regarded as the most highly organized behavioral activity of early infancy.

For term infants, oral feeding is a "natural physiologic process" that proceeds with minimal difficulty during the first days of life. However, the transition to oral or bottle-feedings in preterm infants might be significantly delayed, as a result of anatomic and functional immaturity of the gastrointestinal system, PCA, acute and/or chronic illness, neurobehavioral maturation, oral-motor dysfunction, and behavioral aversion (Box 17-4).

The development and physiologic process of infant oral feeding has been extensively discussed in numerous clinical and research-based publications. Conceptually, oral feeding is defined as a multi-faceted series of events involving the activities of food seeking, ingestion, and deglutition (swallowing) (Rudolph, 1994). Additionally, oral feeding is described as a highly integrated neurobehavioral process whereby the evolution of oral-motor skills parallels the general sequence of fine and gross motor skill acquisition during infancy (Rudolph, 1994; Tuchman, 1994). Developmentally, it is suggested that the early primitive and reflex patterns of infant oral feeding are sequentially extinguished and replaced by mature feeding patterns as a result of maturational changes within the brain and CNS (Rudolph, 1994; Tuchman, 1994). Research has documented a positive correlation between brain maturation and the emergence of higher-level behavioral skills (Fischer & Rose, 1994). Oral feeding is commonly portrayed as a three-stage process (Box 17-5).

Although neonates and young infants rely on parents and other caregivers to provide the nutrients needed for adequate growth and development, the establishment of competent oral feeding skills requires an intact and functioning brain and CNS, as well as the ability to rhythmically coordinate the neuromotor activities of sucking, swallowing, and breathing (Gryboski, 1969; Koenig, Davies, & Thach, 1990; Mathew, 1991). During infancy, sucking, swallowing, and breathing are the essential motor components of the oral feeding process (Mathew, 1991). The following sections will discuss each of these components in greater detail.

## Sucking

Investigations of the development of oral feeding during infancy have primarily focused on bottle-feeding. Research has primarily focused on describing the neonatal sucking response, a major component of oral feeding. Sucking is a rhythmic action of the tongue and jaw that causes fluid to flow out of a nipple or maternal teat due to changes in intraoral pressure (Glass & Wolf, 1994). Sucking includes both negative (suction) and positive (compression) pressure components (Sameroff, 1968). Sucking has been described as a push-pulling action, whereby the positive pressure changes created by the rhythmic compression of the nipple between the tongue and palate acts to push fluid out of a nipple into the oral cavity, and negative pressure changes function to draw fluid from the nipple (Sameroff, 1968; Tuchman, 1994; Glass & Wolf, 1994). Negative or suction pressure is generated through rhythmic contractions of jaw muscles and tongue movements working in concert to pull fluid out of the nipple into the mouth (Mathew, 1991; Sameroff, 1968). In bottle-feeding, the tongue appears to move in a piston-like fashion; whereas in breast-feeding, there is more of a rolling movement of the

---

Box **17-5**   Oral Feeding: A Three-Stage Process

| Stage | I | Entails the recognition of hunger by the infant or caregiver; acknowledgment of infant hunger cues; the process of obtaining food substances; and ingestion |
| --- | --- | --- |
| Stage | II | Involves the complex motor activities of deglutition (swallowing); deglutition is a complex series of neuromotor activities functioning to transport food and fluids from the mouth to the stomach while preventing the aspiration of food substances into the trachea and lungs |
| Stage | III | Entails the activities of esophageal swallowing and gastrointestinal absorption |

Modified from Tuchman, D.N., & Walter, R.S. (Eds.). (1994). *Disorders of feeding and swallowing in infants and children: Pathophysiology, diagnosis, and treatment.* San Diego: Singular.

tongue. Term infants have the capability to regulate the amount of pressure that is generated during sucking (Glass & Wolf, 1994; Rudolph, 1994; Sameroff, 1968). Preterm infants might, however, experience varying degrees of difficulty in generating and maintaining sufficient pressures required for competent oral feeding. Sometimes the infant must be "taught" how to suck correctly (Marmet & Shell, 1984).

There are two types of sucking that have been described in the literature—nonnutritive and nutritive sucking (Wolff, 1968). NNS is defined as a repetitive pattern of mouthing activity on a pacifier (Tuchman, 1994; Wolff, 1968) and is a precursor to NS behavior. From a developmental perspective, NNS and spontaneous mouthing movements have been observed in utero as early as 15 to 18 weeks' gestation, with maturational changes in patterns of NNS noted over time (Hack, Estabrook, & Robertson, 1985). Wolff (1968) described NNS as alternating periods of short sucking bursts and pauses. The rate of sucking is approximately two sucks per second, with a suck-to-swallow ratio of six to eight sucks per swallow (Wolff, 1968). NS occurs spontaneously or might be initiated by the presence of a pacifier in the infant's mouth (Miller, 1986). Furthermore, whereas NS only takes place during oral feeding, NNS has been observed during all sleep-wake cycles (Wolff, 1972), might occur at the end of a feeding, or might be interspersed between bursts of NS (Conway, 1994). NNS just before bottle-feeding is associated with improved oxygen saturations (Pickler, Frankel, Walsh, et al., 1996). One aspect of NNS that is just beginning to be researched is long-term effects on dental formation (Warren & Bishara, 2002). These long-term effects must be part of our considerations when it comes to all aspects of feeding.

## Nutritive Sucking

In contrast, NS is defined as the pattern of sucking that occurs when a bolus of fluid is introduced into the infant's mouth (Conway, 1994). NS is organized as a continuous sequence of long and slow bursts of sucking at pressures sufficient to deliver fluid from a nipple (Medoff-Cooper & Ray, 1995). Research has described the developmental progression and maturation of NS following birth (Gryboski, 1969). Infants born before 32 weeks' gestation demonstrate

mouthing movements not associated with effective sucking. Between 32 and 36 weeks' gestation, preterm infants display an immature pattern of sucking that consists of short sucking bursts occurring at a rate of 1 to 1.5 sucks per second. In this stage of development, swallowing either precedes or follows each sucking burst. A more mature pattern of NS usually emerges by 35 to 36 weeks' gestation and is characterized by prolonged bursts of 10 to 30 sucks per second with a suck-to-swallow ratio of 1:1.

Additionally, physiologic studies of neonatal sucking during bottle-feeding have found that NS is comprised of two distinct phases: a continuous sucking phase and an intermittent sucking phase (Mathew, Clark, Pronske, et al., 1985; Shivpuri, Martin, Carlo, et al., 1983). Continuous sucking patterns occur during the first 2 minutes of oral feeding and are depicted by long, uninterrupted sucking bursts accompanied by brief pauses in sucking (Mathew, Clark, Pronske, et al., 1985; Shivpuri, Martin, Carlo, et al., 1983). As sucking continues, an intermittent pattern of NS emerges, which is characterized by shorter bursts of sucking alternating with three to five periods of sucking pauses.

It also appears that sucking patterns change during the course of breastfeeding. Research suggests that sucking frequency, patterning of bursts and sucking pauses, and ratio of sucks to swallows are significantly influenced by changes in rate of milk flow during maternal "let-down." As noted by Glass and Wolf (1994), slower sucking rates and lower ratios of suck to swallow occur with increased milk flow.

## Milk Volume Intake during Nutritive Sucking

Research suggests that the volume of fluid expressed per suck is regulated by a combination of factors including nipple flow rates, sucking efficiency, sucking patterns, taste, and characteristics of containers used for bottle-feeding (Mathew, 1988, 1990, 1991). In studies investigating the effects of various types of nipple units upon milk flow during bottle-feeding for term and preterm infants, Mathew (1988, 1990) found wide variability in milk flow within and among the various types of nipples that are used for bottle-feeding term and preterm infants. The firmness or pliability of the nipple and size of the nipple hole are important determinants of milk flow during bottle-feeding. High-flow nipple units, such as those used for preterm infants, are generally softer in consistency and have larger feeding holes (Mathew, 1991). Nipples used for term or older preterm infants might be stiffer in consistency, with a wide range of feeding hole sizes. All nipple-unit types have similar flow patterns—the bigger the hole, the larger the flow of milk (Mathew, 1991).

The use of high-flow nipple units for bottle-feeding preterm infants has been based on the assumption that faster milk flow compensates for the preterm infant's limited ability to generate sufficient pressures requisite for oral feeding (Mathew, 1991). However, there are limited empiric data to support this premise (Mathew, 1991). Conversely, in research comparing sucking pressures in term and preterm infants during bottle-feeding, Mathew, Belan, and Thoppil (1992) found that the differences in sucking pressures between the two groups were statistically nonsignificant, although the authors documented a tendency toward lower sucking pressures in preterm infants. Stable respiratory patterns and better oxygenation, and less drooling and choking have been associated with use of orally supportive nipples with low flow (Dowling, 1999; Hill & Rath, 1993, 1999).

Research also suggests that the rate of milk flow might be affected by the characteristics of the containers used during bottle-feeding (Duara, 1989). Collapsible feeding bags were associated with faster feeding rates compared with the slower feeding demonstrated with the use of glass containers (Duara, 1989). It is thought that the vacuum created during sucking from a glass container limits the amount of milk expression from the bottle (Duara, 1989). Duara (1989) suggests that introducing vent holes in the nipple could overcome the vacuum effect created during sucking from glass containers. Most standard nipples used today have vent holes.

Sucking efficiency is another determinant of milk volume expression during oral feeding (Mathew, 1991). The presence of congenital and/or acquired defects of the lip and/or palate and abnormalities in oral-motor muscle tone (paralysis, weakness, hypertonia) can limit both the infant's ability to form an adequate lip seal and the ability to generate sufficient pressure changes required for effective sucking.

VandenBerg (1990) noted that sucking efficiency can also be influenced by characteristics associated with prematurity, including an immature sucking response; low muscle tone; poor state regulation; autonomic instability; disorganized sucking-swallowing and breathing patterning; and the inability to effectively switch from NNS to NS.

In response to these findings, some nurseries choose not to routinely use preemie nipples because of the increased milk flow they provide. They use standard nipples right from the initiation of oral feeding because they will not provide increased flow during a time when the infant is just learning to coordinate the highly organized process of bottle-feeding. However, what might be best of all is choosing a particular nipple for a particular baby and not having any standard process for initiating bottle-feeding. This technique requires accurate assessment and a team of professionals working together to facilitate the infant during this process (see the feeding documentation sheet presented earlier for a way to document this process).

### Swallowing

Swallowing, or deglutition, is also an integral component of infant oral feeding. Swallowing is a complex and coordinated motor activity that functions to transport food and fluids from the mouth to the stomach while preventing the aspiration of food substances into the trachea and lungs (Tuchman & Walter, 1994). There are three distinct phases of swallowing—oral, pharyngeal, and esophageal (Mathew, 1991; Mathews, 1994; Tuchman, 1994). During early infancy, the oral phase of deglutition is a reflex activity that initiates with NS.

The second phase of deglutition, known as the pharyngeal phase, comprises a sequential series of semiautomatic movements that are triggered by the presence of liquid or solid food in the oral cavity (Ichord, 1994). Pharyngeal deglutition involves the preparation of the oral-nasal cavity, airway, and esophagus for the movement of fluid or food bolus into the pharynx and ultimately into the esophagus (Ichord, 1992). As the infant swallows, breathing is "reflexively" suppressed, and the upward movement of the epiglottis closes the airway and laryngohyoid complex, thereby preventing the aspiration of food contents into the tracheobronchial tree (Ichord, 1992; Rudolph, 1994).

Phase III, or esophageal deglutition, entails the delivery of food or liquids into the stomach by the peristaltic contractions of the esophagus and the concurrent automatic inhibition of the upper esophageal sphincter (Ichord, 1992). Esophageal deglutition is activated by the presence of food in the esophagus, and is thought to be a continuation of pharyngeal deglutition (Mathew, 1991).

## Breathing

Breathing is an autonomic process that we seldom acknowledge except when we have a cold or increased work of breathing, such as during exercise. In the full-term infant, the process is much the same. However, the immaturity of the preterm respiratory system impairs the mechanics of breathing. Preterm infants are at increased risk for aspiration, apnea, and periodic breathing, which is increasingly apparent during feeding. The issue of coordination of sucking, swallowing, and breathing is of concern for these infants.

## Sucking, Swallowing, and Breathing

Coordination of sucking, swallowing, and breathing is related to the type of sucking (NNS or NS), the flow of the milk (a little to swallow or a lot), and the neuromaturation of the infant. In general, increasing gestational age and PCA are positively correlated to greater success in this process. A great deal of organization is required for this process; thus, the infant's energy resources, developmental maturation, and the environment will have an impact on the infant's ability to be successful (Mathew & Bhatia, 1989). Evidence to support earlier introduction of oral feedings, requiring coordination of suck, swallow, and breathing in synchronization with improvement of the transition from tube to oral feeding, is growing (Simpson, Schanler, & Lau, 2002). Given these newer findings, it is important to be able to assess feeding readiness accurately.

## ASSESSMENT OF FEEDING READINESS

The questions of when and how to introduce oral feeds to hospitalized preterm infants are controversial issues for which there are still no clear answers. Although the literature and anecdotal reports indicate that several criteria have been used by NICU staff to determine preterm infant readiness for initiating oral feedings, numerous publications report that, for the most part, feeding-related decisions are typically not research based (Kinneer & Beachy, 1994; Medoff-Cooper, Verklan, & Carlson, 1993; Pridham, Sondel, Chang, et al., 1993). For example, it is customary practice for oral feedings to be delayed until the infant reaches a weight of 1500 g and/or is 34 to 35 weeks' PCA (Medoff-Cooper & Ray, 1995; Mason-Wyckoff, McGrath, Griffin, et al., 2003). There is no evidence to support the maturation of suck-swallow coordination, weight, and maturation; however, this parameter traditionally has been used to assess feeding readiness. Indeed, recent research suggests that young preterm infants might be able to initiate and sustain breastfeeding activities as early as 32 weeks' PCA (Meier & Brown, 1996). However, for preterm infants with bronchopulmonary dysplasia (BPD), the impact of increased respiratory effort on breathing patterning during oral feeding should be considered in feeding-related decisions. For these infants, the transition to oral feedings may be significantly delayed.

Generally, the literature suggests that decisions of when and how to introduce oral feedings are primarily guided by: established nursery routines or customs (McCain, 1997; Medoff-Cooper & Ray, 1995); caregiver preference; or what is most convenient for the staff (McCain, 1997). It is also common practice for clinicians to utilize what Dr. Gerald Merenstein, neonatologist in Denver, Colorado, calls a "trial-and-error" approach, whereby specific interventions are introduced, continued, or deleted based on infant response or tolerance (Kinneer & Beachy, 1994). Consequently, feeding practices are likely to vary from nursery to nursery, and might even vary from caregiver to caregiver within the same unit, often based on subjective assumptions of the caregiving team. See Box 17-6 for parameters to be included in an assessment of feeding readiness.

## SETTING THE STAGE FOR FIRST AND SUBSEQUENT FEEDING SUCCESS

Once the decision to provide bottle-feeding has been made, there are many subsequent decisions that must be made by the caregiver. If left to chance, as is often

## Box 17-6   Indications of Neurobehavioral Readiness for Feeding

Neurobehavioral maturation—Conceptualized through Als' Synactive Theory of Development (Als, 1982)
- Gestation age versus postconceptual age (PCA)
- Older than 32 weeks' PCA

Physiologic/behavioral stability
- Respirations fairly regular, rate of 40 to 60 breaths per minute
- Physiologic and behavioral cues—Signs of stress
- Approach versus avoidance cues
- Can the baby manage his environment?

Hunger cues such as mouthing, rooting, and waking for feedings

Behavioral state—Ability to be available, attentiveness
- Smooth behavioral state transitions with a wide variety of states available
- Ability to reach and maintain an alert state

Motor development—Ability to hold him/herself together
- Low versus high tone
  Limp vs. flexed and tucked
- Oral-motor development
  Good facial tone
  Energy resources

From McGrath, J.M., & Conliffe-Torres, S. (2000). *Feeding practices and nursing interventions in the NICU: A self-study module.* Des Plaines, IL: National Association of Neonatal Nurses.

the case in the NICU, these choices can ultimately determine the successful attainment of bottle-feeding by the preterm infant. These decisions focus on how and when caregivers should intervene and support the infant through the process. From a macro- to micro-perspective, the environment of the NICU and, specifically, that infant must first be addressed; both are important in supporting the infant during this process (Box 17-7).

A difficult or immature feeder might display more incoordination of sucking, swallowing, and breathing, requiring more intensive intervention and attention. These infants are often easily overstimulated and tire quickly with bottle-feeding. Careful attention to their individualized needs is required for these infants to become successful with bottle-feeding.

Lastly, infant-caregiver interaction, co-regulation, and caregiver commitment to feeding must be considered. Feeding success for the infant is largely dependent on the care providers' attention to the individualized needs of the infant (Shaker, 1999). Reciprocity must exist between the infant and the caregiver for successful oral feeding to occur. This reciprocity might be difficult to achieve if there is no consistency in care providers; thus, consistency

of care is an issue of concern when promoting feeding success. Documentation of feeding readiness cues and stress behaviors during the feeding, as well as interventions used to support the infant, can promote feeding success when several care providers feed the preterm infant. It is also important to note that not every intervention is necessary for every infant; feeding should be individualized to the infant. When providing intervention, we should never do for the infant what he can do for himself. Box 17-8 contains interventions to promote feeding success, and Box 17-9 contains nursing actions that can detract from the infant's ability to achieve success. Many preterm infants have trouble with reflux related to oral feeding. GI reflux is abnormal frequent passage of gastric contents into the esophagus. Reflux can detract from feeding success as well as delay growth and development. Remember that more than 70% of preterm infants have reflux, although only a few are symptomatic enough to require intervention. Interventions should be only provided as needed and should be related to the symptoms (Box 17-10). Pharmacologic interventions should be reserved for when all other interventions have failed and should

Box **17-7**   STEPS TO CONSIDER WHEN PREPARING FOR BOTTLE-FEEDING

Assess the infant's neurobehavioral readiness for feeding
- Use Als' Synactive Theory of Development as a framework for intervention
- Respiratory stability

Is there a time of day when this infant is more awake?

Consider the environment
- Light, noise, activity, space: How do these affect *this* infant?
- What else has happened in this infant's day or the past 24 hours that could affect feeding success?
- What in the environment facilitates state transition for *this* infant?

Preparation of the care provider
- Does this care provider know *this* baby?
- Commitment of this care provider to the infant's success: Does she or he have the time to provide the support *this* infant will need?

Data from Als, H. (1982). Toward a synactive theory of development: Promise for the assessment of infant individuality. *Infant Mental Health Journal, 3,* 229-243.

be monitored closely; these medications are not without their own issues and concerns.

## Scheduled Versus Demand

There are now several published studies to support the feeding of preterm infants on a demand schedule (Collinge, Bradley, Perks, et al., 1982; Pridham, Kosorok, Greer, et al., 1999; Saunders, Freidman, & Stramoski, 1990). Researchers have found that the staff must be trained to recognize the subtle signs of feeding readiness in the preterm infant. In addition, coordination and support of the caregiving team is important to the successful implementation of demand feeding in the NICU. Demand feeding does, however, better support the preterm infant in reaching alert states that have been repeated, correlated with increased feeding success (McCain, 1995, 1997; McGrath, 1999; McGrath & Medoff-Cooper, 2002; Medoff-Cooper & Brooten, 1987; Medoff-Cooper, McGrath & Bilker, 2000).

## PSYCHOSOCIAL AND FAMILY ISSUES: PREPARING FOR DISCHARGE

As soon as possible, parents must be facilitated to provide as much of the routine caregiving as they are available and willing to do. Participating in feeding increases the parents' feelings of involvement and contribution to their infant's well being. During gavage feeding, parents should be encouraged to hold the infant, provide Kangaroo care, or support the infant who is learning to integrate NNS (supporting the pacifier). Social interaction during gavage feeding should be based on the infant's availability and behavioral cues. Whenever possible, the parents should provide the bottle-feeding. This might mean the feeding schedule is adjusted to the visiting schedule of the parent. Careful attention should be focused on the parents' and infant's success during the feeding and relayed to the parent. Parents should not be denied the opportunity to feed even the most difficult infant; remember, this is their baby!

## FUTURE RESEARCH IMPLICATIONS AND CONCLUSIONS

Understanding the interaction between preterm infant, the care provider, and the environment during bottle-feeding has been studied systematically in parts, but the dynamics of the entire holistic process remains basically untouched. Hill (2002) systematically explained the literature to design a theory of feeding efficiency for preterm infants; however, as yet this theory is untested. For example, coordination of sucking, swallowing, and breathing has been systematically studied, yet all the factors that contribute or diminish feeding success appear ambiguous (Ashland, 1995; Case-Smith, Cooper, & Scala, 1989; Medoff-Cooper & Brooten, 1987; Medoff-Cooper, Verklan, & Carlson, 1993; Medoff-Cooper, Weininger, & Zukowsky, 1989). Few interventions have been

**Box 17-8** INTERVENTIONS THAT FACILITATE FEEDING SUCCESS

| Intervention | Rationale |
|---|---|
| Decreasing environmental stimulation | Allows the infant to be focused on the feeding. This can include dimming bright lights, choosing a place that is quiet and away from activity. This might be difficult in the environment of the NICU, but should be a priority in preparation. (Hill, 2002; Shaker, 1999) |
| Oral support of chin and cheeks | Has been shown to positively affect feeding success. The facial muscles of the preterm infant are underdeveloped, and the infant has no buccal pads to support the intensity of sucking needed to generate milk flow. (Einarsson-Backes, Deitz, Price, et al., 1994; Hill, Kurkowski, & Garcia, 2000) |
| Type of nipple | Must be individualized to the infant. The care provider must continuously assess sucking, milk flow, and seal for determination of appropriateness of nipple type. There should be no set routine for what nipple to use first or when, but should be individualized based on the infant's behaviors and cues. (Bu'Lock, Woolridge, & Baum, 1990; Matthew, 1990, 1991; Schrank, Al-Sayed, Beahm, & Thach, 1998) |
| Swaddling the infant | Supports flexion with hands up and into body; supports development of flexion as well as decreases disorganized behaviors that could detract from feeding success. Positioning the infant so that the head is higher than the torso and holding the infant close to your body, supporting flexion and organization. (Shaker, 1999) |
| Burping | Can be very stressful for most preterm infants; however, there are ways to make this intervention less stressful. When possible, infants should be placed on the shoulder for support, and rubbing of the back is less stressful than patting. If a shoulder position is not tolerated, holding the infant upright on your lap with his head curled forward over your hand and rubbing the back should facilitate burping. |
| Infant-paced feeding | Allow the infant to decide when to suck and when to pause. Pausing allows the infant who has difficulty coordinating sucking, swallowing, and breathing to reorganize and continue with the feeding. Pausing is not the time for intervention; allow the infant to pace the feeding. (Jordan, 1998; Lau & Schanler, 2000; Hill, 2002; Medoff-Cooper, Verklan, & Carson, 1993) |
| Temperature | Temperature of the formula or breastmilk has been shown to have no real effect on feeding success; however, most believe that extremes should be avoided and that as close to room temperature as possible is most likely best for most infants. Infants who also go to breast might do better with bottle-feedings that are slightly warmer than room temperature. Consistency is an issue that needs to be considered. (Blumenthal, Lealman, & Shoesmith, 1989; Holt, Davies, Hasselmeyer, et al., 1962) |
| Kangaroo care | Kangaroo care before bottle-feeding might facilitate alertness and transition to quieter states, which could promote feeding success. Kangaroo care does not tire the infant and should not be avoided because the infant needs to rest for bottle-feeding. (Bohnhorst, Heyne, Peter, et al., 2001; Hurst, Valentine, Renfro, et al., 1997; Conde-Agudelo, Diaz-Rosello, & Belizan, 2001) |
| Non-nutritive sucking | Has been found to increase alertness during the feeding by calming the infant before the feeding. (McCain, 1995, 1997; McCain, Gartside, Greensberg, & Lott, 2001; Pickler, Mauck, & Geldmaker, 1997; Wolff, 1972) |

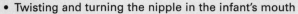

Box **17-9**    Caregiver Actions That Can Detract from Feeding Success

- Twisting and turning the nipple in the infant's mouth
- Pushing/pulling the bottle in and out of the infant's mouth
- Using a nipple with too large a hole, or one that is too soft
- Pushing infants to suck when they tire or are pausing, taking a break
- Putting vitamins or medications into the feeding, which might alter the taste. Preterm infants have been found to have a keener sense of taste than previously thought.

Modified from Shaker, C.S. (1990). Nipple feeding premature infants: A different perspective. *Neonatal Network, 8*(5), 9-16.

Box **17-10**    Interventions to Support Infant with Symptomatic Reflux or Feeding Intolerance

- Elevating the head of the bed at least 30 degrees.
- Positioning the infant in prone or sidelying position.
- Providing frequent feedings of small volumes to decrease gastric distention.
- Many care providers choose to thicken feedings with cereal; however, this practice must be done with consistency to be successful. The research that suggests thickening of feedings found that pre-thickened infant formulas (by the manufacturer) worked best. However, because these are seldom available, a consistent approach that guarantees uniformity is required (Vandenplas, Lifshitz, Orenstein, et al., 1998).
- Do not add cereal to formula until just before that feeding; cereal left in formula for extended periods becomes very thick and chunky in nature, diminishing the infant's ability to extract it from the nipple.
- Cross-cut nipples or large, single-hole nipples are suggested. Nipples that are cut by nursing staff at each feeding are inappropriate because the inconsistent size of the cut detracts from the infant's ability to regulate his/her own feeding. Sometimes the flow is too fast (large cuts in nipples increases chances for reflux), sometimes too slow (small cuts in nipple hole tire the infant quickly).
- Pharmacologic interventions should be reserved for when all other interventions have failed and should be monitored closely; they are not without their own issues and concerns.
- Gastrointestinal reflux is abnormal frequent passage of gastric contents into the esophagus. Reflux is experienced by many preterm infants and might detract from feeding success as well as delay growth and development.

systematically studied, but chin and cheek support appears to be effective (Einarsson-Backes, Dietz, Price, et al., 1994; Hill, Kurkowski, & Garcia, 2000); still, more research with other interventions is needed. Assessment of bottle-feeding success before discharge from the NICU is essential, so that infants and, thus, families are not at risk for feelings of failure, poor attachment, and/or re-hospitalization related to failure to thrive. More research is needed on aspects of breast-feeding, including use of an interdisciplinary, family-centered approach; factors that enhance breastfeeding success; and physiologic aspects on infant outcomes.

Another important area of research is the impact on methods of feeding on long-term consequences of development beyond the NICU and infancy periods.

## CONCLUSION

Feeding is a routine task that is often not considered a priority, especially given the critical care ambiance of the NICU. Research that holistically examines the dynamic process of bottle-feeding the preterm infant will enhance the feeding and transition of these infants from hospital to home. More importantly, it must be noted that bottle-feeding is an interactive process that requires reciprocity between the caregiver and infant; *both* members of the feeding dyad must be competent. Yet, no definition or set of objective components could be found in the literature that clearly delineated all the criteria that care providers use to describe "successful bottle-feeding." In one national survey study (Siddell & Froman, 1994), less than 50% of the nurses identified specific guidelines utilized in the nurseries where they worked for initiating bottle-feeding, and little to no explicit criteria were used for evaluating successful bottle-feeding. Therefore, given the recognized importance of successful bottle-feeding of preterm infants before discharge from the NICU, the lack of identified guidelines and criteria in regard to successful bottle-feeding and the lack of research in this area are serious concerns. Research that examines all the aspects of the NICU that impact this process will provide a better understanding of what is needed to further facilitate the transition from hospital to home for these high-risk infants and families. Feeding practices and their promotion in the NICU environment constitute a benchmark that is now a part of many parent-satisfaction surveys as well as a method of benchmarking for quality improvement regarding individualized, family-centered, developmental care (IFDC) (Saunders, Abraham, Crosby, et al., 2003). Feeding is one aspect of IFDC that requires a commitment to using infant and family cues to set up a plan of care. Feeding is a critical element in determining morbidity and mortality of infants, and we must recognize that use of IFDC is as well.

## ACKNOWLEDGMENT

Modified from McGrath, J.M., & Conliffe-Torres, S. (2000). *Feeding practices and nursing interventions in the NICU: A self-study module.* Des Plaines, IL: National Association of Neonatal Nurses.

## *REFERENCES*

Ahluwalia, I.B., Morrow, B., Hsia, J., et al. (2003). Who is breast-feeding? Recent trends form the pregnancy risk assessment and monitoring system. *Journal of Pediatrics, 142*(5), 486-491.

Als, H. (1982). Toward a synactive theory of development: Promise for the assessment of infant individuality. *Infant Mental Health Journal, 3*, 229-243.

American Academy of Pediatrics (AAP). (1996–1997). Work group on breastfeeding: Breastfeeding and the use of human milk. *Pediatrics, 100*(6), 1035-1039.

Ashland, J. (1995). *Successful feeding performance for premature infants: Qualitative and quantitative indicators* (doctoral dissertation). Arizona State University, Tempe, AZ.

Berseth, C.L. (1990). Neonatal small intestinal motility: Motor responses to feeding in term and preterm infants. *Journal of Pediatrics, 117*(4), 777-782.

Berseth, C.L., Bisquera, J.A., & Paje, V.U. (2003). Prolonging small feeding volumes early in life decreases the incidence of necrotizing enterocolitis in very low birth weight infants. *Pediatrics, 111*(3), 529-534.

Bishop, B.E. (1995). Infant feeding: Preventing the pitfalls. *American Journal of Maternal Child Nursing, 20*, 295.

Blackburn, S. (2003). *Maternal fetal and neonatal physiology: A clinical perspective* (2nd ed.). St Louis: W.B. Saunders.

Blumenthal, I., Lealman, G., & Shoesmith, D. (1989). Effect of feeding temperature and phototherapy on gastric emptying. *Archives in Disease in Childhood, 55*(1), 562-574.

Bohnhorst, B., Heyne, T., & Peter, C.S., et al. (2001). Skin-to-skin (kangaroo) care, respiratory control, and thermoregulation. *Journal of Pediatrics, 138*, 93-197.

Bu'Lock, F., Woolridge, M.W., & Baum, J.D. (1990). Development of coordination of sucking, swallowing and breathing: Ultrasound study of term and preterm infants. *Developmental Medicine and Child Neurology, 32*(8), 669-678.

Burrin, D.G., & Stoll, B. (2002). Key nutrients and growth factors for the neonatal gastrointestinal tract. *Clinical Perinatology, 29*(2), 65-96.

Case-Smith, J., Cooper, P., & Scala, V. (1989). Feeding efficiency of premature neonates. *American Journal of Occupational Therapy, 43*(4), 245-250.

Clark, R.H., Wagner, C.L., Merritt, R.J., et al. (2003). Nutrition in the neonatal intensive care unit: How do we reduce the incidence of extrauterine growth restriction? *Journal of Perinatology, 23*(4), 337-344.

Collinge, J.M., Bradley, K., Perks, C., et al. (1982). Demand vs. scheduled feedings for premature infants. *Journal of Obstetric, Gynecologic, and Neonatal Nursing (JOGNN), 11*, 362-367.

Conde-Agudelo, A., Diaz-Rosello, J.L., & Belizan, J.M. (2001). Kangaroo care to reduce morbidity and mortality in low birthweight infants (Cocherane review). In *Cochrane library* (issue 2). Oxford: Update Software.

Conway, A. (1994). Instruments in neonatal research: Measuring preterm infant feeding ability, Part 1: Bottle-feeding. *Neonatal Network, 13*(4), 71-73.

de Pipaon, S., VanBeek, R.H., Quero, J., et al. (2003). Effect of minimal enteral feeding on splanchnic uptake of leucine in the postabsorptive state in preterm infants. *Pediatric Research, 53*(2), 281-287.

DiGirolamo, A.M., Brummer-Strawn, L.M., & Fein, S.B. (2003). Do perceived attitudes of physicians and hospital staff affect breastfeeding decisions? *Birth, 30*(2), 94-100.

Dowling, D. (1999). Physiological responses of preterm infants to breastfeeding and bottle feeding with the orthodontic nipple. *Nursing Research, 48*(2), 78-85.

Duara, S. (1989). Oral feeding containers and their influence on intake and ventilation in preterm infants. *Biology of the Neonate, 56*(5), 270-276.

Einarsson-Backes, L.M., Deitz, J., Price, R., et al. (1994). The effect of oral support on sucking efficiency in preterm infants. *American Journal of Occupational Therapy, 48*(6), 490-498.

Fischer, K.W., & Rose, S.P. (1994). Dynamic development of coordination of components in brain and behavior: A framework for theory and research (pp. 3-66). In G. Dawson & K.W. Fischer (Eds.), *Human behavior and the developing brain.* New York: Guilford.

Fletcher, M. (1998). *Physical diagnosis in neonatology.* Philadelphia: Lippincott-Raven.

Glass, R.P., & Wolf, L.S. (1994). A global perspective on feeding assessment in the neonatal intensive care unit. *American Journal of Occupational Therapy, 48*(6), 514-526.

Griffin, T.L., Meier, P.P., Bradford, L.P., et al. (2000). Mothers' performing creamatocrit measures in the NICU: Accuracy, reactions, and cost. *Journal of Obstetric, Gynecologic, and Neonatal Nursing (JOGNN), 29*(3), 249-257.

Gryboski, J. (1969). Suck and swallow in the premature infant. *Pediatrics, 43,* 96-102.

Hack, M., Estabrook, M.M., & Robertson, S.R. (1985). Development of sucking rhythm in preterm infants. *Early Human Development, 11,* 133-140.

Hill, A.S. (2002). Toward a theory of feeding efficiency for bottle-fed preterm infants. *The Journal of Theory Construction & Testing, 6*(1), 75-81.

Hill, A.S., Kurkowski, T.B., & Garcia, J. (2000). Oral feeding support measures used in feeding the preterm infant. *Nursing Research, 49*(1), 2-10.

Hill, A.S., & Rath, L.S. (1999). The relationship between drooling, age, sucking pattern characteristics, and physiological parameters of preterm infants during bottlefeeding. *Research and Nursing Practice.* Available online at *www.graduateresearch.com.*

Hill, A.S., & Rath, L. (1993). The care and feeding of the low-birth-weight infant. *Journal of Perinatal and Neonatal Nursing, 6*(4), 56-68.

Ho, M.Y., Yen, Y.H., Hsieh, M.C., et al. (2003). Early versus late nutrition support in premature neonates with respiratory distress syndrome. *Nutrition, 19*(3), 257-260.

Holt, L.E., Davies, E.A., Hasselmeyer, EG., et al. (1962). A study of premature infants fed cold formulas. *Journal of Pediatrics, 61,* 556-561.

Hurst, N.M., Valentine, C.J., Renfro, L., et al. (1997). Skin-to-skin holding in the Neonatal Intensive Care Unit: Influences on maternal milk volume. *Journal of Perinatology, 17*(3), 213-217.

Ichord, R.N. (1992). Advances in neonatal neurology. *Pediatric Annals, 21*(6), 339-345.

Jordon, S. (1998). The controlled or paced bottle feeding. *Neonatal Network, 3*(2), 21-24.

Kenner, C., Bagwell, G.A., & Torok, L.S. (2003). Transition to home (pp. 893-901). In C. Kenner & J.W. Lott (Eds.), *Comprehensive neonatal nursing: A physiologic perspective* (3rd ed.). St. Louis: W.B. Saunders.

Kenner, C., & Lott, J.W. (2004). *Neonatal nursing handbook.* St. Louis: W.B. Saunders.

Kinneer, M.D., & Beachy, P. (1994). Nipple feeding premature infants in the neonatal intensive-care unit: Factors and decisions. *Journal of Obstetric, Gynecologic, and Neonatal Nursing (JOGNN), 23*(20), 105-112.

Kliethermes, P.A., Cross, M.L., Lanese, M.G., et al. (1999). Transitioning preterm infants with nasogastric tube supplementation: Increasing likelihood of breastfeeding. *Journal of Obstetric, Gynecologic, and Neonatal Nursing (JOGNN), 28*(3), 264-273.

Koenig, J.S., Davies, A.M., & Thach, B.T. (1990). Coordination of breathing, sucking, and swallowing during bottle feedings in human infants. *Journal of Applied Physiology, 69*(5), 1623-1629.

Lau, C., & Schanler, R.J. (2000). Oral feeding in premature infants: Advantage of a self-paced milk flow. *Aceta Paediatrics, 89,* 453-459.

Marmet, C., & Shell, E. (1984). Training neonates to suck correctly. *American Journal of Maternal Child Nursing: MCN, 9,* 401-407.

Mason-Wyckoff, M., McGrath, J.M., Griffin, T., et al. (2003). Nutrition: Physiologic basis of metabolism and management of enteral and parenteral nutrition (pp. 425-447). In C. Kenner & J.W. Lott (Eds.), *Comprehensive neonatal nursing: A physiologic perspective* (3rd ed.). St. Louis: W.B. Saunders.

Mathew, O.P. (1988). Nipple units for newborn infants: A functional comparison. *Pediatrics, 81*(50), 688-691.

Mathew, O.P. (1990). Determinants of milk flow through nipple units: Role of hole size and nipple thickness. *American Journal of Disease in Children, 144*(2), 222-224.

Mathew, O.P. (1991). Science of bottle-feeding. *Pediatrics, 119*(4), 511-519.

Mathew, O.P., Belan, M., & Thoppil, C. (1992). Sucking patterns of neonates during bottle-feeding: Comparison of different nipple units. *American Journal of Perinatology, 9,* 265-269.

Mathew, O.P., & Bhatia, J. (1989). Sucking and breathing patterns during breast- and bottle-feeding in term neonates. *American Journal of Disease in Children, 143,* 588-592.

Mathew, O.P., Clark, M.L., Pronske, M.L., et al. (1985). Breathing pattern and ventilation during oral feeding in term newborn infants. *Journal of Pediatrics, 106,* 810-813.

Mathews, C.L. (1994). Supporting suck-swallow-breathing coordination during nipple feeding. *American Journal of Occupational Therapy, 48,* 561-562.

McCain, G.C. (1995). Promotion of preterm infant nipple feeding with nonnutritive sucking. *Journal of Pediatric Nursing, 10*(1), 3-8.

McCain, G.C. (1997). Behavioral state activity during nipple feedings for preterm infants. *Neonatal Network, 16*(5), 43-47.

McCain, G.C., Gartside, P.S., Greensberg, J.M., & Lott, J.W. (2001). A feeding protocol for healthy preterm infants that shortens time to oral feeding. *Journal of Pediatrics, 139*(3), 374-379.

McGrath, J.M. (1999). *Maturation of alertness in extremely early born preterm infants: Prior to caregiving and during a feeding protocol in the NICU* (unpublished doctoral dissertation). University of Pennsylvania, School of Nursing, Philadelphia, PA.

McGrath, J.M., & Medoff-Cooper, B. (2002). Alertness and feeding competence in extremely early born preterm infants. *Newborn and Infant Nursing Reviews, 2*(3), 174-186.

Medoff-Cooper, B., & Brooten, D. (1987). Relation of the feeding cycle to neurobehavioral assessment in preterm infants: A pilot study. *Nursing Research, 36*(5), 315-317.

Medoff-Cooper, B., McGrath, J.M., & Bilker, W. (2000). Nutritive sucking and neurobehavioral development in preterm infants from 34 weeks PCA to term. *American Journal of Maternal Child Nursing: MCN, 25*(2), 64-70.

Medoff-Cooper, B., & Ray, W. (1995). Neonatal sucking behaviors. *Image: Journal of Nursing Scholarship, 27*(3), 95-200.

Medoff-Cooper, B., Verklan, T., & Carlson, S. (1993). The development of sucking patterns and physiologic correlates in very-low-birthweight infants. *Nursing Research, 42*(2), 100-105.

Medoff-Cooper, B., Weininger, S., & Zukowsky, K. (1989). Neonatal sucking as an assessment tool: Preliminary findings. *Nursing Research, 38*(3), 162-164.

Meier, P., & Anderson, G.C. (1987). Responses of small preterm infants to bottle- and breast-feeding. *American Journal of Maternal Child Nursing: MCN, 12*, 97-105.

Meier, P., & Brown, L. (1996). State of the science: Breastfeeding for mothers and low-birthweight infants. *Nursing Clinics of North America, 31*(2), 351-365.

Meier, P.P. (2001). Breastfeeding in the special care nursery: Prematures and infants with medical problems. *Pediatric Clinics of North America, 48*(2), 425-442.

Meier, P.P., & Mangurten, H.H. (1993). Breastfeeding the preterm infant. In J. Riordan & K. Auerbach (Eds.), *Breastfeeding and human lactation*. Boston: Jones & Bartlett.

Merritt, T.A., Piller, D., & Prows, S.L. (2003). Early NICU discharge of very low birth weight infant: A critical review and analysis. *Seminars in Neonatalogy, 8*, 95-115.

Miles, M.S., Funk, S.G., & Kasper, M.A. (1991). The neonatal intensive care unit environment: Source of stress for parents. *American Association of Critical Care Nurses (AACN): Clinical Issues, 2*(2), 346-354.

Miller, A.J. (1986). Neurophysiological basis of swallowing. *Dysphagia, 1*, 91-100.

Moore, K.L., & Persaud, T.V.N. (2003). *The Developing human: Clinically oriented embryology* (7th ed.). St. Louis: W.B. Saunders.

Morriss, F.H. Jr., Moore, M., Weisbrodt, N.W., et al. (1986). Ontogenic development of gastrointestinal motility: IV. Duodenal contractions in preterm infants. *Pediatrics, 78*(6), 1106-1113.

Nascimento, M.B., & Issler, H. (2003). Breastfeeding: Making the difference in the development, health and nutrition of term and preterm newborns. *Reviews of Hospital and Clinical Faculty of Medicine Sao Paulo, 58*(1), 49-60.

Pereira, G.R., & Balmer, D. (1996). Feeding the critically ill neonate. In A.R. Spitzer (Ed.), *Intensive care of the fetus and neonate* (pp. 823-833). St. Louis: Mosby.

Pickler, R.H., Frankel, H.B., Walsh, K.M., et al. (1996). Effects of nonnutritive sucking on behavioral organization and feeding performance in preterm infants. *Nursing Research, 45*(3), 132-135.

Pickler, R.H., Mauck, A.G., & Geldmaker, B. (1997). Bottle-feeding histories of preterm infants. *Journal of Obstetric, Gynecologic, and Neonatal Nursing (JOGNN), 26*(4), 414-420.

Pinch, W., & Spielman, N. (1990). The parents' perspective: Ethical decision-making in neonatal intensive care. *Journal of Advanced Nursing, 15*, 712-719.

Premji, S., & Chessell, L. (2001). Continuous nasogastric milk feeding versus intermittent bolus milk feeding for premature infants less than 1500 grams. *Cochrane Database Systematic Reviews, 1*, CD001819.

Pridham, K., Kosorok, M.R., Greer, F., et al. (1999). The effects of prescribed versus ad libitum feedings and formula caloric density on premature infant dietary intake and weight gain. *Nursing Research, 48*(2), 86-93.

Pridham, K.F., Sondel, S., Chang, A., et al. (1993). Nipple feeding for preterm infants with bronchopulmonary dysplasia. *Journal of Obstetric, Gynecologic, and Neonatal Nursing (JOGNN), 22*(2), 147-154.

Rudolph, C.D. (1994). Feeding disorders in infants and children. *Journal of Pediatrics, 125*(6)(Pt 2), S116-S124.

Sameroff, A.J. (1968). The components of sucking in the human newborn. *Journal of Experimental Child Psychology, 6*, 607-623.

Saunders, R.P., Abraham, M.R., Crosby, M.J., et al. (2003). Evaluation and development of potentially better practices for improving family-centered care in neonatal intensive care units. *Pediatrics, 111*(4)(Pt 2), e437-e449.

Saunders, R.B., Friedman, C.B., & Stramoski, P.R. (1990). Feeding preterm infants: Schedule or demand. *Journal of Obstetric, Gynecologic, and Neonatal Nursing (JOGNN), 20*(3), 212-218.

Schrank, W., Al-Sayed, L.E., Beahm, P.H., & Thach, B.T. (1998). Feeding responses to free-flow formula in term and preterm infants. *Journal of Pediatrics, 132*(3)(Pt 1), 426-430.

Shaker, C.S. (1990). Nipple feeding premature infants: A different perspective. *Neonatal Network, 8*(5), 9-16.

Shaker, C.S. (1999). Nipple feeding preterm infants: An individualized, developmentally supportive approach. *Neonatal Network, 18*(3), 15-22.

Shiao, S.P.K., Youngblut, J.M., Anderson, G.C., et al. (1995). Nasogastric tube placement: Effects on breathing and sucking in very-low-birth-weight infants. *Nursing Research, 44*(2), 82-88.

Shivpuri, C.R., Martin, R.J., Carlo, W.A., et al. (1983). Decreased ventilation in preterm infants during oral feeding. *Journal of Pediatrics, 103*, 285-289.

Siddell, E.P., & Froman, R.D. (1994). A national survey of neonatal intensive care units: Criteria used to determine readiness for oral feedings. *Journal of Obstetric, Gynecologic, and Neonatal Nursing (JOGNN), 23*(9), 783-789.

Simpson, C., Schanler, R.J., & Lau, C. (2002). Early introduction of oral feeding in preterm infants. *Pediatrics, 110*(3), 517-522.

Slater-Myer, L.P., Saslow, J.G., & Stahl, G.E. (1996). Development of the gastrointestinal tract (pp. 843-856). In A.R. Spitzer (Ed.), *Intensive care of the fetus and neonate.* St. Louis: Mosby.

Symington, A., Ballantyne, M., Pinelli, J., et al. (1995). Indwelling versus intermittent feeding tubes in premature neonates. *Journal of Obstetric, Gynecologic, and Neonatal Nursing (JOGNN), 24*(4), 321-326.

Timms, B.J., DiFiore, J.M., Martin, R.J., et al. (1993). Increased respiratory drive as an inhibitor of oral feeding of preterm infants. *Journal of Pediatrics, 123*(1), 127-131.

Troche, B., Harvey-Wilkes, K., Engle, W.D., et al. (1995). Early minimal feedings promote growth in critically ill premature infants. *Biology of Neonate, 67*(30), 172-181.

Tuchman, D.N. (1994). Physiology of the swallowing apparatus (pp. 1-25). In D.N. Tuchman & R.S. Walter (Eds.), *Disorders of feeding and swallowing in infants and children: Pathophysiology, diagnosis, and treatment.* San Diego: Singular.

Tuchman, D.N., & Walter, R.S. (Eds.). (1994). *Disorders of feeding and swallowing in infants and children: Pathophysiology, diagnosis, and treatment.* San Diego: Singular.

VandenBerg, K.A. (1990). Nippling management of the sick neonate in the NICU: The disorganized feeder. *Neonatal Network, 9*(1), 10-11 .

Vandenplas, Y., Lifshitz, J.Z., Orenstein, S., et al. (1998). Nutritional management of regurgitation in infants. *Journal of the American College of Nutrition, 17*(4), 308-316.

Vidyasagar, D., Theorell, C., & Peters, B. (2003). *Guideline for breastfeeding for the newborn infant in the NICU/ICN.* Chicago, IL: University of Illinois Medical Center at Chicago Women's and Children's Nursing Services.

Warren, J.J., & Bishara, S.E. (2002). Duration of nutritive and nonnutritive sucking behaviors and their effects on the dental arches in the primary dentation. *American Journal of Orthodontics & Dentofacial Orthopedics, 121*(4), 347-356.

Wolff, P.H. (1968). The serial organization of sucking in the young infant. *Pediatrics, 42*, 943-955.

Wolff, P.H. (1972). The interaction of state and nonnutritive sucking. *Third symposium on oral sensation and perception.* Springfield, IL: Charles C. Thomas.

# 18 Family Issues/Professional-Parent Partnerships

Lois V. S. Gates, Jacqueline M. McGrath, and
Katherine M. Jorgensen

Because the focus of this text is individualized family-centered, developmental care (IFDC), many concepts related to the family and implementation of developmental strategies that support family outcomes are found in several chapters throughout the text. First, we see families as the primary co-regulator of their infant within the echo niche that families create for their infant; that fosters that infants' humanness (see Chapter 3). We acknowledge that the trust that must form between the infant and the primary caretaker is essential to this developmental process. Then we see families in terms of the influence a mother and the maternal environment has on the infant's development prior to birth (see Chapter 9), acknowledging the importance of not only the in utero environment but also the relationship already beginning to form between the infant and family. From there, we explore the developmental influences of families as the primary animate environment for the infant/child in the context of the neonatal intensive care unit (NICU) (see Chapter 14). Lastly, we explore the relationship of parents and families with their infants as the ideal place for developmentally appropriate caregiving and intervention to occur (see Chapter 15).

In this chapter, the issues related to parents/family are explored through the belief that forming a *partnership* with families is the ideal way to foster their role as "expert" in relationship to their child, and to better equip them with the skills they will need to be their child's best advocate after they leave the confines of the NICU.

Parenting is a proving ground under the most idyllic setting and greatly challenged when life begins in the NICU. Traditionally, nurses, physicians, and therapists have designated themselves as NICU primary caregivers. This is changing and, to some extent,

we encourage parents to visit and participate in care, but mostly on our terms of timing and activity, and more in the areas of tasks or caregiving they can provide than in building relationships.

However, there is an increasing appreciation that parenting has a profound impact on long-term outcomes for NICU graduates. Furthermore, parenting is a very complex role. There are many influences on parenting style: these include, but are not limited to, the life experiences, expectations, cultural values and beliefs, social support, and emotional status of the parents. Interactions and vulnerabilities among parents and children as well as among family and community support systems influence parenting style and substance (Minde & Minde, 1998).

Within the context of parenting as a very complex and influential role, NICU professionals have an opportunity to recognize that parents are not visitors. They are *partners* in the care of their infant. We need to partner with parents throughout the hospital stay. Such a partnership has the potential to stabilize and strengthen the family unit toward positive parenting behaviors that nurture child development. In this chapter, we review various aspects of parenting as related to developmental outcomes within the context of a partnership.

## PROFESSIONAL-PARENT PARTNERSHIPS

A partnership exists when there is a relationship between two or more parties that have a shared goal. A professional-parent partnership must be contingent and supportive, contain both independent and dependent variables, and share risks and benefits (Bruns & McCollum, 2002). The contingent and supportive aspect embraces the reality that every parent-professional dyad has a slightly different hue, based

on the strengths and understanding of each participant. The independent and dependent variables flex
according to the issue at stake—be it ventilator management, the type of nutrition provided, or the
infant's feeding schedule. Effective partnerships
between professionals and families must be based on
mutual respect, valuing family expertise, fully shared
information, and joint decision-making (Hobbs &
Sodomka, 2000). Finally, there are shared benefits
and risks. Potential benefits include decreased length
of stay (LOS), increased satisfaction for both staff and
parents, and enhanced neurodevelopmental outcomes for the infant. Both professionals and parents
must view the partnership as a commitment to the
needs of the infant. Failure to trust and work together
adds potential social risk for the infant. A partnership
of integrated medical and parent care offers the
infant the best opportunity for developmentally
sound outcomes (Cusson & Lee, 1994; Costello &
Chapman, 1998).

To be successful in partnership toward a shared
interest or goal, we sometimes have to step outside
of our roles as health professionals to more fully
understand the world of the other party (the parents). We as professionals feel "at home" in the
NICU, familiar with the sights, sounds, and smells
all around us as we focus on the assessment, ventilation, feeding, medication administration, or procedure at hand. However, the parents often enter a
bewildering, unfamiliar environment, still exhausted from delivery, and emotionally drained by their
current crises. It is when professionals step out of
their scientific, technical realm and peer into the
social and emotional sphere of the parents that they
can more effectively engage in care planning and
problem solving with the family (Bruce & Ritchie,
1997; Speedling, 1997).

Another issue to consider in the development of
this partnership is the belief that professionals have
about the role of families in the NICU. For a true
partnership to form, families must be on an equal
playing field with the professionals. They must not be
*visitors*. They must be active players in the caregiving
team and, as such, they are essential participants in
the decision-making process (Stainton, Prentice,
Lindrea, et al., 2001). Members of the caregiving team
are welcome at anytime. They are not asked to leave

for rounds or report. They are not asked to leave for
procedures or in crisis situations. They are encouraged to actively participate as their child's advocates
in all of these events. They can choose who visits their
child, and they are not included in the count if there
is to be a limited number of visitors at the bedside
because of space. In this partnership, parents can
choose when to bring in "well" siblings. They can
make decisions about caregiving schedules, such as
when their infant will be bathed, when the bottle-
feedings will occur, and in which parts of these caregiving interventions they will be involved. Not all
parents/families want to be involved or be present in
all these situations, but it should be their choice to
choose which they will participate in and how much
(Mason, 2003).

Implementing this concept is not easy, given the
existing culture and environment of the NICU. Despite the growing evidence to support family-centered
care interventions, most healthcare providers want to
implement the strategies only when it is convenient
for them. Fear about what families might encounter as
well as fear from the healthcare team about the efficacy of this practice is associated with the resistance to
implementation (McGahey, 2002). Proposed advantages and disadvantages of family presence are outlined in Box 18-1. Major arguments against family
presence include (Mason, 2003):

- There is not enough research to support this
  change in practice. The truth is there is also little
  evidence to support the tradition of keeping parents and families out of the room during invasive
  procedures.
- Family presence increases the number of malprac-
  tice suits. Again, evidence does not support this
  belief. Family presence during these events allows
  the development of strong bonds between families and professionals. Families also see first hand
  that everything possible was done for their child
  (MacLean, Guzzetta, White, et al., 2003).
- Nurses and physicians disagree on the issue, and
  this disagreement can deepen the chasm between
  these two professionals. Educating physicians,
  administrators, and all health professionals is the
  key to overcoming this consideration. Few institutions have policies or procedures to address this
  practice, making implementation at this time, for

Box 18-1 PROPOSED ADVANTAGES AND DISADVANTAGES OF FAMILY PRESENCE DURING RESUSCITATION AND INVASIVE PROCEDURES

**Advantages**

Bonding between family members healthcare provider is facilitated.

Family members can observe the efforts of the healthcare team, and the mystery of activities behind closed doors is reduced.

Family members can provide comfort to their infant speak words of encouragement, and touch their infant.

Family freedom to obtain closure, accept outcome of efforts, are facilitated.

Families perceive that they are actively involved, participating in the resuscitative efforts or the invasive procedure.

Being present during resuscitation or an invasive procedure, rather than hearing a verbal accounting, might dispel the family's doubts about the course of events.

Family-centered care with holistic approach with acknowledgment of family as part of the infant is fostered.

**Disadvantages**

Family members might disrupt the resuscitation and efforts.

Healthcare staff might not be able to control their emotions in front of families.

Fear of litigation might inhibit staff from performing necessary tasks well.

Potential exists for emotional scarring of family or staff, with violent emotional memories of the event.

Long-term effects on family's emotional status are unknown.

Family might not understand the tasks or procedures that are being performed.

Having the family present might influence the decision about the duration of the resuscitation efforts.

Modified from McGahey, P.R. (2002). Family presence during pediatric resuscitation: A focus on staff. *Critical Care Nurse, 22*(6) 29-34.

the most part, haphazard. MacLean, Guzzetta, White, et al. (2003) found that less than 5% of the nurses who responded to their study had policies to support family presence during resuscitation and invasive procedures, although more than 50% of them worked on units that allowed this practice.

- Having family members present during invasive procedures will make the healthcare team nervous and, thus, could negatively affect the care of the infant/child. There is no compelling evidence to support this argument, and most healthcare professionals would argue that often the positive affects of this situation outweigh the negative affects.

- Not enough is known about the psychosocial impact on the family who is present during these events. Only one randomized trial has addressed this issue (Robinson, Mackenzie-Ross, Campbell-Hewson, et al., 1998), and no negative effects were found; in fact, the trial was stopped because the effects were so positive for families.

Parents must be well informed of their infant's needs and care and, for the most part, we do that.

What we do not do is always keep them informed of the *implications*, both short- and long-term, of the issues at hand (King, 1992). In an observational study of 18 infants and families in the NICU, it was found that although we often provide families with information about their infant and the here and now, we often do not provide them with the "so what" of this information (King, 1992). What was noted was that parents were given all the information needed to legally make informed consent decisions for the child, but they often were not told all the possible implications. This was where professionals showed an overall hesitance to generalize because of the uncertainties of the situation, and, therefore, parents were not always provided with all the information they needed to understand the whole situation for their child.

This kind of problem can be alleviated when parents are considered part of the caregiving team. They are involved in decision-making discussions. They are active participants in nursing/medical rounds, and they have full disclosure and understanding of the medical record. Parents/families have begun to be included in medical rounds in many NICUs around the country; however, this inclusion does not meet the criteria of a professional-parent partnership if they are not an active part of the discussion and decision-making process for their child. Just being present without true understanding of the discussion is not enough (Mason, 2003). Parents must be truly educated, and have confidence in both their knowledge and their role to believe that their input will be acknowledged as equal in the decision-making for true membership in the caregiving team to exist.

Thorne and Robinson (1988a, 1988b, 1989) conducted a qualitative study with family members of chronically ill patients who were actively involved in healthcare relationships. The researchers found three stages families progressed through in developing relationships with their healthcare providers. Families initiated the relationship, engaging in *naïve trust.* They began their relationships with the healthcare professionals passively believing everyone would act in the best interest of their family member. They believed they would always be informed of care and would be included in decision-making.

Predictably, over time, differences in needs began to surface, and family members became *disenchanted* (the second stage) with the healthcare providers. The more unmet expectations the family encountered, the less trust they had in the healthcare system. *Guarded alliance,* the final stage, was established because of the families' need to somehow be involved and in control of their family member's care. Families became more informed and able to maneuver the healthcare system because of their past experiences. They knew who to trust, and began to know what questions to ask, and although they were not completely satisfied with all the relationships, they began to form trusting relationships with a few healthcare professionals. They chose these professionals not because they were the most

medically competent, but because they treated their family member with the most compassion. They appeared to really care. This caring was greatly valued by family members.

Additionally, the researchers were able to sort the families who had progressed to guarded alliance into four distinct categories (Figure 18-1). These categories portrayed how the participants reconstructed trust with the healthcare professionals. The first category was "hero worship." Families chose one particular healthcare provider they could depend on for information and support. This healthcare provider is trusted above other professionals. The family member's choice of healthcare

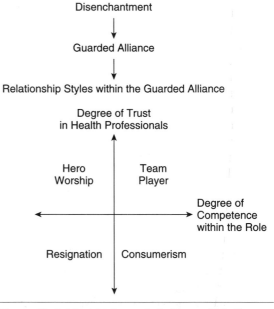

Figure **18-1**  Model of guarded alliance. This figure demonstrates the relationship between the degree of trust and competence within the model. (*Adapted from Thorne, S.E., & Robinson, C.A. [1989]. Guarded alliance: Healthcare relationships in chronic illness.* Image: Journal of Nursing Scholarship, 21[3], 156.)

provider was often based on a particular personality trait of the professional that family members found made the professional seem more like themselves. This sort of relationship was uncertain and difficult to maintain because it placed a high degree of dependency on one particular health professional. It also did not place as much responsibility for decision-making on the family member.

Some families were unable to establish any trust with healthcare providers. They were skeptical of everyone. They continued to stay involved with the healthcare provider because they felt they had no choice and had no control over the situation. However, they did not appear responsible for their healthcare choices either. Sometimes, it appeared as if they chose "resignation" (the second category) because it was less draining and required less energy compared with other choices.

Other families chose to deal with the system through "consumerism" (the third category). These families saw their role as one in which they needed to become expert consumers. They learned to maneuver the system and became excellent at finding ways to get their needs met. They became well informed and used the information about their infants' illness to increase manipulation of the system. They were in control of their health care, but they were completely responsible, also. This increased burden required increased energy expenditure on the part of the family.

The last category, "team playing," occurred when the family and the healthcare professional worked together, both acknowledging the strengths of the family as well as the limitations of medical science and deficits of the system to meet the needs of the family and ill family member. There was collaboration and a reciprocal trusting relationship with ownership shared by both participants. Responsibilities and limitations were clear and shared.

Although some family members consistently chose one type of relationship for interacting with healthcare professionals, most fluctuated between types and chose different styles of communication in different relationships and at different times. The four relationships can also be described in terms of the degree of trust and competence displayed by each participant. Family members with low trust in the healthcare provider and low competence (knowledge and understanding) related to the illness would most likely rely on resignation as a way to maneuver the system whereas family members who had developed a trusting relationship and understood the illness of their family member as well as the limitations of medical science would function more as a team player. Each of the four types can be valuable in a given situation because a family member cannot always have all the information; consequently, healthcare professionals need to be flexible and aware of the decisions families might make to best meet their needs. Although this research was not done in the NICU, the model does have application in our interactions with families (McGrath, 2001). More research needs to be done that addresses not only the needs of families but also the needs of health professionals, especially in the environment of the NICU.

## CORE VALUES

As in any partnership, the core values supporting the mission and philosophy shared within the partnership drive decision-making and implementation of strategies. The core values are the expected outcomes for which we are striving. One component of any NICU mission is to promote/maintain excellence in health care for neonates and young infants. Historically, in the NICU, science and technology have often propelled the medical management of the infant (McGrath, 2000). Newer developmental and psychosocial values, based on the increasing evidence that IFDC is not only good for the infant but is also good for families, are the basis for the implementation of IFDC. Therefore, core values that are the foundation for the professional-parent partnership in the NICU include the following:
- Bonding is critical to positive parenting.
- The parent is the single constant in the child's life.
- Parents are the "experts" on their child's characteristics and needs.

When we incorporate these values into a philosophy of action, we engage in communications and activities that nurture the family. Flexible times and spaces for parents support the bonding and caring process between parent and infant. Frequent inter-actions between the parent and infant support the primary developmental task of the infant: that of establishing trust with the environment. Remember this trust is what provides the infant the freedom to explore and experience the environment. Through these interactions, the parent's love and attention sets the stage for nurturance and protection. The long-term developmental and health needs of the child are contingent on the parent's ability to care for and nurture the child; that parental ability is based on a strong bond of love and a sense of duty toward the child. This relationship must be both supported and expected in the NICU.

## PARTNERSHIP BENEFITS

Professional-parent partnerships have the potential to form a solid bridge across the chasm between the NICU and home for high-risk infants and families. The foundation of such a bridge is a relationship based on respect and trust and becomes a working alliance toward healthy discharge where parents become confident in their role as parent of this child (Speedling, 1997).

### Potential Benefits

There are several potential benefits for infants and families in a working professional-parent alliance:
• Supports the parent-infant bond
• Enhances parent-infant communication
• Supports the integrity of the family unit
• Eases the transition home (Lawhon, 2002; Pearson & Anderson, 2001)

## PARENT-INFANT BOND

Kennell and Klaus (1998) define bond as "a unique relationship between two people that is specific for those two and endures through time." The parent-child dyad is influenced by both intrinsic and extrinsic factors within and between parents, child, family and community. The addition of a caregiver makes this a triadic relationship and can create a barrier to the bonding and interacting process. The NICU presents a number of challenges to the parent-infant bond (Haut, Peddicord, & O'Brien, 1994). Poor visibility of the infant coupled with unfamiliar sights and sounds

leads to barriers to holding. These factors can hinder bonding. However, this process must take place.

Haut, Peddicord, and O'Brien (1994) identify three distinct levels of bonding that can affect families in the NICU. The first traverses labor and delivery and admission into the NICU. This first level of bonding can be lengthened by both preterm labor and prolonged stabilization. The family "hangs" in the world of the unknown during this stage. Fretful about the possibilities related to the potential birth, stabilization, or even death of their child, families might pull away at this time and be afraid to think in terms of the child yet to be born as real or something they can hold on to.

The second level of bonding occurs during the long hospitalization. During this period, the initial look and touch by the parent advances to beginning care giving. Although the child is now born, the parents might feel more separated and distant (and this might be real) than they did during the first phase. Attempts at early bonding during this stage are often frustrated by: the length of time parent and child are separated, machines surrounding the infant, inconsistent infant progress, and the demands of family and work lives. As hospitalization lengthens, the momentum of bonding is threatened by the very lack of infant progression. Parents might feel they are unable to parent as they would like, or they might not be confident in their care compared with the care provided by the professionals in the NICU. If the child is very ill, they might also feel as if what they provide is meaningless, especially when they cannot hold or comfort their infant or when they must stand by and watch their child in pain. When the scope of parent care cannot be advanced, it is important to vary the activity of parenting, according to the infant's developmental status, to maintain an intact thread of bonding.

Finally, as discharge approaches and parents prepare to assume complete care of the infant, a new angst threatens the bonding process. This third level of the bonding process occurs as the parents prepare and transition from the hospital to the home with their infant. Often discharge comes so long after birth, and follows a plateau of balancing hospitalization and family lives, that parents experience difficulty in learning the tasks of caring for their infant and assuming the responsibility for decision making about the infant's care.

Throughout hospitalization, parents need support as they adapt to not only their role as new parents of this infant (even if they have other children), but as parents to a hospitalized infant. Such support should include providing parents with both the rights and responsibilities of the parent of a hospitalized infant (Box 18-2). Using developmental time-

lines and activities, a professional-parent partnership supports both the infant and parent needs.

## PARENT-INFANT COMMUNICATIONS

Successful parenting is relationship based. The ability of parents to establish a caring relationship with their child is influenced by many social factors. However, following preterm birth, this relationship is also compromised by the infant's limited ability to

---

**BOX 18-2    CONSUMER BILL OF RIGHTS AND RESPONSIBILITIES: FAMILY-CENTERED CARE**

| | |
|---|---|
| Information disclosure | Families as consumers have the right to receive accurate, easily understood information, and some might require assistance in making informed healthcare decisions about their health plans, professionals, and facilities. |
| Choice of providers and plans | Families have the right to a choice of healthcare providers that is sufficient to ensure access to appropriate high-quality health care. |
| Access to emergency services | Consumers have the right to access emergency healthcare services when and where the need arises. Health plans should provide payment whenever the consumer has reasonably and appropriately used these services. |
| Participation in treatment decisions | Families have the right and responsibility to full participation in all decisions related to the care of their child. |
| Respect and nondiscrimination | Families have the right to considerate, respectful care from all members of the healthcare system at all times and under all circumstances. An environment of mutual respect is essential to maintain a quality healthcare system. |
| | Families might not be discriminated against in the delivery of healthcare services or healthcare plan benefits as required by law based on race, ethnicity, national origin, religion, gender, age, mental or physical disability, sexual orientation, genetic information, or payment source. |
| Confidentiality of health information | Families have the right to confidentiality. Families have the right to review and copy the medical records of their child and request amendments to those records. |
| Complaints and appeals | Families have the right to a fair and efficient process for resolving differences with health plans, healthcare providers, and the institutions that serve them, including a righteous system for internal review and an independent system for external review. |
| Consumer responsibilities | In a healthcare system that protects consumer/family rights, it is reasonable to expect and encourage families to assume reasonable responsibilities. Greater individual involvement by consumers in their care increases the likelihood of achieving the best outcomes and helps support a quality improvement, cost-conscious environment. |

Adapted from Leyden, C.H. (1998). Consumer bill of rights: Family-centered care. *Pediatric Nursing, 24*(1). 72-73.

give positive feedback to parents. Reciprocity between infant and parent has long been known to fuel this relationship and add to the growth and development of the child as well as the positive parenting skills of the parent. When we educate parents about their infant's communicative resources and the parent activities that can benefit the infant, we foster the development of a relationship that produces positive parenting (Lawhon, 2002; Thomas, 1999). There are three components of such a practice (McGrath & Conliffe-Torres, 1996):

- Model contingent behavior
- Educate about and help interpret infant cues
- Affirm the importance of the parenting role

When the relationship of parenting is established before the tasks of care are transferred to the parents, the parents can begin to understand and appreciate the individual developmental pathway of their child. Modeling contingent caregiving is probably the most powerful tool in parent education. When we provide developmentally sound handling, positioning, and response to cues, the parents can observe that which is difficult to "picture" from unfamiliar language. Words such as midline, containment, and flexion, are not familiar parent words. Our actions toward and communication with the infants demonstrate the "how to" and affirm the potential of even a preterm or ill infant to communicate with parents and caregivers.

Parents have an acute need for education and information. It is important to remember that many parents come to us as informed consumers with strong treatment preferences (Hobbs & Sodomka, 2000). The number of medically related "hits" on the Internet is astounding; parents are looking everywhere for information that will help them better understand this situation. Always begin by assessing where the parent is in his/her understanding (Woodwell, 2002). What was clear yesterday might seem unclear today. It might be important to help them with their exploration of the available resources so they have the best understanding of their child and the implications of decisions. Knowledge about their infant's medical status and individual developmental needs can empower them to become active partners with the NICU staff (Brazy, Anderson, Becker, et al.,

2001; Loo, Espinosa, Tyler, et al., 2003). We educate parents by modeling appropriate behaviors and using the many videos and booklets available for parent education. Armed with knowledge, they are likely to experience less anxiety and be better able to provide care for and interact with their infant (Pearson & Anderson, 2001). As they employ learned techniques of handling, bathing, and feeding, their infant will respond positively, and affirm their efforts. It is this positive interaction that gives parents confidence, comfort, and joy in parenting. All of these activities facilitate the parenting process even in a high-risk environment. In addition, effective parenting can have a beneficial effect on neurodevelopmental outcomes. (McGrath & Conliffe-Torres, 1996; McGrath, 2001; Thomas, 1999).

## FAMILY-UNIT INTEGRITY

Having an infant in the NICU is a great stressor for not only the parents individually but on the entire family unit, regardless of size or configuration. Families are psychologically vulnerable after the birth of a sick infant. Their sense of helplessness yields to a heightened receptivity to accepting help and responding positively to this challenge in their lives (Siegel, Gardner, & Merenstein, 2002).

In the course of daily rounds and caregiving, there are many opportunities for NICU staff to support a healthy family and parent-child relationship:

1. Adopt and practice a welcoming attitude toward families.
2. Communicate with the parents on a regular basis—not just in crises.
3. Ask parents for their observations about their baby, and affirm their comments.
4. Educate parents about their infant's medical and developmental status.
5. Discuss the baby's comfort/pain management with parents.
6. Discuss the anticipated LOS and how parents are preparing for transfer home.
7. Resist the "parents updated" approach, and work toward parent understanding and participation in care.
8. Appreciate the family's dynamics and response to stress and crises. Remind parents to recognize

and provide for their own needs as well as those of the infant and extended family.

9. Offer opportunities for parent-to-parent support.

Parent assessment is critical to supporting their evolving parental role. Parents' first need is to have confidence that their infant is getting all the best care he/she requires. Once assured, they can respond to encouragement to care for themselves enough to actively participate in their infant's care (Hurst, 2001). The professional "model" of care often seeks a "diagnosis," something that is weak and wrong and needs treatment. The family-centered model recognizes strengths and builds on the assets that the family brings to the relationship (McGrath, 2001). Needs must be acknowledged and resources provided, but the overall partnership must build on the strengths within the family unit. The scope and progression of the parental role must match the infant's developmental and medical timeline toward discharge.

## TRANSITION EASE

Scharer and Brooks (1994) describe the transfer of care from NICU to home in 4 stages.

**Stage I**: Nurses are the primary care providers. The focus is on stabilizing the infant and doing a baseline family assessment of strengths and vulnerabilities. Mothers are concerned about nursing competence, and nurses about the mother's ability to learn to care for her infant.

**Stage II**: Nurse and mother begin to share in the care of the infant. Professionals provide the technical care and assess response to interventions, and the parent establishes a relationship with the infant and begins to learn about the infant's developmental and medical status. The touching, seeing, and talking stages of bonding happen.

**Stage III**: Professionals and parents share in both the normal and technical aspects of the infant's care. Parents learn the technical components of care, and how to evaluate changes in the infant's response to care. Increasing autonomy at this stage facilitates transfer home.

**Stage IV**: Parents provide care. It is often helpful to have a day or nighttime rooming-in situation available to parents to psychologically transfer care before actual discharge to home. Throughout hospitalization, a program that educates and affirms parenting in an expanding role with increasing autonomy eases the anxiety of taking a high-risk infant home (Costello & Chapman, 1998).

## BENEFITS FOR THE NICU

In a review of 29 studies over 10 years that focused on parental interventions, Cusson and Lee (1994) suggested that supporting and educating parents and facilitating early interactions with their infants might be the most cost-effective intervention available to us. Parents' readiness for discharge is contingent upon the completion of the bonding process and transfer of care from professionals to parents. Developing a partnership with parents that incorporates them into the plan of care in a very tangible, supportive, and progressive manner, decreases role confusion, inconsistency, and both staff and parent frustration. The result of such a program can increase both parent and staff satisfaction and decrease cost by decreasing LOS—significant markers in health care today.

## CAREGIVER CHALLENGES

Implementation of every program presents a challenge. The stance of the participants should reflect a desire to embrace this opportunity to change the focus of family caregiving such that families become our patients with the babies. First, the approach has to include an open mind and attitude. Professionals have to be willing to re-evaluate their significance in the life of the infant and family. They also have to develop a greater understanding of the infant's need for the presence and care of the parent and the parent's need to process the NICU experience. To relate to the parent's situation, it helps to explore what might frighten us to hear: to peak into the world of fear and uncertainty; to be stunned by a sudden change in events and plans; to be overwhelmed by a strange environment; to feel loss of control. We cannot wave a magic wand, but we can repeat explanations, listen to their fears, and affirm their role. We need to understand and accept that we do not have all the answers, but work as a team of professionals and parents to individualize the plan of care to support the long-term outcomes for both infants and families.

## PARTNERSHIP STRATEGIES

Partnership strategies that we should consider when formulating a family-centered developmental care plan include our ability to:

1. Establish and build a relationship based on trust. Family focus groups report that central to trust is the feeling of belonging and inclusion (Espenshade, 1999). Parents need to feel that their presence is both legitimate and beneficial to their children. Both research and experience demonstrate that parents want to be recognized as capable providers of direct care for their infant, and when offered information in the manner that they prefer, can make appropriate decisions for their infant (Bruns & McCollum, 2002). There has to be physical space dedicated to parents as well as the "warmth" of a family atmosphere. Professionals need to accent the positive, listen carefully, and always be aware of gender and cultural differences.

2. Facilitate collaboration. When we validate and empower parents, we grant them a measure of control over the care process. Parents' values and desires must be explored and incorporated into the plan of care. No one model fits all parent-professional dyads. Extravagant communication is essential to collaboration; this includes both formal and informal communications. An individualized approach will facilitate parenting as an active process with generous opportunity for parents to communicate with their infant and with caregivers. Freedom to ask questions and an expanded role in the hospital facilitate decision-making at home.

3. Create an environment that honors the role of parenting. System continuity and flexible boundaries support the parent-child dyad from one shift and one day to another and from one unit to another. A key component is to assess the family resources, explore the family needs and desires, and then work with the family to develop a care plan that supports their infant's long-term health and developmental goals.

## RESOURCES

Our most important resource in partnering with parents is the infant's own developmental timeline.

When we apply parent education and activities along this pathway, we establish a parent-child relationship pattern that will serve them for the rest of their lives. A sample parenting pathway is included in Box 18-3. There are many excellent videos, books, and Internet resources for parent education. When we stay focused on the infant's care and development, we are less likely to develop team friction about the details of care. Using developmental care as a basis for the parent-infant care keeps the partnership focused on the infant.

## EVALUATION

We should never underestimate the power and influence we have over families at this very vulnerable segment of their lives. We have this partnership for a brief time that soon ebbs from memory. Parents carry this partnership into the rest of their lives. Whether their child expires after a short stay or thrives under our long or short period of care, how we support and affirm parents will influence them for a long time. Our NICUs are replete with letters from parents that include comments such as the following:

- You helped us to feel competent and comfortable in caring for our baby . . .
- You supported us and showed us compassion and were sensitive to the needs of our family . . .
- You enabled us to make decisions in the care of our baby . . . even small decisions made a difference in helping us to feel like parents . . .

Many institutions use standardized "patient satisfaction" surveys as a quality outcome measure and benchmarking tools. Less frequently used, but perhaps more important are family focus groups and informal parent coffees or pizza nights. Sometimes an informal setting with other parents and away from the bedside provides a "safe" opportunity for parents to share their fears, concerns, or needs. We can use these occasions to continually learn from parents, to gain a better understanding of their needs as NICU parents, and to ascertain how we can empower them as parents of a high-risk infant.

## PRETERM PARENTS AND GRIEF CONCEPTS

The transition into the role of parenting is a major task for all new parents. Many factors come into play

Box 18-3 PARTNERING WITH PARENTS IN DEVELOPMENTALLY SUPPORTIVE CARE FOR HIGH-RISK INFANTS

**PENN STATE CHILDREN'S HOSPITAL, THE MILTON S. HERSHEY MEDICAL CENTER**
**PROGRAM OVERVIEW**
**DEVELOPMENTAL CARE GUIDELINES FOR CAREGIVERS AND PARENTS**
**Creating a Very Specific Role for Parents**

1. Supports the bonding and caring process between parent and child.
2. Recognizes that parents are the single constant in the child's life. A parent's love and attention is a grounding and stabilizing force in the child's world.
3. Supports the long-term developmental and health needs of the child; the parent's ability to care for and nurture a child is contingent upon a strong bond of love and a sense of duty toward the child.

**Goals of Developmental Care**

1. Preserve energy; promote growth and recovery.
2. Reduce stress and prevent agitation; facilitate regulatory capabilities.
3. Facilitate neurobehavioral organization based on the infant's capabilities.
4. Promote caregiver and parent understanding of individual infant's behavior.
5. Normalize the environment to the extent that medical and nursing care permit.

**Key Points**

1. The developmental care team has developed these tools to help us all advance the quality and consistency of our developmentally supportive and family-centered care.
2. The tools include *Health Care Provider's Guide to Developmental Care* and *Parent's Guide to Developmental Care*.
3. The content in the parent's guide is included in the *Health Care Provider's Guide*.
4. The timelines represent the sequential nature of development. They are not restricted to a certain gestational age or adjusted age. A very ill, near-term infant might require the treatment and handling of a very preterm infant. For any infant, start at the most fragile stage, and advance according to infant's status and capabilities. A very preterm infant might follow the time line very closely. A 34-week-old infant might start at the most fragile stage but advance to stage 4 within 4 or 5 days.
5. How to use and apply these tools
   • Take time to read through carefully.
   • Introduce the tool to parents and help them to select parenting activities that work for them and their infant.
   • Document on the Plan of Care (in the Teaching/Discharge Plan Section) the mutually developed nursing/parent plan.
   • Document teaching and activities on the Patient Education Record—Neonatal.
   • Document the parents' interactions/participation and plan in the Progress Notes.
6. Resources for staff: If you are feeling uncomfortable about your own understanding of developmental care and/or parent support, please use the following resources:

**NEW RESOURCES**

• Parent Tape 1: Parenting the Acutely Ill Child
• Parent Tape 2: Parenting the Growing Preemie
• NICU Staff Development Tape 1: Preemie Development: An Overview
• NICU Staff Development Tape 2: The Preemie and the NICU Environment

*Continued*

**Box 18-3**   Partnering with Parents in Developmentally Supportive Care for High-Risk Infants—cont'd

- NICU Staff Development Tape 3: Positioning and Handling the High-Risk Infant
- NICU Staff Development Tape 4: The Growing Preemie
- NICU Staff Development Tape 5: Helping Families in the Special Care Nursery
- "Kangaroo Care" tape
- Booklet: "My Special Start."
- New self learning booklet, "Feeding Transition for the Preterm Neonate," by B. Noerr.

**OTHER RESOURCES**
- Videotape: "Getting to Know Your NICU."
- Videotape: "Prematurely Yours."
- Videotape: " . . . To make a Difference."
- Videotape: "Behavior of the Premature Infant."
- Booklet: "Developmentally Supportive Care: Theory and Application," by P.K. Hiniker and L.A. Moreno

Used with permission from Penn State Children's Hospital, The Milton S. Hershey Medical Center, Hershey, PA; copyright 2003 by Pennsylvania State University.

that can either enhance this transition or hamper the process. Some of these factors include parental age and the amount of time together as a couple. Extremes of parental age might affect the ability to care for a new infant due both to maturity and knowledge. Adolescent parents often do not have the maturity to take on the magnitude of care required. In addition, they might lack resources and knowledge about infant care (Thurman & Gonsalves, 1993). Older parents might have additional resources but can find this huge life change very stressful as they leave the lifestyle patterns to which they are accustomed. Time together as a couple can be very helpful during the stress that can accompany this period. Experience together through other stressful events can enhance the "team" approach as they work together for mutual support.

Additional factors include support systems and coping skills. Support systems might be available via a large extended family or through a close network of friends. This support system is helpful during the stress of change as well as providing some relief to tired parents. Coping skills are necessary to deal with the associated stress and to survive the unexpected events that might occur.

This transition period occurs not only after delivery, but throughout the pregnancy as the parents plan for the upcoming addition to the family. During the pre-delivery time, the parents begin to visualize their "dream" infant, discuss parenting styles, and begin to make life-style changes. These activities are important to initiate and carry out the parenting role.

When this process is interrupted by a preterm delivery, in essence the parents as well as the infant are preterm. The period needed for psychological preparation has been abruptly shortened. In addition, the parents are thrown into a high-stress period with many fears and unknowns. They certainly did not achieve the dream infant, and the infant might actually look very different from those mental images that were so important during the preparation phase (Bialoskurski, Cox, & Hayes, 1999).

The parents of a preterm infant are thrust into the very foreign environment of the NICU. At times it might seem to be very unfriendly as well. Control over the situation is lost. They are forced to learn about many complex and frightening medical diagnoses and interventions. They fear for their infant's survival. They are concerned about the pain the many interventions might be inflicting upon the infant. Decisions must be made that can have long-term consequences. It all becomes very overwhelming (Miles & Holditch-Davis, 1997).

The birth of a preterm infant might be experienced very differently between the parents (Doering, Dracup, & Moser, 1999). Mothers concentrate on the health status of their infant rather than their own condition. They have many questions about the why's and how's of the early birth with much guilt associated with the event. Mothers are anxious to demonstrate caregiving competence to "make up" for not producing the perfect infant (Kenner, 1995). Fathers will be much more focused on the well-being of their partner, and conflicts can arise between them regarding the amount of time spent in the unit with the infant. Fathers might feel ignored or neglected. This feeling is due to our communication style as professionals wherein the emphasis is on the maternal role or the infant's activity (Kenner, 1995). Support for the father as well as the mother is important to keep them both involved throughout the hospitalization. Inclusion of fathers when information is provided is critical for future decision-making and consistency. Early physical contact must be encouraged to enhance attachment that can be delayed in the father (Sullivan, 1999). The mother is much more likely to initiate early physical contact whereas the father might be more apprehensive and reticent.

Parents need to be included in all aspects of care based on their ability and desire. Parents do not visit their infants. Instead, they are an important part of the care team providing parenting versus medical care. Parents provide comfort and calming with a soft familiar voice and positive tactile stimulation. Access needs to be ensured to meet the parent's needs to be with their infant. This is important for the development of attachment that is integral to their ongoing relationship after discharge.

Parents often experience a number of emotions as they go through the NICU hospitalization due to the grief caused by this event. They must first grieve the loss of the dream before they can accept the current situation (Gardner, Hauser, & Merenstein, 2002; Siegel, Garner, & Merenstein, 2002). Because of this, they might not always exhibit rational behavior and can feel very stressed and out of control. Understanding the etiology of some of these behaviors can assist the professional in supporting the family. This will facilitate a much more positive relationship between the family and the hospital staff.

Parents might experience several stages of grief. They can move through these stages with relative ease or become stuck within a stage without progression. Clinical setbacks can reactivate a previously experienced stage. The pattern will be very different given the uniqueness and individuality of each couple.

Upon the delivery of the infant, the parents might exhibit shock. This shock can be related to the infant's unexpected birth; his/her appearance; or just the chain of events leading up to the NICU stay. They might feel helpless, hopeless, out of control, and guilty that this early delivery has occurred. Anger might also surface as they review the circumstances and realize they did everything they were supposed to and yet still have this less than desired pregnancy outcome.

Sadness and anxiety often follow. This generally occurs a few days after the delivery as the parents begin to experience the uncertainty and unpredictability of the infant's course. This might be demonstrated in two different ways. The parents might begin to withdraw from the situation and fail to attach to the infant. They might spend less time with the infant. They often describe symptoms of depression. However, they might become increasingly more anxious. This anxiety might interfere with the processing of information and appropriate interactions with those around them, including the infant. Friction between the two parents might be noted. In either case, the parents will require additional support. A social worker, member of the clergy, or psychiatric professional might be very instrumental in assisting the family through this difficult stage.

Conflicts can arise as parents deny receiving information or choose not to believe the information provided. This is yet another stage in their grief. Information might need to be repeated or reinforced several times. It needs to be provided in a direct manner using language the parents understand rather than medical terms. Consistency in the information is important, as conflicting messages will only add stress to the parents. Family meetings conducted on a regular basis, not just during times of crisis, can provide this consistency as all members of the team come together and communicate in a unified manner. Parents can hear all of the perspectives, and ask questions. This gives them more control over the situation, as they possess the necessary information to make decisions and plans for the coming weeks and months.

Establishing equilibrium is a time during the grief process when the parents become more comfortable with the situation. They are beginning to let go of the dream and accept the reality. Stress will decrease, enhancing the interactions with their infant and the staff providing care. This stress might return as they prepare for discharge, and they fear they will not be able to provide the care required by their infant. Early integration of the parents into caregiving and ongoing infant care education can alleviate some of this stress and prepare the parents for successful, independent caregiving at home.

Reorganization is the last stage of the grief process. Often it does not occur until well after the current hospitalization. It might become evident as parents return to the unit with the infant or send a photo around the first birthday or the anniversary of the discharge date.

The NICU experience is a very difficult time for any parent. Early support and integration into the parenting role often eases much of the distress. Promoting positive experiences, such as Kangaroo care, supports the parent and their important role during the hospitalization (Affonso, Bosque, Wahlberg, et al., 1993). Staff's understanding of this irrational and stressful time can promote positive relationships that enhance the experience for all involved.

## CONCLUSION

Prolonged hospitalization in the NICU is a difficult place to establish family-professional partnerships. However, because families are the constant in the child's environment, assisting families to have a positive outcome from their NICU experience should be a priority when providing care. Using a framework that supports the development of a partnership in which all members are respected, as equals, should facilitate healthcare providers in acknowledging and supporting family needs and expectations that will ultimately benefit the development of the child. In this chapter we have discussed parent partnerships; however, research in the area of NICU parents often focuses on maternal concerns and comments. The next chapter explores one qualitative study done with NICU fathers. This study is used as an exemplar to examine the issues of the *Father's Role in NICU Care* (see Chapter 19).

## REFERENCES

Affonso, D.D., Bosque, E., Wahlberg, V., et al. (1993). Reconciliation and healing for mothers through skin-to-skin contact provided in an American tertiary level intensive care nursery. *Neonatal Network, 12*(3), 25-32.

Bialoskurski, M., Cox, C.L., & Hayes, J.A. (1999). The nature of attachment in a neonatal intensive care unit. *Journal of Perinatal Neonatal Nursing, 13*(1), 66-77.

Brazy, J.E., Anderson, B.M.H., Becker, P., et al. (2001). How parents of premature infants gather information and obtain support. *Neonatal Network, 20*(2), 41-48.

Bruce, B., & Ritchie, J. (1997). Nurses' practices and perceptions of family-centered care. *Journal of Pediatric Nursing, 12*(4), 214-222.

Bruns, D.A., & McCollum, J.A. (2002). Partnerships between mothers and professionals in the NICU: Caregiving, information exchange, and relationships. *Neonatal Network, 21*(7), 15-23.

Costello, A., & Chapman, J. (1998). Mothers' perceptions of the care-by-parent program prior to hospital discharge of their preterm infants. *Neonatal Network, 17*(7), 37-42.

Cusson, R.M., & Lee, A.L. (1994). Parental interventions and the development of the preterm infant. *Journal of Obstetric, Gynecologic, and Neonatal Nursing (JOGNN), 23*(1), 60-69.

Doering, L.V., Dracup, K., & Moser, D. (1999). Comparison of psychosocial adjustment of mothers and fathers of high-risk infants in the neonatal intensive care unit. *Journal of Perinatology, 19*(2), 132-137.

Espenshade, S. (1999). *Family focus group report.* Hershey, PA: The Milton S. Hershey Medical Center.

Gardner, S.L., Hauser, P., & Merenstein, G.B. (2002). Grief and perinatal loss (pp. 754-786). In G.B. Merenstein, & S.L. Gardner (Eds.), *Handbook of neonatal intensive care* (5th ed.). St. Louis: Mosby.

Haut, C., Peddicord, K., & O'Brien, E. (1994). Supporting parental bonding in the NICU: A care plan for nurses. *Neonatal Network, 13*(8), 19-25.

Hobbs, S.F., & Sodomka, P.S. (2000). Developing partnerships among patients, families, and staff at the medical college of Georgia hospital and clinic. *The Joint Commission: Journal of Quality Management, 26*(5), 268-276.

Hurst, I. (2001). Mother's strategies to meet their needs in the newborn intensive care unit. *Journal of Perinatal Neonatal Nursing, 15*(2), 65-82.

Kennell, J.H., & Klaus, M.H. (1998). Parent-infant bonding: Biologic, psychologic, and clinical aspects (pp. 290-304). In J.D. Noshpitz, P.L. Adams, & E. Bleiberg (Eds.), *Handbook of child and adolescent psychiatry. Vol. 1. Infants and preschoolers: Development and syndromes.* New York: John Wiley and Sons.

Kenner, C. (1995). Transition to parenthood (pp. 171-184). In L.P. Gunderson, & C. Kenner (Eds.), *Care of the 24-25 week gestational age infant: A small baby protocol* (2nd ed.). Petaluma, CA: NICU Ink.

King, N.M.P. (1992, May-June). Transparency in neonatal intensive care. *Hastings Center Report*, 18-25.

Lawhon, G. (2002). Facilitation of parenting the premature infant in the newborn ICU. *Journal Perinatal Neonatal Nursing, 16*(1), 71-82.

Leyden, C.H. (1998). Consumer bill of rights: Family-centered care. *Pediatric Nursing, 24*(1), 72-73.

Loo, K.K., Espinosa, M., Tyler, R., et al. (2003). Using knowledge to cope with stress in the NICU: How parents integrate learning to read the physiologic and behavioral cues of the infant. *Neonatal Network, 22*(1), 31-37.

MacLean, S.L., Guzzetta, C.E., White, C., et al. (2003). Family presence during cardiopulmonary resuscitation and invasive procedures: Practices of critical care and emergency nurses. *American Journal of Critical Care, 12*(3), 246-257.

Mason, D.J. (2003). Family presence: Evidence versus tradition. *American Journal of Critical Care, 12*(3), 190-192.

McGahey, P.R. (2002). Family presence during pediatric resuscitation: A focus on staff. *Critical Care Nurse, 22*(6) 29-34.

McGrath, J.M. (2000). Developmentally supportive caregiving and technology: Isolation or merger of intervention strategies? *Journal of Perinatal and Neonatal Nursing, 14*(3), 78-91.

McGrath, J.M. (2001) Building relationships with families in the NICU: Exploring the guarded alliance. *Journal of Perinatal and Neonatal Nursing, 15*(4), 74-83.

McGrath, J.M., & Conliffe-Torres, S. (1996). Integrating family-centered developmental assessment and intervention into routine care in the neonatal intensive care unit. *Nursing Clinics of North America, 31*(2), 367-383.

Miles, M.S., & Holditch-Davis, D. (1997). Parenting the prematurely born child: Pathways of influence. *Seminars in Perinatology, 21*(3), 254-266.

Minde, K.K., & Minde, R. (1998). Parenting and the development of children (pp. 265-283). In J.D. Noshpitz, P.L. Adams, & E. Blieberg (Eds.), *Handbook of child and adolescent psychiatry. Vol. VII Advances and new directions.* New York: John Wiley and Sons.

Pearson, J., & Anderson, K. (2001). Evaluation of a program to promote positive parenting in the neonatal intensive care unit. *Neonatal Network, 20*(4), 43-48.

Robinson, S.M., Mackenzie-Ross, S., Campbell-Hewson, G.K., et al. (1998). Psychological effect of witnessed resuscitation on bereaved relatives. *Lancet, 352*, 614-617.

Scharer, K., & Brooks, G. (1994). Mothers of chronically ill neonates and primary nurses in the NICU: Transfer of care. *Neonatal Network, 13*(5), 37-47.

Siegel R., Gardner, S.L., & Merenstein, G.B. (2002). Families in crisis: Theoretic and practical considerations (pp. 725-753). In G.B. Merenstein, & S.L. Gardner (Eds.), *Handbook of neonatal intensive care* (5th ed.) St. Louis: Mosby.

Speedling, E. (1997). *Family focus group report.* Hershey, PA: The Milton S. Hershey Medical Center.

Stainton, C., Prentice, M., Lindrea, K.B., et al. (2001). Evolving a developmental care culture in a neonatal intensive care nursery: An action project. *Neonatal Paediatric and Child Health Nursing, 4*(1), 6-14.

Sullivan, J.R. (1999). Development of father-infant attachment in fathers of preterm infants. *Neonatal Network, 18*(7), 33-39.

Thomas, D. (1999). Parenting education. *Journal of Child and Family Nursing, 2*(5), 322-331.

Thorne, S.E., & Robinson, C.A. (1988a). Health care relationships: The chronic illness perspective. *Research in Nursing & Health, 11*, 293-300.

Thorne, S.E., & Robinson, C.A. (1988b). Reciprocal trust in health care relationships. *Journal of Advanced Nursing, 13*, 782-789.

Thorne, S.E., & Robinson, C.A. (1989). Guarded alliance: Health care relationships in chronic illness. *Image: Journal of Nursing Scholarship, 21*(3), 153-157.

Thurman, S.K., & Gonsalves, S.V. (1993). Adolescent mothers and their premature infants: Responding to double risk. *Infants and Young Children, 5*(4), 44-51.

Woodwell, W.H. Jr. (2002). Perspectives on parenting in the NICU. *Advances in Neonatal Care, 2*(3), 161-169.

# 19 Father's Role in NICU Care: Evidence-Based Practice

## Shawn Pohlman

Developmentally supportive care must be implemented in the context of the family. The family is central to the infant's development, and families must participate in their infant's care (National Association of Neonatal Nurses [NANN], 2000). Family-centered caregiving empowers families to confront and more successfully manage the demands and challenges of having a critically ill newborn (Harrison, 1993). However, family-centered caregiving implies a focus on the entire family—mother, father, baby—and their needs. Fathers are sometimes ignored once the mother is well enough to be present at the bedside (Holditch-Davis & Miles, 1997). This tendency to place more emphasis on mothering is reflected in the sparse amount of research on fathers. Fathers are often left out of the study sample altogether and, when included, are compared with mothers, as though mothers are the "gold standard" (Holditch-Davis & Miles, 1997).

Most research on fathering has focused on fathers and healthy infants and children. These research findings suggest that father-infant interactions are shaped by a complex web of relationships—between fathers, their children, and between their children's mothers (Federal Interagency Forum on Child & Family Statistics, 1998; Volling & Belsky, 1991). According to Jordan (1990), mothers and infants are "key recognition providers," meaning that their attitudes, actions, and interactions can either promote or impede the evolving father relationship and role development. In addition to the mother and the baby, other key players that impact fathering include healthcare providers, friends, co-workers, and other family members. Extending beyond the immediate circle of family and friends, men's motivation to parent responsively is also powerfully shaped by cultural images of father-

The "F" designations (F01, F02, and so on) preceding many quotations in this chapter refer to specific fathers from the author's study.

hood, as well as men's socioeconomic background, social circumstances, and earlier experiences, especially with their own parents (Federal Interagency Forum on Child & Family Statistics, 1998). In addition, research suggests that fathers and mothers get to know their babies differently. For example, fathers hold and touch infants differently than mothers. A qualitative study of 14 fathers and term infants revealed that fathers held their infants "like a football" because they wanted them to exist as separate beings, but holding produced the feelings of closeness they desired (Anderson, 1996). Research has repeatedly shown that fathers interact more playfully with both term and preterm infants than mothers. Mothers, however, are usually the primary caregivers (Field, 1981; Lamb, 1997).

This chapter is based on the findings of one qualitative study to be used as an exemplar of the father's role in the neonatal intensive care unit (NICU) because few researchers have exclusively focused on fathers and preterm infants. The purpose of this study was to deepen the understanding of fathering after an early birth and make fathers' experiences more visible. To provide family-centered caregiving, nurses must have a better understanding of the experience from a father's perspective. Fathers, as mothers, are a part of individualized, family-centered, developmental care (IFDC); however, they are often secondary in the discussions. Therefore, the emphasis in this chapter is to highlight the fathering from the father's perspective and to build on the preceding chapter in which the need for partnerships with families to promote developmental care is discussed.

The philosophic framework for the study was based in interpretive phenomenology, which assumes that humans dwell in a meaningful world. The use of the first person pronoun "I" throughout this chapter is reflective of this methodologic approach. As noted by Webb (1992), use of the first person is essential to qualitative research because researchers influence, exercise choices, and make decisions about the directions of their research and the conclusions they draw.

Findings from this interpretive study form the basis of this chapter. Three themes best captured the demands of fathering a preterm infant: The juggle between work, hospital, and home; the struggle to "get to know" their infants; and communication barriers between fathers and healthcare professionals. The chapter concludes with how fathers nurtured relationships with their infants through their voices.

One important theme that emerged from the study findings was that fathers found that juggling the time for hospital visits and home activities around their work was the most stressful aspect of having a preterm infant in the NICU. This finding is significant because a father's stress might lie outside the NICU doors and, therefore, be relatively invisible to neonatal healthcare providers.

## STUDY'S SAMPLE/DEMOGRAPHICS

The study sample consisted of 8 fathers, between the ages of 22 and 40 years, who had preterm infants between 25 and 32 weeks' gestation (27 weeks average). Fathers' annual incomes ranged from 11,000 to more than 100,000 dollars. Seven of the fathers were married, and, for all except one father, this was their first fathering experience.

## DATA COLLECTION

Interviews began within a month after birth and continued at home for 3 to 4 months after discharge. In total, 63 interviews were conducted. While the baby was in the NICU, interviews occurred every 2 to 3 weeks; once at home, they took place every month. Each interview was tape-recorded and transcribed verbatim. The narrative data were analyzed in the interpretive tradition that evolved as my understanding of their lives deepened from numerous readings of the narrative texts and several written interpretations.

## FINDINGS

As mentioned, three themes emerged from this study: (1) the primacy of work, (2) fathering in the hospital: from expert to novice, and (3) managing the home front: life outside the NICU.

## The Primacy of Work

Fathers returned to work quickly after birth out of necessity, because they were providing financially for their families. One father expressed his thoughts about working; words that could easily serve as their motto: "My family is important, that's why I go to work every day. When you have a baby, it's kind of a must, isn't it? Work every day." Fathering propelled them to approach their mandate with a greater sense of urgency. One father discussed how his thoughts about work have changed since the birth of his daughter:

. . . I guess I'm a little more serious about it . . . now I've got some responsibility . . . I think I always did a good job but now I really want to make sure I do a good job and try to work through a little more of the politics and stuff to try to get somewhere.

During this study, four fathers were hired into new positions that were promotions in terms of salary and/or insurance. Fathers often changed jobs to replace their wives' lost income after their baby's arrival. Although these fathers accepted their breadwinner roles, they were ambivalent about the primacy of that role in their lives. I asked each father whether he was primarily work or family oriented. This father's response exemplified their feelings:

*F06:* . . . my priority would be my family, but, obviously, waking hours-wise, you spend more time at work than you do at home . . . Yeah, if it came down to a choice between the two, if you look at it that way, it would be family.
*I:* So feeling-wise it's family, but practically . . .
*F06:* Yeah, practically speaking, I'm at work a lot.

These narratives depicted the power of tradition as fathers attempted to carve out the shape of their own fathering. Fathers missed only a couple days of work after their infant's birth, returning right back once both mother and baby were in stable condition.

## Fathering in the Hospital: From Expert to Novice

Fathers had limited experiences with infants of any size, let alone small ones, which is in direct contrast to the vast array of skills they had accumulated in their various occupations. By listening carefully to their words as they described being "experts" at work, insight was gleaned regarding the difficulties they experienced in being demoted to "novices" in the NICU. One father noted that "it's really comforting to know that I'm good at this. There's no one else out there [who] can do this job better than what I can." He described his feelings about getting a promotion at work: "When I'm getting recognized, I guess I take that to heart. And when I'm not getting recognized, I sort of feel let down." Fathers felt confident at work: " . . . at work I have a lot of confidence, I know what's expected of me. I know what I've gotta do to get where I want to go."

Fathers felt as though there was nothing they could "do" during their infant's hospital stay, which was in contrast to the sense of productivity I gleaned from their work narratives. A father discussed his feelings about being an observer:

*F08*: There were some people [who] would go down there for hours on end . . . You feel bad, but what do you do? You can't sit there in the NICU for eight hours a day. I couldn't do anything to help. So, we'll go down there for a couple of hours every day and call a couple times a day. That was it . . . I mean, it's kind of out of your control, obviously, what goes on there . . . I probably should've spent more time down there when he was in the NICU all that time . . . I felt guilty at first because I saw other parents there [who] were always there . . . I'm coming in after work, you know. It kind of puts you on a guilt trip kind of thing I guess, self-guilt trip.

*I*: You felt guilty.

*F08*: Yeah, but what could you do? . . . You sit there and look at him in an incubator for hours on end. I wasn't making a difference being there. At the end, when he was bigger, when we could start feeding him or get him out and hold him for awhile, then that made a difference, but still, you're limited with how much of that you could do so . . .

Fathers visited the NICU almost every day after work, but stayed only a few hours. Fathers visited because they wanted to see their infants and support their partners, not because they were "doing" something for their baby. Because they perceived themselves as somewhat extraneous, they struggled with the grind of daily visits.

Fathers often mentioned the importance of "doing" in the narratives. This strengthens Freud's (1995) notion that fathers might feel "completely superfluous" in the NICU because they are not actively involved in caregiving. I would argue that their notion of "doing" involved caregiving and playing, in the future when their infants were much older and interactive.

Many of the fathers were relieved to return back to work after the birth: "In some ways I felt happy to be back, get back into a routine and get my mind on some things that were going on. It wasn't a bad thing." Another father recalled:

It was my decision. They [his employer] were understanding. They knew what was going on. They said take as much time as possible or as needed. But, I guess I sort of had the mentality that the place was going to fall apart without me . . . what can I do here, I really can't do nothing here. It will get my mind off it, so I might as well just go back to work.

Although going to work helped fathers cope, it also conjured up a host of worries, guilty feelings, and struggles. When I asked one father what had been difficult, he noted:

Just dealing with being at work everyday, you know, worrying about him . . . I'll be just working and then all of a sudden I'll just stop and . . . he'll just come through my mind . . . I just kind of wonder if something's wrong with him . . .

Spending time in the NICU was not a top priority for these fathers. They focused their sights on a target outside the NICU—their work, which was satisfying, because they were providing financially, and comforting, because they were good at it. The NICU environment does not nourish a father's need to feel secure and appreciated because the focus is on the baby and mother. Fathers quickly ascertain that the real "experts" in this setting are often the nurses, who are primarily female, relegating the fathers to the sidelines. One father described his experience of going from expert to novice in an interview just after his infant was discharged:

This here [having a preterm infant] has just been a pretty, just a frightening ordeal more or less . . . you're sort of walking on pins and needles the whole time in the NICU, and, I mean, at work, I'm in a position where I pretty much snap my fingers and it should happen . . . I get my way quite a bit there. And at home, she [his wife] is the boss. (He laughed). And she snaps her fingers, I do it.

## Managing the Home Front: Life Outside the NICU

Although fathers were upset when their infants developed a medical complication, the most difficult aspects of the experience were positioned outside of the NICU. Not only did fathers have to balance their time between work and the hospital, they had to find time to keep their households running smoothly. One father, whose infant was born at 28 weeks' gestation, recalled this difficult scenario during our first interview:

> *I:* . . . Can you tell me about a recent event that stands out as . . . difficult?
>
> *F01:* . . . the whole last week has just been difficult for some reason. It's just almost like a spiral . . . I invited some of my friends over to give them cigars and all that good stuff . . . we were drinking and one of my girl friends was kidding around with one of the guys out in the front yard and she decided to jump off the porch after him and she broke her ankle . . . so that's been on my mind, what's going on with that . . . if I'm liable and if I'm not liable . . . And with my son and my wife being in the hospital for so long, you know, the bills start piling up . . . And the other day when it was icy, I pulled into a [parking] spot and . . . I get out of my car and the car slides into the drain . . . It wasn't bad. We got it out and everything was fine. And then the other day, my check, I have direct deposit and for some reason it didn't go in, and they took my car payment out and her car payment and the house payment all out and it wasn't in there . . . It's been a rough week . . .

Obviously, he was stressed, but all the examples he gave me had little to do with the NICU—they revolved around his life outside of the hospital. His reply was significant because the question was open-ended, and he chose his own response.

The fact that his response lacked NICU scenarios might be insightful in terms of his attachment to his son who was only 12 days old at the time. Sullivan (1999) explored the development of attachment between fathers and preterm infants and reported that fathers did not experience feelings of attachment until their babies were older, between 1 and 5 months.

Another stressful aspect for fathers was their role as a "go-between." Not only did they have to satisfy the demands of work and the hospital, they were confronted with the needs of their partners, their pets, and their children who longed for their attention.

Fathers tried to hide their own emotions from their partners, which might have made coping harder. Clark and Miles (1999) reported a similar finding in their study on fathers of infants diagnosed with severe congenital heart disease: Fathers struggled to remain strong while hiding their own emotions. In the following excerpt, a father talked about suppressing his fears regarding his son's medical outcome:

> *F05:* It's just like a touch and go thing. He's like sitting at a yellow light and you're wanting to know: Should I go on through it or should I stop?
>
> *I:* Every day you probably have that feeling.
>
> *F05:* Every day, the emotions, stress . . . not to say that I don't cry, because I do and I feel better. I try not to do it around my wife.

## "IT'S REALLY HARD TO GET TO KNOW HER"

These are the words of one father whose daughter was born at 26 weeks' gestation. Fathers often found that "getting to know" their infant was a very complex and thorny process, filled with many emotions: jubilation, frustration, anxiety, and fear. Three exemplars depicted their varied experiences.

### Getting to Know: In the NICU

Dan was a happily married man who worked as a financial analyst. His daughter, Mary, was born at 26 weeks. Although small, her medical course was uneventful. Dan had little experience with infants or children. He considered his own father to be a very good father and an important influence in his life: "I'd say he's pretty much a role model for dads, always around, always doing stuff with us." When I asked him what made him a great father, he noted: "A lot of patience . . . If something went wrong or someone was hurt, he was always the one who was calm and would talk through what to do."

Dan's first impression of his daughter after birth was typical:

> It's kind of scary looking . . . They're hooked up to all these different machines . . . The worst part of coming to visit was . . . all the monitors that she's hooked up to and you find yourself just watching the monitors constantly.

When he first held Mary, he remarked how he "couldn't feel her. She was so tiny that it was like I had a towel in my hand." Holding felt "awkward" at first:

I remember feeling a little awkward, a lot awkward . . . I didn't really know how to hold her . . . I just didn't know what to do. I'm holding her, and I think alarms are going off . . . She'd squirm, and I guess they can put their head down and cut off their circulation, so I'm trying to fiddle with her but I don't want to move her too much because I don't want to break her.

By the third interview, Dan was already quite comfortable caring for Mary. He was able to get her out of the isolette by himself (something most fathers feared) and remarked:

Actually, right now, I think I feel comfortable doing just about anything with her . . . I think it's just because she's getting bigger.

By the next interview, Dan was holding his daughter for up to 2 hours at a time on a regular basis.

Of the eight fathers, Dan was the most confident providing caregiving for his tiny daughter. His comfort level was especially notable because he had no experience with children, and Mary was a temperamentally difficult infant. He described his daughter as "sassy" and "irritable." I attribute Dan's ability to quickly become comfortable caring for Mary to his inherent self-confidence, which emanated from him during interviews both verbally and nonverbally. His upbringing, which was shaped by his own father's dependable presence and calm demeanor, enabled him to feel secure enough to attempt caregiving despite feeling scared and intimidated on the inside because he had virtually no practical experiences to draw upon.

Kyle is a 26-year-old man who worked as a manager at an electronics store. His wife gave birth to a son named Carl at 27 weeks' gestation. Carl had an unremarkable medical course. Unlike Dan, this father had quite a bit of experience with older children because he was an involved uncle. He described his own father as "quiet" and "a little distant." When asked if he was a good father to him growing up, he noted:

I'd have to say that's a little questionable. He wasn't bad by any means but I definitely missed the involvement that either my mom or my grandpa gave to me. I was really involved with sports . . . and my mom would be the one who would take me to the practices and pick me up . . . And my grandpa, he was the one to go outside and play with me, if I was at their house. And those things are really meaningful now that I look back at it . . . That's definitely the path that I don't want to go down. I want to be involved with him as much as I can. It's tough.

When Kyle first visited the NICU, he described his thoughts:

He looked really, really red and they had the lights on him . . . and it was just a very emotional moment . . . He was never on any breathing machine . . . just all the things hooked to him . . . was a little overwhelming. The weight wasn't even an issue anymore, just seeing him hooked to all those things.

Kyle, however, was scared and ambivalent about holding his son:

I'm really excited about it, to tell you the truth, just being able to feel his skin up against mine and know that I created this . . . But on the other hand, I'm scared because he's still so small and I don't want to do nothing wrong . . . I've never really had to deal with anything that small before. I've never changed a diaper before. I've never done any of that stuff before . . . There's a lot of things going through my mind and what if I do this wrong, what if I do that wrong. I guess I start questioning myself on those things, and maybe that's why I haven't held him yet.

He finally held Carl when he was 3 weeks old, but did so under pressure:

. . . the nurse forced me into it to tell you the truth. I really wasn't ready for it . . . I was still pretty nervous as far as actually doing it. They told me I wasn't leaving until it happened so they got a gown and I ended up holding him. I held him for about an hour and a half . . . (pause). I guess it was all that I expected.

Although Kyle described holding as "almost breathtaking," at the same time, he noted that it was "a relief" because he was "overcoming a fear." Holding was more of a task he had to accomplish to satisfy doubts emanating from within, not necessarily a tender, fulfilling moment. In our next interview, he talked about the fact that the "fear is gone" but yet he refrained from holding his son because he "didn't want to take that time away from Lisa [his wife] and she really gets into that." Kyle seemed wary of making a mistake and looking inept. In the words of Gray (1992), "A man's deepest fear is that he is not good enough or that he is incompetent.... A man is particularly vulnerable to this incorrect belief.... He wants to give but is afraid he will fail, so he doesn't try." (p. 56)

Kyle ventured into fatherhood on shaky grounds. He was attempting to recreate fathering in a way that was different from what he had experienced, but he lacked the self-confidence needed to fulfill his desires of being an "involved" dad. Although Carl was an easy baby, Kyle hesitated to provide caregiving independently and was afraid to feed his son. Shortly after his son's discharge, he applied for a promotion at work that helped to ease the family's financial strains, but demanded more time away from home with less time for fathering.

Larry was a 22-year-old, temporarily unemployed father of a daughter born at 25 weeks' gestation. Although he left the study after only one interview, I surmised that his relationship with his family was strained. When asked what his daughter, Leah, was like, he responded:

She's very active. You touch her and she'll squint her eyes and she'll kick... She's got to learn to adjust to who she is cause she doesn't really know. If something touches her ...she tries to kick away...she is always leaned up against something and if she gets too squirmy, her eyes start moving around.

Because Larry was able to spend every day with Leah, he studied her behaviors and talked about them in details that I did not hear from other fathers. He had none of the typical distractions: work and home (they were from out-of-town and lived next to the hospital in a special residence). As a result, he got to know his daughter quite intimately and spoke most lovingly about her: "She's very, very sweet...I don't see her as she's really low birthweight or anything like that. I just see her as my baby. I see her just the way she is." Larry's biggest fear was not being able to protect Leah, whom he was already quite attached to:

I don't like not being around her. If it was up to me, I'd take her and keep her down here [in the residence] ...

cause I don't like her being up in the NICU around people that doesn't care about her...it's not their baby, so they don't know how it feels to be close to her like I am.

Larry's strong emotional ties to Leah may have been fueled by his own emotional emptiness left over from frayed past family relationships.

These exemplars illustrate the powerful influence of one's past, particularly one's own father, on a man's ability to trust himself enough to venture out and "get to know" his infant. Self-confidence was an asset in an environment that is more threatening than soothing, and typically more focused on the needs of the infants and mothers. Researchers have repeatedly noted that a father's childhood experiences with his own father shape his fathering practices (Belsky, 1984; Daly, 1993; Hyman, 1995; Klitzing, Simoni, Amsler, & Burgin, 1999).

## Getting to Know: At Home

When their infants are in the NICU, fathers yearn to have them home. They do not "feel" like fathers while their infants are in the hospital. One father told me that fathering "is still not real, in a sense, but I think a lot of that is just because he's in the NICU and not at home... I've thought Father's Day is coming up and I'm a dad now, but I don't feel like a dad yet. I haven't been the one taking care of him or anything." Even after their infants are discharged home, fathers seem uneasy about labeling themselves as fathers—just yet. When I asked one father what had been the most surprising aspect of becoming a dad, he responded:

I don't know if I know what that term is yet, because she's so young... she doesn't do anything. It's just like you feed her, and it's not like you can give her advice.

In some ways, it was easier to "father" at home because they no longer had to visit the hospital, which enabled them to have more control over time spent with their infants. However, several fathers discovered that, after hospital discharge, the rank of "expert" was passed from the nurse to the mother, bypassing them altogether. After all, mothers typically spend much more time in the NICU caring for their infants and know them better. This phenomenon seemed most prevalent in the one realm most crucial to infant survival and cherished by mothers: feedings. Kyle, a father who was very hesitant about doing feedings, discussed his thoughts:

I just don't feel comfortable doing it, honestly. I don't know why . . . if she's gone . . . and I know it's time to feed, I know what's expected of me and I jump right to it. I guess if she's here, I just sort of assume that she's gonna do it and I let her take care of it . . . I guess it's just that I feel more comfortable seeing her holding him than me personally holding him. I don't know how exactly to hold him or what [bottle] angle . . . and she usually comes over, 'No, you're not holding him right, you're not doing this right, you're not doing that right' and sometimes it gets a little frustrating . . . it's easier just to let her do it.

Later, I asked Kyle about his son's feeding schedule, but his answer to my question was preempted by his wife, who was sitting in an adjacent room. Her interruption is further evidence that feedings were her "turf":

I: So, when do you actually feed him then [at night]?
F01: It's been around . . .
Mother: 12:00 AM, 2:00 AM, 5:30-6:00 AM
F01: I usually don't get to bed until 11:30-12:00 AM, and then he wakes back up at 2:00 AM. Then I've got to get back up at 5:00 AM to go to work. So I'm sort of running on about four cylinders right now.

This father was reluctant to feed his son, especially in his wife's presence, because he lacked confidence; confidence that can only be realized by "doing." Kyle was left standing in the sidelines and not fully participating in his son's care, which, as you may recall, was particularly salient for him because he feared walking down his own father's "uninvolved" path. These narratives illustrate how a mother can shape (positively or negatively) the caregiving experiences of a father.

Fathers found meaning in their infants' growing sense of awareness. Fathers could not wait for the day they could play with them; playing helped to fulfill their need for "doing." When I asked one father to describe a recent meaningful event, he noted:

I've been playing with him a lot more . . . reading to him, some of his books . . . He's got a few new toys . . . So playing with him with those, and I roll around with him a little

bit now . . . We play tackle . . . I just lay on my back on the floor and have him like on my chest and roll one side to the other, he seems to like that.

When I asked another father what it was like so far being a father, he responded:

I guess I'm anxious for him to grow. Right now he's sort of a mama's boy, more or less. I mean I can't wait to get to the point [of] getting down on the floor and playing with him with his playpen . . . What I'd really like to do is just get outside and throw a ball with him or go fishing. That's what I can't really wait for.

Fathers seemed comfortable projecting their "fathering" off into the future. They all seemed willing to bide their time during their children's "infancy" stage, dreaming of the day they could really "do" fathering.

Five fathers expressed concerns over spoiling their infants. They reported that their partners were "jumping" at the slightest whimper, and that was contributing to the problem. One father noticed doing things differently with his daughter than his wife:

. . . sometimes she will cry for no reason and Debbie will jump up. Every time, she jumps up . . . Well, I'll jump up most of the time, but there's sometimes when she's crying where I won't, just to see if she'll shut up. And Debbie gets mad at me for that . . . And it's like 'well, just wait and see if she'll shut up' because it's not a 'she's in pain' cry . . . It's just a little 'waa,' she's pissed about something.

Another father reported a similar scenario:

We had . . . grabbed him every time he made a little noise . . . I knew that was going to come back to bite us, but I couldn't convince my wife of that. It has come to pass . . . She can't put him down. He can't sleep on his own . . . he's gotta be held all the time. If he's not, he's screaming.

This father felt that the reason they had trouble putting their son down was because "he was in the hospital for 3 weeks so he really wasn't being held all the time . . . So you want to kind of make sure that he's got that psychological security and that somebody is there for him." Miles and Holditch-Davis (1997) studied mothers 3 years after the birth of a preterm infant and found that they adopted a "compensatory" parenting style that included providing increased stimulation, attention, protection, and difficulty with limit setting. Fathers seem to find it easier to distance themselves from their infant's appeals for attention because they are more separate, whereas mothers are more connected by virtue of giving birth (Ehrensaft, 1990).

Fathers expressed four concerns in caring for their infants at home: fear of relapse, negative behavioral cues, development concerns, and home apnea monitors. One father became alarmed when his son caught a cold after being home for 3 months because " . . . he's been through so much already and any little thing that he gets could maybe have a relapse . . . you're just afraid." Although there are no studies that have examined father's worries related to infant hospitalization, researchers who examined mothers' concerns have reported that they remain worried about their child's health after discharge (Docherty, Miles, & Holditch-Davis, 2002; Miles & Holditch-Davis, 1997). In my study, fathers' worries were warranted: Four fathers had infants who were rehospitalized—two for serious respiratory illnesses and two for reflux.

One father, Dan, found his daughters' behavioral cues difficult to handle. The first behavior he noticed was gaze aversion:

I'll feed her or try to talk to her and she'll kind of be looking off into the distance, almost like avoiding looking at me. I noticed she does that a lot and . . . It was kind of getting a little frustrating.

Dan also had to deal with Mary's back arching:

I almost couldn't get her to bend at the waist . . . she's a little stubborn. Her face was red and she was not going to let me do it.

Dan admitted that she had "really tested my patience sometimes." One night she vomited up her formula, and he lost his patience:

I kind of lost it a little bit . . . kind of screamed a little bit. It was just out of total frustration . . . I kind of felt bad because I was still holding her and I was letting my frustration out . . . It's not her fault, and I shouldn't yell at her . . . I'm sure, especially talking about overstimulation, [that] I pushed her to the limit right there.

In our last interview, I asked Dan how he felt about Mary's affect on his time:

Sometimes I'd rather not be taking care of her. Sometimes you just want to do your own thing, and she takes up a lot of time. That's just part of the deal. I love her, but . . . I don't always have to like her, you know.

Many of the fathers were on the "lookout" for developmental problems and somewhat surprised that their infants were doing better than expected. One father noted that "everybody says he's going to be behind because of all this [prematurity], but it seems to me he's already ahead because of all this." They did seem to notice little things:

We just noticed that he wasn't noticing his own hands out in front of him and they were more at his sides . . . not pulling them up. And then just last night we noticed when we were feeding him that he was playing with his hands.

Another father talked about how his son's development could "haunt us for quite some time." He had been told that his son should be caught up by age 2, but he added: "That's a long time to think about something like that."

Fathers found their infants' home apnea monitors a source of security and an annoyance. Although they admitted their initial necessity, they were anxious to return them. One father labeled the monitor "that stupid box" because "if I pick him up and take him with me, I've gotta take that [monitor] with me . . . That makes it a pain in the butt." These words, by the way, are coming from a father who rushed his son to the hospital because of accurate monitor alarms. Another father noted that the monitor was the "only stress thing that's left right now." The monitor symbolized the stress of the preceding months, and its removal marked the beginning of normalcy. Fathers found dealing with the monitor distasteful because; for them, learning infant caregiving was very challenging without incorporating an electronic device into the picture.

Fathers often found it difficult to relax even at home. One father's words reflected all their experiences quite well:

It's like . . . you've got this little fire going over there and you got the smoke detector in the room. But this little fire . . . ain't setting it off. But, at any time, it could catch something else on fire.

# COMMUNICATION BARRIERS

Recent studies underscore the fact that, when it comes to nurse-mother relationships, there is more "than meets the eye" transpiring in the NICU (Fenwick, Barclay, & Schmied, 2001; Hurst, 2001; Lupton & Fenwick, 2001). One theme was the imbalance of power between the mother and nurse: Mothers struggled to attain the role of "mother," whereas nurses attempted to maintain their roles as the "experts." Although these studies were focused on mothers, I discovered, inadvertently, that fathers were also scrutinizing NICU caregivers. Fathers were sometimes frustrated with their observations and interactions with health professionals; however, they kept quiet about their displeasure—silent, but waiting with a watchful eye.

## "I'm Sort of the Second Ears"

Several fathers were annoyed with their lack of communication with healthcare providers, especially physicians. One father's story, in particular, illustrates the problems busy fathers face as they strive to keep informed amidst a traditional medical system:

F09: ... [it was] frustrating because you're trying to figure out everything that's going on and, of course, it would just happen that, as soon as I'd leave, one of the doctors would come in. And ... normally I'd be the one asking a bunch of questions. I don't know if it was just because Kelly [his wife] was just so bombarded with everything ... She wasn't thinking straight ... So, I'd be the one asking most of the questions ... They'd come in and tell her all this stuff, and she'd try to relay it the best she could to me, but still, I wasn't there to hear it, so it's kind of like you're missing information. So, it's like you want to be there all the time in case the doctor came in, but you never knew when they were gonna come in.

I: Yeah, so that was hard.

F09: Actually, I had her hold the phone up ... one time because the doctor had just gotten there when I was at home. So, I kind of listened in.

Although this father spent every night sleeping on a cot next to his wife's bed, he was unable to get his information first-hand because he had to leave for work before doctor's rounds.

Four fathers expressed disappointment about receiving information through the nurses, not the doctors. One father was "apprehensive about asking the nurses" because he wanted to get information straight from the physicians. He noted: "I kind of thought that with different nurses, things we'd ask, there were sometimes inconsistencies." Another father noted that it:

... wasn't meaningful until the doctors came around and actually said 'hey, well, this is what we found, this is what we think it is. And, of course, it was pretty much the same thing as the nurses said and, not saying that I don't trust any of the nurses, because they have done an outstanding job, but it felt a little more meaningful coming from the doctor.

The number of fathers who had not spoken to a physician for several weeks was an unfortunate finding. Fathers lost contact with physicians because they were often at work in the mornings when physicians made their rounds. However, one father resisted speaking to a physician because the doctor on call that particular evening was less familiar to him.

Most fathers received information about their infant's progress from their wives, who had more time to spend in the NICU. One father recalled: "she talks to them [doctors] and finds out most of the information ... and she usually relates it to me when I get home from work." Although getting information second hand was not as meaningful, it was still valuable, because they really wanted to stay informed.

## "We Don't Push"

Fathers refrained from comment when bothered by observations in the NICU. When I asked one father to describe his caregiving, he noted:

She ... has changed his diapers a couple of times. It depends on the nurse, we don't push, you know. I don't like to get on the bad side of a nurse that's watching my kid, and she's the same way ... If they say 'do you want to change his diaper?,' she'll change his diaper.

Freud (1995) first reported this hesitancy in fathers with premature infants. He wrote "fathers know that one had better not be openly critical of them [health caregivers] lest they take it out on the baby (a common ever-present fear)" (p. 238). Hurst (2001) noted that mothers feared being labeled as difficult because they did not want to jeopardize their babies' care in the NICU.

In my conversations with Dan, he recalled several situations in which he was frustrated by the nurses' actions, yet he seemed reluctant to confront them. Initially, he did not understand why the nurses were so nonchalant about monitor alarms. He recalled:

. . . They go off, and sometimes it doesn't feel like Mary gets enough attention. I'm not sure why things are going on, like her saturation was dropping down, and it keeps dropping down. It's like 'hold on, something's going on, somebody do something.' Nobody seems to get excited. It's kind of tough to see because I'm sure they know what they're doing, but it's my baby.

He noted that he "can't really tell the nurses how to do their job and stuff, but I think if . . . I notice that it's bothering me that much, then I'll say something." He acknowledged that he was "walking a fine line" in the NICU. Perhaps fathers remained quiet because of their novice status in the NICU or perhaps they are not as attached to their infants at that point in time and might lack the vigor that is needed to bring their concerns to the surface.

## "She's Yours, But . . . "

Fathers are in a precarious position in the NICU. They have had to learn that it is the nurses who are the experts—a fact that they accept, but not without trepidation. However, they are new fathers, a role that normally is accompanied by the privilege of ownership. But, as long as their infants are in the NICU, their parental rights are in suspension. They often feel as though they have to ask permission to provide caregiving for their own children. One father noted:

We didn't feel as informed as we could have about our boundaries. I mean it was like our own child, but we didn't know what we could do with her. It's kind of a strange feeling where she's yours, but you have to ask permission to do things.

Several fathers reported that nurses sometimes attached "rules" with infant caregiving. One father recalled an episode in which he "was coerced by the nurses":

I was in there by myself . . . They said 'do you want to hold him?' And I said 'yes' and they said 'have you changed his diaper?' And I said 'no,' and they said 'oh, if you don't change the diaper, you can't hold him. That's a rule.' They all got a big kick out of that.

Perhaps nurses have found that coercion is an effective way to motivate fathers. Although quite innocent on first glance, upon closer examination, their rules emanate dominance, much like the relationship a parent would have with a child. Rules, subtly, but powerfully, keep fathers in their place—as novices. Fathers might "obey" these rules because they are threatened, and, frankly, they often need the nurse's help.

## "It Depends on the Nurse"

Another finding was how carefully fathers watched the nurses and how thoughtfully they described those interactions. There was definitely a sense of better and worse in terms of how well nurses communicated with them. Dan described a "good" nurse as someone who would initiate a verbal exchange with him regarding his daughter's progress. A good nurse would:

. . . come up and tell you everything . . . They saw you come in and, as soon as they got a chance, they would come over and fill you in on what's going on with your baby, if anything changed. They'd ask you if you want to do this with her. A lot of times we didn't know we could do that. So then we'd know we should've been doing that.

The nurses that he labeled as "bad" communicators would initially ignore him, even when not busy. This was significant because his usual routine was to "just wait for the nurse to come in and give us kind of a report. Then we try to get her out and hold her . . . " He recalled "sometimes when you'd come in, I [wondered] . . . why aren't they coming to tell us things? I know they saw us come in." He might have been abiding by the unwritten rule that parents must seek permission before entering their infant's bedside space. When his presence was not acknowledged, and he had to wait for a period of time to be granted permission, he got frustrated.

Larry saw nurses as either caring or uncaring, depending on their nonverbal communication. He described his second skin-to-skin holding experience:

*F03*: . . . The nurse . . . was all right, but she wasn't too good about it . . . She didn't get the drape and put it around us and she just gave us the rocking chair and said 'take off your shirt and sit down there.' We didn't like it too much. The other nurse, she was really cool about it.

*I*: Oh, so it varies by nurse.

*F03*: Yeah, I guess. Like the nurse out there today, she's a real nice woman. She's really caring about the baby and stuff . . . I like the nurses that care about the baby, see who they are and that they're a baby, that they're a premature baby, not just go over there, do your job, pull the tubes, you know, suction them out, do this, do that, hurry up and get it done with the baby . . . I like the people that you know take care of her, be nice to her and stuff. You know, it's not really being nice to her. It's just trying to take your time.

*I*: So you can tell that pretty quickly about a nurse do you think?

*F03*: Yeah, pretty much. Almost every day there's a different nurse in there. Ever since I've been going up there, there has been almost a different nurse every day . . . And I can tell just by how the nurse acts and everything whether she's gonna be gentle. Usually they are pretty rough, they all are pretty much, and I just get nervous. It's not that she don't care about the baby or anything, it's just that she wants to get her job done. That's how I feel. She just wants to hurry and get her job done.

Although Larry was very protective of Leah, and it upset him to watch nurses care for his daughter in a hurried fashion, he kept his thoughts to himself. Although I was not present during his interactions with nurses, I doubt if they had any idea how carefully he was watching them, and the intensity of the feelings he harbored inside.

Larry brought up a very problematic practice that several fathers commented on: inconsistency of caregivers. One father remarked that the lack of consistency of nurses was "discomforting" because:

You get a rapport with somebody, and it's hard to switch because you can't just assume you can talk to this person about the same subject and they're going to understand how you're talking to them or what you're talking about or what you mean.

He felt that having consistent nurses allowed him the opportunity to get to know the nurses "a little bit better . . . which made it easier to talk with them, makes it easier for you to think 'well, what can I ask this person?'" Building rapport with nurses was important to fathers, but a real challenge because they saw a new face every day.

## MAKING A CONNECTION: THE FATHER'S VOICE

These fathers faced barriers few must contend with: small, medically fragile infants housed in Plexiglas boxes, devices that have the words "caution" and "do not touch" invisibly, yet indelibly, scribbled all over them. During my early interviews, I recall being astounded at how much fathers talked about using their voices when describing interactions with their infants. Fathers often did not feel comfortable touching and holding their tiny infants, and talking was a way to connect without getting physical. It is simple, easy, safe, and distinct—men's voices are instrumentally different than women's voices—a perfect fit.

The story of one 40-year-old father, Kenny, is remarkable in terms of the way he used his voice when communicating with his son, who was born at 25 weeks' gestation. One year before his son's birth, his wife, Denise, had a miscarriage due to an incompetent cervix. As a result, she had a cerclage placed during this pregnancy. Kenny initiated conversations with his unborn son from early on with a definite purpose: To keep him inside as long as possible. He coached his son: "I've been telling him 'come up here, son' because I knew we had time. She was on bed rest, so I kept telling him, talking to her belly, 'come up here, son, come up here.' So he really did . . . She started having pain and stuff in her ribs, and she said that was because the baby was up there, probably kicking her in the ribs." Once Denise was in active premature labor, the doctors discovered that the baby was positioned at a very high station. This news prompted Kenny to initiate a new set of instructions to his son:

When she was dilated in there [labor and delivery], they couldn't get him out because he was way up there. So . . . I'd talk down low to her belly and I said 'come down here son, it's time, come on out, don't worry, daddy'll catch you.' And then . . . I went out and smoked a cigarette. As soon as I got back, they was on their way to get me. The baby was already down there and ready to go.

When I asked him if he felt he had something to do with his son's sudden descent, he remarked: "Basically, yeah. Probably. I would talk to him all the time when she was pregnant." I discovered that the reason he told his son to "come up here" was to prevent him from somehow "kicking that stitch and breaking it." Whether his words influenced the delivery outcome or not, there is no doubt that this father had already established a connection to his son using his voice.

This voice connection only grew stronger with the passage of time. When I asked him to describe his thoughts just after birth, he recalled: "It was just an eerie feeling. He was alert and knew that we was there because he recognizes our voices." Later in that same interview, he described early visits in the NICU:

> F05: . . . he opens his eyes when he hears my voice and mama's voice.
> I: That's pretty neat.
> F05: He glances at us and watches us. He followed my voice as soon as I talked. I told her 'watch his eyeball' and I kind of moved a little bit and he'd watch my shadow.

The words of another father, Larry, touched me in a special way. I think it might have been the love he expressed for his young daughter, despite the fact he had only known her for 3 weeks. This little girl filled a void in his life created by a turbulent past. Because he adored her so, he gallantly struggled to connect with her as a father:

> F03: I try to get her used to my voice. That's pretty much what I do. I just talk stupid stuff to her, you know, just like you normally do to a baby . . . Just try to get her used to my voice. She knows her mom's voice real well.
> I: . . . Is there anything in particular that you do . . . to see if Leah can learn that you're the dad?
> F03: I get really close to her, by her face, and talk to her, not real deep or anything. I just talk my normal voice to her, real close to her. You know, cause all the other nurses are standing back, and she hears their voices but it's a loud voice when the nurses are talking to us . . . I know none of the nurses get real close to her and try to talk real sweet to her or anything, but that's what I mainly try to do.
> I: . . . Okay, so there really isn't anything you've figured out yet that is specific to her reacting to you, but you think she is doing it to mom. She knows mom's voice.
> F03: . . . I know she pretty much knows my voice but you know, she just doesn't react to it as well. But that's all right. I'll stick my mouth through that [isolette porthole] and 'oooh' like that and try to get her used to my vocal cords or whatever. And talk to her like that, sticking my mouth to her so that she can feel the vibration.

Although Larry had little formal education, he seemed to be quite perceptive. He recalled his thoughts about his daughter's emerging smile:

> I think I seen her smile, but the nurses say it's some kind of . . . reaction in her face that might make her look like she's smiling . . . But, I don't care, I still think she's smiling.

My purpose in including this quote is not to wrangle with the validity of the nurse's explanation of smiling, but to discuss the emotional implications of the nurse's response. The nurse overlooked an important aspect of their interaction: Larry was seeking positive affirmation from his daughter. By offering a scientific rebuttal, the nurse lost the opportunity to provide him positive feedback. According to VandenBerg (2000), providing positive meaning for parents is crucial because it gives them credit for being parents, and "even tiny expressions can be supportive" (p. 63).

## RECOMMENDATIONS FOR CHANGE IN PRACTICE

The needs of fathers must be considered in the implementation of nursing care for high-risk infants—that is, developmentally supportive and family-centered, especially if we are to individualize our care. The following recommendations for practice are based on the study findings. We have little evidence to support the father's role in the NICU or its relationship to the implementation of IFDC. The study reported in this chapter is just a start on this journey. More research is needed to validate these findings and evaluate the following suggested interventions, which were developed to reflect the father's point of view.

- The fundamental foundation for nursing practice in the NICU should be built upon a consistency of caregiving model. Fathers need to establish rapport with a small team of nurses to feel safe enough to proceed with learning caregiving and begin building a strong father-infant relationship.
- Approach interactions with mothers and fathers differently because they are coming to parenthood from two different perspectives. Providers who interface with male and female clients must be sensitive to gender roles and how they factor into client-provider interactions (Ringheim, 2002). Nurses must remain open to potential gender

differences and ascertain the particular interests and goals of individual fathers, rather than make the assumption, for example, that mastering diapering is a mandatory requirement for infant discharge.

- Refrain from judgment based on fathers' visiting patterns, reluctance to provide infant caregiving, and so on. Fathers' stressors might lie well outside of the NICU, and, therefore, be invisible to NICU healthcare professionals.

- Offer frequent positive affirmation to fathers regarding their baby's behavior and/or appearance and the father's accomplishments, no matter how small. Elevate fathers to the status of an expert in their role as parents, with the goal being to incorporate fathers as partners in caregiving.

- Give fathers as much choice and control as feasible with infant interactions. Refrain from coercion; instead, discuss their goals for learning caregiving. Fathers are often not as comfortable as mothers with holding their infants and might not be as interested in learning caregiving while in the NICU.

- Evaluate unit policies, especially visitation policies and other policies that limit parental access to information (availability of charts, ability to listen to medical rounds, timing of physician rounds, etc.). It might be helpful to refer to *NANN's Infant and Family-Centered Developmental Care Guideline for Practice* (NANN, 2000) to determine if the unit is meeting the needs of the families.

- Talk with fathers, although they might be hard to engage initially. As you build rapport with them, they will usually relax and open up. I found that talking was a therapeutic intervention in itself for fathers in my study.

- Keep fathers well informed. Good communication with them is essential to building rapport. Consistency in caregiving is the key to good communication.

- Provide quality information related to their infant's medical condition and developmental needs. Learning developmental caregiving is much more than providing knowledge as often occurs in a teaching session (Lawhon, 2002). Facilitate parents emerging competence while they are at the bedside with their baby. Practice makes perfect.

- Strive to never lose sight of the experience from the eyes of a first-time visitor to the NICU. Often the

aspects of the environment that are inconsequential to you (monitor alarms, etc.) are very frightening for them.

## CONCLUSION

The family (infant, mother, and father) must be the core of developmental caregiving. These study findings deepen our understanding of the family because they illuminate the father's perspective after an early-birth experience. Fathers noted that juggling their time between work, hospital, and home was stressful—a finding that may go unnoticed by neonatal health caregivers because these stressors often lie outside the NICU. Fathers returned to work quickly after their infants' birth because they could "do" something at work; work boosted their feelings of confidence and competence. A father's ability to get to know his preterm infant was shaped by past and present relationships, specifically with his own father and his wife/partner. It takes self-confidence to "try on" fathering in a threatening environment like the NICU.

Fathers were sometimes frustrated with their interactions with neonatal healthcare providers because they felt they were overlooked. Fathers, however, kept quiet about their displeasure because they were novices in this environment and feared repercussions. Fathers appreciated nurses who readily communicated with them and treated their infants with loving care. Fathers made a connection with their infants using their voices—an approach that is safe, easy, and distinct.

Once at home after discharge, fathers discovered that the rank of expert had been passed from the nurse to the mother. Mothers could either draw fathers closer to their infants with their attitudes or actions or keep them more on the periphery. Fathers voiced concerns about their infants' health and development at home, including their fears of spoiling and their discontentment with home monitors.

Findings from previous research studies that examined the experiences of fathers of term and preterm infants assisted my interpretation of these study findings. More research is needed, however, to broaden our understanding of fathering a preterm infant. Future studies on fathering after an early birth need to be designed to include mothers and nurses, because their voices would offer significant insight into the father's world. For nurses to provide expert, developmentally sound caregiving, they must have a better understanding of the fathers of their tiny patients. Without such an understanding, meaningful family-centered caregiving is impossible.

## ACKNOWLEDGMENT

The research in this chapter was supported by a grant from the Foundation for Neonatal Research and education, Santa Rosa, California.

## *REFERENCES*

Anderson, A. (1996). The father-infant relationship: Becoming connected. *Journal of the Society of Pediatric Nurses, 1*(2), 83-92.

Belsky, J. (1984). The determinants of parenting: A process model. *Child Development, 55,* 83-96.

Clark, S., & Miles, M. (1999). Conflicting responses: The experiences of fathers of infants diagnosed with severe congenital heart disease. *Journal of the Society of Pediatric Nurses, 4,* 7-14.

Daly, K. (1993). Reshaping fatherhood: Finding the models. *Journal of Family Issues, 14*(4), 510-530.

Docherty, S.L., Miles, M.S., & Holditch-Davis, D. (2002). Worry about child health in mothers of hospitalized medically fragile infants. *Advances in Neonatal Care, 2*(2), 84-92.

Ehrensaft, D. (1990). *Parenting together.* Chicago: University of Illinois Press.

Federal Interagency Forum on Child & Family Statistics (1998). *Nurturing fatherhood: Improving data and research on male fertility, family formation, and fatherhood.* Available online at *www.aspe.os.shhs.gov/fathers/cfsforum/front.htm.*

Fenwick, J., Barclay, L., & Schmied, V. (2001). Struggling to mother: A consequence of inhibitive nursing interactions in the neonatal nursery. *Journal of Perinatal and Neonatal Nursing, 15*(2), 49-64.

Field, T. (1981). Fathers' interactions with their high-risk infants. *Infant Mental Health Journal, 2,* 249-256.

Freud, W. (1995). Premature fathers: Lone wolves? In J. Shapiro, M. Diamond, & M. Greenberg (Eds.), *Becoming a father* (pp. 234-242). New York: Springer.

Gray, J. (1992). *Men are from Mars, women are from Venus: A practical guide for improving communication and getting what you want in your relationships.* New York: HarperCollins.

Harrison, H. (1993). The principles for family-centered neonatal care. *Journal of Pediatrics, 82,* 643-650.

Holditch-Davis, D., & Miles, M. (1997). Parenting the prematurely born child. *Annual Review of Nursing Research, 15,* 3-34.

Hurst, I. (2001). Vigilant watching over: Mothers' actions to safeguard their premature babies in the newborn intensive care nursery. *Journal of Perinatal and Neonatal Nursing, 15*(3), 39-57.

Hyman, J. (1995). Shifting patterns of fathering in the first year of life: On intimacy between fathers and their babies. In J. Shapiro, M. Diamond, & M. Greenberg (Eds.), *Becoming a father: Contemporary social, developmental, and clinical perspectives* (pp. 256-267). New York: Springer.

Jordan, P. (1990). Laboring for relevance: Expectant and new fatherhood. *Nursing Research, 39,* 11-16.

Klitzing, K., Simoni, H., Amsler, F., & Burgin, D. (1999). The role of the father in early family interactions. *Infant Mental Health Journal, 20*(3), 222-237.

Lamb, M. (1997). The development of father-infant relationships. In M. Lamb (Ed.), *Role of the father in child development* (3rd ed., pp. 104-120). New York: Wiley & Sons.

Lawhon, G. (2002). Facilitation of parenting the premature infant within the newborn intensive care unit. *Journal of Perinatal and Neonatal Nursing, 16*(1), 71-82.

Lupton, D., & Fenwick, J. (2001). 'They've forgotten that I'm mum': Constructing and practicing motherhood in special care nurseries. *Social Science and Medicine, 53,* 1011-1021.

Miles, M., & Holditch-Davis, D. (1997). Parenting the prematurely born child: Pathways of influence. *Seminars in Perinatology, 21*(3), 254-266.

National Association of Neonatal Nurses (NANN). (2000). *Infant and family-centered developmental care: Guideline for practice* (Document 1201). Glenview, IL: NANN.

Ringheim, K. (2002). When the client is male: Client-provider interaction from a gender perspective. *International Family Planning Perspectives, 28*(3), 170-175.

Sullivan, J. (1999). Development of father-infant attachment in fathers of pre-term infants. *Neonatal Network, 18*(7), 33-39.

VandenBerg, K.A. (2000). Supporting parents in the NICU: Guidelines for promoting parent confidence and competence. *Neonatal Network, 19*(8), 63.

Volling, B., & Belsky, J. (1991). Multiple determinants of father involvement during infancy in dual-earner and single-earner families. *Journal of Marriage and the Family, 53,* 461-474.

Webb, C. (1992). The use of the first person in academic writing: Objectivity, language and gatekeeping. *Journal of Advanced Nursing, 17,* 747-752.

# 20 Early Intervention beyond the Newborn Period

**Deborah Winders Davis, Jane K. Sweeney, Carol Spruill Turnage-Carrier, Chrysty D. Graves, and Linda Rector**

All newborns have the potential to experience events that will alter their developmental trajectory. It is important for healthcare professionals who work with infants to understand the complex nature of human development. We can provide individualized care to optimize each infant's potential, if the normal process of human development is considered within the context of the infant's gestational age, postconceptual age, healthcare needs, and environment. Although much remains unknown about the numerous developmental processes that influence an infant's outcome, it is clear that human development involves complex interactions between the child and his/her environment. Only through a better understanding of these processes and the factors involved, can we hope to alter and improve development.

Unfortunately, predicting outcome is a more difficult task than it was once thought to be. Children who have experienced major insults during the newborn period sometimes survive with remarkably intact nervous systems, whereas children who appear to be free from risk have developmental delays and deficits. In this chapter, we discuss the need for early intervention (EI) strategies beyond the newborn period to decrease complications of a neonatal intensive care unit (NICU) stay. First, we review some theoretic perspectives that contribute to our understanding of developmental risk.

## OVERVIEW OF RELEVANT DEVELOPMENTAL CONCEPTS

For EI to be successful, one must have a clear understanding of the many factors that can influence outcome for individual children and the interaction between those factors. Due to the complex nature of human development, we have been unable to adequately predict specific outcomes for specific children. More importantly, the selection of and expectations for developmental interventions must be based on an understanding that children and their environments have unique qualities. Intervention programs can no longer be designed with the idea that one program "fits all." Therefore, as healthcare professionals, before we can design appropriate interventions to enhance developmental outcomes or minimize negative trajectories, we must identify the factors that are working at several levels to produce less than optimal outcomes (Sameroff & Fiese, 2000). Before discussing specific factors that can influence outcome, a review of important concepts related to developmental outcome are presented.

One important model that has had a major impact on our thinking about development is known as the *bioecological model* (or sometimes simply the *ecological model*) of development (Bronfenbrenner & Crouter, 1983; Bronfenbrenner & Morris, 1998; Sameroff & Fiese, 2000). Although it is beyond the scope of this chapter to thoroughly discuss this model, a summary of the critical concepts are presented. (See Bronfenbrenner & Morris, 1998 for a comprehensive review.) The ecological model of human development is described as consisting of four major components, which are *Process, Person, Context,* and *Time* (Bronfenbrenner & Morris, 1998). Process involves the specific way in which the organism interacts with the environment or it can be thought of as the mechanism of development. To fully understand development, one should study "how" (Process) the organism (Person) performs a specific skill within a naturalistic setting (Context) and how the behavior changes with age (Time). Although this view of development is not new, researchers have been slow to employ methods that adequately address all aspects of the model (Bronfenbrenner & Morris, 1998). The challenge for researchers is to find new methods that include all the dimensions of this complex model of human development.

*Dynamic systems theory* is another model that identifies the complex nature of human development (Thelen & Smith, 1996). Before the emergence of these contemporary systems theories, development was often viewed in terms of traditional dichotomies such as "nature versus nurture," "structure versus function," or "brain versus behavior," to name a few, but it is no longer acceptable to consider development in such simplistic terms (Thelen & Smith, 1996). Rather, in a dynamic view of development, structure determines function and function determines structure within a context-specific environment. Not all functions or structures develop at the same rate. Therefore, although some aspects of development might have critical periods or optimal periods for development to occur, other processes can continue to unfold into adulthood.

Another important concept inherent in a systems view of development is that experience can alter brain organization (Kolb, 1995). Experience can include external events such as those provided by the physical environment, but it can also include internal events such as alterations in hormone release, development itself, and even thought processes (Kolb, 1995). The capacity of the brain to change in response to such experiential events is known as *brain plasticity* or *neuropruning*.

Plasticity is an important concept in normal development, but it is even more important in understanding outcomes and processes that occur as a result of abnormal development; brain insults due to prematurity, hemorrhage, trauma; and other medical and biologic risk factors. Plasticity adds to our understanding not only of how the brain is affected by adverse events, but also how the brain responds to intervention. At birth, the dendritic growth in the deepest layers of the human cortex has reached about 60% of maximum while the dendritic growth in the more superficial layers has reached

only 30% of maximum (Kolb, 1995). Although dendritic growth varies with the cortical layer and location, it is clear that intense dendritic growth occurs during the first 18 postnatal months (Kolb, 1995). Although cortical reorganization may be greatest during infancy and early childhood, recent evidence indicates that it continues into adulthood (Nelson, 2000). With an understanding of the continued brain growth and differentiation occurring in early development and the dynamic nature of developmental processes, it is easier to understand how experience can affect structure.

Although providing a developmentally optimal environment might not compensate for the most severe structural insults, it can lessen the effect of the early insult. Conversely, children who are born with intact neurologic systems can have less than optimal outcomes if they do not have experiences that stimulate dendritic growth and differentiation. Balbernie (2002) explains that a single risk factor "is not directly psychopathogenic; it is a representation of probability, so that a cluster can bias toward an unfavorable developmental outcome" (p. 330). Outcome is determined by numerous dynamically interacting factors, which include number, type, frequency, and duration of adverse events or risk factors. Therefore, a child who is born at 26 weeks' gestation to an alcohol-dependent mother who is living in poverty and has few social support networks might have a very different outcome from a child born at 26 weeks to a healthy woman who received frequent prenatal care, is married, and has a supportive family network. However, knowing that a child has been exposed to factors that place him/her at risk for adverse developmental outcomes is not enough. Understanding "how" the risk factors produce the adverse outcome will provide a foundation for intervention.

## DEVELOPMENTAL FOLLOW-UP

A systems approach to development provides a useful foundation upon which to organize developmental follow-up. Although the systems models described earlier were designed for use in the study of developing systems, the concepts can form the basis for assessment and intervention. Specifically, in a *systems model*, one must consider the child within his/her environment over time, keeping in mind that the child and the environment are dynamically interacting. In addition, as the child changes over time, the impact of specific factors might change. Therefore, developmental follow-up that is designed to assess not only the child, but also the physical and psychosocial environments within which he/she develops, is most advantageous. Because some aspects of brain development occur up to the age of 15 to 20 years, long-term follow-up is essential to identify some disabilities, especially those that involve higher-level cognitive skills that might not emerge until late childhood or adolescence.

Who should receive such comprehensive evaluations? Although, ideally, all children would benefit from developmental follow-up, it is not fiscally possible. Therefore, developmental follow-up is usually available for those children who have been exposed to factors that place them at significant risk for developmental problems. Box 20-1 lists some of the factors that should be considered as potential mediators of

## Box **20-1**  Neonatal Follow-up Assessments: Potential Mediators of Outcome

**Child Biologic Factors**

Prenatal and neonatal risks
Current health status
Chronic health conditions
Child's temperament
Mental capacity
Nutrition

**Physical Environmental Factors**

Availability of resources
Organization of the home

**Psychological/Social/Educational Environment**

Family structure
Family support systems
Parental education
Parent-child interaction
Parental beliefs
Parental mental health status
Parental temperament
Parental mental capacity

development. Although this list is not exhaustive, it reminds us that we are dealing with a very complex system. Multidisciplinary and comprehensive assessments are needed to identify individual strengths and weaknesses.

## DEVELOPMENTAL INTERVENTION

Sameroff and Fiese (2000) summed up the major problem that has plagued interventionists when they said, "Unfortunately, there are no universal treatments for all children" (p.135). They go on to say that most intervention programs are not comprehensive enough to address all of the potential factors that could influence development (Sameroff & Fiese, 2000). In addition, generally, intervention programs lack the specificity to modify developmental trajectories for individual children.

The primary reason for the lack of specificity is that much is still unknown about the underlying processes responsible for many developmental delays and disabilities. It has been well documented that medically high-risk infants, especially those born prematurely, are particularly vulnerable to such delays. In addition, adverse environments, such as those associated with extreme poverty, have been shown to have a negative influence on developmental competence (Bradley, Corwyn, Pipes McAdoo, & Garcia Coll, 2001; Watson, Kirby, Kelleher, & Bradley, 1996). However, much research is still needed to identify all of the factors that might be responsible for these delays and the process by which these factors interact to produce the deleterious outcome. Once we adequately understand the processes and mechanisms underlying these delays and deficits, *specific* interventions can be developed to facilitate adaptation of a remarkably pliable nervous system (Jobe, 2001).

## COGNITIVE SKILLS: ATTENTION, SELF-REGULATION, AND PERCEPTION

Although the following section focuses on the development of cognitive skills, keep in mind that from a bioecological framework, cognitive development does not occur in isolation from other developmental systems nor can it be removed from the environmental context in which it occurs. In fact, much early learning occurs within social interactions between the child and significant adults in his/her environment, especially the mother (Landry, Miller-Loncar, Smith, & Swank, 2002; Landry, Smith, Swank, et al., 2001; Landry, Smith, Swank, & Miller-Loncar, 2000; Rowe & Wertsch, 2002). It is through these interactions that the child learns about the environment and the relations that occur between objects and people in the environment (Smith, Landry, & Swank, 2000). Keep in mind, too, that while cognitive development will be discussed separately, it does not occur independently from development in other domains such as motor, social, and emotional development.

*Cognition* has been defined as the act or process of knowing. Therefore, although cognitive development has been discussed as though it were a single entity, many processes are working together as one develops the ability "to know." As stated earlier, cognitive development does not occur separately from development in other domains nor is it a unitary process. Cognitive development occurs as the result of the child's emerging and interactive skills in areas such as perception, memory, attention, and problem solving. Of particular interest in relation to cognitive development, especially the development of attention skills, is the development of self-regulation.

*Self-regulation* is a term that has been used to describe a variety of functional skills. Although the various ways in which self-regulation has been described and measured seem very different, there might be some connection between the seemingly discrepant views, which will be discussed in more detail later. First, however, let us examine the self-regulation of cognitive skills, especially attention regulation. In that context, it can be thought of as an individual's ability to make adjustments in the intake and use of information to appropriately respond to the demands of his/her environment. Attention control, selective attention, attention allocation, attention regulation, and executive function are a few terms that imply self-regulation of cognition. Control or regulation of attention is important because it allows the child to select relevant perceptual and conceptual information that permits adaptation to the environment, and it facilitates the storage of important information, which forms the basis for the child's development of self and world representations (Derryberry & Reed, 1996).

*Self-regulatory skills* emerge as a function of the interaction between biologic factors, such as the child's temperament and variations in physiologic and neurologic processes, and environmental factors, such as the quality of the physical and social contexts within which development occurs (Ruff & Rothbart, 1996). Temperament might directly impact attention regulation or it might have an indirect impact by altering the caregiving environment.

Researchers have identified links between the development of attention regulation skills and the quality of the environment. In a longitudinal study of children who were born of low birthweight (LBW), Robson and Pederson (1997) used a multidimensional and multivariate approach to examine attention problems in infancy and early childhood. They found that attention was correlated with the quality of the environment during infancy and childhood. In addition, they found that both infant characteristics and environmental factors were related to attention problems and suggest a multidimensional, transactional model for studying attention problems (Robson & Pederson, 1997). Additionally they suggest that a safe, organized physical environment and a responsive, nurturant social environment can facilitate the development of self-regulatory abilities (Robson & Pederson, 1997).

Some children, such as those born prematurely or who are medically fragile, are more at risk for problems related to the development of attentional skills. Because preterm infants are less responsive to their environment and are more at risk for deficits in attention regulation in infancy, their cognitive development might continue to be directly and indirectly impeded throughout childhood. It is easy to see how problems with the self-regulation of attention could influence academic success for these high-risk children. It has also been suggested that a group of cognitive, social, behavioral, and academic problems reported in children born prematurely might best be viewed as alterations in self-regulatory functioning rather than as separate problems (Davis & Burns, 2001; Sykes, Hoy, Bill, et al., 1997). Failures of self-regulatory functioning, particularly self-regulation of attention, could explain why children in this population require a disproportionate amount of special education services, even in the absence of major disability or general cognitive deficits (Davis & Burns, 2001).

Much is still unknown about exactly how deficits in attention and perception affect cognitive development, but it is clear that there is a relationship that needs to be explored further. One way that perceptual defects can lead to cognitive delays relates to the earlier discussion about neuronal growth and differentiation. If, for example, a child has a visual impairment that goes undetected and untreated, the result might be structural changes in the brain. Structural changes can occur as the result of a lack of stimulation to the visual pathways. Depending on the critical period for specific pathways, timing and severity of the insult, and timing and appropriateness of the intervention, permanent alterations in structure and function can result.

Self-regulation has been examined in the context of emotion and physiologic regulation as well as self-regulation of cognitive processes such as attention and learning. Until recently, these types of regulations were considered totally separate entities. Blair (2002) reviewed the literature linking the development of cognition and emotionality and proposed a developmental neurobiologic model for school readiness. In this model, Blair (2002) proposes that "school readiness can be seen as influencing and being influenced by developmental processes occurring at the neurobiologic, physiologic, behavioral, family, classroom, school, and community levels" (p. 118). In the neurobiologic model, self-regulation is a key factor in school readiness, and self-regulation is viewed from a variety of domains. Related to the ecological model for developmental processes, the neurobiologic model for school readiness supports the notion that the child is viewed within a context—in this case, the classroom. Specific self-regulatory skills are needed to successfully make the transition from the home environment to the school environment. Blair (2002) emphasizes the importance of understanding the development of self-regulation and the interconnections between self-regulation, temperament, cognitive, emotional and social development, and the environment. Based on the neurobiologic model of conceptualizing school readiness, it appears that the lines between these seemingly separate systems cannot be clearly determined. With the idea that there is

an interconnection between the development of physiologic regulation and self-regulatory processes in emotionality, attention, and cognition, it might be important to assess infants and young children for indications that a child might have difficulties in physiologic self-regulation. Regulatory disordered infants have been described to have disturbances or difficulties in sleep regulation, self-consoling, feeding, and arousal (disorganization and distractibility) (Ruff & Rothbart, 1996). These early behaviors might be precursors for later attention and learning problems as well as social competence.

Another concept that can no longer be considered to have a unitary origin is temperament. Blair (2002) suggests that some aspects of temperament can be constitutionally determined whereas others might be environmentally induced. Although temperament is generally considered to be biologically based; it is not "hardwired" and therefore can be altered by environmental influences. Others have suggested that temperamental characteristics develop and change over time (Posner & Rothbart, 2000; Rothbart, 1989; Rothbart & Bates, 1998). Furthermore, temperament is not simply related to reactivity and self-regulation, but has been defined as the individual difference in one's expression of these constructs (Posner & Rothbart, 2000; Rothbart & Bates, 1998). Others have linked early physiologic measures of stability to later social competence at school age in children born prematurely (Doussard-Roosevelt, McClenny, & Porges, 2001). It is becoming very clear that these systems are not easily separable and that more data are needed to determine the exact mechanism by which they interact and how all of these processes relate to optimal developmental outcomes, especially related to academic success and social competence. More importantly, understanding mechanisms of self-regulation in normally developing children could lead to advances in diagnosis, prevention, and treatment of developmental problems such as attention deficit hyperactivity disorder (ADHD) and learning disabilities (Posner & Rothbart, 2000).

As developmentally appropriate care in the NICU is becoming standard practice, more data are emerging that explore the relationship between various types of intervention and self-regulatory processes. For example, one such study describes the physiologic stability gained by premature infants who were exposed to kangaroo care as compared with a control group (Feldman, Weller, Sirota, & Eidelman, 2003). Based on the information presented previously, we can hypothesize that interventions, such as Kangaroo care that support physiologic self-regulation in infancy will have a positive impact on later cognitive, behavioral, and emotional self-regulation.

## EARLY INTERVENTION

Early intervention (EI) is often discussed as if it were a unitary concept and a concept that is universally understood by everyone. However, neither conceptualization of EI is correct. The purpose of EI programs is to promote childhood health and development for children who are vulnerable due to a variety of reasons, including prematurity, neurologic insults, and less than optimal home environments. The efficacy of the program depends on the location, the treatment target, the timing for initiating treatment, the intensity, the duration, and the curriculum or intervention provided (Brooks-Gunn, 2003). Healthcare professionals often think of EI simply in terms of a medical model that includes services such as nutritional support, occupational and physical therapy, and medical and nursing intervention (Hitzfelder, 1996). However, the literature describes numerous early intervention programs that are designed to assist environmentally vulnerable children to achieve academic success equal to that of children from less vulnerable environments (Brooks-Gunn, 2003). For example, Head Start and Early Head Start are two early-intervention programs that focus on improving academic success for children living in poverty or near-poverty conditions. Other programs seek to provide interventions for multiple factors that place them at risk for developmental problems. Not all EI is the same, and availability of specific programs is often determined by the available resources in each community. EI programs designed to promote health and development for children from vulnerable environments are often administered through state health departments and other agencies supported by federal, state, and local public funding sources.

In the remainder of this chapter, we describe the history and implementation of early intervention programs that were initiated in response to a federal mandate and are often referred to as infant-toddler programs. In 1986, the U.S. Congress passed a law known as PL 99-457, Part H, to begin a new era for infants and young children with disabilities and their families. The signing of this law brought major changes to the way services were provided by placing the focus of care within the context of the family and the home environment and by encouraging collaboration between various healthcare disciplines and agencies (Bishop, 1999). The law was reauthorized in 1991 as PL 102-119, the Individuals with Disabilities Education Act (IDEA), and again in 1997 as the IDEA Amendments of 1997 (PL 105-17, Part C). The regulations resulting from this legislation are extensive and cannot be fully described in this chapter, but the important components are summarized, especially those most relevant to healthcare professionals. The law and related regulations are public information and are readily available for review, if more detail is needed.

The purpose of PL 105-17, Part C, is to enhance development of infants and toddlers with disabilities. The law made federal funding available to states that voluntarily implemented the EI program (Bishop, 1999). According to the regulations, the purpose of the EI program for infants and toddlers with disabilities is to provide financial assistance to the States to:

1. Maintain and implement a statewide, comprehensive, coordinated, multidisciplinary, interagency system of EI services for infants and toddlers with disabilities and their families;
2. Facilitate the coordination of payment for EI services from Federal, State, local, and private sources (including public and private insurance coverage);
3. Enhance the State's capacity to provide quality early-intervention services and expand and improve existing EI services being provided to infants and toddlers with disabilities and their families; and
4. Enhance the capacity of the State and local agencies and service providers to identify, evaluate, and meet the needs of historically underrepresented populations, particularly minorities, low-income, inner-city, and rural populations.

For healthcare professionals, the two most important elements of the implementation of the law relate to the mandated service coordination component and the Individualized Family Services Plan (IFSP). As discussed earlier, lawmakers changed the focus of the new EI system from a child-centered to a family-centered philosophy (Bishop, 1999). All aspects of the new system are focused on supporting families to obtain all the services needed to optimize the child's functional capacity within the home environment.

As summarized by Bishop (1999), the IFSP "is a family-directed assessment of resources, priorities, and concerns of the family and the identification of the supports and services necessary to enhance the family's capacity to meet the developmental needs of the infant or toddler" (p. 187). Note the heavy emphasis on *family*. It is important to recognize that the IFSP process was designed to assist families in the identification of the child's strengths and weaknesses, the family and community resources, and, most importantly, the family's priorities and concerns. It is the role of the healthcare professional to enhance the capacity of the members of the family to recognize and communicate their concerns. The family must be an integral part of every IFSP.

Part C states that the IFSP must identify the service coordinator from the profession most immediately relevant to the infant's or toddler's or family's needs (or who is otherwise qualified to carry out all applicable responsibilities under this part) and who will be responsible for the implementation of the plan and coordination with other agencies and persons. The role of the service coordinator is an essential element of the legislation. The service coordinator is responsible for all aspects of the development, implementation, and ongoing evaluation of the IFSP. When the child reaches the age of 3 years, it is the responsibility of the service coordinator to assist the family in the transition to a school-based program, if appropriate. Although a multidisciplinary team of professionals will provide the needed services, it is the service coordinator who ensures that the needs of the family are met and the services are provided in a timely manner. In the ongoing service coordination process, the ever-changing needs of the child and the family are assessed, and alterations are made in the IFSP to address new concerns.

Eligibility to participate in the EI system is partly mandated by the federal law and partly determined by each individual State. A child is eligible if he/she is younger than 3 years of age and needs EI services because the individual is experiencing developmental delays, as measured by appropriate diagnostic instruments and procedures in one or more of the following areas: cognitive development, physical development, communication development, social or emotional development, and adaptive development, or if the child has a diagnosed physical or mental condition that has a high probability of resulting in developmental delay. In addition, at the discretion of each State, at-risk infants and toddlers might be included. The most problematic aspect for each State in the implementation of the law is defining eligibility criteria for children who are biologically, socially, emotionally, medically, and/or environmentally at risk for developmental delays. Children born prematurely, for example, are one group of children who have had to have special consideration. Although many children born prematurely have diagnoses that clearly make them eligible for EI services, others are simply "at risk" for developmental delays. Each State is responsible for identifying the procedure for determining eligibility.

The federal regulations clearly describe the required content for the IFSP. For example, the IFSP must be written, and it must include a multidisciplinary assessment of the child's current strengths and needs and the identification of the appropriate services to meet such needs. An assessment of the family's resources, priorities, and concerns, along with the identification of the supports and services necessary to enhance the family's capacity to meet the developmental needs of the infant or toddler, must be included. The family is provided a review of the IFSP at 6-month intervals (or more often, when appropriate, based on infant or toddler and family needs). The regulations state that the IFSP must be developed and implemented in a timely manner. The content of the IFSP is clearly defined by the regulations and must include the following:

1. A statement of the infant's or toddler's present levels of physical development, cognitive development, communication development, social or emotional development, and adaptive development, based on objective criteria;
2. A statement of the family's resources, priorities, and concerns relating to enhancing

the development of the family's infant or toddler with a disability;

3. A statement of the major outcomes expected to be achieved for the infant or toddler and the family, and the criteria, procedures, and timelines used to determine the degree to which progress toward achieving the outcomes is being made and whether modifications or revisions of the outcomes or services are necessary;

4. A statement of specific EI services necessary to meet the unique needs of the individual child and family, including the frequency, intensity, and method of delivering services;

5. A statement of the natural environments in which EI services shall appropriately be provided, including a justification of the extent, if any, to which the services will not be provided in a natural environment;

6. The projected dates for initiation of services and the anticipated duration of the services;

7. The identification of the service coordinator from the profession most immediately relevant to the infant's or toddler's or family's needs (or who is otherwise qualified to carry out all applicable responsibilities under this part) who will be responsible for the implementation of the plan and coordination with other agencies and persons; and

8. The steps to be taken to support the transition of the toddler with a disability to preschool or other appropriate services.

The plan must be discussed with the parents and written, informed consent must be obtained before the provision of EI services described in the plan. Only those services to which the parent provides consent will be implemented.

The federal regulations also established State Interagency Coordinating Councils to coordinate the state EI programs. The composition of the Councils is regulated by the federal law, and each governor appoints the Council members. A full description of the mandated Council composition can be found in the federal regulations, but must include representation from parents of infants or toddlers with disabilities.

Any healthcare professional who is involved in the follow-up of children who might be eligible for such early-intervention services is responsible for familiarizing herself/himself with the appropriate state eligibility definitions and procedures and available services and service providers, as well as all aspects of the federal law under which the states are operating. Many states have websites to assist parents and professionals in obtaining information specific to that state's EI system. This above description provides only a general overview of the EI program components.

The importance of any EI program, whether it is the one mandated by PL 105-17, Part C, or other agency-specific programs, is to assess each child within the context of that child's specific family environment and to assist each family in developing a plan of care that optimizes that specific child's developmental potential. The family-centered plan should assess and provide interventions, as needed, across domains to include physical growth and development, cognitive development and school readiness, behavioral regulation, and psychosocial and emotional well-being. Support of the family or caregivers is a crucial part of health care after hospital discharge. Nurses are in an important position to identify potential problems, facilitate parental involvement in meeting the child's developmental needs, and in minimizing long-term developmental sequelae.

In addition to the role of the nurse and other healthcare providers in developing and implementing the IFSP, these professionals can also serve to support and educate parents of children who might not qualify for services under the PL 105-17, Part C, mandate, but who require special care. These children might have minor neurologic or cognitive deficits that do not meet the requirements to receive special services. However, these parents might benefit from learning ways in which they can manipulate the environment and structure activities to best support the developmental needs of their children.

## SUMMARY

In the previous sections, we address some specific issues related to developmental follow-up. Empirical support is not available to recommend a specific program for EI. It is clear from the theoretic data available that EI is important. However, the exact composition of the intervention is not clear, and additional research is required. Some things that must be kept in mind are that the intervention should be child- and family-centered, interdisciplinary, and comprehensive and should be based on a bioecological view of development such that the environment in which the child develops is a critical component of assessment and intervention. The program should not only provide services to meet the medical needs of the child, but must also provide family support, education, and empowerment so that the family can continue to support the child's optimal development throughout childhood and possibly into adulthood. For more information on EI from a legislative perspective, please see Chapter 23.

Because of the integral role that physical and occupational therapy plays in EI, the role of each is described in the following sections. Each discipline has a specific and important role as a member of the multidisciplinary team of professionals involved in EI evaluation and treatment. Depending on the specific needs of each child and family, a physical or an occupational therapist can serve as the primary service coordinator.

The final section describes the challenging situation for families and healthcare professionals when children are discharged from the NICU who remain dependent on ventilators and/or other sophisticated medical technologies. Caring for the technology-dependent child in the home environment requires skilled professionals who can evaluate the needs of the child and the family and effectively communicate with the family to educate and support the family members in not only meeting the child's medical and healthcare needs, but also to support growth and development across multiple domains.

## ROLE OF THE PHYSICAL THERAPIST

In this section, an overview is presented on essential aspects of neonatal physical therapy practice: theoretical framework, clinical training, professional roles, and intervention options for neonates during the NICU and outpatient phases. Physical therapists (PTs) became members of newborn medicine teams in the early 1970s, to contribute diagnostic data

through musculoskeletal, neurologic, and developmental examinations and to participate in early collaborative management of extremity deformities, movement impairment, feeding delay, adaptive equipment needs, and long-term interdisciplinary follow-up (Sweeney & Swanson, 2001). In 1973, pediatric physical therapy became a recognized specialty by the American Physical Therapy Association (APTA), and the development of advanced practice board certification, in pediatric physical therapy, was finalized in 1986 by the American Board of Physical Therapy Specialties (Tecklin, 1994). Unlike nursing, subspecialty certification in neonatal physical therapy is not yet available on the national level, but NICU practice guidelines from APTA Task Forces were first reported in 1989 and revised in 1999 (Scull & Deitz, 1989; Sweeney, Heriza, Reilly, et al., 1999). Competencies for pediatric PTs working in EI settings with NICU graduates and others with motor impairment were developed in 1991 (APTA Task Force, 1991).

### Theoretic Framework

Many theoretic concepts guide physical therapy practice in NICU and early-intervention settings by creating a framework for optimizing posture and movement of neonates and infants and for promoting development of the infant-family system. Concepts reviewed in this section are dynamic systems, collaborative care, and musculoskeletal plasticity. Other common physical therapy theoretic frameworks used in neonatal and EI practice are the following models: (1) enablement and disablement; (2) preventive care; (3) neurodevelopmental treatment; and (4) motor control and motor learning (Bradley, 2000; Heriza & Sweeney, 1994; Howle, 2002; Larin, 2000; Sweeney, Heriza, Reilly, et al., 1999). As posture and movement specialists, the underlying movement science base for pediatric physical therapy is derived from developmental biomechanics, developmental kinesiology and pathokinesiology, motor control, motor learning, and motor development. In NICU and early-intervention settings, physical therapists rely uniquely on principles of movement science, supported by other clinical, behavioral, and basic (anatomy, physiology, neuroscience, physics) sciences in pediatric physical therapy (Sweeney, Heriza, Reilly, et al., 1999).

### Dynamic Systems

Although neonatal PTs have a primary role in the examination and intervention of postural control and movement, there are many other interacting systems and environments that influence neonatal functional performance. Figure 20-1 illustrates the many systems and environments interacting simultaneously as the infant responds to the task (examination or intervention) of the PT in the NICU, home, or community environment. Therapy procedures are conducted within multiple, interacting contexts of physiologic and behavioral stability of the infant, learning style and grief level of the parents, quality of collaborative relationship with neonatal nurses, and environmental constraints and modifications of the NICU and follow-up settings. Because of this complexity, neonatal practice is considered to be on the advanced, subspecialist level, and inappropriate

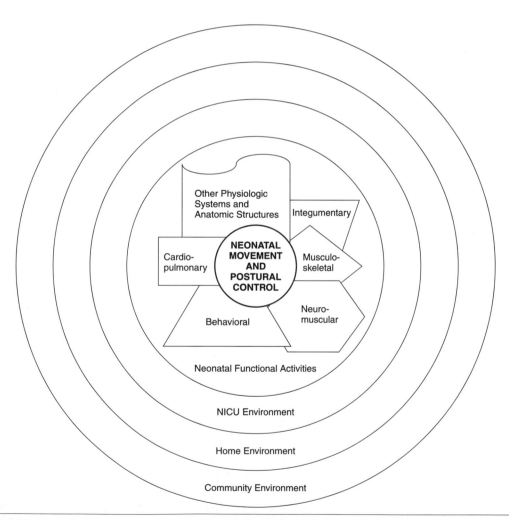

Figure **20-1** Dynamic systems and interactive environments influencing neonatal functional performance. (*From Sweeney, J.K., Heriza, C.B., Reilly, M.A., et al. [1999]. Practice guidelines for the physical therapist in the neonatal intensive care unit [NICU]. Pediatric Physical Therapy, 11, 119-132.*)

for physical therapy paraprofessionals, students, or adult-oriented generalists. Only during precepted practicum experiences in the NICU can therapists learn the simultaneous monitoring of several, interacting physiologic, behavioral, and sensori-motor systems of infants while judiciously selecting and administering a physical therapy or developmental procedure appropriate to the NICU environment and to family dynamics (Sweeney & Chandler, 1990; Sweeney, Heriza, Reilly, et al., 1999).

## Collaborative Care

A framework of interdisciplinary and family collaboration is essential for physical therapy procedures to be effective in NICU and follow-up settings. Building strong therapeutic relationships with families and professional caregivers requires role transition of the PT from a consultant or guest to an integrated team member (Sweeney, 1993). When this transition occurs, creative, collaborative partnerships can develop from combined expertise, creative energy, commitment, and mutual problem solving. Stages of transitions in collaborative partnership development between PTs and neonatal nurses are described in Figure 20-2. The good intentions and excellent clinical skills of the PT are insufficient without the critical

ingredient of high-quality therapeutic relationships with parents and neonatal caregivers.

## Musculoskeletal Plasticity

Theoretic concepts of plasticity apply to the immature musculoskeletal system as well as to development of the brain and neurologic system described earlier. Although preterm infants' organ systems continue to mature, the musculoskeletal system is being shaped by the effects of gravity and by environmentally imposed immobility in the NICU. Neonatal PTs analyze forces that shape the contour and alignment of infant skulls, spinal curvatures, and extremities to create opportunities for strategic positioning and to take advantage of peak skeletal system plasticity and muscular tissue elasticity in the neonatal period. Due to transplacental transmission of maternal relaxin, the first month of life is described as the highest period of musculoskeletal elasticity (Hensinger & Jones, 1981). Neonatal practitioners can play a powerful role in minimizing or preventing plagiocephaly, torticollis, and extremity malalignment by supporting skeletal integrity and postural alignment. Conversely, inattention to neonatal musculoskeletal plasticity and alignment can contribute quickly to positional deformity, asymmetry, and sensorimotor disorganization (Sweeney & Gutierrez, 2002).

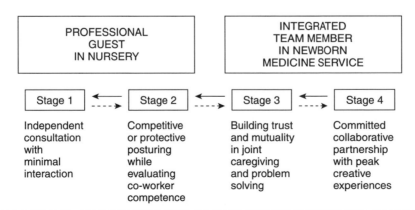

Figure **20-2** Stages and transitions in developing collaborative partnerships between physical therapists and neonatal nurses. (*From Sweeney, J.K. [1993]. Assessment of the special care nursery environment: Effects on the high-risk infant. In I.J. Wilhelm (Ed.),* Physical therapy assessment in early infancy *[pp. 13-44]. New York: Churchill Livingstone.)*

## Subspecialty Training

Neonatal physical therapy is an advanced level, subspecialty area within pediatric physical therapy. As with all neonatal practitioners, precepted training in NICU settings is also required for PTs. NICU practice guidelines from both the APTA (Sweeney, Heriza, Reilly, et al., 1999) and the American Occupational Therapy Association (AOTA, 1993) indicate that the NICU is not an appropriate practice area for paraprofessionals, student therapists on clinical affiliations, or entry-level therapists. Even with supervision, the PT or occupational therapist (OT) assistant and student therapist or new graduate are not prepared to "provide moment-to-moment examination and evaluation of the infant and have the ability to modify or stop preplanned interventions when the infant's behavior, motor, or physiologic organization begins to move outside the limits of stability with handling or feeding" (Sweeney, Heriza, Reilly, et al., 1999). Because level II and III nurseries might be located in medical centers without pediatric therapy services, it is critical for neonatal nurse managers and practitioners to analyze the neonatal subspecialty training of therapists working in neonatal care. It is not uncommon for adult-oriented generalist therapists to provide consultation to NICUs in hospitals where no pediatric therapists are employed and outpatient pediatric therapy services are referred to community agencies.

Neonatal nurses might become involved in mentoring pediatric therapists in neonatal care because fellowship training opportunities in neonatal physical therapy are not easily accessible. An eased entry to neonatal practice is advised where gradual, sequential, precepted experience occurs with medically fragile, hospitalized children on feeding lines, ventilators, or supplemental oxygen, and physiologic monitoring equipment. Following this experience, examination of term infants and participation in NICU follow-up clinics (including exposure to family stresses and culturally diverse caregiving practices) are recommended before a precepted practicum in intermediate and intensive care units. Precepted experiences offer the best preparation for appropriate, accountable, and ethical practice in neonatal therapy (Semmler, 1990; Sweeney

& Chandler, 1990), but discrepancies exist on best practice and actual practice preparation for therapists working in NICUs (Rapport, 1992). Neonatal nurses can play a significant role in guiding and advocating for specialized training for therapists interested in neonatal care and interdisciplinary NICU follow-up.

## Physical Therapy Roles and Services

### Professional Roles and Competencies

Task-force members from the Section on Pediatrics, APTA, developed practice guidelines and professional competencies for NICU and early-intervention settings. The competencies include screening, examination, intervention, consultation, scientific inquiry, administration, clinical education, and self-learning/professional development. Roles and clinical proficiencies for NICU practice are outlined in Appendix A of the APTA guidelines. Major roles for PTs working with infants and preschool children in early-intervention settings are listed in Box 20-2.

### Neonatal Physical Therapy Services

In collaborative caregiving with neonatal nurses and parents, PTs participate in neonatal care through examination of neurologic, neuromotor, oral-motor, and musculoskeletal function within the context of each infant's physiologic and behavioral tolerance. Indications for referral include infants with the following conditions:

- Impaired movement, postural control, or body alignment
- Brachial plexus injuries
- Positional deformities of extremities
- Myelodysplasia
- Chromosomal/genetic abnormalities with established neuromotor risk
- Impaired behavioral state regulation during routine caregiving
- Very-low birthweight (VLBW) with need for baseline neurodevelopmental examination at discharge for NICU follow-up
- Impaired oral-motor and feeding function

Based on examination findings, cardiopulmonary stability, and caregiver collaboration, the following

Box 20-2 ROLES FOR PHYSICAL THERAPISTS WORKING WITH INFANTS AND PRESCHOOL CHILDREN WITH PHYSICAL DISABILITIES OR AT DEVELOPMENTAL RISK

- Screen for neuromusculoskeletal, cardiopulmonary, and general developmental dysfunction.
- Identify with the family their priorities, strengths, and needs.
- Examine children's neuromusculoskeletal status and motor skills for differential diagnosis.
- Examine and monitor children's cardiopulmonary status and response to physical handling during testing and intervention.
- Examine and monitor infant neurobehavioral organization and stability during testing and intervention.
- Develop family recommendations and monitor implementation.
- Design, implement, and monitor therapeutic interventions.
- Recommend or implement environmental modifications.
- Recommend or fabricate adaptive equipment, mobility devices, and orthotics.
- Participate in interdisciplinary planning.
- Serve as case manager or service coordinator.
- Consult with and refer to community agencies and professionals.
- Evaluate intervention effectiveness and modify programs.

From Cochrane, C.G., Farley, B.G., & Wilhelm, I.J. (1990). Preparation of physical therapists to work with handicapped infants and their families: Current status and training needs. *Physical Therapy, 70,* 372-380. Reprinted with permission from the American Physical Therapy Association.

interventions can be integrated into an infant's care plan (Heriza & Sweeney, 1994; Sweeney & Swanson, 2001):

- Environmental modification to reduce noise, light, and excessive handling
- Body and extremity positioning, including customized modifications for reflux wedges, bath tubs, swings, and seats
- Facilitation of gestational age-specific postural control, alignment, and movement if absent, delayed, or asymmetric
- Judiciously applied tactile and kinesthetic stimulation contingent on physiologic, behavioral, and motor responses as well as on postconceptual age
- Extremity taping of foot deformities and splinting of wrist and hand to improve alignment
- Neonatal hydrotherapy (therapeutic bathing) to promote extremity movement and enhance behavioral readiness for feeding and interaction
- Oral-motor therapy and feeding trials
- Parent education and support
- Discharge planning for continuity of developmental monitoring and potential referral for infant therapy services

## Physical Therapy Early Intervention Services

Regardless of the pediatric practice setting (home, community agency, public school, private clinic), many PTs follow a management plan similar to the processes illustrated in Figure 20-3 (Heriza & Sweeney, 1994). Guided by family concerns and priorities, preliminary goals are established and examination processes are begun to analyze components of impaired sensorimotor function. The examination includes (1) developmental and functional levels; (2) neuromuscular, sensory, musculoskeletal, and cardiopulmonary impairments and functional limitations; and (3) physical therapy diagnosis of movement impairment. Common standardized examination procedures used by PTs are outlined in Table 20-1. Based on the evaluative findings, therapeutic interventions are selected or referrals are made to other professionals and therapy settings. The interventions are focused on preservation and enhancement of functional mobility and prevention of deformity and pain. Ongoing collaboration is essential for identifying and modifying goals and objectives with the family and for enhancing continuity and avoiding duplication of services

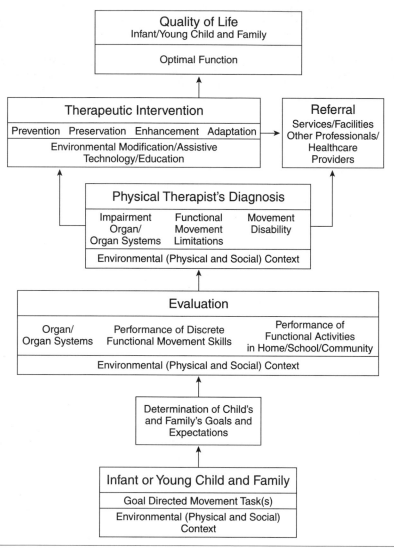

Figure **20-3** Practice model of pediatric physical therapy for infants and young children. (*From Heriza, C.B., & Sweeney, J.K. [1994]. Pediatric physical therapy: Part I. Practice scope, scientific bases, and theoretical foundations.* Infants & Young Children, 7[2], 20-32.)

with other professionals. Transdisciplinary service-delivery models are not considered appropriate for infants and children with specific postural control and movement impairments because the therapy role is likely released to a professional without movement science expertise.

In summary, the pediatric PT is a movement scientist using combinations of neuromuscular, musculoskeletal, cardiopulmonary, and developmental approaches and procedures in both NICU and early-intervention outpatient settings for neonates and young children with physical or developmental disabilities. Guiding the approach to movement dysfunction are concepts of dynamic systems theory, collaborative care, and musculoskeletal plasticity. The primary focus in clinical practice is interdisciplinary, collaborative, and family-centered with expanded roles in teaching, administration, consulting, and

Table **20-1**   SELECTED PEDIATRIC PHYSICAL THERAPY MEASUREMENT INSTRUMENTS

| Instrument | Age Range | Purpose |
| --- | --- | --- |
| Alberta Infant Motor Scale (Piper & Darrah, 1994) | 0-18 months | Identify delayed or typical gross motor development |
| Bayley Scales of Infant Development (motor scale) (Bayley, 1993) | 0-42 months | Quantify gross and fine motor development |
| Gross Motor Function Measure (Russell, Rosenbaum, Gowland, et al., 1993) | 0-5 years | Measure gross motor change in children with cerebral palsy |
| Neurological Assessment for Preterm and Full-Term Newborn Infants (Dubowitz, Dubowitz, & Mercuri, 1999) | Not stated | Examine posture, tone, reflexes, and neurobehavioral and behavioral state abilities |
| Neonatal Oral Motor Assessment Scale (Braun & Palmer, 1985) | Not stated | Examine movement of oral structures during nonnutritive and nutritive sucking and identify pathologic versus disorganized sucking patterns |
| Peabody Developmental Motor Scales (Folio & Fewell, 1983) | 0-83 months | Establish gross and fine motor performance levels |
| Test of Infant Motor Performance (Campbell, Osten, Kolobe, & Fisher, 1993) | 32 weeks' postconceptual age; 13 weeks postterm | Evaluate postural control, spontaneous movement, head control |

research. Neonatal nurses and neonatal nurse prac-tioners (NNPs) can play a major role in orienting and mentoring pediatric PTs in the unique culture, tech-nologic, and caregiving aspects of the NICU. This collaborative partnership is critical to the success and safety of neonatal physical therapy procedures and to the effectiveness of discharge planning in referring infants with sensorimotor risk or impairment to follow-up teams and community resources.

# ROLE OF THE OCCUPATIONAL THERAPIST

Advances in medical technology have resulted in increased survival of the premature baby. Smaller (<500 g), younger (<26 weeks' gestational age) infants are surviving, but with more complex med-ical conditions and increased lengths of stay in the NICU. This evolution has lead to the need for increased use of interdisciplinary services, often including the use of occupational therapy. The prac-tice of occupational therapy in the NICU seems to vary across the country, with several factors defining specific roles and functions (AOTA, 1993).

## Evolving Role

Occupational therapists traditionally provided rehabilitative services to those hospitalized infants identified as high risk or infants with certain diag-noses or problems. Historically, the OT's role was a rehabilitative model. For example, if a problem was identified (example: cleft palate), an order was writ-ten, an evaluation was performed, and direct treat-ment was provided.

Research in the 1980s described the traditional NICU environment and possible adverse effects to the developing neonate (Lawhon & Melzar, 1988). Increased levels of light and sound, inappropriate handling, and interruptions in behavioral state were shown to be initially stressful often with long-term negative outcomes (Als, 1982). Als' research related to co-regulatory developmental caregiving chal-lenged the OT to modify her traditional role of a problem-based model and examine typical treatment approaches as they relate to the infant. Therefore, the model of caregiving became proactive rather than reactive.

## Competency

In general, the training of the OT does not include substantial theory or practicum with the high-risk infant; therefore, it is essential that the OT practicing in the area of neonatology have additional or specialized training, which might include advanced workshops and a mentoring relationship. The AOTA (AOTA, 2000) official document on knowledge and skills for the OT in the NICU describes best practice. Clinical expertise in pediatrics and neonatology are additional requirements for competency. OTs must also develop advanced clinical reasoning skills to make appropriate decisions regarding the infant and the family (Mattingly, 1991a, 1991b; Anzalone, 1994).

Occupational therapies are challenged to develop a model for practice in the NICU. Gorga (1994) states: "occupational therapists are challenged to continue to develop a practice model that considers what is common to all neonatal units: an approach to prevent or minimize physical disability and developmental problems of infants within the context of the family." The role of the OT in the NICU is difficult to describe, owing to the varied practices throughout the country. However, one can define the OTs role using Gorga's model, which includes minimizing physical disabilities and developmental problems within the context of the family.

The neonatal therapist must have knowledge and skills necessary to assess the premature infants physical abilities (AOTA, 2000). Evaluation of movement, tone, reflexes, and posture in the developing infant provides the team and family with critical information. Individual treatment plans and intervention strategies can be developed and taught to caregivers. Additional physical factors can be evaluated by the OT and include range of motion (passive and active), strength, and orthopedic status. Through evaluation and treatment planning, the OT might develop recommendations on positioning and handling as well as strategies for activities (feeding, bathing, dressing) that support development or prevent physical disabilities.

## Prevent or Minimize Developmental Problems

The neonatal OT also has the knowledge and skills necessary to assess the developmental course, abilities, and vulnerabilities of the infants in the NICU (AOTA, 2000). Evaluation might include differences/variances in the developmental progression, neurobehavioral skills, sensory development, motor development, social-emotional development, and daily-life activities. Feeding, bathing, and additional caregiving activities are examples of daily-life activities. Assessment and understanding of additional factors that influence the infant's development, such as environment, medical course, and family issues, are also essential to treatment planning. The OT must then formulate an individualized plan with collaboration of other team members and the family to develop goals that ultimately support and optimize the infant's development.

### Prevention within the Context of the Family

The competent neonatal therapist has a responsibility to understand the unique needs of the families of the infants in the NICU. OTs must not only be skilled and knowledgeable about the infant's abilities and their developmental issues, but also be sensitive to each family's unique set of values, expectations, culture, and history. The experience of having a baby in the NICU creates an increased level of stress and anxiety for the family unit. The OT must be able to establish therapeutic relationships with the families to act as a collaborative team member in fostering the infant's development (Dunst, Trivette, & Deal, 1988; Holloway, 1998). Supporting the family and promoting their roles as the primary caregivers is optimal and a primary role of the OT. The OT must work collectively with the additional staff or team members to ensure consistent approach for the families and to avoid confusion. Integrating family-centered care principles into routine care in the NICU is a challenge to the caregiver as well as to the OT. To intervene with families requires knowledge of grief, attachment/bonding, and family dynamics.

The OT must apply a holistic philosophy of practice into this setting. Neonatal OT practice should also include the ability to anticipate future needs for intervention with the infant and family. The OT can offer suggestions for follow-up, environmental adaptations, and/or transition to home.

## Prevention through Education

The neonatal OT has the responsibility to provide education to the family, staff, and any other team member who interfaces with the NICU. A clear understanding of the OTs role is essential for nursing and medical staff to work collaboratively as a team. Direct intervention with the infant and family, consultation with other team members, and implementation of a collaborative plan is, in summary, the OTs role.

When an infant experiences difficulties at birth, his or her chances for developmental difficulties are increased, and a high-risk or follow-up program might be recommended at discharge for the NICU. These programs follow the progress of babies who have an increased likelihood of developmental delay. Occupational therapy might be recommended by the follow-up team or by a physician.

Occupational therapy services beyond the NICU might include evaluation of motor development, self-care skills, sensory-integrative skills, cognitive development, and/or upper-body strength and coordination. The OT might also evaluate the home setting for adaptive equipment, appropriate toys, and safety. OTs can also evaluate infants with cerebral palsy, Down syndrome, autism, coordination/motor difficulties, orthopedic issues, apraxia, sensory-integration dysfunction, or difficulty in the area of activity of daily living skills.

Motor development can be evaluated to ensure the infant is reaching appropriate developmental milestones. The OT can assess movement patterns, reflexes, and postural tone, and their influence on motor development. Self-care skills for the infant include feeding, bathing, and dressing. Often the premature infant is discharged with oral/motor difficulties requiring the expertise of the OT to ensure feeding milestones progress. The infant might require specialized techniques for bathing and dressing, and the OT can work with the parents or caregivers to employ appropriate strategies. Evaluation of sensory-integrative skills includes assessing the infant's ability to receive, process, and respond to sensory stimulation of touch, taste, smell, hearing, and vision. The OT might refer infants with hearing deficits to speech therapy. Cognitive development encompasses the infant's ability to process incoming information and development of critical thinking skills. Concrete and abstract thinking skills can be formally assessed with standardized tests. Finally, the OT must evaluate range of motion, upper body strength/coordination, and hand function.

Treatment is based on age-appropriate activities and can be provided in the infant's home or daycare center. Treatment might be direct, with hands-on demonstration with the infant, and modeling interventions for the parent. Treatment might be consultative, with education and recommendations given to the parent or caregiver in the form of a home program. Treatment might include techniques to improve self-care, developmental milestones, cognition, sensory-integrative skills, strengthening for upper body, and postural activities. Through routine weekly or monthly visits, the OT can determine whether the baby is reaching proper developmental milestones, such as achieving head control or rolling over. Functional activities such as feeding might also be included in a treatment session if the infant is found to have oral/motor difficulties. Often the OT recommends age-appropriate toys, games, or activities that facilitate development. Evaluation of the infant's home setting is essential in making suggestions for various positions, for play and sleep. The parent might require education in adapting the home to meet the needs of the child. Some infants require specialized positioning devices or other adaptive equipment (example: feeding equipment such as a special nipple or adaptive spoon). OTs might also provide services for those infants requiring upper-extremity splinting.

Families of infants who require special services such as occupational therapy require support and education to continue the treatment plan and recommendations between therapy visits. The OT must collaborate with additional therapists to ensure continuity of care and lessen any confusion for the parent. Many states offer services through early-childhood intervention programs and are funded on a state/local level. Parents might qualify for these services or might hire private pediatric occupational therapists to evaluate and treat their infant.

The role of the OT is to support the primary caregiver and establish clear goals with the family that are obtainable for both the family and the child. Education and support of the family members on how to help the infants develop to their highest potential is the challenge for the pediatric OT.

## DEVELOPMENTAL ISSUES FOR THE TECHNOLOGY-DEPENDENT INFANT

Increased survival of infants with a variety of diseases, including prematurity, has brought with it a rising inpatient population of infants who are virtually growing up in the NICU. Heart disease, bronchopulmonary dysplasia, congenital anomalies, malabsorption syndrome secondary to necrotizing enterocolitis (NEC), and central nervous system (CNS) abnormalities are but a few reasons these infants are considered at risk and remain hospitalized. Frequently, other complications occur along with the primary diagnosis to further cause physiologic stress, such as hypoxia, bronchospasm, gastroesophageal reflux (GER), and ventilator dependency. Respiratory treatments, complex pharmacologic regimens, ventilator and oxygen management, and physical and occupational therapy treatments are but a few of the ongoing, complex interactions that occur throughout the day in the life of the technology-dependent child. The hospital environment and routine can significantly impact long-term developmental outcomes if the length of stay is prolonged, especially during sensitive periods of brain development and sensory integration. (Hitzfelder, 1996).

Infants with chronic illness or dependency on technology often remain hospitalized for prolonged periods of time. Due to their illness or fragility, these infants frequently do not get the opportunities for normal experiences that enhance developmental progress and functional organization of the CNS. Intervention must begin as soon as possible to facilitate optimal outcomes for NICU graduates. Ongoing assessment, support, and guided intervention should be based on each infant's thresholds, sensitivities, competencies, and tolerance.

## EARLY INTERVENTION IN THE NICU

As discussed previously in this chapter, EI services have been initiated in the NICU and beyond, based on Part C of the IDEA. Most states have developed programs to meet the requirements of the federal mandate, although many states have not yet developed a plan for children who remain in the NICU for an extended period. Colorado, for example, developed one such program called "Beginnings," which adapted the IFSP to meet the developmental needs of newborn infants and families while in the NICU setting (Browne, Langlois, Ross, & Smith-Sharp, 2001). Before the program began, EI was initiated late in the hospital stay or after discharge, although many infants in the NICU meet the legal eligibility criteria for EI from birth. Typically, EI has meant providing services to children from birth to 3 years in a community setting. NICU infants and their families often meet eligibility criteria for early-intervention services under Part C of the IDEA that guarantees services and rights to families with children who have special needs from birth to 3 years of age. In Colorado, these criteria (see Appendix E) include congenital syndromes associated with developmental delay, sensory impairment (hearing loss, visual impairment), metabolic disorder, pre- and perinatal infections, and VLBW ($\leq$1200 g). The process starts with identifying an infant who meets eligibility criteria and gaining consent from the family for EI services. Developmentally supportive care is started at birth, and the IFSP is developed no later than 7 to 10 days after admission. A flowchart of the IFSP process for intervention by the OT is seen in Figure 20-4. Although this flowchart is for the OT, any early interventionist could use this process. Many hospitals have already initiated a developmental plan from admission; the IFSP formalizes the plan for eligible infants and recruits key individuals (see Appendix E) along with the bedside nurse and family to begin the continuum of EI. Staff and family to support the infant during the hospital stay and provide the link to the community to ensure that developmental needs of high-risk infants continue to be addressed after discharge from the NICU use this ongoing plan. Parents see that developmental issues are important from the very "Beginning," and might be more compliant with developmental follow-up after discharge.

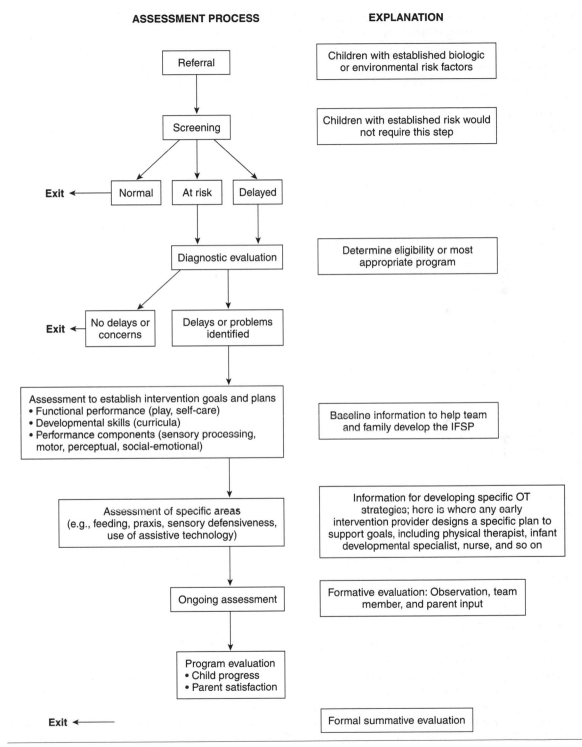

Figure 20-4 The assessment process. *IFSP*, Individualized family service plan; *OT*, occupational therapy.

Box 20-3    Family-Focused Early Intervention beyond the Newborn Period
in the Hospital and Community Setting

- Service coordination
- Developmental assessment/screening
- Audiology
- Ophthalmology
- Physical therapy
- Occupational therapy
- Speech and language therapy
- Infant mental health services
- Social services
- Medical/nursing services
- Nutrition (including feeding disorders)
- Family counseling and education
- Assistive technology services and devices

Early childhood intervention services are available in most clinical settings, although the terms used to describe the services might vary from state to state and between different communities. Community EI is federally and state funded and provides the same services in the home after discharge. Box 20-3 lists the various services available in both hospital and community EI programs. The hospital setting has not been recognized as the ideal place to begin such services and rarely do the state- and federal-funding entities reimburse the hospital for providing EI services. For infants growing up in the hospital setting, EI has to start when they are medically stable and can tolerate some normalized activities.

Service coordination is key to ensuring that all needs are identified early and high-risk infants receive appropriate services; that must start in the inpatient setting. Therefore, a person must be assigned and accountable to the high-risk infant and family for optimal needs assessment, service coordination, and liaison with family for the entire hospital stay. Any number of staff could fill this role including therapists, nurses, or infant developmental specialists.

## DEVELOPMENTAL DOMAINS

Developmental domains required by law for the IFSP include the physical, cognitive, communication, social/emotional, and adaptive. Although the Colorado "Beginnings" IFSP domains are different (feeding, sleeping, being with people, calming,

movements, response to environment, and health or medical condition), one can easily place each of these indicators within one of the legally required categories. Goldberger and Wolfer (1991) created a matrix framework for potential environmental threats to development in the hospital and NICU setting and suggested the relationship of these threats to the developmental domains. Instead of the term *threats*, the word *challenges* should be used, because most individuals more readily perceive it as relating to a situation that can be overcome. The word *threat* seems more final and irreversible. The matrix (see Appendix E) can be used to identify specific hospital challenges to an individual infant's development and trigger appropriate interventions toward the developmental domains that might be affected. An additional domain, the regulatory/sensory category has been added, although this aspect could fall under the emotional domain. As a separate entity, it might be easier to assess for developing problems with self and external regulation and sensory integration difficulties that evolve in infants during long-term hospitalization. The matrix can be used during developmental rounds when nurses, therapists, development specialist, and/or EI representative, physicians, practitioners, and families, if present, review and update the developmental plan of care. There are other appropriate methods of planning, besides the matrix or Colorado "Beginnings" format, but these methods provide a structure, which is critical to ensure that all developmental domains are included as a frame of reference for intervention.

## GOALS OF DEVELOPMENTAL PROGRAM FOR INFANTS BEYOND THE NEWBORN PERIOD

General goals for infants with prolonged hospital stays include promoting self-regulation that can reduce agitation, preserve energy to promote growth, support CNS organization (Holditch-Davis, Blackburn, & VandenBerg, 2003), facilitate normal acquisition of developmental skills, and foster parent-infant attachment all within the context of the infant's individual tolerance and coping abilities

during recovery. Facilitating normal progress does not require a highly aggressive stimulation program that could prove harmful physiologically, emotionally, and developmentally to a recovering infant. Goldberger (1990) recommends that the goals of stimulation programs for infants requiring prolonged hospitalization include environmental modification to provide adequate and appropriate developmental opportunities along with considerations that maximize the infant's comfort. Parents must be included during all phases of planning, implementing, and evaluating the developmental support of their infants. Their participation builds knowledge, skills, and attitudes (Figure 20-5) that

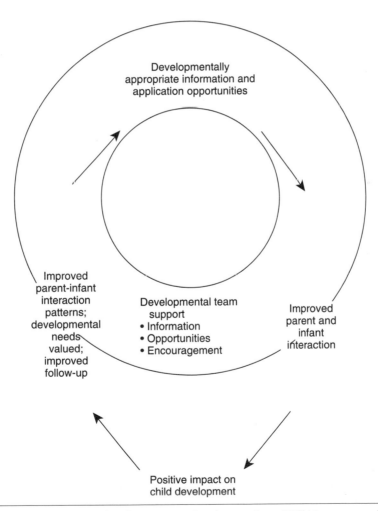

Figure **20-5** Developmental intervention for parents: Continuum from NICU to community.

will help them provide developmental support for their infants after they leave the NICU.

## PARENTS SHAPE LONG-TERM OUTCOMES

A longitudinal, prospective follow-up study (Gross, Mettleman, Dye, & Slagle, 2001) of former premature infants compared with term, control children examined the effects of family structure and stability on academic performance at 10 years of age. The term children were more likely to have better academic performance, defined as appropriate grade level without additional educational services, than the former premature children (odds ratio 3.4; 95% confidence interval, 1.9-6.0). Improved school outcomes for the premature children were significantly associated with family conditions such as higher parent education, two parents (married or unmarried) or consistent caregivers, stable family composition, and stable geographic residence over the 10 years. The family factors were more predictive of school outcomes than perinatal complications. The former premature children in this study, who had consistent contact with both biological parents, were three times more likely to be at appropriate grade level than the preterm children having regular contact with only one parent. Although unstable family conditions existed in both the term and preterm children, family instability had a greater impact on the prematurely born children. Studies such as this one reinforce the need to support families of high-risk children while they are in the hospital setting, and, following hospital discharge, to emphasize to parents the integral role they play in providing a developmentally supportive environment. The developmentally supportive environment, including parent-child interactions, has been shown to influence developmental outcomes.

A pilot study with 42 mothers of LBW premature infants was conducted in a NICU with mothers randomized to two groups: (1) four-phased educational program starting 2 to 4 days after birth and continuing through 1 week after discharge, and (2) comparison mothers who were given education on audiotape over the same time frame. Follow-up was conducted at 3 and 6 months postconceptual age for all infants in the study. The COPE (Creating Opportunities for Parent Empowerment) program is an educational-behavioral intervention consisting of infant behavior information and parent role information, and parent activities with workbook to help parents apply their knowledge. COPE infants had significantly higher scores (t[39] = 2.0, $P < 0.05$) on the Bayley Scales of Infant Development-II Mental Development Index at 3 months postconceptual age than comparison infants, and the difference was greater at 6 months (t[38] = 2.0, $P < .05$). Twenty percent of the comparison infants (4 of 20) had developmental delays identified at 6 months postconceptual age, with none of the COPE infants demonstrating delay. COPE mothers reported significantly stronger beliefs about expectations concerning their premature infants' behaviors/characteristics and their role as parents, and these beliefs were strongly correlated with infant development outcomes at both 3 (r = .62, $P < 0.001$) and 6 months (r = .62, $P < 0.001$).

Shore (2001) postulates that infants who do not experience the emotionally charged interactive experiences with familiar caregivers that are associated with attachment might be at risk for chronic relationship difficulties. Parents must be involved at all levels in planning and implementing the developmental plan. Their assessment of their infant's responses also provides valuable behavioral data concerning reliable individual cues. Developmental goals can be met through play, with help from parents. Play also helps the parent in assuming the parenting role and enhancing the interactions between parent and child. Opportunities for interactions that will be successful can reinforce the bond between the infant and family and improve the transition to home. Parents learn to synchronize interactively with their infant to support cognitive processing by adapting the type, amount, variability, and timing of activity/stimulation according to their infant's vulnerabilities, thresholds, and capabilities. Parents have the opportunity to practice rhythmic coordination of interaction, tempo of interaction, reading infant signals/cues, and modifying/adapting behavior that is contingent and responsive to their infant. They can also learn when their infant is actively engaged or giving "disengagement" signals when needing a "time out." Figure 20-5 is a visual representation of how parent intervention is an ongoing process that can ultimately lead to improved patterns of parent-infant interaction and improved developmental outcomes. Parents who see themselves as active learners who can make a positive impact on their child's development might continue to seek information, apply their learning, and advocate for a better outcome for their NICU graduate during and after discharge from the hospital.

## INFANT CHARACTERISTICS

Physiologic and behavioral characteristics of these infants can also cause problems with developmental and emotional progress when they are hospitalized. Some infants who have moved from acute to chronic recovery might already be in a negative response cycle, which includes irritability; crying; hyperarousal or under-arousal; defensiveness; regurgitation; prolonged, persistent crying; disorganized state behaviors; feeding problems; sleep problems (Hofacker & Papousek, 1998); poor self-regulation; repetitive motor patterns with a predominance of extensor movement; frantic activity; and overreactivity to stimuli (Holditch-Davis, Blackburn, & VandenBerg, 2003). These infants might become overstimulated to even benign, familiar routine care and respond dramatically without the gradual buildup of irritability to crying or other subtle stress cues to alert the caregiver. The caregiver might not easily discern ill-defined cues. Gross physiologic distress cues can be the first signs of stress requiring immediate medical support. It is frequently difficult to separate whether the physiologic sequelae or the behavioral response was the first in the sequence of spiraling events in one of these episodes. All of these characteristics define an unpredictable infant who can easily frustrate caregivers and parents. Other infants simply do not seem to have the energy to attend and interact. A general cookbook approach will not work with these infants with special needs. Familiar caregivers and parents will achieve the skill needed to read subtle cues and prevent some of the stressors that evoke such responses by these vulnerable, susceptible infants. Regular positive interaction with a familiar caregiver provides a sense of safety and security that supports an infant's natural curiosity and exploration of familiar and novel or new social-emotional experiences and the physical environment (Shore, 2001).

## HEARING AND VISION SCREENING

Periodic sensory screening and neurobehavioral evaluation is especially important for the high-risk or developing premature infant during and after their NICU stay. Nurses are often the first to notice an infant's failure to respond normally to sensory stimulation. Pediatric audiologists and ophthalmologists currently screen in the NICU for hearing and vision impairment and continue follow-up for those infants with ongoing problems or who are at risk for later development of sensory impairment (American Academy of Pediatrics [AAP], 2001a; Erenberg, Lemons, Sia, et al., 1999; Hall, 2000; Johnson, 2002; Joint Committee on Infant Hearing [JCIH], 1995; JCIH, American Academy of Audiology, American Academy of Pediatrics, American Speech-Language-Hearing Association, & Directors of Speech and Hearing Programs in State Health and Welfare Agencies, 2000; Mehl & Thomson, 2002; Rose, 1999; Saunders & Hutchinson, 2002). Specialized developmental support to compensate for the infant's impairment should start as early as possible. The hearing-impaired infant will not benefit from a musical mobile, but might enjoy objects with colored lights, vibrating objects, watching their caregiver's face, and different textures or activities that facilitate development of other senses, such as smell and taste. It is very important for the staff and family to fully understand the degree of impairment and the infant's true limitations and to base interactions with the child on those limitations. Sensory-impaired infants might become highly agitated when staff members begin care or treatments, because they cannot see or hear staff approach the bed. Infants with multiple disabilities require an even more thoughtful approach to care. A change in approach might mean letting the infants capture a person's smell before touch rather than speaking to the infant before care. In the developmental philosophy, these infants would be gently aroused for care even before sensory deficits are identified; this minor difference to the plan can help minimize the effects of intrusion into their space without warning. Developmental/child life specialists and OTs should be included in planning an appropriate environment and activities for these infants' complicated needs.

Nurses might also be required to monitor and care for infants who wear or use assistive devices such as hearing aids or speaking valves for tracheotomies. When the infant is fitted for a device, the dispensing specialist (audiologist or speech therapist) should provide the necessary training and written materials for both staff and parents so that the assistive technology is used and cared for correctly. Studies from data collected over 30 years showed 27% to 92% of children's hearing aids were malfunctioning during random evaluation (Rigo, 1998). It is recommended that the condition and performance of a hearing aid be monitored at least daily (Rigo, 1998). Any information specific to an infant should also be written on the developmental plan. Boxes 20-4 and 20-5 are examples of written plans for use of hearing aids and speaking valves for infants.

One must remember that not all hearing or vision problems are obvious or associated with genetically linked conditions. Some conditions are nongenetic and require a thorough screening and physical examination to detect the problem and prevent long-term consequences. An example is nongenetic causes of hearing loss.

## Nongenetic Causes of Hearing Loss

Before the 1970s, LBW and perinatal factors were associated with about 2% of children with hearing loss. With an increase in survival of LBW infants, increased numbers of NICUs, and universal newborn hearing screening, that percentage has risen. Former LBW infants account for 19% of children with hearing loss, while 8% of hearing loss is associated with perinatal factors (Roizen, 1999). Six of the risk factors for sensorineural hearing loss (SNHL) or conductive hearing loss (CHL) indicated by the JCIH are associated frequently with the NICU

---

Box **20-4**   Use and Care of Hearing Aids

1. Hearing aids to be worn 10 to 15 minutes, 4 times per day.
2. Gradually increase as tolerated until using during awake periods over 6 to 8 weeks.
3. Decrease ambient noise especially when hearing aids are worn.
4. Talk to infant; provide socially relevant sounds, call by name.
5. Know the parts of the hearing aid, and reinforce teaching of same to parents.
6. Correctly insert batteries.
7. Correct insertion of earmold; methods of cleaning.
8. Correct position of volume.
9. Understand acoustic feedback and how to troubleshoot.
10. Extreme temperature changes, moist, damp environment, dirt, hairspray, and dust can damage hearing aids
11. Hearing aid condition and performance is checked daily
    a. Hearing aid, tubing, and earmold for:
        1. Hearing aid switches
        2. Cracks or stiffened tubing
        3. Cerumen or moisture on the earmold
    b. Battery for:
        1. Voltage
        2. Corrosion
        3. Compartment is completely closed
    c. Listen for:
        1. Quality of amplification and sound
        2. Acoustic feedback, excessive noise levels, or signals when volume control is rotated or tapping the hearing aid
        3. Smooth increase in volume as control is rotated

**Box 20-5   USE AND CARE OF PASSY MUIR/SPEAKING VALVE FOR INFANTS WITH TRACHEOTOMIES**

1. Speaking valve (SV) trial successful and plan for wearing valve is on chart.
2. Frequency, duration, and indications for wearing valve are specific.
3. Speech therapy sessions are scheduled.
4. Respiratory therapy assists when patient is on a ventilator during SV sessions.
5. Specific monitoring parameters before, during, and after SV session include:
    a. Heart rate
    b. Respirations
    c. Respiratory pattern
    d. Work of breathing
    e. Oxygenation (pulse oximeter)
    f. Breathing pattern when valve is removed
    g. Behavior when valve is placed for:
        1. Agitation
        2. Sweating
        3. Color change
        4. Breath holding
        5. Frantic movement
        6. Panicked, worried expression
        7. Increased secretions
    h. Ventilator pressures (might need to adjust positive end expiratory pressure [PEEP] after SV is placed)
    i. Ability to produce sounds
6. Remove SV for physiologic or behavioral indications of intolerance and report to M.D., respiratory therapist, and speech therapist.
7. Monitor SV and do not use if the following observations are made:
    a. One-way valve is stiff or cracked.
    b. Hub is cracked.
8. Clean with soap and water; rinse, and air dry when soiled, or once a day.
9. Use is usually limited to about 2 months wear.
10. Spend time face to face talking with infant, calling by name, read stories, make funny noises, sing simple songs.

experience. These are (1) birthweight of 1500 grams or less, (2) hyperbilirubinemia at the exchange transfusion level, (3) Apgar scores of 0 to 4 at 1 minute and 0 to 6 at 5 minutes, (4) 5 days or more of mechanical ventilation, (5) ototoxic medications, and (6) bacterial meningitis. Many NICU graduates fall into high-risk categories, including those with congenitally acquired infections, craniofacial anomalies with abnormalities of the pinna and ear canal, syndromes associated with SNHL or CHL (e.g., trisomy 21, CHARGE), hypoxemia, and congenital hypothyroidism. Timing of onset is important because some infants may not demonstrate hearing loss until after discharge. Nursing staff will need to inform parents of the risk factors for late onset or delayed hearing loss so the family will understand and comply with follow-up hearing screenings.

Hypoxia and hyperbilirubinemia are frequent risk factors associated with SNHL. Studies of NICU graduates have shown that a history of transcutaneous oxygen less than 50 mmHg, Apgar score less than 6 at 5 minutes (Roizen, 1999), pneumothoraces, bronchopulmonary dysplasia (BPD), and renal failure (Borradori, Fawer, Buclin, & Calame, 1997) is associated with hearing loss. Any illness associated with hypoxemia must be considered a major risk factor for hearing loss. Congenital diaphragmatic hernia, PPHN, and ECMO are a classic triad that includes many factors related to SNHL. Developmental support to minimize oxygen consumption and conserve energy is considered a part of the plan for vulnerable infants physiologically reactive to their environment.

The incidence of hyperbilirubinemia is 2.5 times greater in children with SNHL (Roizen, 1999). Higher bilirubin concentrations combined with one or more of the following: (1) apnea, (2) bradycardia, (3) cyanosis, and (4) hypothermia, were associated with increased risk of hearing loss ($p < 0.001$).

NICU graduates have often been exposed to ototoxic medications such as aminoglycosides (gentamycin, kanamycin) and diuretics (furosemide). Prolonged administration of pancuronium bromide (pavulon) has been associated with higher incidence of SNHL thought to be related to the cumulative dose and duration of therapy (Cheung, Tyebkhan, Peliowski, et al., 1999). Borradori, Fawer, Buclin, and Calame (1997) found ototoxicity to be associated with prolonged administration and a higher total dose with aminoglycosides and furosemide. Use of ototoxic drugs during the prenatal period is thought to result in CHL due to malformation of the ossicles (bones) of the inner ear.

Vaccinations for rubella and HIB have reduced the incidence of hearing loss from infectious causes. Hearing loss associated with meningitis has been significantly decreased with the HIB vaccine. Cytomegalovirus still remains a common cause of hearing loss.

Prenatal exposure to alcohol resulting in fetal alcohol syndrome (FAS), trimethadione, methyl mercury, and iodine deficiency has been associated with hearing loss. Delayed maturation of the auditory system, SNHL (7% to 29% with FAS), intermittent CHL resulting from recurrent serous otitis media (RSOM), and central hearing loss comprise four types of hearing loss due to prenatal exposure to alcohol (Church & Abel, 1998). Delayed language acquisition and expressive and receptive language are typical with FAS children. This means they have poor comprehension of single words and verbal commands, difficulty with grammar, and poor auditory memory (i.e., storing words and sentences). Expressive and receptive language delays may occur in as high as 86% of children with FAS. Speech disorders associated with FAS include lack of fluency, speaking in monotone, slurred speech, and articulation problems.

The clinical features of CHARGE include ocular coloboma, heart defects, atretic choanae, retarded growth and development, genital hypoplasia, and ear anomalies associated with a high incidence of moderate to severe hearing loss. Cumulative data from five studies (n = 140) showed that 80% of patients with CHARGE have moderate to severe hearing loss (SNHL and mixed), and when mild hearing loss is included, the figure rises to 87% (Edwards, Kileny, & Van Riper, 2002).

Infants with hearing loss meet eligibility criteria of the Individuals with Disabilities Education Act (IDEA). If services are begun in the hospital setting, an individualized family service plan (IFSP) can be initiated and systems mobilized to meet the family/infant needs during the hospitalization. The IFSP becomes the ongoing record of needs and services that is valuable in transitioning an infant with identified hearing loss to the community with no loss of monitoring, habilitation, and services (JCIH, American Academy of Audiology, American Academy of Pediatrics, American Speech-Language-Hearing Association, & Directors of Speech and Hearing Programs in State Health and Welfare Agencies, 2000). The IFSP service coordinator from the hospital and community is responsible for getting needed services and assisting the family in either setting.

### Developmental Screening

Developmental screening is defined as "identifying children who may need more comprehensive evaluation" (AAP, 2001b). Outcomes of developmental evaluations are listed in Box 20-6. Primary pediatric follow-up for high-risk infants requires periodic developmental and neurobehavioral assessment. The Pandora's box has been opened, and the expectation for developmental screening, evaluation, sup-

---

**Box 20-6**    OUTCOMES OF DEVELOPMENTAL EVALUATION

1. Diagnosis
2. Interdisciplinary plan for intervention and supportive services
3. No problem identified
4. Additional observation required

port, and intervention is no longer seen as limited to the primary pediatrician or community setting.

Neurobehavioral assessment tools (Box 20-7), such as the Brazelton Neonatal Behavioral Assessment Scale (BNAS), Neonatal Individualized Developmental Care and Assessment Program (NIDCAP®) (Boston,

MA) and Assessment of Preterm Infant Behavior (APIB) are used to assess full-term and preterm infant behavior and form the basis for interventions. During the acute illness phase, these interventions are focused on minimizing the effects of the environment, reducing stress, promoting rest, providing appropriate levels

---

## Box 20-7    NEONATAL ASSESSMENTS REQUIRING CERTIFICATION FOR ADMINISTRATION

| Assessment | Time to Administer | Training Contact |
|---|---|---|
| **NEONATAL BEHAVIORAL ASSESSMENT SCALE (NBAS)** | | |
| For healthy term infants up to 2 months, Scale comprises 28 behavioral and 18 reflex items for assessing infant capabilities in the autonomic, motor, state, and social-interactive systems within the dynamic context of interaction with caregivers and the environment (never standardized). Served as model for Assessment of Preterm Infant Behavior (APIB). Requires recertification every 3 years. | 20-30 minutes | The Brazelton Institute 1295 Boylston Street Suite 320 Boston, MA 02215 E-mail: *brazelton.institute@tch. harvard.edu www.brazelton-institute.com* |
| **NEONATAL BEHAVIORAL ASSESSMENT SCALE— REVISED (2000) (NBAS-R)** | | |
| 26 behavioral and 14 reflex items. Crying, consolability, and threshold for stimulation are documented along with current functioning in the autonomic, motor, state, and social-interactive systems. Performance norms are being collected in a large population of healthy neonates to standardize this instrument. | 12-15 minutes | The Brazelton Institute |
| **CLINICAL NEONATAL BEHAVIORAL ASSESSMENT SCALE (CLNBAS)** | | |
| Brief neurobehavioral examination comprising 18 behavioral and reflex items for describing the newborn's physiologic, motor, state, and social capabilities from birth to 2 months. It is a joint observation by family and caregiver designed to help parents learn their infant's cues and understand their infant. Two goals of the examination include promoting relationships between both infant and family and caregiver and family. It is always conducted with the parents to provide | Variable | The Brazelton Institute |

*Continued*

**Box 20-7    Neonatal Assessments Requiring Certification for Administration—cont'd**

| Assessment | Time to Administer | Training Contact |
|---|---|---|
| a structured observation that captures their infant's strengths, challenges, individuality, adaptive capacity, and temperament. | | |

### NATURALISTIC OBSERVATION OF NEWBORN BEHAVIOR (NONB)

| Assessment | Time to Administer | Training Contact |
|---|---|---|
| Based on Als' Synactive Theory of Neurobehavioral Organization.<br>For preterm and term infants to 44 weeks too fragile for handling; formal observation of behaviors repeated at 2-minute intervals before, during, and after caregiving events over 60 minutes or more to assess the interplay of the infant behavioral subsystems (autonomic, motor, state that includes attention-interaction and self-regulation) to the environment or caregiving events. These observations are usually repeated in 2-week intervals until discharge. Signs of stress, stability, and thresholds, strengths, and sensitivities are used to form the basis for ongoing developmental support for each infant. Certification required and recertification is every 2 years. NIDCAP® Level I. | Minimum of 1 hour | National NIDCAP® Center Heidelise Als, PhD, Director Boston, MA (617) 355-8249 *www.nidcap.com* |

### ASSESSMENT OF PRETERM INFANT BEHAVIOR (APIB)

| Assessment | Time to Administer | Training Contact |
|---|---|---|
| Based on Als' Synactive Theory of Neurobehavioral Organization.<br>For stable preterm (>30 to 32 weeks) and term infants Complex assessment that provides a profile of the integrated subsystem of an infant's current functioning within the context of dynamic environmental demands. Structured test items are conducted by an APIB certified therapist who handles and observes the infant while assessing neurobehavioral organization, self-regulatory capabilities, type, and amount of caregiver facilitation required by the infant to maintain organized behavior. Used more in research than the clinical setting. NIDCAP® Level II. | | National NIDCAP® Center |

### Family Infant Relationship Support Training (FIRST)

| Assessment | Time to Administer | Training Contact |
|---|---|---|
| Continuing education program for parents and community-based professionals, created to promote participants' skills in developmental | | Center for Family and Infant Interaction Denver, Colorado |

*Continued*

**Box 20-7**  NEONATAL ASSESSMENTS REQUIRING CERTIFICATION FOR ADMINISTRATION—CONT'D

| Assessment | Time to Administer | Training Contact |
|---|---|---|
| support for high-risk or former premature infants, infants with special needs, disorganized infants, or high-risk families as they move to the community setting. The program was adapted from NIDCAP®, and the workshops are available for public health nurses, early interventionists, community service providers, private therapists, NICU graduate parents, and anyone who serves infants and their families in the community setting. | | *www.uchsc.edu/sm/ peds/cfii* (This site also includes information on Colorado's "Beginning" program of Early Intervention in the NICU and Part C IDEA) |
| **INFANT BEHAVIORAL ASSESSMENT AND INTERVENTION PROGRAM** | | |
| For birth to 6 months of age. Includes the following training on Infant Behavioral Assessment (IBA) and Neurobehavioral Curriculum for Early Intervention (NCEI). Als' Synactive Theory of Neurobehavioral Organization provides the framework for the assessment using observation to facilitate understanding of the infant while the NCEI helps early interventionists learn and implement neurobehavioral strategies to support infant development. | | Rodd Hedlund, MEd Mary Tatarka, MS, PT Washington Research Institute (206) 285-9317 E-mail: *rhedlund@ wri-edu.org* *www.wri-edu.org/infant/* |

Adapted from Hunter, J.G. (1996). The neonatal intensive care unit. In J. Case-Smith, A.S. Allen, & P.N. Pratt (Eds.), *Occupational therapy for children* (p. 609). St. Louis: Mosby; and Holditch-Davis D., Blackburn S.T., & VandenBerg, K. (2003). Newborn and infant neurobehavioral development. In C. Kenner & J.W. Lott (Eds.), *Comprehensive neonatal nursing: A physiologic perspective* (p. 241). St. Louis: W.B. Saunders.

of stimulation, and supporting the family/infant relationship within the NICU. For infants who cannot tolerate handling, naturalistic observations can be used. For older preterm infants who can tolerate handling, interventions that involve handling can be used if the infant's stress signals are respected.

There are no formal developmental assessments that have been developed for this unique population of infants growing up in the NICU or pediatric unit. Some developmental specialists or psychologists adapt standard tools such as the Bayley Scales of Infant Development; however, stress or fatigue might be significant factors in completing standardized tests. A variety of instruments is available to assist the practitioner/specialist in understanding the level of current developmental functioning of a hospitalized infant. Two types of standardized tests are available (Table 20-2) for use with infants past the neonatal period: norm-referenced and curriculum-based, criterion-referenced. Developmental assessment instruments should be chosen with the purpose of the test in mind (Table 20-3). Although many tests are available to assess infants and toddlers, developmental professionals, based on the needs of each infant, should make test selections. In general, the purpose of the testing is to understand an infant's functional capacity in each developmental domain to optimize interventions and strategies. Involving the parents in the assessment process allows them to become active participants and set realistic goals for the child's progress.

Table 20-2   COMPARISON OF NORM-REFERENCED AND CRITERION-REFERENCED TESTS

| Characteristic | Norm-Referenced Test | Criterion-Referenced Test |
| --- | --- | --- |
| Purpose | Comparison of child's performance with normative sample | Comparison of child's performance with a defined list of skills |
| Content | General; usually covers a wide variety of skills | Detailed; might cover specific objectives or developmental milestones |
| Administration | Always standardized | Can be standardized or nonstandardized |
| Psychometric properties | Normal distribution of scores; means, standard deviations, and standard scores computed | No score distribution needed; a child can pass or fail all items |
| Test development | Items chosen for statistical performance; might not relate to functional skills or therapy objectives | Items chosen for functional and developmental importance; provides necessities for developing therapy objectives |
| Examples | Bayley Scales of Infant Development revised, Peabody Developmental Motor Scales (PDMS), Bruininks-Hawaii Early Learning Profile (HELP), Oseretsky Test of Motor Proficiency, Pediatric Evaluation of Disability Inventory (PEDI) | PDMS, PEDI, Early Intervention Developmental Profile, Gross Motor Function Measure |

From Richardson, P.K. (1996). Use of standardized tests in pediatric practice. In J. Case-Smith, A.S. Allen, & P. Pratt (Eds.), *Occupational therapy for children* (p. 206). St. Louis: Mosby.

The norm-referenced test is used to evaluate how an infant performs relative to the average performance of a normative sample of infants. Some tests, like the Bayley Scales of Infant Development II, also use reference groups with specific diagnoses for comparison, but care must be taken when interpreting the data from such groups because the sample size varies widely between groups.

The criterion-referenced test is used to glean information on how well an infant performs on specific tasks; therefore, the performance is compared with a particular criteria or skill. The goal of this type of test is to evaluate what skills the infant can perform to provide guidance toward appropriate intervention. Table 20-4 describes some standardized tools available for infant screening. Table 20-5 describes some of the criterion-referenced tools that identify areas of ability and provide strategies to support development in specific areas. These interventions are usually family-friendly, and parents can easily use them when they interact with their child in the hospital. Nurses,

developmental specialists, or occupational or PTs together evaluate the infant to identify developmental domains needing support or intervention. These data provide valuable information to help parents or family members understand developmental goals and to be active participants in caring for their child. Empowering the parents to support the growth and development of their child will enhance the quality of the caregiving environment and promote optimal developmental outcomes.

Criterion-referenced tools are used to help the specialist and staff members to understand an infant's current abilities and provide recommended activities for improving functional abilities (see Table 20-5 for the Hawaii Early Learning Profile, which is curriculum-based and criterion-referenced). Because these screening tools were not designed for use with high-risk infants in a hospital setting, infant developmental specialists, therapists, psychologists, or nurses who are knowledgeable about signs of stress and fatigue should administer

Table **20-3** EXAMPLES OF DEVELOPMENTAL ASSESSMENTS BY TESTING PURPOSE

| Purpose | Type of Test | Examples |
|---|---|---|
| Screening | Standardized | Denver Developmental Screening Test II |
| | | First STEP |
| | | Milani Comparetti Motor Development Screening for Infants and Young Children |
| Diagnostic tests | Norm referenced | Bayley Scales of Infant Development |
| | Criterion referenced | Movement Assessment of Infants |
| Program planning | Curricula | Developmental Programming for Infants and Young Children |
| | | Hawaii Early Learning Profile |
| | | Carolina Curriculum for Infants and Toddlers with Special Needs |
| | | Battelle Developmental Inventory |
| | | Assessment, Evaluation, and Programming System for Infants and Children |
| | Informal scales | Scales developed by individual therapists |
| Program evaluation | Standardized | Toddler and Infant Motor Evaluation |
| | | Peabody Developmental Motor Scales |
| | Criterion based | Hawaii Early Learning Profile |

From Case-Smith, J. (1998). Assessment. In J. Case-Smith (Ed.), *Pediatric occupational therapy and early intervention* (p. 51). Boston: Butterworth-Heineman.

them. For optimal developmental progress, the activity plan should be implemented consistently and reinforced frequently by professionals and/or family members.

In some situations, it might be necessary to use a tool that provides information about the quality of interaction between the parent and infant. Instruments such as the Parent Child Interaction Feeding and Teaching Scales from the Nursing Child Assessment Satellite Training (NCAST) (Seattle, WA: University of Washington) provide information about the quality and abilities of both infant and parent interaction within a dynamic feeding and teaching interaction (Box 20-8).

It is important to remember that most screening instruments do not have normative references for all infants in the NICU setting. However, valuable information concerning strengths and areas needing intervention can support developmental progress in the hospital setting. These screening instruments can be used in many settings, including the home, hospital, follow-up clinic, daycare centers, and later,

in schools. Instruments vary considerably in the amount and type of training required for administration, expense, and time to complete. Instrument selection depends on a number of factors including unit size, composition, level of care, numbers of eligible infants, funding, personnel, patient population characteristics and cultural and system dynamics. Regardless of the instrument selected, assessments should be conducted professionally with expertise in testing and measurement.

Hospitalized infants can be very difficult to test and should not experience stress from developmental screening. Often the parent or nurse can provide good information on an infant's abilities, thresholds, and vulnerabilities. Screening might have to be done in more than one session or over time to avoid stressing an infant. Naturalistic observations during a therapy session with OT/PT or child life specialist might help when using a criterion-based assessment tool. Developmental domains can be assessed through interdisciplinary collaboration with other specialists, such as a PT for evaluating

Table 20-4    STANDARDIZED DEVELOPMENTAL ASSESSMENTS

| | Test Title | | |
| --- | --- | --- | --- |
| | Bayley Scales of Infant Development (Bayley, 1993) | Peabody Developmental Motor Scales (Folio & Fewell, 1983) | Battelle Developmental Inventory (Newborg, et al., 1988) |
| Age range | 2-42 months | Birth-83 months | Birth-8 years |
| Testing time | 45 minutes | 45-60 minutes | 45-120 minutes |
| Materials available in the testing kit | X | X (partial) | — |
| Primary purpose | Diagnosis | Eligibility Documenting motor delay | Program development |
| **Major areas tested** | | | |
| Personal-social | X | — | X |
| Communication | — | — | X |
| Cognition | X | — | X |
| Self-help | — | — | X |
| Fine motor | X | X | X |
| Gross motor | X | X | X (motor) |
| Visual motor | | X | X (motor) |
| **SCORES OBTAINED** | | | |
| Age level | X | X | X |
| Percentile | — | X | X |
| Standard | X | X | X |

From Case-Smith, J. (1998). Assessment. In J. Case-Smith (Ed.), *Pediatric occupational therapy and early intervention* (p. 53). Boston: Butterworth-Heineman.

motor development; a developmental specialist evaluating cognitive, emotional, language; and the primary nurse assessing social, self regulatory strengths, and physiologic stability.

Developmental progress is not only a function of the infant's innate abilities but is also dependent upon opportunities provided to the infant. Within the NICU setting, normalizing the environment for age-appropriate activity is a challenge. The developmental domains can be assessed for the purpose of guidance toward areas in which an infant might need more support and intervention. The intent of these assessments is not to predict outcomes, but to document progress, identify potential areas of delay, plan specific interventions, and/or refer an infant for specialized services, such as speech; occupational and physical therapy; feeding interventions; child life therapy; or, possibly, pediatric psychological consultation (Ritchie, 2002). Traditional milestone achievement focuses primarily on capabilities, whereas developmental intervention in the NICU centers around ongoing support to nurture developmental progress within the context of each infant's thresholds, vulnerabilities, and abilities.

## DEVELOPMENTAL INTERVENTION

General suggestions for developmental support for infants during prolonged hospitalization are shared in Box 20-9. Emphasis is on knowing each infant's current level of functioning in all developmental domains to provide appropriate developmental support. Supporting parents in providing developmental interventions is important to their overall view of their infant by allowing them opportunities for parent-child interaction. These skills form the foundation for attachment, reciprocity, mutual exploration, and developmental interaction between infants and parents long after leaving the NICU.

Table 20-5   DEVELOPMENTAL CURRICULA

| | Curriculum Type | | | |
|---|---|---|---|---|
| | Assessment, Evaluation, and Planning System for Infants and Children (0-3 years) (Bricker, 1993) | Hawaii Early Learning Profile (Furuno et al., 1985; Parks, 1992) | Carolina Curriculum type for Infants and Toddlers with Special Needs (Johnson-Martin et al., 1991) | Developmental Programming for Infants and Young Children (Schafer & Moersch, 1981); Early Intervention Developmental Profile (Rogers & D'Eugenio, 1981) |
| Age range | Birth through 36 months | Birth through 36 months | Birth through 24 months | Birth through 36 months |
| Strengths | Comprehensive assessment of six domains | Chart and checklist provided; activity guide; seven domains | Includes 24 domains; guide provides activity suggestions | Includes activity guide; five separate volumes |
| Major areas evaluated | X | X | X | X |
| Social-emotional | X | X | X | X |
| Communication | X | X | X | X |
| Cognition | X | X | X | X |
| Self-help and adaptive | X | X | X | X |
| Fine motor | X | X | X | X |
| Gross motor | X | X | X | X |
| Visual motor | — | — | X | X |
| Includes intervention activities | X | X | X | X |
| Includes adapted methods | X | X | X | — |
| Field tested | X | X | X | X |
| Validity studies | — | — | X | X |

From Case-Smith, J. (1998). Assessment. In J. Case-Smith (Ed.), *Pediatric occupational therapy and early intervention* (p. 55). Boston: Butterworth-Heineman.

## DEVELOPMENTAL TEAMS

Developmental teams include a group of individuals from several disciplines who have relevant knowledge and skills to assess, plan, and implement a program for developmental surveillance and evaluation in the clinical setting. Teams might include, but are not limited to, the following professionals: physicians, infant mental health or development specialists, child life specialists, physical and occupational therapists, clinical nurse specialists, nurses, nurse practitioners, and/or pain-team representatives. The family is welcome and invited to participate in planning, implementation, and evaluation. Developmental issues are discussed during daily rounds, but more comprehensive developmental planning can occur during developmental rounds, which concentrate on issues related to specific domains, including emotional, social, motor, cognitive, language, physiologic, sensory integration, self-regulation, and comfort/pain. Developmental care plans are reviewed and modified on an ongoing basis.

## Box 20-8    PARENT-INFANT INTERACTION

**NURSING CHILD ASSESSMENT SATELLITE TRAINING (NCAST)**

Kathryn Barnard
University of Washington
Box 357920
Seattle, WA 98195-7920
(206) 543-8528
*www.ncast.org*

The Parent-Child Interaction Feeding and Teaching Scales are used for describing caregiver-child communication and interaction during a feeding (birth to 1 year) or teaching situation (birth to 36 months). Scales are used in research, clinical, or home setting for observing parent-child interaction. Describes behavior of both parent and child during interactions, contingency of responses, strengths, and challenges of the dyad's communication. The parent-child interaction observations are recognized by the legal system in child custody and abuse cases.

## Box 20-9    GENERAL INTERVENTIONS BEYOND THE NEWBORN PERIOD

1. Limit number of caregivers.
2. Encourage development of day-night rhythms.
3. Respond rapidly, appropriately, and consistently to crying/cues.
4. Enhance sensory experience to foster enjoyment and pleasure (i.e., tube feeding with accompanying sensations of being held and sucking a pacifier).
5. Provide planned multisensory opportunities that let the infant participate rather than passively experience the activity (i.e., pat-a-cake with caregiver rather than hanging an object in front in visual field).
6. Provide predictable routines (daytime schedule, bedtime ritual) and people who are familiar.
7. Offer age-appropriate activities that include familiarity, variety, change, and both new and familiar situations.
8. Respect the infant's personal space—avoid painful or uncomfortable procedures in their bed, and let infant know at all times when you are approaching to avoid startling.
9. Provide developmentally appropriate play materials that are within reach.
10. Support opportunities for exploration and motor development (i.e., floor play on mat, variety of positions).
11. Ensure quiet nurturing experiences as daily events with parents or staff if parents cannot be available.
12. Design developmental plan in collaboration with parents that includes planned activities with parents/family.

Nurses are an integral part of the developmental team because of their in-depth knowledge of the infants in their care. Although these developmental assessments are valuable, they provide only a snapshot of the child's abilities. Therefore, it is important for the child to be evaluated over time to identify the specific areas of progress and areas in which new interventions might be needed.

## THE PLAN

Collaboration with each infant's health team and family is necessary in determining the best way to maximize the infant's developmental potential through the comprehensive plan. Depending on the behaviors observed, the team might decide a developmental specialist or infant psychologist should be involved. This might be particularly important when repetitive cycles of negative physical or behavioral response are observed. It is then very important that everyone follows through with the plan that evolves, so that the infant receives consistent feedback and reinforcement. This is true of plans by any team member including the physical or occupational therapist, speech language therapist, child life specialist, clinical nurse specialist, nurse practitioner staff nurse, and others.

A pervasive theme with hospital care is the lack of consistency, unpredictable nature of experiences, and the environment and multiple caregivers. Following through with the developmental plan can provide a means of providing consistency and predictability within the hospital setting. Reducing the number of caregivers through organized teams and strategic assignment planning must be tackled at the managerial level of support, but consistency in delivering the plan of care is based on the accountability and responsibility of the bedside caregiver and other direct-care providers.

## LINK TO COMMUNITY

Finally, the infant is ready to transition to the community. Referral to a developmental follow-up center and/or community EI program is made. The IFSP follows the infant to provide history and current information to the next provider for early-intervention services. The changeover to community-based intervention is further supported when representatives from the community visit the hospital setting to meet the infant and family and smooth the transition and services into the home. Connecting with the family before they become "lost" in the community might help to alleviate the parent's unease with a new "system" of services. Nurses can collaborate with the infant's health team to tailor a discharge conference with the family and developmental representatives that cultivate use of community developmental follow-up services.

## HOSPITAL-BASED EARLY INTERVENTION

EI does not have to wait until discharge from the hospital. Developmental delay can occur when there is an absence of developmental supports through normative experiences and opportunities for the NICU or hospitalized infant. An infant developmental or child life specialist, nurse, and/or OT/PT can initiate regular neurobehavioral and developmental screening for complex infants to provide a basis for the developmental plan. Language must be carefully considered when discussing any developmental assessment with a family to avoid predicting future outcomes. It is more appropriate to discuss an infant's goals and activities to support reaching those goals in terms of opportunities for the infant/family rather than elaborating on delays that are most likely transient. Intervention is geared to enhance potential, and it is important to emphasize the parents' significance in fostering their infant's optimal developmental outcome. If parents are involved early on, they will be more likely to see the significance of even the smallest achievement of their infant. Continued teaching by staff, specialists, and therapists can help parents become knowledgeable in the developmental support of their infant and informed advocates for their child in the community after discharge. Evaluating the effectiveness of such programs might include measures of infant developmental progress both short- and long-term, parent satisfaction, quality of parent-child interaction, cost of program, and return to follow-up. Although not an exhaustive list, outcomes must be tracked for continual improvement of the program and often as a means to obtain funding/reimbursement.

## CONCLUSION

In this chapter, we reviewed the principles of EI that extend beyond the NICU and the newborn period. We explored an area that is very important for support of optimal growth and development. EI is a good example of an interdisciplinary coordination of care and an area in which many neonatal health professionals are not very knowledgeable. Typically, the focus of most neonatal care is during the NICU stay, but, as this chapter points out, our ultimate goal is to discharge an infant and family that will reach their optimal level of well-being. To reach that goal, EI is a cornerstone of care that reaches beyond the hospital realm and the newborn stage of life.

# REFERENCES

Als, H. (1982). Toward a synactive theory of development: Promise for the assessment of infant individuality. *Infant Mental Health Journal, 3*, 229-243.

American Academy of Pediatrics (AAP). (2001a). Screening examination of premature infants for retinopathy of prematurity. *Pediatrics, 108*(3), 809-811.

American Academy of Pediatrics (AAP). (2001b). Committee on Children with Disabilities: Developmental surveillance and screening of infants and young children. *Pediatrics, 108*(1), 192-196.

American Occupational Therapy Association (AOTA). (1993). Knowledge and skills for occupational therapy practice in the neonatal intensive care unit. *American Journal of Occupational Therapy, 47*, 1100-1105.

American Occupational Therapy Association (AOTA). (2000). Specialized knowledge and skills for the occupational therapy practice in the neonatal intensive care unit. *American Journal of Occupational Therapy, 54*, 641-648.

American Physical Therapy Association Task Force on Early Intervention, Section on Pediatrics (APTA). (1991). Competencies for physical therapists in early intervention. *Pediatric Physical Therapy, 33*, 77-80.

Anzalone, M.E (1994). Occupational therapy in neonatology: What is our ethical responsibility? *American Journal of Occupational Therapy, 48*(6), 563-566.

Balbernie, R. (2002). An infant in context: Multiple risks, and a relationship. *Infant Mental Health Journal, 23*, 329-341.

Bayley, N. (1993). *Bayley Scales of Infant Development* (2nd ed.). San Antonio, TX: Psychological Corporation.

Bishop, KK. (1999). Services to families of infants and toddlers with disabilities. In R. Constable, S. McDonald, & J.P. Flynn (Eds.), *School social work: Practice, policy, and research perspectives* (4th ed.). Chicago: Lyceum Books.

Blair, C. (2002). School readiness: Integrating cognition and emotion in a neurobiological conceptualization of children's functioning at school entry. *American Psychologist, 57*, 111-127.

Borradori, C., Fawer, C.L., Buclin, T., & Calame, A. (1997). Risk factors for sensorineural hearing loss in preterm infants. *Biology of the Neonate, 71*(1), 1-10.

Bradley, N.S. (2000). Motor control: Developmental aspects of motor control in skill acquisition. In S.K. Campbell (Ed.), *Physical therapy for children*, (2nd ed., pp. 45-87), Philadelphia: W.B. Saunders.

Bradley, R.H., Corwyn, R.F., Pipes McAdoo, H., & Garcia Coll, C. (2001). The home environments of children in the United States Part I: Variations by age, ethnicity, and poverty status. *Child Development, 72*, 1844-1867.

Braun, M.A., & Palmer, M.M. (1985). A pilot study of oral-motor dysfunction in "at risk" infants. *Physical and Occupational Therapy in Pediatrics, 5*, 13-20.

Bronfenbrenner, U., & Crouter, A.C. (1983). The evolution of environmental models in developmental research. In W. Kessen & P.H. Mussen (Eds.), *Handbook of child psychology: Vol 1. History, theory, and methods* (4th ed., pp. 357-414). New York: Wiley.

Bronfenbrenner, U., & Morris, P.A. (1998). The ecology of developmental processes. In W. Damon & R.M. Lerner (Eds.), *Handbook of child psychology: Vol. 1. Theory* (5th ed.). New York: Wiley.

Brooks-Gunn, J. (2003). Do you believe in magic? What we can expect from early childhood intervention programs. *Social Policy Report, Society for Research in Child Development, 17*(1), 1-14.

Browne, J.V., Langlois, A., Ross, E.S., & Smith-Sharp, S. (2001). Beginnings: An interim individualized family service plan for use in the intensive care nursery. *Infants and Young Children, 14*(2), 19-32.

Campbell, S.K., Osten E., Kolobe, T.H.A., & Fisher, A. (1993). Development of the test of infant motor performance. *Physical Medicine and Rehabilitation Clinics of North America, 4*, 541-551.

Cheung, P.Y., Tyebkhan, J.M., Peliowski, A., et al. (1999). Prolonged use of pancuronium bromide and sensorineural hearing loss in childhood survivors of congenital diaphragmatic hernia. *Journal of Pediatrics, 135*(2)(Pt 1), 233-239.

Church, M.W., & Abel, E.L. (1998). Fetal alcohol syndrome. Hearing, speech, language, and vestibular disorders. *Obstetrics & Gynecology Clinics of North America, 25*(1), 85-97.

Cochrane, C.G., Farley, B.G., & Wilhelm, I.J. (1990). Preparation of physical therapists to work with handicapped infants and their families: Current status and training needs. *Physical Therapy, 70*, 372-380.

Davis, D.W., & Burns, B.M. (2001). Problems of self-regulation: A new way to view deficits in children born prematurely. *Issues in Mental Health Nursing, 22*, 305-323.

Derryberry, D., & Reed, M.A. (1996). Regulatory processes and the development of cognitive representation. *Developmental Psychopathology, 8*, 215-234.

Doussard-Roosevelt, J.A., McClenny, B.D., & Porges, S.W. (2001). Neonatal cardiac vagal tone and school-age developmental outcome in very low birth weight infants. *Developmental Psychobiology, 38*, 56-66.

Dubowitz, L., Dubowitz V., & Mercuri, E. (1999). *Neurological assessment of the preterm and full-term newborn infant.* London: MacKeith Press.

Dunst, C.J., Trivette, C.M., & Deal, A.G. (1988). *Enabling and empowering families: Principles and guidelines for practice.* Cambridge, MA: Brookline Books.

Edwards, B.M., Kileny, P.R., & Van Riper, L.A. (2002). CHARGE syndrome: A window of opportunity for audiologic intervention. *Pediatrics, 110*(1)(Pt 1), 119-126.

Erenberg, A., Lemons, J., Sia, C., et al. (1999). Newborn and infant hearing loss: Detection and intervention. American Academy of Pediatrics. Task Force on Newborn and Infant Hearing, 1998-1999. *Pediatrics, 103*(2), 527-530.

Feldman, R., Weller, A., Sirota, L., & Eidelman, A.I. (2003). Testing a family intervention hypothesis: The contribution of mother-infant skin-to-skin contact (kangaroo care) to family interaction, proximity, and touch. *Journal of Family Psychology, 17*, 94-107.

Folio, M.R., & Fewell, R. (1983). *Peabody Developmental Motor Scales and Activity Cards.* Itasca, IL: Riverside Publishing.

Goldberger, J. (1990). Lengthy or repeated hospitalization in infancy: Issues in stimulation and intervention. *Clinical Perinatology, 17*, 197-206.

Goldberger, J., & Wolfer, J. (1991). An approach for identifying potential threats to development in hospitalized toddlers. *Infants and Young Children, 3*(3), 74-83.

Gorga, D. (1994). The evolution of occupational therapy practice for infants in the neonatal intensive care unit. *American Journal of Occupational Therapy, 48*(6), 487-489.

Gross, S.J., Mettleman, B.B., Dye, T.D., & Slagle, T.A. (2001). Impact of family structure and stability on academic outcome in preterm children at 10 years of age. *Journal of Pediatrics, 138*, 169-175.

Hall, J.W. III. (2000). Screening for and assessment of infant hearing impairment. *Journal of Perinatology, 20*(8 Pt 2), S113-121.

Hensinger, R.N., & Jones, E.T. (1981). *Neonatal orthopedics,* New York: Grune & Stratton.

Heriza, C.B., & Sweeney, J.K. (1994). Pediatric physical therapy: Part I. Practice scope, scientific bases, and theoretical foundations. *Infants & Young Children, 7*(2), 20-32.

Hitzfelder, N.J. (1996). Occupational and physical therapy: Guide for families and professionals about types of therapy service and delivery models. Dallas, TX: Easter Seals Foundation.

Hofacker, N.V., & Papousek, M. (1998). Disorders of excessive crying, feeding, and sleeping: The Munich Interdisciplinary Research and Intervention Program. *Infant Mental Health Journal, 19*, 180-201.

Holditch-Davis, D., Blackburn, S.T., & VandenBerg, K.A. (2003). *Newborn and infant neurobehavioral development* (3rd ed.). St. Louis: W.B. Saunders.

Holloway, E. (1998). Relationship-based occupational therapy in the neonatal intensive care unit. In J. Case-Smith (Ed.), *Pediatric occupational therapy and intervention* (pp. 111-127). Boston: Butterworth Heinemann.

Howle, J.M. (2002). *Neuro-developmental treatment approach: Theoretical foundations and principles of clinical practice.* Laguna Beach, CA: Neurodevelopmental Treatment Association.

Jobe, A.H. (2001). Predictors of outcome in preterm infants: Which ones and when? *Journal of Pediatrics, 138*, 153-156.

Johnson, A.N. (2002). Update on newborn hearing screening programs. *Pediatric Nursing, 28*(3), 267-270.

Joint Committee on Infant Hearing. (1995). 1994 Position statement. *Pediatrics, 95*(1), 152-156.

Joint Committee on Infant Hearing, American Academy of Audiology, American Academy of Pediatrics, American Speech-Language-Hearing Association, & Directors of Speech and Hearing Programs in State Health and Welfare Agencies. (2000). Year 2000 position statement: Principles and guidelines for early hearing detection and intervention programs. *Pediatrics, 106*(4), 798-817.

Kolb, B. (1995). *Brain plasticity and behavior.* Mahway, NJ: Erlbaum.

Landry, S.H., Miller-Loncar, C.L., Smith, K.E., & Swank, P.R. (2002). The role of early parenting in children's development of executive processes. *Developmental Neuropsychology, 21*, 15-41.

Landry, S.H., Smith, K.E., Swank, P.R., et al. (2001). Does early responsive parenting have a special importance for children's development or is consistency across early childhood necessary? *Developmental Psychology, 37*, 387-403.

Landry, S.H., Smith, K.E., Swank, P.R., & Miller-Loncar, C.L. (2000). Early maternal and child influences on children's later independent cognitive and social functioning. *Child Development, 71*, 358-375.

Larin, H.M. (2000). Motor learning: Theories and strategies for the practitioner. In S.K. Campbell (Ed.), *Physical therapy for children* (2nd ed., pp. 170-197). Philadelphia: W.B. Saunders.

Lawhon, G., & Melzar, A. (1988). Developmental care of the very low birth weight infant. *Journal of Perinatal and Neonatal Nursing, 2*(1), 56-65.

Mattingly, C. (1991a). What is clinical reasoning? *American Journal of Occupational Therapy, 45*(11): 979-986.

Mattingly, C. (1991b). The narrative nature of clinical reasoning. *American Journal of Occupational Therapy, 45*(11), 998-1005

Mehl, A.L., & Thomson, V. (2002). The Colorado newborn hearing screening project, 1992-1999: On the threshold of effective population-based universal newborn hearing screening. *Pediatrics, 109*(1), E7.

Msall, M.E., & Tremont, M.R. (2002). Measuring functional outcomes after prematurity: Developmental impact of very low birth weight and extremely low birth weight status on childhood disability. *Mental Retardation and Developmental Disabilities Research Reviews, 8*(4), 258-272.

Nelson, C.A. (2000). The neurobiological bases of early intervention. In J.P. Shonkoff, & S.J. Meisels (Eds.), *Handbook of early childhood intervention* (2nd ed., pp. 204-227). New York: Cambridge University Press.

Piper, M.C., & Darrah, J. (1994). *Motor assessment of the developing infant.* Philadelphia: W.B. Saunders.

Posner, M., & Rothbart, M. (2000). Developing mechanisms of self-regulation. *Development and Psychopathology, 12*, 427-441.

Rapport, M.J.K. (1992). A descriptive analysis of the role of physical and occupational therapists in the neonatal intensive care unit. *Pediatric Physical Therapy, 4,* 172-178.

Rigo, T.G. (1998). Habilitation and Communication Development in Hearing-Impaired Infants and Toddlers. In F.P. Billeaud (Ed.), *Communication disorders in infants and toddlers* (2nd ed., pp. 187). Boston: Butterworth-Heinemann.

Ritchie, S.K. (2002). Primary care of the premature infant discharged from the neonatal intensive care unit. *Maternal Child Nursing (MCN), 27,* 76-85.

Robson, A.L., & Pederson, D.R. (1997). Predictors of individual differences in attention among low birth weight children. *Developmental and Behavioral Pediatrics, 18,* 13-21.

Roizen, N.J. (1999). Etiology of hearing loss in children: Nongenetic causes. *Pediatric Clinics of North America, 46*(1), 49-64.

Rose, V.L. (1999). AAP recommends the development of universal newborn hearing screening programs. American Academy of Pediatrics. *American Family Physician, 60,* 1020.

Rothbart, M. (1989). Temperament and development. In G.A. Kohnstamm, J.E. Bates, & M.K. Rothbart (Eds.), *Temperament in childhood* (pp. 187-247). New York: Wiley.

Rothbart, M., & Bates, J. (1998). Temperament. In W. Damon & N. Eisenberg (Eds.), *Handbook of child psychology: Vol. 3. Social, emotional, & personality development* (5th ed., pp. 105-176). New York: Wiley.

Rowe, S.M., & Wertsch, J.V. (2002). Vygotsky's model of cognitive development. In U. Goswami (Ed.), *Blackwell handbook of childhood cognitive development* (pp. 538-599). Malden, MA: Blackwell Publishing.

Ruff, H.A., & Rothbart, M.K. (1996). *Attention in early development* (pp. 174-198). New York: Oxford University Press.

Russell, D., Rosenbaum, P., Gowland, C., et al. (1993). *Gross motor function measure manual* (2nd ed.). Hamilton, Canada: McMaster University.

Sameroff, A.J., & Fiese, B.H. (2000). Transactional regulation: The developmental ecology of early intervention. In J.P. Shonkoff & S.J. Meisels (Eds.), *Handbook of early childhood intervention* (2nd ed., pp. 135-159). New York: Cambridge University Press.

Saunders, R.A., & Hutchinson, A.K. (2002). The future of screening for retinopathy of prematurity. *Journal of American Association for Pediatric Ophthalmology and Strabismus, 6*(2), 61-63.

Scull, S., & Deitz, J. (1989). Competencies for the physical therapist in the neonatal intensive care unit (NICU). *Pediatric Physical Therapy, 1,* 11-14.

Semmler, C. (1990). Neonatal therapy. In C.J. Semmler & J. Hunter (Eds.), *Early occupational therapy intervention.* Gaithersburg, MD: Aspen.

Shore, A.N. (2001). Effects of a secure attachment relationship on right brain development, affect regulation, and infant mental health. *Infant Mental Health Journal, 22*(1-2), 7-66.

Smith, K.E., Landry, S.H., & Swank, P.R. (2000). Does the content of mothers' verbal stimulation explain differences in children's development of verbal and nonverbal cognitive skills? *Journal of School Psychology, 38,* 27-49.

Sweeney, J.K. (1993). Assessment of the special care nursery environment: Effects on the high-risk infant. In I.J. Wilhelm (Ed.), *Physical therapy assessment in early infancy* (pp. 13-44). New York: Churchill Livingstone.

Sweeney, J.K., & Chandler, L.S. (1990). Neonatal physical therapy: Medical risks and professional education. *Infants and Young Children, 2,* 59-68.

Sweeney, J.K., & Gutierrez, T. (2002). Musculoskeletal implications of preterm infant positioning in the NICU. *Journal of Perinatal and Neonatal Nursing, 16*(1), 58-70.

Sweeney, J.K., Heriza, C.B., Reilly, M.A., et al. (1999). Practice guidelines for the physical therapist in the neonatal intensive care unit (NICU). *Pediatric Physical Therapy, 11,* 119-132.

Sweeney, J.K., & Swanson, M.W. (2001). Low birth weight infants: Neonatal care and follow up. In D.A. Umphred (Ed.), *Neurological rehabilitation* (pp 203-258). St. Louis: Mosby.

Sykes, D.H., Hoy, E.A., Bill, J.M., et al. (1997). Behavioural adjustment in school of very low birthweight children. *Journal of Child Psychology and Psychiatry, 38,* 315-325.

Tecklin, J.S. (1994). A brief history of the Section on Pediatrics of the American Physical Therapy Association. *Pediatric Physical Therapy, 6,* 109-112.

Thelen, E., & Smith, L.B. (1996). *A dynamic systems approach to the development of cognition and action.* Cambridge, MA: MIT Press.

Watson, J.E., Kirby, R.S., Kelleher, K.J., & Bradley, R.H. (1996). Effects of poverty on home environment: An analysis of three-year outcome data for low birth weight premature infants. *Journal of Pediatric Psychology, 21,* 419-431.

# 21 NICU and beyond Benefits: Benchmarking with Measurable Outcomes

## Rita H. Pickler, Barbara A. Reyna, and Jacqueline M. McGrath

Individualized, family-centered, developmental care (IFDC) for preterm and sick infants has resulted in both revolutionary and evolutionary changes in neonatal care practices. Unfortunately, there is no universal definition of the term "developmental care." Rather, IFDC incorporates many interventions, some of which have not been fully tested through well-designed research studies, although they have been implemented (Byers, 2003). Some developmental care programs have been designed primarily to affect changes in the neonatal intensive care unit (NICU). Other programs of developmental care are aimed at mediating the effects of too much, too little, or inappropriate forms of stimulation. This confusion over terms and methods makes evaluation of both short- and long-term outcomes difficult. However, there has been some specific research focused on short-term outcomes and postdischarge benefits of programs that fall under the umbrella of developmental care. Although the methodologic quality of much of this research has been, for the most part, unfavorably critiqued (Jacobs, Sokol, & Ohlsson, 2002; Symington & Pinelli, 2002), there are some findings that warrant consideration. In this chapter, we review four potential areas of short-term benefits of developmental care in the NICU: medical outcomes, length of hospitalization, feeding outcomes, and family satisfaction; and three areas of potential post-NICU benefits of developmental care: morbidity after discharge, developmental milestones and neurobehavioral performance, and family well-being.

## IMPROVED MEDICAL OUTCOMES

Improved medical outcomes during initial hospitalization have been associated with NICU care that is based on developmental care models. In particular, there is documentation that use of IFDC results in the reduction of numbers of days requiring mechanical ventilator and need for oxygen therapy (Als, Lawhon, Duffy, et al., 1994; Als, Lawhon, Brown, et al., 1986); which is associated with a decrease in severe lung disease and in the incidence of intraventricular hemorrhage (Als & Gilkerson, 1997; Als, Lawhon, Brown, et al., 1986; Als, Duffy, McAnulty, 1996; Buehler, Als, Duffy, et al., 1995). However, two other controlled trials in which IFDC protocols were instituted did not find a difference in the need for respiratory support among the groups (Becker, Grunwald, Moorman, & Stuhr, 1991; Westrup, Kleberg, & von Eichwald, 2000).

In an attempt to begin to design and compare benchmarking criteria for family-centered care, 11 centers within the Vermont Oxford database voluntarily outlined and collected variables and outcomes measures (Box 21-1). However, even with this planned initiative to implement a change in practices, data collected from the centers that participated in this project in 1998 and 2000 demonstrated an overall increase in the incidence of chronic lung disease (CLD) from 27.3% in 1998 to 31.4% in 2000 (Saunders, Abraham, Crosby, et al., 2003). The incidence of CLD increased in seven centers and decreased in four. Statistical correlations or analysis for relationships was not done in this project, and there was no report of correlation between the degree of family-centered care initiated and the outcomes; however, all centers reported having moved to greater implementation of family-centered care by then, as opposed to when they had started the course of this project. The differences in these results and the previously reported results can be explained by the degree of control for initiation of the IFDC

Box 21-1    Impact of Changes in Visitation Policies on Parents' Satisfaction at DeVos Children's Hospital

**Aim:**

Promote family visitation to allow siblings to visit when most convenient for parents and the patients.

**Measure:**

The parent satisfaction survey question, "The visitation policy met my family's needs" will show an improvement from previous surveys.

**CYCLE #1**

**Plan:**

Home Sweet Home committee will evaluate current sibling visitation practice and compare current practice to information gained at site visits for the family-centered care focus group.

**Do:**

- Do a literature search of visitation practices in NICUs.
- Share current visitation policy information from site visits, and results of a literature search to nursing staff at the policy retreat, and in the interdisciplinary team meeting.
- Present same information to the Infection Control Department.

**Study:**

Staff agreed the sibling visitation policy needed to change. The policy should be more convenient to families but also be respectful to patient conditions. Infection Control has concerns regarding introduction of communicable diseases and wants more time to review the literature.

**Act:**

New sibling visitation policy created. Continue to work with Infection Control to address their concerns.

**CYCLE #2**

**Plan:**

Write a new sibling visitation policy based on input from staff, information from benchmark centers, and literature.

**Do:**

- Inservice staff to new policy.
- Post new policy on the First Board.
- Inform families of the change by posting signs in the parent scrub room and letters at the bedside.

**Study:**

Initial reaction from staff was mixed. Many staff members noted less stress when visitation times are not concentrated to two designated time periods during the week. Other staff expressed more stress with families able to visit at their convenience and the interruption in workflow. Staff expressed frustration with poorly supervised toddlers, experiencing an incident when a sibling was noted to be pulling on critical tubing. Families' feedback will be assessed on the parent satisfaction survey.

**Act:**

Adjustments were made in the policy based on feedback. Siblings under 3 years of age will visit only once a week for a brief period.

Box 21-1 IMPACT OF CHANGES IN VISITATION POLICIES ON PARENTS' SATISFACTION AT DEVOS CHILDREN'S HOSPITAL—CONT'D

**CYCLE #3**

**Plan:**

A sibling health screening form acceptable for neonatal services and infection control will be developed.

**Do:**

- Health screen created based on prior literature search, information from benchmark centers and other centers in the We Are Family Focus Group.
- Present draft health screen to interdisciplinary practice council and infection control.
- Identify unit secretaries to administer health screen.
- Educate staff of process and implement health screening.
- Send a letter to families and place a poster in the parent scrub room to inform families of the new sibling health screening.

**Study:**

Initially the process was stressful for secretaries. Secretaries did not feel qualified to administer a health screen.

**Act:**

Work with the secretaries to refine the screening process. Add the managers and charge nurses as a resource for the secretary when he/she has a concern regarding the health of the child.

**CYCLE #4**

**Plan:**

Discontinue announcing families and visitors over the intercom.

**Do:**

- Obtain a sign-in book with dividers for each room for families and visitors to enter their names, time of arrival, and time of departure.
- Post welcoming signs for families and visitors guiding them to the main desk.
- Keep the doors to the patient care rooms closed to help identify when people are entering the nurseries.

**Study:**

Parents with infants in the unit were initially confused by the change, but no family complained about the change. Maintaining closed doors was a hassle and did not seem to add a benefit to identifying when a parent or visitor arrived. Staff fears of parents walking in during a procedure were unfounded. Discussions with staff about comfort level of doing procedures, such as an IV insertion, with parents present enabled staff to feel more comfortable. Decreased noise levels were enhanced by eliminating the announcement.

**Act:**

Evaluate parent satisfaction survey. Discontinue closing doors unless the unit noise level becomes a problem.

From Moore, K.A.C., Coker, K., DuBuisson, A.B., et al. (April 2003). Implementing potentially better practices for improving family-centered care in neonatal intensive care units: Successes and challenges, *Pediatrics, 111*(4).

interventions. In the research protocols, there was a great deal of rigor in the degree and kind of developmental care provided. This is most likely quite different from the environments in which the Vermont Oxford data were collected. Each center was at a different place in the implementation of IFDC and, thus, comparisons are difficult to make. Much still needs to be learned as we begin to benchmark and establish better family-centered care practices in the NICU.

## LENGTH OF HOSPITALIZATION

Length of hospitalization or stay (LOS) has been demonstrated to decrease with implementation of the Newborn Developmental Care and Assessment Program (NIDCAP®) (Boston, MA) approach (Als, Lawhon, Brown, et al., 1986; Als, Lawhon, Duffy, et al., 1994; Fleisher, VandenBerg, Constantinou, et al., 1995) and within other research protocols for which the staff was trained in the observation of behavioral cues as a means for providing IFDC intervention (Becker, Grunwald, Moorman, & Stuhr, 1991; Brown & Heermann, 1997). However, in a more recent controlled trial in Sweden where the NIDCAP® approach was used, there was no change in the LOS for intervention versus control infants (Westrup, Kleberg, von Eichenwald, et al., 2000). This was also the conclusion within the Vermont Oxford family-centered care benchmarking report (Saunders, Abraham, Crosby, et al., 2003), where there was no change found in the LOS across the 11 centers. The mean LOS decreased in seven of the centers and increased in four. It might be that the LOS is affected by too many factors for IFDC to have an overall effect. However, when IFDC is found to be successful, the decreased LOS has also decreased the cost of newborn intensive care (Als, Lawhon, Duffy, et al., 1994; Fleisher, VandenBerg, Constantinou, et al., 1995; Petryshen, Stevens, Hawkins, & Stewart, 1997).

## FEEDING OUTCOMES

Improved weight gain with decreased time to enteral feeding has been demonstrated as an outcome of some of the IFDC research protocols (Als, Lawhon, Brown, et al., 1986; Als, Lawhon, Duffy, et al., 1994; Becker, Grunwald, Moorman, & Stuhr, 1991; Brown & Heermann, 1997; Fleisher, VandenBerg, Constantinou, et al., 1995). However, initiation of earlier enteral feeding for the very low birthweight (VLBW) infant has been studied as a separate intervention and had favorable results unrelated to the initiation of developmental care

(Meetze, Valentine, McGuigan, et al., 1992; Troche, Harvey-Wilkes, Engle, et al., 1995).

Sucking behaviors are thought to be an ideal barometer of central nervous system maturation as well as overall organization of behaviors and have been used as a measure for neurodevelopment outcomes (Medoff-Cooper, Verklan, & Carlson, 1993); however, no research that involved IDFC interventions has directly measured sucking outcomes. This is an outcome variable that needs further evaluation.

In the Vermont Oxford project (Saunders, Abraham, Crosby, et al., 2003) no differences were found in the mean corrected gestational age (36.2 weeks at each data point) when infants attained full oral feedings between 1998 and 2000. However, the median corrected age varied among centers from 34.7 to 36.6 weeks. Another feeding variable was evaluated in the Vermont Oxford project that was not previously described in other research protocols. They asked families in the first 48 hours of admission to the NICU what was their preferred discharge-feeding plan. Families were given the option of choosing bottlefeeding, breastfeeding, or some combination of the two. Then they examined VLBW infants at discharge and whether they were receiving the identified feeding plan or not. They found that with infants for whom the plan was bottlefeeding, 94% were discharged on this plan; however, when the identified plan was breastfeeding or a combination of breast and bottlefeeding, the concordance was only 67% and 74%, respectfully. It appears that much still needs to be learned about how to better facilitate breastfeeding in this high-risk population.

One feeding related intervention often found within developmental care protocols that has demonstrated positive outcomes, is the initiation of nonnutritive sucking (NNS). The beneficial effects of providing NNS during intermittent gavage feeding have been described for LBW preterm infants and include fewer number of gavage feedings; accelerated maturation of the sucking reflex related to increased experience with sucking, with subsequent earlier initiation of bottle feedings; greater daily weight gain; shorter hospital stay; and decreased hospital costs (Pinelli & Symington, 2000). However, in a well-controlled prospective study, NNS was not associated with improved growth outcome for VLBW preterm infants. Therefore, the data on outcome measures with respect to offering NNS during gavage feeding are inconclusive, and further study is needed (Bernbaum, Pereira, Watkins, & Peckham, 1983). However, no published studies have reported adverse outcomes associated with NNS when safe pacifiers are used (Pinelli & Symington, 2000).

## PARENT SATISFACTION

Most research protocols in which the NIDCAP® approach has been used to deliver IFDC to infants and their families have reported improved satisfaction with care, decreased parental stress, increased parental comfort, and competence at discharge from the NICU (Als, Lawhon, Brown, et al., 1986; Als, Lawhon, Duffy, et al., 1994; Fleisher, VandenBerg, Constantinou, et al., 1995). However, no objective measures were used to demonstrate these outcomes with families, thus making them difficult to duplicate in other centers. Institutions most often assess parental satisfaction after discharge with generalized questionnaires related to satisfaction with overall hospitalization that seldom include items related to IFDC. In the Vermont Oxford benchmarking report (Saunders, Abraham, Crosby, et al., 2003), parent-reported outcomes were collected with a web-based tool that took most parents 10 to 15 minutes to complete *(www.howsyourbaby.com)*. Questions from four categories were included: the baby's stay in the hospital; leaving the hospital; the baby at home; and special questions from the health team. Examples of questions asked include: (Saunders, Abraham, Crosby, et al., 2003)

- How well do you know your infant (personality; likes and dislikes; ways my infant uses to calm himself/herself)?
- During your infant's hospital stay, how often did you feel like a parent?
- How ready do you feel you are to care for your infant after discharge from the hospital?
- How do you feel about feeding your baby?
- How have you felt about breastfeeding? (for mothers planning to breastfeed)

No outcome results of the survey were published in the benchmarking report, but objective measurement of these variables looks promising and appears to be an ongoing process for the centers participating in the project. Understanding the components of parent satisfaction with family-centered care strategies is an area in which we are gaining understanding; inclusion of families in the development of these criteria will only serve to strengthen the partnership that is forming between the healthcare providers and the parents.

## MORBIDITY AFTER DISCHARGE

Morbidity is the incidence of disease and complication. From the mid-1970s through the mid-1990s, morbidity as well as mortality rates for preterm infants steadily declined. Since the mid-1990s, however, morbidity and mortality rates have been static (Horbar, Badger, Carpenter, et al., 2002). Preterm infants continue to have a relatively high incidence of morbidity related to ongoing medical problems. Major morbidity can result from complications of chronic lung disease and intraventricular hemorrhage, which are themselves morbidities of prematurity. In children born preterm, these conditions contribute to the higher incidence of cerebral palsy and developmental delay as well as problems associated with vision and hearing, speech and language, and learning and school performance (Blackburn, 1998).

As noted earlier, improved medical outcomes during initial hospitalization have been associated with NICU care that is based on developmental care models, such as reduction in severity of CLD and the incidence of intraventricular hemorrhage (Buehler, Als, Duffy, et al., 1995). However, only recently has there been any effort to specifically examine the effects of developmental care practices on long-term morbidity outcomes, including those related to respiratory function. For example, individualized care, such as that provided through the NIDCAP® approach, has been found to result in improved pulmonary function, behavior organization, and improved developmental and social skills at 8 months of age in infants who were born preterm (Feldman & Eidelman, 1998).

### Readmissions and Emergency Room Visits

There is limited current information on rehospitalization rates of infants who were born preterm.

Infants with chronic conditions, such as bronchopulmonary dysplasia and short bowel syndrome, might require rehospitalization for exacerbation of their chronic disease. Other infants might require rehospitalization or emergency room care for acute respiratory illness, gastroenteritis, dehydration, and sepsis. Surgical repair of an inguinal hernia also contributes to the post-NICU discharge rehospitalization rate (Termini, Brooten, Brown, et al., 1990).

There are no data correlating developmental care practices to either acute care visits or rehospitalization rates. For example, although published data exist detailing rates of readmission following NICU discharge, the data have not kept up with changing trends in either preterm infant care (e.g., postsurfactant data) or changes in healthcare trends. Moreover, while comparisons to current rates of readmission might be useful as developmental care becomes more widely practiced, it will be difficult to distinguish the impact of developmental care on those rates from other changes in NICU care. Research that accounts for the interactions of all these variables must be developed so that long-term implications of developmental care practices in the NICU can be better assessed, and recommendations for future practices can be made.

## DEVELOPMENTAL MILESTONES AND NEUROBEHAVIORAL PERFORMANCE

Preterm birth places a child at a greater risk for poor developmental outcomes of long-term duration (Hack, Flannery, Schluchter, et al., 2002). Infants born preterm have a historically high incidence of poor neurodevelopmental outcome, including low intelligence quotient, cerebral palsy, visual impairment, hearing impairment, and learning disabilities. Close to 20% of preterm infants develop major cognitive disabilities by middle-school age. Therefore, although survival of preterm infants has improved dramatically over the past three decades, depending on year of birth, birthweight, and birth gestation, the incidence of major disability in these children ranges from 20% to 50% in the first years of life (Ment, Vohr, Allan, et al., 2003). In addition, although the incidence of major motor, sensory, and intellectual handicaps in preterm infants who do not have sig-

nificant medical complications has declined, there are continuing concerns that the physical and social characteristics of the NICU environment might delay or distort optimal developmental patterns. In fact, improved survival rates of the gestationally youngest preterm infants might place these children at greater developmental risk, because they typically remain hospitalized for extended periods, at a time when their neurologic and behavioral systems are immature and unstable (Als & Gilkerson, 1997; Wolf, Koldewijn, Beelen, et al., 2002). The risk for crippling sequelae in these youngest and most fragile preterm infants ranges from 15% to 25% (Kleberg, Westrup, Stjernqvist, & Lagercrantz, 2002).

Numerous neurobehavioral and temperament deviations have been noted in children who were born preterm. Individualized developmental care during hospitalization has been found to have positive short-term effects on autonomic, motor, behavioral, and attentional organization in these children (Becker, Grunwald, & Brazy, 1999). Neurobehavioral improvements in the period immediately following discharge have also been documented (Buehler, Als, Duffy, et al., 1995). For example, 73 preterm infants who received skin-to-skin care in the NICU were studied at 37 weeks, 3 months, and 6 months. Compared with the control group, the infants who received skin-to-skin care scored higher on the Bayley Mental Developmental Index (MDI) and the Psychomotor Developmental Index (PDI) at 6 months of age (Feldman & Eidelman, 1998). In another small study involving infants with birthweights ranging from 1501 to 2099 g, the infants who received skin-to-skin care had significantly higher Bayley MDI scores at 12 months than did infants in the control group (Ohgi, Fukuda, Kusumoto, et al., 2002). Assessing the longer-term benefits of developmental care has proven more difficult, especially in such areas as cognition and motor outcomes.

Cognitive development is an important outcome to consider when evaluating the benefits of interventions based on models of developmental care. Although IQs might be normal for most children who were born preterm, an estimated 10% to 40% have IQs that are borderline or low. In addition, children who were born preterm are reported to be less adaptable and more impulsive and to have shorter attention spans than children who were born at term. Children born preterm also display decreased social competence and need more environmental structure than do children who were born at term (Blackburn, 1998). In addition, language delays are especially common in children who were born preterm, with incidence rates ranging from 20% to 40%. The delays are both expressive and receptive in nature and correspond to learning and school problems, which are also high in children born preterm. Incidence rates of school difficulties in children born preterm range from 20% to 65% during the early school years, with rates increasing as the children get older (Bhutta, Cleves, Casey, et al., 2002).

Some researchers have reported statistically significant improvement in cognition at 9 and 12 months corrected age following NIDCAP® or similar intervention (Als, Lawhon, Brown, et al., 1986; Als, Lawhon, Duffy, et al., 1994; Resnick, Armstrong, & Carter, 1988). These results did not persist at 2 years of age. Moreover, other researchers have not found cognitive improvements following NIDCAP® or like interventions (Ariagno, Thoman, Boedikker, et al., 1997; Westrup, Kleberg, von Eichwald, et al., 2000). Although other studies have been undertaken to test the effects of various interventions on long-term neurobehavioral outcomes, these studies either have serious methodologic flaws or the reports from the studies lack sufficient data for full evaluation (Symington & Pinelli, 2002).

Despite the paucity of research findings demonstrating clear effects of developmental care on long-term neurodevelopmental outcomes, there are some studies that suggest important benefits to more contingently patterned caregiving. For example, research has shown that a preterm infant at 20 weeks' postconceptual age, who has had individualized developmental care during hospitalization, has more differentiation of brain tissue than a full-term counterpart (Buehler, Als, Duffy, et al., 1995). This differentiation shows particularly interesting changes in the frontal lobe functioning of preterm infants. Although further research is needed to substantiate these findings, results such as these are promising.

Another outcome of major concern for infants born preterm is motor function. Birthweight is a major predictor of motor development; the lower the birthweight, the greater the likelihood of delays in motor development. In particular, cerebral palsy, especially spastic diplegia, is more common in infants born preterm. The incidence of cerebral palsy ranges from 3% to 8% in children who were born preterm (Blackburn, 1998). Improved motor milestone achievement at 12 and 24 months of age following intervention with developmental care approaches has been reported (Resnick, Armstrong, & Carter, 1988). Research has failed to substantiate a relationship of developmental care to short-term precursors of motor disorders, such as decreasing the incidence of intraventricular hemorrhage.

## FAMILY WELL-BEING

Family disruption and financial stress during the hospitalization of a preterm infant are common. The incidence of separation, divorce, abuse, and neglect are high among families of preterm infants. Research has repeatedly documented high levels of stress, anxiety, depression, distress, and grief in mothers of preterm infants (Affleck, Tennen, & Rowe, 1990; Gennaro, 1996; Miles, Holditch-Davis, & Shepherd, 1998). Post-discharge, families of preterm infants might be required to make unexpected lifestyle changes. Preterm infants can be more difficult to parent, less adaptable, less predictable, and fussier than the normal weight, term infants (Gennaro, 1996; Hughes, Shults, McGrath, et al., 2002).

Several studies have examined the long-term concerns of parents of preterm infants. Lengthy hospital stays in NICUs can jeopardize the development of maternal/parental-infant attachment by impeding close contact between mothers, fathers, and their babies (Miles, Funk, & Kasper, 1991). It is well known that prolonged hospitalization of preterm infants has detrimental effects on family functioning and parent-child interaction. In particular, disruptions of the parent-child relationship and not feeling like a parent are significant sources of stress for parents of hospitalized preterm infants (Hughes, McCollum, Sheftel, et al., 1994). Alterations in parental role functions, including being unable to hold or feed their infant, are part of the disrupted relationship experienced by parents (Miles, Funk, & Kasper, 1991). In addition, parenting styles can be affected by global concern regarding the health and well being of their infant. The anxiety and worry over whether an infant will survive, and then thrive after discharge, might lead a parent to compensate for what the child had been through in the early months of life (Docherty, Miles, & Holditch-Davis, 2002).

Parental stress is increased by not being able to clearly predict when a child will be discharged home. Hospital discharge often brings relief to parents, but it can also bring anxiety related to assuming total responsibility for their infant. When parents take their child home, the transition is often traumatic (Brooten, Kumar, Brown, et al., 1986) with parents feeling incompetent to perform even the most basic of childcare tasks (Affleck, Tennen, Allen, et al., 1986). Parenting stress includes concerns regarding the potential for illness, and whether the infant is feeding enough and achieving adequate weight gain.

Advances in neonatal care have resulted in the survival of VLBW infants. Many of these infants are discharged home with chronic health problems that require continued dependence on technology and require close medical surveillance for an extended period of time. This adds an additional financial and emotional stress for the family (Youngblut, Brennan, & Swegart, 1994). Throughout the continuum from hospital to discharge and postdischarge, the largest concerns of parents are related to infant health, with the next largest area of concern being infant weight and development (Gennaro, Zukowsky, Brooten, et al., 1990). The need to develop interventions and strategies to promote parenting and reduce the distress experienced by parents of preterm infants during hospitalization is apparent and can have long-term implications. Parents should be provided the opportunity to "room-in" with their infant and assume full responsibility for their infant's care prior to discharge. This can help reassure parents about their infants' readiness for discharge, teach them how to respond to their infant's pattern of behavior, and test the reality of caregiving (Costello & Chapman, 1998).

Two critical components for a mother to achieve a sense of personal growth, despite having a medically fragile infant, is feeling as though she is a mother to her infant and developing a physical closeness with her infant (Miles, Holditch-Davis, Burchinal, et al., 1999). Mothers who participate in "kangaroo care" with "kangaroo nutrition" (breastfeeding or formula-feeding provided during skin-to-skin holding) express greater competence than mothers who do not participate in these interventions (Tessier, Cristo, Velez, et al., 1998). Parental participation in caregiving might reduce guilt and sadness that often is not manifested until after discharge (Griffin, Wishba, & Kavanaugh, 1998). Family functioning appears to be improved, as parents feel less stressed and depressed and more effective following NICU care that is developmentally individualized (Als & Gilkerson, 1997). Infant outcomes and home environment show improvement in low-income mothers who have participated in NICU-based developmental programs (Parker, Zahr, Cole, et al., 1992). Fathers who participate in skin-to-skin care, either actively or through support of the mother have been noted to provide a more optimal environment for their infants following discharge (Feldman, Eidelman, Sirota, et al., 2002).

However, despite measures to reduce parental stress during hospitalization, parents might continue to view their infant as fragile or chronically ill for some time following discharge (Miles & Holditch-Davis, 1997). The development of support systems postdischarge to provide opportunities for reflective "debriefing" for parents might be helpful. Both during and after hospitalization, mothers should be given information and hope that realistically reduces worry about their child's health (Miles, Holditch-Davis, Burchinal, et al., 1999)

## CONCLUSION

At present, there are some data that demonstrate modest improvement in both short- and long-term outcomes in preterm infants following developmental care programs. Although NIDCAP® and similar programs have been used in the NICU setting for more than 10 years, little research has been done outside of major NIDCAP® centers to demonstrate the long-term effect of these programs or of specific interventions included in the programs. That, coupled with the relatively short time that developmental care has been used, contributes to the paucity of data. What research has been done has involved small samples in select settings. However, some interventions studied in the past 30 years have been shown to have a favorable effect on later development (Feldman & Eidelman, 1998).

Long-term follow-up studies of children born preterm and hospitalized in NICUs before the widespread use of developmental care programs clearly demonstrates the serious, enduring sequelae to preterm birth and lengthy stays in NICUs. In addition, new theoretic frameworks, such as Als' synactive theory, and new basic science research about brain and neurologic development, support the use of new models of care over traditional caregiving practices.

As research on the effects of developmental care on both short- and long-term outcomes in preterm infants continues, investigators and clinicians should also be aware of the mediation of the home environment on these outcomes. The effects of the early social environment and parent-infant interactions over time can influence later development and need to be considered when examining the long-term benefits of developmental care practices (Magill-Evans & Harrison, 1999; Miceli, Goeke-Morey, Whitman, et al., 2000). In addition, the neuroplasticity of the human brain allows for at least some mediation of the adverse effects of the NICU environment.

As research continues to improve our understanding of the effect of neonatal intensive care, attention will need to be given to ensuring adequately sized and diverse samples from many settings. In addition, clinicians and researchers will need to clarify language regarding the type and character of developmental care being provided and studied. Environmental and individually directed interventions that reduce or modify the adverse characteristics of NICU based on developmental care models require much further study before recommendations can be made for universal adoption. Research about these interventions must be methodologically sound, and measures of effectiveness should incorporate short- and long-term biologic and behavioral outcomes (Perlman, 2001). As research in this area proceeds, the underlying mechanisms by which developmental care interventions result in improved outcomes will be revealed and incorporated into routine caregiving in the NICU.

## REFERENCES

Affleck, G., Tennen, H., Allen, D.A., et al. (1986). Perceived social support and maternal adaptation during the transition from hospital to home care of high-risk infants. *Infant Mental Health Journal, 7*, 6-17.

Affleck, G., Tennen, H., & Rowe, J. (1990). Mothers, fathers, and the crisis of newborn intensive care. *Infant Mental Health Journal, 11*, 12-25.

Als, H., Duffy, F.H., & McAnulty, G.B. (1996). Effectiveness of individualized developmental care in the newborn intensive care unit (NICU). *Acta Pediatrics Supplement, 416*, 21-30.

Als, H., & Gilkerson, L. (1997). The role of relationship-based developmentally supportive newborn intensive care in strengthening outcome of preterm infants. *Seminars in Perinatology, 21*, 178-189.

Als, H., Lawhon, G., Brown, E., et al. (1986). Individualized behavioral and environmental care for the very low birth weight preterm infant at high risk for bronchopulmonary dysplasia: Neonatal intensive care unit and developmental outcome. *Pediatrics, 78*, 1123-1132.

Als, H., Lawhon, G., Duffy, F.H., et al. (1994). Individualized developmental care for the very low-birth-weight preterm infant: Medical and neurofunctional effects. *Journal of the American Medical Association (JAMA), 272*, 853-858.

Ariagno, R.L., Thoman, E.B., Boedikker, B., et al. (1997). Developmental care does not alter sleep and development of premature infants. *Pediatrics, 100*, 1-7.

Becker, P.T., Grunwald, P.C., & Brazy, J.E. (1999). Motor organization in very low birth weight infants during caregiving: Effects of a developmental intervention. *Journal of Developmental and Behavioral Pediatrics, 20*, 344-354.

Becker, P.T., Grunwald, P.C., Moorman, J., & Stuhr, S. (1991). Outcomes of developmentally supportive nursing care for very low birthweight infants. *Nursing Research, 40*(3), 150-155.

Bernbaum, J.C., Pereira, G.R., Watkins, J.B., et al. (1983). Nonnutritive sucking during gavage feeding enhances growth and maturation in premature infants. *Pediatrics, 71*, 41-45.

Bhutta, A.T., Cleves, M.A., Casey, P.H., et al. (2002). Cognitive and behavioral outcomes of school-aged children who were born preterm. *Journal of the American Medical Association (JAMA), 288*, 728-737.

Blackburn, S. (1998). Environmental impact of the NICU on developmental outcomes. *Journal of Pediatric Nursing, 13*, 279-289.

Brooten, D., Kumar, S., Brown, L.P., et al. (1986). A randomized clinical trial of early hospital discharge and home follow-up of very-low-birth-weight infants. *New England Journal of Medicine, 315*, 934-939.

Brown, L.D., & Heermann, J.A. (1997). The effects of developmental care on preterm infant outcome. *Applied Nursing Research, 10*(4), 190-197.

Buehler, D.M., Als, H., Duffy, F.H., et al. (1995). Effectiveness of individualized developmental care for low-risk preterm infants: Behavioral and electrophysiologic evidence. *Pediatrics, 96*, 923-932.

Byers, J.F. (2003). Components of developmental care and the evidence for their use in the NICU. *Journal of Obstetric, Gynecologic, and Neonatal Nursing (JOGNN), 28*(3), 174-180.

Costello, A.M., & Chapman, J.S. (1998). Mothers' perceptions of the care-by-parent program prior to hospital discharge of their preterm infants. *Neonatal Network, 17*, 37-42.

Docherty, S.L., Miles, M.S., & Holditch-Davis, D. (2002). Worry about child health in mothers of hospitalized medically fragile infants. *Advances in Neonatal Care, 2*, 84-92.

Feldman, R., & Eidelman, A.I. (1998). Intervention programs for premature infants: How and do they affect development? *Clinics in Perinatology, 25*, 613-625.

Feldman, R., Eidelman, A.I., Sirota, L., et al. (2002). Comparison of skin-to-skin (kangaroo) and traditional care: Parenting outcomes and preterm infant development. *Pediatrics, 110*, 16-26.

Fleisher, B.E., VandenBerg, K., Constantinou, J., et al. (1995). Individualized developmental care for very low birthweight premature infants. *Clinical Pediatrics, 34*(10), 523-529.

Gennaro, S. (1996). Family response to the low birth weight infant. *Nursing Clinics of North America, 31*, 341-350.

Gennaro, S., Zukowsky, K., Brooten, D., et al. (1990). Concerns of mothers of low birthweight infants. *Pediatric Nursing, 16*(5), 459-462.

Griffin, T., Wishba, C., & Kavanaugh, K. (1998). Nursing interventions to reduce stress in parents of hospitalized preterm infants. *Journal of Pediatric Nursing, 13*, 290-295.

Hack, M., Flannery, D.J., Schluchter, M., et al. (2002). Outcomes in young adulthood for very-low-birth-weight infants. *New England Journal of Medicine, 346*, 149-157.

Horbar, J.D., Badger, G.J., Carpenter, J.H., et al. (2002). Trends in mortality and morbidity for very low birth weight infants, 1991-1999. *Pediatrics, 110*, 143-151.

Hughes, M., McCollum, J., Sheftel, D., et. al. (1994). How parents cope with the experience of neonatal intensive care. *Children's Health Care, 23*, 1-14.

Hughes, M., Shults, J., McGrath, J.M., et al. (2002). Temperament characteristics of premature infants in the first year of life. *Developmental and Behavioral Pediatrics, 23*, 430-435.

Jacobs, S.E., Sokol, J., & Ohlsson, A. (2002). The newborn individualized developmental care and assessment program is not supported by meta-analyses of the data. *Journal of Pediatrics, 140*, 699-706.

Kleberg, A., Westrup, B., Stjernqvist, K., & Lagercrantz, H. (2002). Indications of improved cognitive development at one year of age among infants born very prematurely who received care based on the Newborn Individualized Developmental Care and Assessment Program (NIDCAP®). *Early Human Development, 68*, 83-91.

Magill-Evans, J., & Harrison, M.J. (1999). Parent-child interactions and development of toddlers born preterm. *Western Journal of Nursing Research, 21*, 292-307.

Medoff-Cooper, B., Verklan, T., & Carlson, S. (1993). The development of sucking patterns and physiologic correlates in very-low-birth weight infants. *Nursing Research, 42*(2), 100-105.

Meetze, W.H., Valentine, C., McGuigan, J.E., et al., (1992). Gastrointestinal priming prior to full enteral nutrition in very low birth weight infants. *Journal of Pediatric Gastroenterology and Nutrition, 15* (2), 163-170.

Ment, L.A., Vohr, B., Allan, W., et al. (2003). Change in cognitive function over time in very low-birth-weight infants. *Journal of the American Medical Association (JAMA), 289*, 705-711.

Miceli, P.J., Goeke-Morey, M.C., Whitman, T.L., et al. (2000). Birth status, medical complications, and social environment: Individual differences in development of preterm, very low birth weight infants. *Journal of Pediatric Psychology, 25*, 353-358.

Miles, M.S., Funk, S.G., & Kasper, M.A. (1991). The neonatal intensive care unit environment: Sources of stress for parents. *American Association of Critical Care Nursing (AACN) Clinical Issues in Critical Care Nursing, 2*(2), 346-354.

Miles, M.S., & Holditch-Davis, D. (1997). Parenting the prematurely born child: Pathways of influence. *Seminars in Perinatology, 21*, 254-266.

Miles, M.S., Holditch-Davis, D., Burchinal, P., et al. (1999). Distress and growth outcomes in mothers of medically fragile infants. *Nursing Research, 48*, 129-140.

Miles, M.S., Holditch-Davis, D., & Shepherd, H. (1998). Maternal concerns about parenting: Prematurely born children. *MCN, American Journal of Maternal Child Nursing, 23*, 70-75.

Ohgi, S., Fukuda, H., Kusumoto, T., et al. (2002). Comparison of Kangaroo care and standard care: Behavioral organization, development, and temperament in healthy, low-birth-weight infants through 1 year. *Journal of Perinatology, 22*, 374-379.

Parker, S.J., Zahr, L.K., Cole, J.G., et al. (1992). Outcome after developmental intervention in the neonatal intensive care unit for mothers of preterm infants with low socioeconomic status. *Journal of Pediatrics, 120*, 780-785.

Perlman, J.M. (2001). Neurobehavioral deficits in premature graduates of intensive care: Potential medical and neonatal environmental risk factors. *Pediatrics, 108,* 1339-1348.

Petryshen, P., Stevens, B., Hawkins, J., & Stewart, M. (1997). Comparing nursing costs for preterm infants receiving conventional vs. developmental care. *Nursing Economics, 15*(3), 138-145.

Pinelli, J., & Symington, A. (2000). How rewarding can a pacifier be? A systematic review of nonnutritive sucking in preterm infants. *Neonatal Network, 19*(8), 41-48.

Resnick, M.B., Armstrong, S., & Carter, R.L. (1988). Developmental intervention program for high-risk premature infants: Effects on development and parent-infant interactions. *Developmental and Behavioral Pediatrics, 9,* 73-78.

Saunders, R.P., Abraham, M.R., Crosby, M.J., et al. (2003). Evaluation and development of potentially better practices for improving family-centered care in neonatal intensive care units. *Pediatrics, 111*(4), e437-e444.

Symington, A., & Pinelli, J. (2002). Distilling the evidence on developmental care: A systematic review. *Advances in Neonatal Care, 2,* 198-221.

Termini, L., Brooten, D., Brown, L., Gennaro, S., & York, R. (1990). Reasons for acute care visits and rehospitalizations in very low-birthweight infants. *Neonatal Network, 8,* 23-26.

Tessier, R., Cristo, M., Velez, S., et al. (1998). Kangaroo mother care and the bonding hypothesis. *Pediatrics, 102,* e17.

Troche, B., Harvey-Wilkes, K., Engle, W.D., et al., (1995). Early minimal feedings promote growth in critically ill premature infants. *Biological Neonate, 67,* 172-181.

Westrup, B., Kleberg, A., von Eichwald, K., et al. (2000). A randomized, controlled trial to evaluate the effects of the newborn individualized developmental care and assessment program in a Swedish setting. *Pediatrics, 105*(1)(Pt 1), 66-72.

Wolf, M.J., Koldewijn, K., Beelen, A., et al. (2002). Neurobehavioral and developmental profile of very low birthweight preterm infants in early infancy. *Acta Paediatrica Scandinavica, 91,* 930-938.

Youngblut, J.M., Brennan, P.F., & Swegart, L.A. (1994). Families with medically fragile children: An exploratory study. *Pediatric Nursing, 20,* 463-468.

# 22 Organizational Climate, Implementation of Change, and Outcomes

Carol Spruill Turnage-Carrier, Charlotte Ward-Larson, and Lois V.S. Gates

The organizational climate and social structure of each neonatal intensive care unit (NICU) is as individual as the different personalities of the people who work there. Climate takes into account the temperament, attitudes, and outlook of the members within an organization. It is important to consider these areas when trying to understand the behaviors and responses of the individuals or groups in the NICU. The climate allows members to understand the general direction of the team, what it means to be part of the group, what actions are appropriate or inappropriate, how others are likely to react, and other information that helps guide behavior and relationships within the group (Folger, Poole, & Stutman, 1997).

Characteristics of organizational climate (Folger, Poole, & Stutman, 1997) include:

- More than the beliefs or feelings of one individual member
- A shared, common experience for members (implies common theme for interactions/atmosphere experienced)
- No one person is responsible for forming the climate
- Climates persist for extended time spans

Because the climate is a reinforcing pattern of interactions, the longer it persists, the more entrenched and enduring the same patterns are likely to become. Changes that "break the spell" by affecting interactions, are needed to redirect the group. In this chapter, we discuss what constitutes an organizational climate and how that impacts on the implementation of developmental care and then provide strategies for fully implementing individualized, family-centered, developmental care (IFDC) into the NICU. Change is never easy, but with some understanding, it can be a little less torturous. The final sections will be devoted to organizational and unit-based outcomes once IFDC is implemented.

## OVERVIEW OF GENERAL PRINCIPLES OF ORGANIZATIONAL CLIMATE

Climates are general themes that underlie all interactions in the social (NICU) unit. Four important categories of climate themes have been identified in Box 22-1. Implementing developmental and family-centered care might be a small step for some organizations and a giant leap for others. The rate of diffusion and acceptance of developmental and family-centered care strategies is related to the social and organizational climate that already exists. How does one determine the climate?

## EXAMINING CURRENT ORGANIZATIONAL CLIMATE

Observation is the first step in examining an organizational climate. It is necessary to diagnose the NICU climate through observing interactions among the individuals in the environment. Talking with interdisciplinary groups and focusing on interaction among members on the same and different levels, such as physician to nurse, nurse practitioner to nurse, nurse manager to secretary, respiratory therapist to nurse and so on, is another important aspect of ascertaining the climate. For example, taking the time to answer the questions in Box 22-2 might provide members a sense of the current work climate and the relative:

- Safety in the social setting
- Level of commitment to one another
- Tolerance for disagreement; voicing issues
- Trust within the group
- Cooperation and approach to problems

## Box 22-1    FOUR IMPORTANT CATEGORIES OF CLIMATE THEMES

| Type of Theme | Examples of Issues Associated with Each Type of Theme |
| --- | --- |
| 1. Dominance and authority relations | Is power concentrated in the hands of a few leaders or is it shared? |
| | How important is power in group decisions? |
| | How rigid is the group's power structure? Do members shift among roles? |
| 2. Degree of supportiveness | Are members friendly or intimate with one another? |
| | Can members trust one another? |
| | Can members safely express emotions in the group? |
| | To what degree does the group emphasize task versus socio-emotional concerns? |
| 3. Sense of group identity | Does the group have a definite identity? |
| | Do members feel ownership of group accomplishments? |
| | How great is a member commitment to the group? |
| | Do members share responsibility for decisions? |
| 4. Interdependence | Can members all gain if they cooperate, or will one's gain be another's loss? |
| | Are members pitted against one another? |

From Folger, J.P., Poole, M.S., & Stutman, R.K. (2001). *Working through conflict: Strategies for relationships, groups, and organizations* (4th ed.). New York: Addison Wesley Longman.

## Box 22-2    EVALUATING YOUR PRACTICE ACCORDING TO FOUR STANDARDS OF DEVELOPMENTAL CARE

| Standard | Questions for Evaluation |
| --- | --- |
| Standard 1: A flexible and individualized approach is taken toward all hands-on caregiving interactions, with continual responsiveness to each infant's competencies, vulnerabilities, and thresholds. | If an infant has an individualized developmental care plan, do I read it carefully and use it as a guide for timing and structuring my care? |
| | Am I mentally and emotionally engaged with each infant in my care, continually guided by the behavior of the infant? (Do I pace my care mindfully and provide positioning and physical supports that bring out the best in the baby, based on his or her individual competencies, vulnerabilities, and thresholds?) |
| | Do I stay attuned to every baby between care periods, so that: (1) I respond promptly if a baby needs attention or added support to stay relaxed and restful, even if I am not the child's assigned caregiver?, and (2) I am ready to begin care when the baby is showing a natural change of state, recognizing that state changes are often very subtle? |
| | Am I flexible in timing my care to support and protect a quiet sleep state? |
| | Do I carry out care that can be flexibly timed (e.g., nursing and medical assessment, weighing, bathing) together with procedures for which timing is less flexible, being careful to avoid overwhelming the baby? |
| | Do I make ongoing judgments about the necessity of interventions for each infant and make collaborative decisions to delay or eliminate interventions that might create unnecessary stress? |

**Box 22-2** EVALUATING YOUR PRACTICE ACCORDING TO FOUR STANDARDS OF DEVELOPMENTAL CARE—CONT'D

For scheduled interventions, such as feedings, medications, or pulmonary treatments, do I identify and make use of appropriate "leeway" to ease timing pressures to the greatest extent possible?

If I have decided that it is necessary and appropriate to awaken a sleeping baby, do I approach the baby gently with a soft touch or whisper, and spend the necessary moments to help a baby move smoothly and comfortably into a higher state before doing any assessment or procedure?

Do I avoid doing any procedures, assessments, or caregiving tasks with an infant in a prone (sleep only) position, where he is unlikely to be able to use self-comforting abilities?

Do I think through my caregiving and collect everything I need before approaching an infant, so that I do not leave the baby on his own or unsupported once my hands-on care has begun?

Am I mindful of the powerful influence of the feeding experience on the infant's emotional development and structure my approach so every feeding is a positive, pleasant, and nurturing time, regardless of the size or age of the baby, or the route or volume of the feeding?

Am I continually aware of the vulnerability of infants' fragile digestive systems during hands-on care before feedings, and work to carefully avoid fluctuations in perfusion that might influence how the gut accommodates and digests feedings?

If an infant has difficulty remaining stable and organized in spite of my careful handling, do I slow down or stop, help the baby recover completely, and reconsider my approach before continuing?

Do I respond to and support the child's efforts to spend time quietly awake in relaxed engagement with his caregivers, recognizing the development of quiet alertness as the necessary foundation for each infant's formation of social relationships?

After helping an infant stay relaxed and wakeful during hands-on care, do I stay with the infant and support a smooth transition back to a restful sleep before stepping away from the bedside?

**Standard 2: Parent-infant relationships are supported form birth.**

Is my manner toward families and their supports warm, respectful, and welcoming?

Is my manner toward families consistent with my words?

Do I maintain flexibility to welcome and support families consistently, at all times of the day?

Do I accommodate the presence of families in the nursery during rounds or shift-change by sharing information in a location and tone of voice that preserves confidentiality?

Do I model careful, nurturing, and supportive caregiving for families?

Do I form relationships with families, show genuine interest in their experience, and respect their central role in the life of their child?

Do I include families in caring for their child in a meaningful way from the time of birth and document their caregiving activities so that other caregivers can support them in a consistent way?

If colleagues have provided inclusive caregiving opportunities for a family during previous shifts, can I be counted on to support the same family inclusion?

*Continued*

Box 22-2    EVALUATING YOUR PRACTICE ACCORDING TO FOUR STANDARDS OF DEVELOPMENTAL CARE—CONT'D

| | |
|---|---|
| | Do I support families in understanding and supporting their babies' behavioral and developmental goals from the earliest possible time, and nurture their confidence in supporting their infant's goals? |
| | Do I support parents in supporting their babies during potentially stressful procedures? |
| | Do I reserve parenting activities (e.g., bathing) for parents? |
| | When I am helping a family care for their infant, do I help them understand how their child's behavior communicates how the baby is handling the experience, and help them use their child's behavior as their guide for pacing, positioning, and interacting with their baby? |
| | Do I explore every family's interest in skin-to-skin holding, and make myself available to support skin-to-skin holding according to the family's needs? |
| | Do I explore opportunities to include and support siblings? |
| | Do families see all infants consistently treated with the support and respect they would want for their own child when they are not around? |
| Standard 3: All caregivers practice collaboratively. | Do I stay at the bedside to support infants in my care through stressful procedures or examinations? |
| | If I need to perform an examination or procedure on an infant who is also in the care of another person at the bedside (e.g., nurse or parent), do I respectfully discuss the need with that person and agree on a time that is in the mutual interest of all? |
| | Do I talk with the other person about how to proceed and what the baby needs before we begin? |
| | Do I show flexibility whenever possible, by gently completing my own caregiving or assessments while the infant is available for another procedure, rather than disturbing the infant again later? |
| | Do I seek another person to support an infant in my care during a potentially stressful experience, including common things, such as bathing and weighing? |
| | Am I willingly available to my colleagues to provide support for infants in their care during potentially stressful procedures? |
| | Do I consistently share information about infants' behavioral competencies, vulnerabilities, and thresholds when communicating with colleagues during rounds or shift changes? |
| | Do I respect and support the roles of other individuals and disciplines in the lives of infants in my care? |
| Standard 4: A developmentally appropriate environment is provided for every infant and family. | Do I adequately support all infants with a consistently calm, relaxing environment, with muted sound and lighting between and during caregiving interactions? (Is this a baby's "home?") |
| | Do I consider all the sources of light, sound, movement, smell, and taste confronting an infant during care and eliminate all inappropriate or unnecessary sources of stimulation? |
| | Am I mindful of my own voice and other sounds I produce in the nursery? |
| | Do I silence alarms as soon as possible, and avoid unnecessary alarms? |
| | If I need to use an over-the-bed light for hands-on care, are the infant's eyes carefully shielded, yet not blindfolded, so I can respond and support the infant if he or she attempts to gaze at me? |
| | Do I provide infants with the bedding and other physical support they need to maintain optimal tone and position, and to remain either in a quiet, restful sleep, or a relaxed, comfortable wakefulness? |

Box 22-2   EVALUATING YOUR PRACTICE ACCORDING TO FOUR STANDARDS
          OF DEVELOPMENTAL CARE—CONT'D

> Am I continually mindful of structuring an infant's visual field to support alert wakefulness as appropriate (without overwhelming), transition to sleep, or quiet, restful sleep?
>
> Do I provide as much space and comfort as possible for family caregiving, keep charts and equipment neatly organized, and avoid clutter?
>
> Do I encourage families to personalize their child's bed space and explore with families ways to make the environment more homelike?
>
> Do I work to minimize moving babies to different bed spaces to accommodate staffing patterns?

From Robison, L.D. (2003). An organizational guide for an effective developmental program in the NICU. *Journal of Obstetric, Gynecologic, and Neonatal Nursing (JOGNN), 32*(3), 382-383.

One of the possible barriers or contributors to negative NICU cultures is the assumption that "it has always been this way." Or "we tried that before, and it did not work." This thinking leads to "trained incapacitation" or a failure of individuals to realize they hold the key to sustaining or changing the climate. When this happens, the members are now controlled by the climate, and the tendency to continue acting the same way is reinforced. The culture usually supports certain shared values and assumptions about how the unit/organization should function (Schein, 1997).

Creating a climate for change can start with examining the current forces in place that support the status quo or change. Climates are created by interactions/social exchanges within an environmental grouping. Changes in interactions or critical events can transform climates by changing social behaviors or setting new expectations. If a change is profound and sustained long enough, a resulting shift in the overall climate can take place (Folger, Poole, & Stutman, 1997). Change is also dependent on the leadership of the organization or unit (Scott, Mannion, Davies, et al., 2003; Robinson, 2003).

A constructive climate that prevents "defensive communication" can facilitate the change in philosophy that respects families by fostering a climate of respect among NICU leaders and staff. The following comparison of a defensive versus a supportive climate might be helpful in setting the stage for a collaborative workforce operating toward the same goals (Box 22-3).

Once the family-centered philosophy has been defined and the vision and purpose created for a particular unit, it is necessary to evaluate existing culture and practice to compare with the new guiding principles and to begin designing an individualized plan for change that will have the power and ability to be successful. Adopting this new philosophy and changing familiar patterns of practice requires careful consideration of the current:

- Leadership
- Culture
- Influence of NICU stressors
- Communication patterns
- Role of parents

## LEADERSHIP SUPPORT AND STYLE

Leadership is a complex social phenomenon. It is easily recognized, but difficult to define. There are almost as many different definitions of leadership as there are people who have tried to define it. Not all leadership theories are applicable to the labor-intensive, professional settings of health care. The ongoing changes that are occurring in the healthcare environment are creating the need for a multidimensional leadership model that incorporates rapidity of change and proactive attitudes as well as enhancing shared leadership and decision making autonomy.

Although there is no one "best" leadership theory, and healthcare providers should always maintain awareness of their own behavior and how the key elements of the leadership situation influence outcomes, there is one model of leadership that supports the reflective process needed for the implication of developmental care and family-centered care models. Transformational leadership is a leadership paradigm that provides a useful model for effective nursing leadership in today's healthcare setting (Robinson, 2003). It is not a set of management techniques but rather a relationship grounded in the leader's values that need to be aligned with the mission of the organization. Transformational leadership is fundamentally a process of motivating others to do more than they originally expected to do (Corrigan, Diwan, Campion, et al., 2002; Kurz & Haddock, 1989, Robinson, 2003). Three factors have been identified as necessary to be an effective transformational leader: charisma, intellectual stimulation, and individual consideration (McDaniel & Wolf, 1992, Robinson, 2003).

Charismatic leaders inspire followers to loyalty to a cause and are seen by followers as possessing qualities that evoke strong emotional reactions. These qualities include visionary abilities, courageousness, and performance abilities consistent with core set of values (McDaniel & Wolf, 1992; Kurz & Haddock, 1989).

The transformational leader provides intellectual stimulation by encouraging followers to be curious, try out new behaviors, or to seek new solutions to old problems (McDaniel & Wolf, 1992). Leaders and followers turn problems into opportunities and challenges. Leaders empower their staff to explore new methods of care, for example. This empowerment is one of the factors related to work environments that is considered to be positive in the face of increasing workforce shortages (Kuokkanen & Katajisto, 2003).

---

**Box 22-3   COMPARISON OF DEFENSIVE AND SUPPORTIVE CLIMATES**

| Defensive | Supportive |
|---|---|
| Staff expend energy protecting self | Accurate information to reinforce supportive behavior in others |
| Focus on defeating an opponent | Focus on achieving common goals; promotes active listening to other views |
| Controlling messages: "You have to do this," "Stop doing that" | Problem-oriented: Defining issues on which group can work toward solutions |
| Evaluative language: "You are positioning that baby wrong" | Descriptive language: "I see one of your baby's goals is directed toward facilitating midline skills. Let's try sidelying with supportive rolls and see how your baby tolerates it" |
| Strategic statements: Message has underlying motivations; tactic using sincere language to get staff to do what you want | Spontaneous: Sincere, open, honest communication; "what we see is what we get"; motivations do not change from day to day |
| Apathetic: Sends message that staff are not important | Empathetic: Acknowledge the legitimacy of the other's emotions and needs; does not suggest one always agree |
| Superiority: Use of power and authority to get own way | Common ground: Shared, problem-solving relationship with opportunity for expressing opinions |
| "Final" word: Others have little real influence over process, decisions, or outcome | Open: Willingness to hear ideas, change one's own position, encourage discussion and participation in decision-making |

Data from Folger, J.P., Poole, M.S., and Stutman, R.K. (1997). Climate and conflict interaction (pp. 178-180). In J.P. Folger, M.S. Poole, & R.K. Stutman (Eds.), *Working through conflict: Strategies for relationships, groups, and organizations* (3rd ed.). New York: Addison Wesley Longman.

Transformational leaders demonstrate to others their openness to self-assessment and willingness to adapt their thinking to new ideas (Kurz & Haddock, 1989). Leaders also help others to reach the "tipping point" towards acceptance of an idea (Gladwell, 2000; Kim & Mauborgne, 2003). The concept of the tipping point is to gain a majority support of an idea to the point of "tipping the balance" of maintaining the status quo.

The third factor necessary for transformational leadership is individual consideration. The transformational leader has concern for followers as individuals and demonstrates an understanding of specific situations of followers. They also attempt to develop followers through delegation, or mentoring. Transformational leaders are described as believers in people (McDaniel & Wolf, 1992; Robinson, 2003).

Because healthcare reform has created resource-constrained environments, nursing care delivery changes, work redesign, problems with patient/family satisfaction, cost-effectiveness issues, and the growing workforce shortage, the need for transformational leaders in nursing has never been so great as it is today. A new vision for health care is needed that will correspond with the strategies for change that are occurring and increase the successful implementation of that change. Talented leaders in nursing will grasp the significance of this reform movement and develop creative solutions to support the vision.

Neonatal intensive care units across the country are not immune to these healthcare changes and the need for new vision. In the face of increased acuity levels, and increased patient census, as well as changing staffing patterns, healthcare providers in NICUs are realizing the need to change the focus of infant care from survival to optimizing long-term health and development and developing a team approach that acknowledges and partners with families (Ohlinger, Brown, Laudert, et al., 2003). Family support goals are changing from crisis intervention, to relationship-based support, with the ultimate goal being to ensure that the family becomes the primary nurturers and advocates for their child. Therefore, the NICU climate needs to increase the competence and security of parents. Transformational leaders in NICUs must attempt and succeed in raising the awareness of colleagues and families of long-term consequence—develo family-centered care issues. Once the ne has been identified, the transformational lea develop ways to overcome the resistance to changes that will occur. The leader must consider the NICU philosophy of care and ask: Is it congruent with developmental care philosophy?

The only way to decide if developmental and family supportive principles guide practice is to take the time to examine current practice in one's own institution and compare those findings with the concepts reflective of family-centered and developmental care philosophy. The key elements of family-centered care are:

- Recognizing the family is the constant in the infant's life
- Facilitating family/professional collaboration is practiced at all levels to enhance
  - Care of the individual infant
  - Program development, implementation, and evaluation
  - Policy formation
- Honoring the racial, ethnic, cultural, and socioeconomic differences of families
- Emphasizing family strengths/individuality and respecting a variety of coping methods
- Sharing complete, consistent information with parents in a supportive manner
- Encouraging and facilitating family-to-family support and networking
- Incorporating developmentally supportive care for infants and their families
- Implementing comprehensive policies and programs that demonstrate commitment to families and include provision of emotional and financial support that meets their needs
- Creating health systems that are accessible by becoming more flexible, culturally competent, and responsive to family-identified needs (National Center for Family-Centered Care, 1990)

In addition to family-centered care principles, there are essential elements that are involved in the implementation of developmental care. These include an individualized, relationship-based approach to care: assessing the environment and intervening to protect the infant against stressors and increasing comfort-positive support for development; encouraging parents as partners in care; and promoting a team approach to care (Holditch-Davis, Blackburn, & VandenBerg, 2003; McGrath, 2003). These principles contrast sharply to the traditional model of NICU care in which the emphasis has been on staff as the experts in a highly-technologic setting that creates psychological and technical barriers that interfere with the developing bond between parent and child. The philosophy appears deceptively simple because the commitment to the principles might require a complete paradigm shift and thorough examination of beliefs, values, and motivations for the way practice is currently applied in the NICU as a system and as individual practitioners.

A checklist for family-centered care in neonatal and pediatric critical care units can be found in *Caring for Children and Families: Guidelines for Hospitals* (Johnson, Jeppson, & Redburn, 1992). Hospital administrators, medical and/or nursing management, staff, and families can use it to evaluate current policies, programs, and practices in the NICU. The move from system-centered care to family-centered care necessitates an evolutionary approach (Hanson, Johnson, & Jeppson, 1994) that:

- Empowers families
- Promotes independence
- Respects family choices
- Recognizes family strengths
- Supports family involvement in caregiving and decision-making
- Respects cultural differences
- Acknowledges the vital role of the family

The concepts invoke changing feelings of "this is nice, but we have patient care to perform, and a hospital to run." How do these lofty ideals become real and applied? The first task is to develop a multidisciplinary group that includes leadership (administrative, medical, and nursing), staff, family representatives and support staff. Family-centered and developmental care must be defined based on research, available literature, needs of patients and families and the community. Once the group is knowledgeable, a vision, mission, and philosophy statements can be agreed upon. These written statements then provide direction for the hospital, department, and staff to move forward with

program design, policy development, facility design change, or renovation, and bedside application. The importance of these written statements cannot be overemphasized because they will be used again and again to keep the focus and vision clear. A philosophy is not usually embraced overnight; therefore, it is best to be prepared for at least 3 to 5 years of reaching toward a vision and implementing small changes over time that are each steps to implementation of the bigger picture. It has been suggested that those who have patience, endurance, and persistence have the best chance of success for changing their philosophy of care as an organization and implementing IDFC successfully (McGrath, 2003; McGrath & Valenzuela, 1994).

An important role for NICU members of family-centered and developmental care committees is ensuring parents have a voice so that the group is not deciding "for" families what they want, but rather, listening to and working together with them. Therefore at least one parent must to be an active, visible member of this group. Parents must be acknowledged as the "expert" when it comes to the needs and characteristics of their infant. Creating a new role in the NICU that acknowledges the parent or family expertise in a paid full- or part-time position is another way of respecting and honoring their time, commitment, and participation.

## NICU CULTURE

When you reach down into the universe and pull something out, you find it is attached to everything else.

John Muir

A family-centered approach challenges old assumptions that healthcare providers should only focus on the treatment of disease and illness. The IDFC philosophy insists that we focus on the holistic perspective that includes the emotional, developmental, social, and economical pressures that impact wellness of the infant and family. In the NICU, this also encompasses important processes of attachment, as well as early emotional and social development of the newly emerging human beings in our midst. The greatest challenge might be in how healthcare providers perceive and deal with their own role, responsibilities, and behavioral changes necessary to reflect the new paradigm. Respecting families and believing they can have a pivotal role in care and decision-making demands a "leap of faith" from traditional system-centered "you're in our arena" mentality to an environment that partnerships with families in all aspects of care.

The NICU has been described (Savage & Conrad, 1992) as:

- Fast-paced
- Technical
- Competitive
- Elitist

It is a very stressful environment because of the pace; the critically ill, fragile patients; and the vast amount of expertise needed to function in the caregiving role. One of the greatest sources of satisfaction and stress to nursing staff can be the feeling of attachment and desire to protect their tiny patients. Staff have developed skills for coping with the particular stresses of their job, and it is no wonder that asking staff to develop a relationship with both an infant and a family constitutes a threat to their own well being. In some cases, distancing from families and babies has allowed the nurse to feel less vulnerable. Relationship-based care with infants and families opens up the possibility for emotionally painful experiences as well as rewarding ones. This can be very scary and stressful for some staff, especially those who are task-oriented and just want to get the tasks of caregiving done.

Traditionally, physicians, nurses, and therapists are considered the experts in the hospital setting and, as such, determine the amount, type, and timing of parent interaction with their infants. Giving up this old paradigm compels caregivers to rethink their comfortable focus of control and view the parents as partners and the "experts" concerning all issues related to their infants.

The NICU culture has placed value on:

- Conformity
- Mastery of technical skills
- Efficiency with tasks
- Control (by the health professionals not families)
- Rapid assimilation of data

This culture, in turn, might have influenced staff to develop attitudes and behaviors based on the old paradigm of thinking. In that environment, health professionals tend to promote themselves as providing caretaking—being the experts and in turn becoming indispensable. They feel compelled to problem-solve for parents instead of empowering them as partners in care. They have a need to exert control rather than relinquish power to parents. In the new paradigm, parents are partners, and control is shared in the NICU. But how does a unit move toward this paradigm shift?

Motivation for adopting new behaviors that are more supportive of infants and families involves acknowledging the staff's previously held values, beliefs, experiences, and needs (McGrath, 2003). It is more positive to create an atmosphere of acceptance in which everyone is learning developmental and family supportive theory and research-based techniques, while at the same time identifying current practice that already exemplifies these concepts. Saving face by acknowledging what is being done well might help to motivate the team to be productive rather than destructive.

The holistic approach to care is at the heart of nursing and has always been one of nursing's greatest gifts to health care. More often than not, the concepts of developmentally supportive care for infants and families are congruent with many nurses' beliefs, and other factors might have more impact on their actions and acceptance. Nurses might cite time as the primary culprit in delaying full implementation. This area will be more fully discussed under Influence of Stressors on the NICU. It is also important to acknowledge that a health professional's need to be acknowledged as the "expert" may be related to his or her own personal struggles with moving from "novice" to "expert" within the peer group or within the greater culture of the NICU. Issues related to the professional's sense of self and self-esteem also need to be considered.

Another cultural factor that can impact progress relates to the reward base in the NICU. Technologic skill and task performance have long been considered the measuring sticks of success in the NICU. Critical thinking is deemed important when centered on physiologic systems. Conformity and reward for skill mastery do not foster a culture accepting of more abstract concepts or relationship building. In this environment, risk taking and creativity might also have been stifled. Key players who hold positions of rank and respect within the NICU should be solicited for their support and participation (McGrath, 2003).

Personal, professional, and organizational change is integral to adopting IDFC successfully. The disruption that takes place during times of change, especially when personal behavior changes are involved, will take sensitive, anticipatory leadership and a clear vision and mission. It is essential that all levels of staff, from a variety of disciplines that practice in the NICU, be involved at the onset, from developing the vision to operationalizing the vision, implementation, and evaluation. As the desire to support infants and families in more meaningful ways spreads throughout the staff, the overall cultural climate of the NICU will follow.

## CONFLICT RESOLUTION STYLES AND AVENUES

Inevitable with any change, is disruption and conflict. Acceptance of change is rarely instantaneous and, generally, there is variability in rates and timing of acceptance. Once the changes are defined that will support developmental and family-centered care, reactions might vary and must be dealt with using positive techniques for diffusing and redirecting energies toward productive goals. Often the recommendation is that leaders should anticipate and plan conscious strategies for dealing with conflict. With this planning, carefully selected tactics would be pre-planned for a variety of situations. This advice, while appearing sensible, suggests the leader has the ability to predict situations in which the well-planned strategy works like a charm. Unfortunately, conflicts arise with two or more participants interacting in a variety of moves and interplays. It is difficult to remember, much less stick to planned conflict resolution tactics. Rather than trying to plan and predict, it is more useful to consider conflict and negotiation styles as a repertoire of options that can be learned and applied to various situations. People have characteristic ways of handling conflict that they tend to apply regardless of the situation. It is important to remember that conflict includes interaction and communication; therefore, really listening to and restating the issue to the person or group is an initial starting point for cooperation. It is often acceptable to ask the person initiating conflict for time to consider the issue they have brought up. Setting a meeting for later in the day or in a few days can allow for time to really consider the problem from several avenues and also provide the other player a little time to gain more control of their emotions.

Five conflict styles (Folger, Poole, & Stutman, 1997) have been identified and are classified as: Assertive behaviors, intended to satisfy one's own concerns; and cooperative behaviors, which satisfy the other individual's concerns. The five conflict styles have been useful for understanding conflict and are listed as:

- Competing: Highly assertive and low in cooperation; great emphasis on individual's own concerns and ignores those of others; there is a desire to defeat the opponent; sometimes called the forcing or dominant style
- Accomodating: Unassertive and cooperative; giving in at the cost of one's own concerns or beliefs; appeasement or soothing; viewed as self-sacrificing and weak
- Avoiding: Unassertive and uncooperative; person withdraws or simply refuses to deal with conflict; person is indifferent to the outcome and might be viewed as apathetic, isolated or evasive; flight instead of fight
- Collaborating: High in both assertiveness and cooperation; seeks solutions that meet the needs of both parties; win-win is sought for outcome; also called *problem-solving style*
- Compromising: Intermediate level of both assertiveness and cooperativeness; both sides give up something to come to agreement; also called *sharing* or *horse trading*

Unfortunately, in the context of the NICU, individual and group styles might be a combination of styles. In any conflict situation, the dynamic nature of the interaction makes it impossible to predict and plan the perfect strategy.

It is impossible to discuss all the possible strategies for dealing with conflict, but a few are worthy of mention such as those in Box 22-4.

The use of conflict styles and tactics to set the stage for integrating change into practice is not

Box 22-4   STRATEGIES FOR DEALING WITH CONFLICT

| Steps in Conflict Resolution | Strategy |
| --- | --- |
| Issue definition | Two-column method: List the pros and cons of an issue, or compare parties' perception of the issue. |
| Conflict process reflection | Meta-communication: Discuss communication patterns with the goal of improving the communication process. |
| Integrative tactics | 1. Propose solution or goals: Identify a common goal or end that both parties agree and can work toward; both sides should value the goal.<br>2. Acknowledge legitimacy of other party's position: Other sides legitimate interests are taken into account, although not always mutually agreed upon.<br>3. Joint fact-finding: Both parties investigate the issues together in an attempt to find evidence base for agreement.<br>4. Single text method: Parties work on a written draft of an agreement and pass back and forth revising until agreement. |
| Change forum | Third party: Parties agree to call in a third party (mediator/facilitator) to help work on conflict resolution. |

simply a matter of which one to choose. The other parties' reactions might cause the tactic to backfire. Use of more productive, problem-solving tactics geared to solicit cooperation and assertiveness seem to be more effective in gaining support and participation from staff involved in dynamic change processes.

## REFLECTIVE PROCESS FOR CONSULTATION

Training staff in a family-centered approach to delivering care can stir emotional responses, challenge personal beliefs and values, and require them to develop or use skills not previously rewarded in the current NICU culture. Training in the traditional sense might only plant ideas, but what actually happens is dependent on many factors. Reflective process is one method leaders can use to nurture staff toward new ways of thinking and provide consistent support over time to help them in the process of integrating developmental and family-centered principles into daily practice with infants and their families. It assumes a long-term commitment to staff to "see them through" a process of change rather than thinking that training programs or a few workshops will provide enough impetus to "get the ball rolling." Key elements of the model are:

- Commitment to security and trust among staff
- Consistent time to meet in safe place for open discussion
- Support for activities that allow reflection on the work at all levels of the organization.

Key elements are needed for effective implementation of the reflective model. The core perspectives serve as the guiding principles with which interactions, relationships, and practice are compared. Three phases of the model (Figure 22-1) depict the progress from development to integration of change. The phases are cyclical, with professionals and organizations moving forward from one to the next phase and then back again in a continuum of growth, development, and integration of new principles into applied practice with infants and families.

The establishment of values, roles, and responsibilities in a setting conducive to trust and security characterizes the *Discovery Phase*. The *Engagement Phase* encourages interaction among staff and discussion of issues that arise when working with families, and facilitates deeper understanding of the principles embraced in the organization. There is a structured format for discussion, and the team is provided regular meeting times with opportunities for individual and group reflection. Experience-based case discussion is one

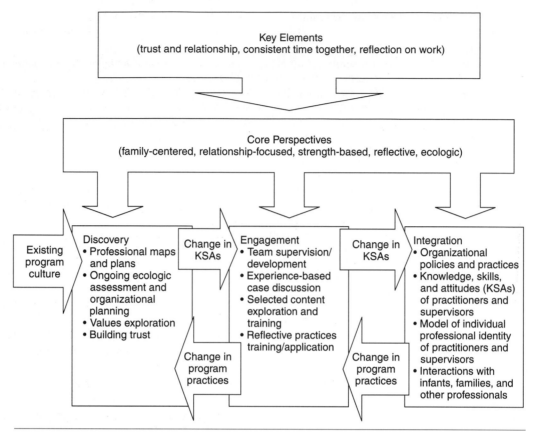

Figure 22-1 A reflective practice model for professional and organizational change. (*Adapted from Copa, A., Lucinski, L., Olsen, E., & Wollenburg, K. (1999). Promoting professional and organizational development: A reflective practice model. Zero to Three, 20[1], 3-9.*)

of the tools used in which staff present individual cases for the purpose of:

- Understanding relationships, clarifying perceptions, acknowledging feelings, asking for group feedback/interpretation
- Gaining deeper understanding from the perspectives of others by exploring and sharing collective experiences with the group
- Summarizing discussion, identifying learning opportunities, and generalizing experience for deeper understanding of the complex relational issues that come up when working with infants and families
- Identifying further education needs of group

The final phase of *Integration* is one that fosters individual growth and change through strong organizational support, program resources and supportive policies (see Figure 22-1).

## ADULT MENTAL-HEALTH PROFESSIONALS FOR STAFF SUPPORT

Not only will staff need support with applying new or different knowledge and skills but attitude adjustments can be challenging to achieve, especially when core values might be challenged or coping styles threatened. Distancing from patients and families can be a coping mechanism for avoiding emotional pain for many staff members. Leaders in the NICU might be ill-equipped to provide the high-level of emotional support that will also be needed when devotion to tasks must become a commitment to people and relationships. Relationships with infants, families, other disciplines, and peers can be rewarding, but until the Knowledge, Skills, and Attitudes (KSA) are balanced, the existing pressures can initially outweigh the compensation or benefits. In addition, nursing staff might have inadequate knowledge and skills related to therapeutic relationships in the context of the NICU. Although they should have the training in their background, they might not have had the opportunities to keep those skills current. Contracting with a mental-health professional for supportive staff sessions might be an option to explore. Sessions for staff could include education, open discussion, and stress management. Some potential topics include:

- Recognizing and reacting appropriately to parent emotional states
- Separating personal needs from the infant's and family's needs
- Ethnic and cultural awareness
- Self-awareness
- Communication techniques with families in and out of crises
- Managing conflict with families and other health-care workers
- Negotiation skills
- Exercise, relaxation, imagery techniques
- Coping with change
- Assertiveness
- Facilitation of infant-family attachment

These are but a few of the kinds of educational sessions that staff might find beneficial as they practice family-centered care. Twenty- or thirty-minute sessions with fun titles such as "Assumption Junction, Not our Function" can minimize negative feelings toward sensitive topics such as making assumptions and jumping to conclusions when families do not call or visit. Anticipatory planning with the use of mental-health professionals during the process of change might also minimize the cost of burnout and turnover.

## INFLUENCE OF STRESSORS ON THE NICU

There are many other factors that influence the implementation of developmentally supportive, family-centered care. Stressors that affect progress and morale of staff include:

- Changes in management policy
  - Increased productivity with few human and material resources
  - Decreased educational hours for staff and managers
  - Reduced orientation hours for new staff
- Staff changes through reduction and reorganization
  - Reduction in number of staff through attrition, layoffs, and reassignment
  - Loss of morale; burnout
- Staff-infant ratios
  - More infants cared for by fewer staff (or it might be a staff mix of professionals with unlicensed personnel)
  - Decreased time for family-centered and developmental-care application
  - Use of patient care assistants for direct care of infants
  - Increased tension and decreased staff satisfaction
- Patient acuity
  - Acuity systems do not account for time to support individual infants and families
  - Task-based systems
  - Trend toward higher acuity levels
- Census patterns
  - Staffing for shifts in census might not capture high census periods
  - Tendency to rotate staff, decreasing continuity for infants and families
  - Use of agency or float personnel unfamiliar with family-centered practice of the institution
- Geography or layout of unit
  - Support of families limited due to unit design that allows lack of privacy, crowding, and large, mammoth units with open layouts
  - Disruption during renovation

Constructive discussions concerning these and other issues influencing the progress of developmentally supportive, family-centered care should take place so that solutions can be generated to address the barriers. Ongoing identification of the stressors that influence care practices is a continuum that can frustrate the most avid advocate for family-centered care. Again, keeping the team working on creative solutions with leadership hearing and responding to valid concerns can maintain focus on the original vision. Looking at issues in light of the "written" vision and mission can help leaders and staff get back on track. It is also acceptable and has been recommended by some that taking a "time out" might help lower tension and give time to recoup energy to continue the struggle.

Acuity systems should be examined and changed to meet the new philosophy expectations. Redesigned acuity systems (Malloch, Neeld, McMurry, et al., 1999) capture family-centered care and developmental planning, education, and interventions as well as adequately estimating clinical needs. One acuity system developed to encompass family-centered principles in the adult setting include domains such as (1) emotional/social/spiritual well-being, (2) family information needs/support status, (3) treatments and interventions, (4) interdisciplinary coordination, (5) clinical condition, and (6) transitions such as readiness of the family to assume responsibility for care (Malloch, Neeld, McMurry, et al., 1999). Domains with descriptors use a rating scale to rate the patient. The system is fully automated for ease of use. There is need for systems-based, automated evaluations that use real information on infant/family holistic needs versus task-based acuity ratings that have been tested for reliability and validity to support the work at the bedside and improve staffing ratios based on individual patient requirements.

Reorganization or redesign often takes the same approach to downsizing both management and staff. Less-skilled workers are frequently added to provide "support" for the more skilled registered nurse (RN) to focus on the patient. The flaw in such thinking is that work processes might stay the same, so that teams are left with more work and fewer people.

Work redesign efforts should be carefully reviewed in light of the scant research to support the changes. Some reports are showing that massive hospital work redesigns are not achieving the desired outcomes (Seago, 1999, 2000, 2002). One medical center reported adopting a patient-focused care model. The nursing care delivery system changed in composition of skill mix by adding patient-care assistants, with RNs managing the team and coordinating all activities of the team. There was no indication that patients received continuity of care teams. The organization's desired outcomes of: (1) improved patient satisfaction and outcomes; (2) improved worker job satisfaction; and (3) increased efficiency and decreased costs through redesigning nursing care delivery, were not realized. Unfortunately, outcomes such as pressure ulcers, falls, and medication errors required an incident report to be included in the measurement (Seago, 1999, 2000, 2002).

Another study (Blegen & Vaughn, 1998) sampling 42 nursing care units found that the proportion of hours of care delivered by RN staff was inversely related to three adverse patient outcomes: (1) medication errors, (2) increased decubiti rates, and (3) complaints by patients or families. Although not significant, trends in data suggested that urinary and respiratory infections obtained from chart review and deaths by morgue report showed an inverse relationship with care by RN staff. These findings suggest that as the hours of RN care increased, adverse patient outcomes decreased.

Other findings are consistent with these reports. Aiken et al. (Aiken, Clarke, Sloane, et al., 2002; Aiken, Clarke, & Sloane, 2001; Aiken, Smith, & Lake, 1994), for almost a decade, have followed patient morbidity and mortality rates in relationship to RN staffing. These studies have supported that mortality rates were significantly lower in hospitals with the highest RN ratios compared with hospitals that had higher licensed practical nurses (LPNs) and unlicensed personnel. In another study (Hartz, Krakauer, Kuhn, et al., 1989), fewer hospital deaths were found in hospitals that had higher RN-to-patient ratios compared with hospitals with lower nurse-to-patient ratios. Moore, Lynn, McMillen, et al. (1999) applied the quality indicators from the American Nursing Association's report card to a convenience sample of 16 medical-surgical units and more than 1500 patients and 300 nurse participants during an 18-month period. They found that the higher percentage of RNs caring for patients was a significant positive indicator of patient satisfaction.

The studies cited indicate that the current trend to reduce RN staff to cut costs might look for the financial "bottom line," but evidence is accumulating that this short-term strategy is not good for patients. Further research is needed to guide nursing leaders in making decisions on nursing-care delivery models. Until then, caution must be exercised when altering skill mix and raising staff-infant ratios. For any change, careful outcome selection, including clinical and financial outcomes, as well as, staff and family satisfaction scores, must be measured. It is a risky trend to trim workforce without the evidence-base to show no harm.

Other changes make sense, such as:

- Increased continuity of care for infants and families (McGrath, 2003; Petryshen, Stevens, Hawkins, et al., 1997)
  - Efficiency of care and coordination
  - Knowledge of infant/family
  - Early identification of problems
- Advanced training for high-level assessment skills and professional development of staff
- Smaller work teams that function for defined periods to enhance collaboration and development of trust and rapport among disciplines
- Nurse liaisons with families to coordinate teaching, information sharing, and continuity
- Critical paths that have specific goals and timelines to support infant/family progress toward discharge
- Regular "town hall" meetings to address staff concerns
- Leadership journal/discussion club to maintain current knowledge and facilitate new skills
- Responsibility and accountability workshops for professional development
- Strong nurse leaders advocating for what is "right" in patient-care staffing ratios and reducing costs of other inefficient processes

There is evidence that individualized developmental care achieves the desired medical, neurobehavioral, cost, and consumer satisfaction outcomes (Als, Lawhon, Duffy, et al., 1994; Fleisher, VandenBerg, Constantinou, et al., 1995; Buehler, Als, Duffy, et al., 1995; Petryshen, Stevens, Hawkins, et al., 1997; Als, 1999; Als & Gilkerson, 1997). To achieve outcomes reported, administrators and NICU leadership must be ready to make the commitment necessary for replicating those outcomes.

## COMMUNICATION PATTERNS

During the last decade, we have begun to realize that the transition to extrauterine life is not without great consequence to premature (and especially very premature) infants. Our challenge as neonatal nurses, as well as other healthcare providers in NICUs, still remains in optimizing the long-term developmental outcomes of these vulnerable infants. The major change that needs to occur during the next decade of care in NICUs will be the move from protocol and procedure-based care to individualized relationship-based developmental care. Quality research documenting the efficacy of developmental and relationship based care is growing. This growing body of research will continue to strengthen the need for accountability of healthcare providers for creating an environment that will support the developmental and emotional well being of vulnerable infants, families, and staff, and not merely meet physiologic needs. As research continues to demonstrate positive short- and long-term outcomes, developmental and relationship-based care should become the standard of practice for all NICUs.

As this shift in practice occurs, quality education programs must also be developed to provide staff with the tools necessary to make appropriate changes in care. Implications for caregiving that could require a change in practice include:

- Precepted clinical training in NICUs, an advanced practice setting for clinicians wanting to develop and refine developmental skills
- Restricted practice for new graduates, generalists, and aids until concepts of developmental and relationship-based care are acquired
- Physiologic and behavioral monitoring before and after handling to establish baselines, acknowledging the individual needs of the infant and recognizing the caregiving styles utilized
- Systematic documentation of physiologic and behavioral effects and modification of care
- Use of a developmental specialists and external consultation as necessary.

All of these changes in practice require changes in the educational process for healthcare providers as well as students choosing to work in NICUs.

Another challenge facing neonatal nurses is the need to support parents of infants in NICUs as the primary advocates and long-term caregivers. Encouraging parents to develop mutual interactive communication with their infant can meet this goal. Another method to acknowledge the role of parents in NICUs is by incorporating families into the decision-making councils and advisory boards of NICUs as developmental care practices are developed. Developmentally supportive care will create a professional alliance that will support the parents' engrossment with their child and the child's neurobiologically based expectations for the nurturance from the family. This alliance listens to the language of the infant's behavior, and uses the dialogue between the infant, family, and caregiver to guide care (Als & Gilkerson, 1997).

## ROLE OF PARENTS IN THE NICU

The parents' presence in the NICU is the most important factor in developing the infant/parent relationship necessary for optimal outcomes during the hospitalization and after discharge from intensive care. They are the constant that will be there when we no longer play a role in their lives. This role must begin immediately with parents as primary nurturers and caregivers at every opportunity. Words or phrases to eliminate from NICU vocabulary include "allowing visitation" and "permission to touch." Expressions such as these imply staff ownership of infants, denying parent's this exclusive relationship with their baby. Language, signs, lack of privacy, and medical/nursing competence separate infants from their parents in a multitude of ways. All of these barriers send a distinct message that parents are not welcomed in the primary role of nurturer and decision-maker until it is time for their infant to go home. In an environment in which IFDC has not been implemented, parents might be required to ask permission to care for their own infant. Then they are required to be available for education, caregiving, and meet physician, staff, and therapist's expectations before discharge. Convenience for the parent might not be considered in scheduling meetings or education.

Family-centered care principles necessitate a change in mindset to incorporate the essential principles espoused in the concept. Parents must have a role in defining the application of the principles in the real world of the NICU and the entire organization.

The five guiding principles (Hanson, Johnson, Jeppson, et al., 1994) are:
- Respect: Choices of families are honored in the belief that they, too, want what is best for their infant
- Information sharing: Complete, accurate information is given to families in a supportive way with respect for individual learning styles

- Collaboration: Both families and professionals have expertise that can be combined to optimize the infant's care; staff have medical and technical expertise, whereas families are the best caregivers and nurturers for their infant
- Family-to-family support: Families in similar situations can be supportive to each other through strength, comfort, friendship, and sharing coping strategies for difficult times
- Confidence building: Occurs through opportunity to care and nurture their infant supported by staff as they become more and more autonomous

In the past, hospital systems have based practices, programs, and policies on the needs and priorities of the system. The work environment and care practices have been created for the convenience of the caregivers rather than the patient and family. Other more patient-centered systems focus on the infant's needs without considering the impact on the family, such as scheduling care routines and medications for the middle of the night prior to discharge. Still others might see the family as needing intervention and refer them to social services or counseling without discussing with or asking the family about their own perception.

With true family-centered care, caregivers seek to understand the families' needs and priorities by asking families what their perspectives are and then attempting to incorporate the families' perspectives in the model of care.

Some examples of family-centered care include (Hanson, Johnson, Jeppson, et al., 1994; Institute for Family-Centered Care, 1994):
- Involvement in developing programs and policies
- Availability of family advisory councils
- Access to information (i.e., patient medical record, communication board/book)
- Open 24-hour welcome on units, including critical care
- Family participation in medical/nursing rounds
- Participation in renovation or design of unit/ hospital
- Family-to-family networking opportunities
- Sibling support
- Exit interviews, surveys, questionnaires
- Suggestion book or "drop box" in waiting area
- Follow-up phone calls
- Family and staff focus groups
- Family panels for in-services

There are many ways for families to become involved. Our job is to broaden our minds to envision expanded opportunities for staff and families to collaborate and build the NICU into a value-driven culture, based on mutual respect and partnership. Listening to families and hearing what they say is integral to the process of building the respect and trust necessary for nurturing family-centered care in the NICU. The parent's role in the NICU is only limited by our ability to "let go" of our need to control and visualize the possibilities. Awareness and knowledge about the need for change is all well and good, but how do we actually implement a change?

## IMPLEMENTATION OF CHANGE

Change is never easy, but it can be accomplished. The implementation of developmental care is an example of a change that is generally supported in theory, but sometimes, due to organizational or unit factors, difficult to achieve, as the previous sections of this chapter have described. This section presents one way developmental care was successfully implemented and strategies that anyone can use to change practice.

## INDIVIDUALIZED FAMILY-CENTERED DEVELOPMENTALLY SUPPORTIVE CARE

Individualized family-centered, developmentally supportive care has emerged as a new paradigm for delivering newborn intensive care. The goal of care is not just survival of high-risk infants, but emphasis is placed on optimal neurodevelopmental outcomes and parenting. During the past 20 years, support for developmental care has gained acceptance and is practiced in one form or another in many NICUs in the United States and globally. The rationale for the Newborn Individualized Developmental Care Assessment Program (NIDCAP®) (Boston, MA) relationship-based paradigm continues to advance through research, standards, and guidelines published by national medical and nursing organizations (Als, Lawhon, Brown, et al., 1986; Als, Lawhon, Duffy, et al., 1994; American Academy of Pediatrics (AAP), 2000; Fleisher, VandenBerg, Constantinou, et al., 1995; Buehler, Als, Duffy, et al., 1995; Westrup, Kleberg, von Eichwald, et al., 2000; National Association of Neonatal Nurses [NANN], 1998, 2000).

Cognitive acceptance of the mortality and logic of this philosophy of care has been easier to gain than actual implementation in the NICU setting (Browne & Smith-Sharp, 1995). Although neonatal nurses have the most opportunity to build relationships with families and apply developmental care principles in practice, an effective program depends on consistent support and effort at all levels of leadership and staff. Browne and Smith-Sharp's (1995) description of the maturational stages toward a developmental nursery (Box 22-5) is useful in understanding where one's own institution might be "stuck" and unable to progress. If developmental care initiatives seem "stuck" in a particular stage of development, it is time to step back and thoughtfully reflect on the implementation process and new ways to move forward and continue to foster a continuum of growth, development, and integration of IFDC, not just in applied practice, but as a philosophic paradigm of NICU care (Browne & Smith-Sharp, 1995). In contrast, Box 22-2 provides a way for individuals to examine and reflect on their own feelings and practices in relationship to IFDC and can provide a basis for individual as well as institutional change (Robison, 2003).

Changing unit philosophy and practice patterns is a dynamic progression that is continually influenced by unit culture. Sustainable change requires attention to both leadership and process. Aspects related to these influencing factors are presented with the understanding that each institution must examine the status of its own IFDC program to identify and overcome obstacles affecting progress.

## EFFECTS OF ORGANIZATION AND/OR UNIT CULTURE

When implementing developmental care, the culture at the unit level must be considered. Unit culture describes the behaviors and responses of the group or individuals within a sector of the organization, in this case, the NICU. The culture allows the members to understand the general direction of the group, what it means to be part of the group, acceptable and unacceptable behavior, how others are likely to react, and other information that guides behavior and

Box 22-5    SIX STAGES OF ACHIEVEMENT TOWARD A DEVELOPMENTAL NURSERY

1. Awareness: Exposed to concept; excited; can see potential impact; expect quick change; inconsistent information and practice leads to frustration and turmoil.
2. Disruption: Staff resistance and apathy from previous frustration; decreased willingness to change practice; some staff might sabotage other staff's developmentally supportive efforts.
3. Organization: Orderly approach to implementation begins; might seek consultative services, attend developmental conferences, visit or contact "developmental" nurseries; formal education is planned.
4. Identity: Policy and procedure development and implementation; might observe a "prescriptive" or procedural approach as in all infants nested without consideration of age or competency; intervention-driven with incomplete understanding of relationship between infant/family behaviors and individualized responsiveness.
5. Integration: Staff recognize areas of refinement but need assistance in moving forward; cognitive acceptance of infant individuality and parent involvement, but unable to see infants as collaborators in their own care and parents as equals; expert consultation and leadership needed to advance.
6. Generation: IFDC is operational and observable in the NICU; the five standards of IFDC are shown at all levels of leadership and staff; IFDC is the "norm" (philosophy) not the option; staff create new approaches to novel situations (no longer rigid or protocol driven); continued growth through reflective processing, evaluation, ongoing education, and strong, effective visionary leadership.

Adapted from Turnage, C.C. (2002). Individualized family-centered developmental care: Reflections on implementation. *Newborn and Infant Nursing Reviews, 2*(1), 28.
*IFDC,* Individualized, family-centered, developmental care; *NICU,* neonatal intensive care unit.

relationships within the group (Folger, Poole, & Stutman, 1997). There are values and beliefs that are held just as in any culture that provides boundaries for behavior.

Unit culture is continually reinforced through persistent patterns of interactions that become entrenched the longer the same patterns endure. This changes, however, as unit leadership changes, if patterns of communication change. Cultural barriers to the implementation or change toward IFDC typically include:

- Rigid power structure
- Unequal distribution of power, influence, and respect among members
- Degree of mistrust
- Decreased autonomy of staff
- Low accountability
- Minimal collaboration
- Lack of ownership for problems or accomplishments

The rate of diffusion and acceptance of IFDC is related to the unit culture that already exists. If the norm is to uphold tradition, it will be difficult to change to developmental care. If blame is placed on the early adopters or intrapreneurs (change agents from within an organization) who want to affect a change, it is not likely that a new mode of care will be adopted. If, however, the norm is to try new perspectives and to look at evidence to support practice changes, developmental care might be easily accepted. The acceptance, however, must have administrative *and* staff support; one without the other will not allow a new idea to flourish.

## DEFINING THE NEW CULTURE

Creating cultural change starts with examining the forces in place that explain the existing environment. Cultural change can begin with changes in interactions and interaction patterns. Critical events, such as "enlightenment through sharing developmental research," can start the transformation by setting new expectations for behavior and practice. It is important to note that a critical event such as massive education will probably not result in permanent change.

The NICU has been described as a "subculture of solidarity" and "decision-making by consensus," an environment that does not support testing of newly acquired knowledge by individual nurses (Spence, Greenwood, McDonald, et al., 1999). A small study of four nurses after a distance education course showed significant acquisition of knowledge and the ability to articulate rationale for nursing interventions. Barriers to application of the theoretic knowledge identified by the nurses included established practices, ritualistic nursing behavior, and resistance to change by some staff who made it difficult for them to implement changes in their care.

Only if the change is profound and sustained long enough will a shift in culture take place (Folger, Poole, Stotman, 1997). Efforts must also take into account any potential negative recollections encountered with previous change projects in the organization. It is probably best to acknowledge prior mistakes and focus on ways to avoid similar outcomes (Ingersoll, Kirsch, Merk, et al., 2000). This process is similar to what most of us do these days for root cause analysis or critical incident reporting. It is important when a root cause analysis is undertaken that it is done without prejudice, without seeking a victim, but rather, focusing on how to learn from the error or problem.

Developing an IFDC council with representation from medicine and nursing leadership, managers, staff, parents, and other disciplines involved in the NICU is instrumental in promoting collaboration and defining the new IFDC cultural expectations or standards. Defining the IFDC standards means setting the expectations for interactions, behaviors, and practice within the new culture. An experienced committee chairperson is valuable in facilitating cooperation, implementing respectful discussion of issues, maintaining appropriate ground rules, and keeping the group focused and respectful. If it seems that the word *respectful* is used a lot, it is, because the only successful way to make a transition to a new approach to practice/care is to have an atmosphere in which questions and concerns can be discussed in an open, above-board manner. If there is a lack of trust or a belief that there is a hidden agenda, then the new approach will most likely be sabotaged.

The first step toward congruence among leaders and staff is defining IFDC as nursery standards that are clearly stated and can be operationalized into everyday practice at every level. If the vision of IFDC is not clearly defined and operationalized, NICU practice reflects the individual philosophy or mood of the caregiver at the bedside (Robison,

2000) or quickly reverts to the old tradition with the onset of any routine NICU stressor. The synactive theory and neonatal individualized care and assessment program (Als, 1982, 1986, 1999; Copa, Lucinski, Olsen, et al., 1999; McGrath, 2000) has been extensively studied and constitutes the model of care many NICUs have adopted for their practice paradigm.

Nursery standards based on the IFDC model highlight key principles that guide practice and serve as a tool for examining whether current practices mirror those principles. These standards are derived from developmental theory, research, published guidelines, and standards for IFDC. Robison (2000) recommends standards that include the following:

1. Individualized, flexible, hands-on care is based on and responsive to each infant's competencies, vulnerabilities, and thresholds.
2. Appropriate developmental environment is provided for each infant.
3. Parent-infant relationships are encouraged and actively supported from birth.
4. Parents are recognized as the rightful owner of their infant with associated privileges, including accurate knowledge concerning their infant and involvement in planning and providing care.
5. A consistent team of caregivers practices collaborative interdisciplinary care.

These principles suggest that prescribed protocols or maps, unless used as a reference or guide, are not advised. The rationale is that each infant and family is an individual unit with unique needs. Although this is good in theory, what happens with the movement toward use of electronic medical records and standardization of language? Are the two diametrically opposed—protocols-standard language, and IFDC? They are not, necessarily, if the staff works collaboratively with parents as partners to individualize the plan of care and identify the measurable outcomes. Another important function of the use of standards or guidelines is that they serve as a way to operationalize IFDC and sustain its adoption. If there is no means of measuring success, there is no way to sustain a change in practice. These standards clearly define the "new" culture of care.

## LEADERSHIP

Confusion over the roles and accountabilities leaders must assume for an effective developmental program can seriously impede progress and send staff a message that leadership is not committed to IFDC. Clarity of role definition and responsibilities can help leadership become better effective-change agents.

Robison (2000) identifies a continuum of leadership defined as those leaders with influence, authority, and power. The influential leaders are most often the visionaries who are educated and/or experienced in IFDC and understand the principles, practice, and potential impact for NICU patients, families, and staff. Examples of this type of leader should include developmental therapists, clinical nurse specialists, unit educators, and parents. Influential leaders are accountable for providing developmental education for both leaders and staff, participating in program development, providing individualized developmental assessments and care plans for high-risk infants, and supporting family and staff in implementing IFDC. These leaders may or may not be a part of the particular NICU environment; they may be researchers, educators, or consultants.

Leaders with authority are the managers and administrators who control resources and evaluate staff performance in maintaining professional competencies and practice standards (Robison, 2000). Leaders in positions of authority are accountable for participating and supporting the process of defining IFDC standards for their units, supporting staff development and ongoing education in IFDC principles and application, holding staff accountable to defined IFDC nursery standards through performance evaluations, and appropriating financial and other resources needed to support IFDC, such as developmental specialist roles, reasonable staffing patterns and skill mix, nursery environment renovation or modification, and supplies (Robison, 2000). A 5-year strategic plan that delineates the time commitment, human and material resources, and budget necessary to support any IFDC initiative is key to successful integration. This plan must include ongoing educational training for staff who work in any aspect of the NICU. The projections are valuable to leaders who must plan ahead to provide the needed resources or to generate dollars to support

new initiatives. All leaders must agree on the terms and commitment delineated in the written implementation plan. Plans must be revisited regularly, as they might change, depending on forces that facilitate or impede the IFDC initiative. For example, today it is very common that a corporate merger might force healthcare delivery systems to integrate. If there is not a written implementation plan that is part of an overall strategic initiative of the organization, this "plan" might get lost in the merger. It might anyway, but a written plan has a better chance of sustaining a corporate change than does a verbal agreement.

Usually the most powerful leaders are the physicians or nurse practitioners who direct the medical plan for individual infants and their families and impact the application of new ideas or caregiving practices (Robison, 2000). Accountability for this group includes acquiring a knowledge base that includes both medical and developmental implications for NICU patients and their families. This must include both short- and long-term outcomes. Collaborating with other staff to incorporate medical care and having defined standards of care, providing visible and consistent support of the program, rewarding staff for implementation efforts, and participating in developing, implementing, and ongoing evaluating of the program are other aspects that must be included in this practice change.

Problems occur most often when leaders with influence meet with a lack of support or outright resistance from leaders with authority and/or power. These leaders with authority may be informal leaders or legitimate leaders. Either barrier can have the same impact on IFDC programs by delaying or halting progress. Managers might not allocate proper resources, such as money for education, staffing patterns, or supportive roles. They might not actively hold nursing staff accountable to IFDC standards, thereby making developmental care an individual caregiver option. Physicians might find it difficult to integrate developmental care within the context of the medical model. They might believe the research is "soft" because behavioral studies do not lend themselves to the rigorous study designs of pharmaceuticals with placebos and blinding to treatment groups. Those with influence might not seek expert consultation as needed or ask leaders with authority and power for resources and support in concrete terms. Education, clearly defined program goals, leadership roles and accountabilities, a written plan for implementation, financial and human resources required, and planned ongoing communication among the leadership and staff representatives with time for reflection and evaluation are important to avoid conflict and facilitate collaboration among IFDC leadership. This does not mean everyone agrees with everyone else all the time. It does mean that important IFDC principles have been agreed on and will be supported by all leadership.

## PROCESS FOR CHANGE

Many developmental specialists or program coordinators recommend that developmental leaders use a reflective process to nurture and support organizations and individuals toward new ways of thinking and acting within a developmental perspective (Copa, Lucinski, Olsen, et al., 1999; Gilkerson & Als, 1995; McGrath, 2000). All levels from leadership to staff can use this process. IFDC philosophy can arouse emotional responses, challenge the beliefs and long-held values of leadership and staff, and require the development of skills that might not have been rewarded in the past. Traditional training with workshops and seminars provides information about IFDC, but what is transferred to the unit and bedside is dependent on many factors. Reflective process is a method leaders can use to nurture and provide consistent support to help staff integrate developmental and family-centered principles into daily practice.

Reflective process in practice is a very different mindset than that of the traditional, fast-paced, action-oriented NICU caregiver. It represents a direct approach to each experience in which one lives in the present and is mindful and attuned to each experience (Gilkerson & Als, 1995; Horns, 1998; Tremmel, 1993). Really being in the present without thoughts of "what I have to do next" allows the caregiver to truly experience the interaction with an infant and family, thoughtfully responding in the moment to the infant and family's ongoing responses as they happen. It means paying attention not only to the experience but also to what the individual thinks and feels during the interaction. For the person or leader that is not attuned to feelings and acts from concrete facts or observations, this point of view or philosophy is difficult to embrace. However, when this philosophy is used, from these thoughtful experiences, knowledge with insight allows individual and group growth and development toward a real change in philosophy. This cannot be taught in a workshop or seminar and might be one of the reasons developmental care seems difficult to implement. Leadership can use reflection to review progress, gain insight, discuss issues, and identify areas of improvement and leadership support. Leaders can also nurture staff toward IFDC standards of practice with specific tools that facilitate reflective process and lead to higher levels of understanding and assimilation of IFDC.

Effective implementation of the reflective model for change include three key elements (Copa, Lucinski, Olsen, et al., 1999): commitment to security and trust among staff and/or leaders; consistent time to meet where open discussion is safe; and activities that allow reflection on work toward IFDC at all unit levels. A forum for working through those issues in a safe, open discussion will help identify barriers and solutions. This forum can serve as a SWOT analysis (strengths, weaknesses, opportunities, and threats analysis) to the actual implementation of IFDC. Leaders and/or staff will meet depending on the "work" or issues on the table. The atmosphere must be one of problem solving, with solutions being directed away from why the change cannot work.

The IFDC standards serve as the guiding principles by which interactions, relationships, and practice are compared. The model marks movement through three stages progressing from (1) exploration or conceptualization of the new paradigm, to (2) mindful practice of IFDC principles, and finally to (3) assimilation of the standards of IFDC as it is applied to NICU practice. Exploration is described as the establishment of values, roles, and responsibilities. It is especially important if leadership and/or staff have widely disparate views concerning IFDC principles. This stage is when IFDC standards for the NICU are agreed upon and accountabilities for their implementation clearly stated. Timelines, with actions, and the parties responsible help to keep the process moving forward toward a positive implementation of IFDC.

Mindful practice supports active interaction among the team members through discussion of issues that arise when IFDC principles are applied to practice with the infants and their families. Technology and tasks can become a safe haven that is concrete and operational, whereas IFDC might seem more abstract for many professionals. Knowledge alone is not sufficient in itself to support application of IFDC. Mastery of clinical reasoning at a higher level is required to organize physiologic and behavioral observation of infants with appropriate ongoing responsiveness in the NICU setting. Experience or case-based learning is used to (1) promote organization of information in a way that is more easily remembered for use in the clinical setting, (2) provide a broad variety of experiences from varying points of view, (3) provide opportunity to reason through IFDC and applications to practice with supportive guidance, and (4) facilitate confidence of the staff and leaders from a range of levels of experience and expertise (Copa, Lucinski, Olsen, et al., 1999; Thomas, O'Connor, Albert, et al., 2001).

Benefits to this method of learning are the active involvement of staff who engage in critical thinking and discussion and the appropriateness of the tool with both novice and experienced nurses (Sudia-Robinson & Walden, 1999). Vignettes (case-based learning) are especially useful as staff present individual experiences with patients and families for the purpose of understanding the experience, gaining insight, sharing thoughts, getting feedback, and identifying further education needs in a respectful, supportive forum for expression. Questions to answer from the various cases reflect the standards; questions may include: (1) Were the infant's cues respected?, (2) Was care modified to support the infant's own abilities, vulnerabilities, or thresholds?, (3) Were parents involved in the experience?, (4) What supports were in place for both infant and parents?, and (5) How would you modify the interaction to incorporate IFDC standards?

Opportunities for reflective sessions with parents can be especially enlightening by providing staff with the parent's perspectives on NICU care, different ways parents might wish to be involved in their infant's care, and barriers to parenting in the highly technologic setting. These sessions can provide new ideas on ways to incorporate families and establish a family-oriented NICU.

A variety of methods for reflection have been described, including vignettes and open forum discussions. Other methods include written cases in a seminar setting, videotaped practice experiences, and Internet learning experiences (Thomas, O'Connor, Albert, et al., 2001). Seminars, small focus groups, or forums, allow active discussion and immediate feedback. Videotaped cases clearly show an experience that can be viewed and reviewed to fully connect to the situation and generate "in the moment" discussion relating the situation to IFDC standards. It is important to focus the filming on the infant's responses and avoid videotape of staff faces, so that the discussion can be open without constraint or hard feelings. Again, group discussion and immediate feedback are available. Standardized situations for web-based learning at an institutional Internet site might allow easy access for some individuals. Pre-structured situations can be described and even video clips inserted for the learner/trainee to evaluate. An electronic bulletin board or chat room provides opportunities for staff to share their understanding of the situation and discuss how IFDC standards can be applied.

In a qualitative study of nurses' experiences, Heerman and Wilson (2000) identified four themes that described the transition from traditional care to IFDC as: (1) negative experiences with IFDC; (2) transitions necessary for partnering with parents, such as acknowledging their preliminary role and fostering competent caregiving; (3) positive experiences with parents; and (4) organizational transitions, such as changing performance expectations. Through open interviews with nurses, important aspects or role transitions were explored, which furthered nurses' insights into the requirements for moving from professional-centered, to shared decision-making and partnering with parents.

One of the health professionals who can be instrumental in a change to IFDC is the advanced practice nurse (APN). APNs from one institution identified barriers during the implementation of a minimal stimulation protocol for VLBW infants (Elser, McIanahan, & Green, 1996). Box 22-6 lists those barriers and possible solutions from an IFDC perspective. The APN change agents discovered that video presentation was an effective tool for implementing the protocol with both physicians and nurses. The APNs assisted with the change process not only through education, but also by providing care to infants using the protocol and serving as highly visible role models. If there are already developmental specialists in the area (might be outside the institution), they can assist with a change, as they already are committed to the principles of IFDC.

There are many innovative ways to keep IFDC standards and practice visible and continually challenge leaders and staff to reason and apply the principles in everyday practice. Assimilation of IFDC into habitual, mindful practice requires sustained efforts over many years. It is easy to tire of the challenge and grow weary with the effort, but if leaders want substantive and sustained change, they must understand that changing from the traditional NICU paradigm that focuses on schedules and tasks and the medical model to IFDC with a focus on family and individualized care, is a long-term initiative. And, in fact, striving for higher levels of excellence with IFDC is a life-long pursuit.

Finally, assimilation is when the IFDC philosophy becomes integrated into practice through strong organizational support, effective leadership, program resources, and supportive policies. Reflective process as a strategy can be very useful when "stuck" at some phase of becoming a developmentally supportive NICU (Browne & Smith-Sharp, 1995). This process is also useful in assisting both leaders and staff in recognizing when practice reflects IFDC standards.

---

**Box 22-6   Possible Barriers and Potential Solutions within the IFDC Perspective**

| Barrier | Solution |
|---|---|
| Anxiety | Focus groups, interview and discussion, mental health professional/counselor, mentoring; variable resources and support professionals such as developmental specialist. |
| Staffing patterns | Support from administrators and managers for adequate staff. |
| Inconsistency of caregivers | Administrators, managers, and staff share responsibility for establishing consistent care teams with fewer numbers of caregivers per patient and family. |
| High staff turnover | Examine reasons for turnover rate, why nurses leave; review exit interview information and work toward solutions specific to findings; open forum discussions or town-hall meetings; staff determined reward systems; IFDC training for all new hires. |
| High census and acuity | Revise acuity and census systems to reflect time spent for IFDC; creative scheduling for high-census seasons; scheduled on-call during high census. |
| Physician/resident rotation | Require IFDC education at the start of the rotation; medical and nursing administrators support IFDC and teach principles to new residents/staff. |
| Staff resistance | On-going education; administrators and managers maintain accountability for IFDC practice through performance appraisal process; leaders visibly support IFDC practice on unit; informal leaders model IFDC principles in practice. |

Adapted from Turnage, C.C. (2002). Individualized family-centered developmental care: Reflections on implementation. *Newborn and Infant Nursing Reviews, 2*(1), 32.

# IMPLEMENTING INDIVIDUALIZED FAMILY-CENTERED DEVELOPMENTAL CARE: CLINICAL PATHWAYS

The team approach to developmental care offers each discipline the opportunity to contribute to the holistic care of the high-risk neonate. Once the new culture is defined, and the change assimilated, the IFDC philosophy needs to be assimilated into practice. One way to achieve this goal is to use an interdisciplinary process to develop clinical pathways (Gaynor, 1999). Clinical pathways that are based on a developmental timeline offer a unique tool to merge the advanced technology of care with the fundamental need for developmentally appropriate family and infant care. Such pathways are based on gestational age at birth and developed along the timeline of adjusted age for each individual baby (Kimberlin & Bregman, 1996). These pathways can serve as a tool to standardize and yet individualize the care of each infant/family unit. As such, they can be used to plan medical and nursing care, educate and integrate the family into the plan of care, and collect data/monitor research protocols/ trend outcomes.

## Pathway Development

Since the mid-1980s, case management using clinical pathways has emerged as a useful tool to gain consistency of care and decrease the cost of care for different groups of patients (Flynn & Kilgallen, 1993). NICU clinical pathways differ from many adult and even pediatric pathways in the area of anticipated progress. In the neonate, developmental capabilities carry equal weight with levels of illness. A very healthy 28-week infant is unlikely to go home in a month, regardless of size or well being because he is not developmentally capable of breathing consistently and taking all food from breast or bottle. Similarly, a 32-week infant with respiratory distress syndrome will likely go home several weeks before the 28-week infant with the same degree of illness. Although there are a number of pathways that have been rigorously developed and are now published (Forsythe, Maney, Ramirez, et al., 1998; Gretebeck, Shaffer, & Bishop-Kurylo, 1998; Malnight & Wahl, 1997; Schwoebel & Jones, 1999; Tobin, Sabatte, Sandhu, & Penafiel, 1998; Vecchi, Vasquez, Radin, & Johnson, 1996),

they remain difficult to transfer from one NICU to another. This phenomenon is probably related to the differences in unit cultures, and the fact that pathways inherently require extensive input from each discipline to secure buy-in from each discipline. Depending on the unit culture, it might be difficult to transition from the medical model of task-directed care to the more holistic model of relationship-based, family-centered care. Pathways can facilitate change but must be consistent with the unit culture and aligned with institutional missions and goals to be useful tools in providing high-quality, economically sound care (Kuhle, 2000).

There are three primary methods of pathway development: (1) pathways can originate from chart reviews that serve to outline current practice and expectations; (2) they can be built up from multiple research-based protocols; or (3) they can include a historical shell into which research-based protocols are superimposed. The third one offers the greatest potential to merge current practice with potentially better practices as technology advances and our understanding of neonates and their families improves.

Table 22-1 is an example of a clinical pathway that is based on a historical shell and has triggers for the initiation of current research-based protocols. It was first developed on the basis of gestational age at birth and adjusted age thereafter (Kimberlin & Bregman, 1996). The timeline is based on the infant's anticipated developmental readiness for transition to home. Nutrition protocols came next and were then followed by testing and screening guidelines, surfactant and ventilator protocols, and transition to home support and care. Developmental care guidelines fit well into pathway development and individualization as they include anticipated capabilities as well as cue-based interventions. One area that lends itself well to pathways is the transition to oral feeding. It has to be individualized for each infant, based on medical stability and readiness as well as infant cues in response to handling and feeding.

Key throughout the hospitalization is the integration of parent planning and care by parents at each stage of development and illness. Figure 22-2, the

*Text continued on p. 452*

Table **22-1** CLINICAL PATHWAY

## 24- TO 26-WEEKS' GESTATION INFANTS
**Designed to Be Applied to the Infant's Individualized Plan of Care**

| Dates | Week 1: Days 1-7 | Week 2: Days 8-14 | Week 3: Days 15-21 | Week 4: Days 22-28 | 30-31 Weeks' Adj. Age | 32-33 Weeks' Adj. Age | 34-35 Weeks' Adj. Age | 36-37 Weeks' Adj. Age | 38 Weeks' Adj. Age | 39 Weeks' Adj. Age |
|---|---|---|---|---|---|---|---|---|---|---|
| Fluids/ nutrition | PIN on day 1 Advance 1-2-3 80 cal/kg/day by day 5 Trophic ASAP See protocol | Continue PIN/IL ? PICC line Advance feeds per protocol | Transition to full enteral feeds Advance calories to 22 and 24/oz Evaluate for reflux | Maintain 110-120 cal/kg/day Vitamins and supplements per protocol | Maintain 110-120 cal/kg/day | Maintain 110-120 cal/kg/day Introduce breast-feeding as tolerated | Maintain 110-120 cal/kg/day Introduce bottle-feeding as tolerated ?DC Na+ supplement | Maintain 110-120 cal/kg/day Encourage all oral feeds as tolerated Transition to DC formula | | |
| Cardio-resp. | Surfactant Gentle vent support Monitor for PDA Monitor for PIE BP support as needed | Wean respiratory support per protocol ? Caffeine | Wean respiratory support ? Diuretics | Wean respiratory support | Wean respiratory support | Wean respiratory support | DC caffeine if stable ? wean diuretics and Na+/K+ supplement | Evaluate home needs: Monitor, oxygen, RSV prophylaxis | | |
| Testing | Metabolic screen | 14-day CUS Check metabolic screen results | | 28-day CUS Nutrition Labs | | ROP exam | Nutrition labs ROP exam Hearing screen | ROP exam F/U CUS | | |
| Family-centered DCGs | 72-hour midline head position Minimal handling Containment Cue-based care | Protective environment Cue-based care DCG Stage I | Protective environment Cue-based care DCG Stage I | Protective environment Cue-based care DCG Stage I-II Family conference | Protective environment Cue-based care DCG Stage II Select / contact pediatrician | Transition to open crib Cue-based care DCG Stage II-III Take CPR and car seat classes | Plan for immunizations Cue-based care DCG Stage III-IV Family conference | Cue-based care DCG Stage IV-V Plan rooming-in with all home-going equipment | | |

*Continued*

Table 22-1  CLINICAL PATHWAY—CONT'D

| | Week 1: Days 1-7 | Week 2: Days 8-14 | Week 3: Days 15-21 | Week 4: Days 22-28 | 30-31 Weeks' Adj. Age | 32-33 Weeks' Adj. Age | 34-35 Weeks' Adj. Age | 36-37 Weeks' Adj. Age | 38 Weeks' Adj. Age | 39 Weeks' Adj. Age |
|---|---|---|---|---|---|---|---|---|---|---|
| **Dates** | | | | | | | | | | |
| | Add humidity to environment; Orient parents: 1. NICU 2. DCG 3. Pain management; Social services referral; Family conference | | | | | See "shaken baby" video | Use discharge checklist | Car seat test before DC; EI referral; Home nursing visits | | |

## 27- TO 29-WEEKS' GESTATION INFANTS
## Designed to Be Applied to the Infant's Individualized Plan of Care

| | Week 1: Days 1-7 | Week 2: Days 8-14 | Week 3: Days 15-21 | Week 4: Days 22-28 | 30-31 Weeks' Adj. Age | 32-33 Weeks' Adj. Age | 34-35 Weeks' Adj. Age | 36-37 Weeks' Adj. Age | 38 Weeks' Adj. Age | 39 Weeks' Adj. Age |
|---|---|---|---|---|---|---|---|---|---|---|
| **Dates** | | | | | | | | | | |
| **Fluids Nutrition** | PIN on day 1; Advance 1-2-3; 80 cal/kg/d by day 5; Trophic ASAP; See protocol | Continue PIN/IL; ? PICC line; Advance feeds per protocol | Transition to full enteral feeds; Advance calories to 22 and 24/oz; Evaluate for reflux | Maintain 110-120 cal/kg/day; Vitamins and supplements per protocol | | Maintain 110-120 cal/kg/day; Introduce breast-feeding as tolerated | Maintain 110-120 cal/kg/day; Introduce bottle-feeding as tolerated; ? DC Na+ supplement | Maintain 110-120 cal/kg/day; Encourage all oral feeds as tolerated; Transition to DC formula | | |
| **Cardio-resp.** | Surfactant; Gentle vent support; Monitor for PDA | Wean respiratory support per protocol; ? Caffeine | Wean respiratory support; ? Diuretics | Wean respiratory support | | Wean respiratory support | DC caffeine if stable; ? Wean diuretics and Na+/K+ supplement | Evaluate home needs: Monitor, oxygen, RSV prophylaxis | | |

| | 72-hour | 14-day | | 28-day | | | |
|---|---|---|---|---|---|---|---|
| **Testing** | Monitor for PIE<br>BP support as needed<br>Metabolic screen | CUS<br>Check metabolic screen results | | CUS<br>Nutrition labs | ROP exam per protocol | Nutrition labs<br>ROP exam<br>Hearing screen | ROP exam<br>F/U CUS |
| **Family-centered DCGs** | midline head position<br>Minimal handling<br>Containment<br>Cue-based care<br>Add humidity to environment<br>Orient parents:<br>1. NICU<br>2. DCG<br>3. Family conference<br>Pain management<br>Social services referral | Protective environment<br>Cue-based care<br>DCG Stage I-II | Protective environment<br>Cue-based care<br>DCG Stage I | Protective environment<br>Cue-based care<br>DCG Stage II<br>Family conference | Transition to open crib<br>Cue-based care<br>DCG Stage III<br>Take CPR and car seat classes<br>See "shaken baby" video | Plan for immunizations<br>Cue-based care<br>DCG Stage IV<br>Use discharge checklist<br>Family conference | Cue-based care<br>DCG Stage V<br>Plan rooming-in with all home-going equipment.<br>Car seat test before DC<br>EI referral<br>Home nursing visits |

*Continued*

Table **22-1** CLINICAL PATHWAY—CONT'D

## 30- TO 33-WEEKS' GESTATION INFANTS
**Designed to Be Applied to the Infant's Individualized Plan of Care**

| | Week 1 Date of Birth/ Gestational Age | Week 2 Date/Adj. Age | 34 Weeks' Adj. Age Date | 35-36 Weeks' Adj Age Date |
|---|---|---|---|---|
| Fluids/nutrition | PIN on day 1 if feeding delay anticipated<br>Advance to 3 g protein and 3 g IL/kg/day<br>80 cal/kg/day by day 5<br>Trophic feed and advance per protocol | Transition to full enteral feeds as tolerated<br>Fortify mother's milk or advance to 22/24-cal formula<br>Advance to 110-120 cal/kg/day<br>Introduce breastfeeding as tolerated | Add vitamins per protocol<br>Maintain caloric intake<br>Introduce oral feeding<br>? Transition to 22 cal at 34-35 weeks | Maintain caloric intake<br>Encourage total oral feeding |
| Cardio-resp. | Support ventilation<br>? Surfactant<br>Observe for PDA<br>Wean vent as tolerated | Wean respiratory support as tolerated<br>? Caffeine | Wean respiratory support as tolerated<br>DC caffeine if stable | Anticipate discharge oxygen and monitor needs<br>? Wean diuretics/Na+ supplement |
| Testing | Metabolic screen | 14-day CUS<br>Check neogen results | Hearing screen | ? ROP exam if birthweight less than 1500 g or unstable course<br>? F/U CUS |
| Family-centered DCGs | Protective environment<br>Minimal handling<br>Containment<br>Cue-based care<br>Orient parents:<br>1. NICU<br>2. Developmental care guidelines<br>3. Family conference<br>Pain management<br>Social services referral | Protective environment<br>Cue-based care<br>Select/contact pediatrician<br>DCG Stage II | Transition to open crib<br>Cue-based care<br>DCG Stage III-IV<br>Parents take CPR and car seat classes.<br>View "shaken baby" video<br>Family conference | Parents provide most of the care<br>Cue-based care<br>DCG Stages IV-V<br>Parents plan rooming-in day/eve or night with all home-going equipment<br>? Home nursing visits<br>? EI referral |

## 34+ WEEKS' GESTATION INFANTS
### Designed to Be Applied to the Infant's Individualized Plan of Care

| Dates | Acute Phase | Recovery Phase |
|---|---|---|
| Fluids/nutrition | PIN on day 1 if feeds delayed more than 48 hours<br>Trophic/protocol feeds ASAP<br>Advance enteral feeds as tolerated | Transition to full oral feeds.<br>Transition to DC formula and supplements |
| Cardio-resp. | Support respiratory system as needed<br>? Surfactant<br>Wean support as tolerated<br>Cardiac echocardiogram as needed<br>Wean support as tolerated<br>Cardiac echocardiogram as needed | Wean respiratory support as tolerated<br>Evaluate home care needs<br>ROP exam per protocol<br>Hearing screen<br>Transition to open crib<br>Transition to parent care |
| Testing | Metabolic screen | DCG Stages IV-V |
| Family-centered DCGs | Protective environment<br>Minimal handling<br>Containment<br>Cue-based care<br>DCG Stages I-IV<br>Orient parents:<br>  1. NICU<br>  2. Developmental care guidelines<br>  3. Family conference<br>Pain management<br>Social services referral | Cue-based care<br>Parents take car seat and CPR classes<br>Evaluate home care needs<br>Car seat testing per guidelines |

Used with permission from Penn State Children's Hospital, Hershey Medical Center, Hershey PA. Copyright 2003 by Pennsylvania State University.

*Adj. age,* Adjusted age; *ASAP,* as soon as possible; *BP,* blood pressure; *cal,* calorie; *CPR,* cardiopulmonary resuscitation; *CUS,* cerebral ultrasound resuscitation; *DC,* discontinue; *DCG,* developmental care guideline; *EI,* early intervention; *IL,* intralipids; *K+,* potassium; *NA+,* sodium; *NICU,* neonatal intensive care; *PDA,* patent ductus arteriosus; *PICC,* percutaneous intravenous central catheter; *PIE,* pulmonary iterstitial emphysema; *PIN,* parenteral intravenous nutrition; *RSV,* respiratory syncytial virus; *ROP,* retinopathy of prematurity.

referenced Developmental Care Guidelines for Parents, is an integral component and is designed to be implemented on an individual basis. Clinical pathways based on developmental care guidelines incorporate very specific interventions/activities/education for both caregiver and parents. This theme recognizes the equally important role that both professionals and parents have in the long-term outcome of high-risk infants (see Family Issues/Professional-Parent Partnerships in Chapter 18).

## Planning Care

Clinical pathways that incorporate developmental care, empower the primary nurse to develop an individualized care plan for each infant/family unit. A written pathway offers even the novice practitioner the framework and knowledge to develop a research-based practice that can be creatively individualized for each infant and family unit. Furthermore, standardized practices traditionally decrease variability and yield savings in cost and improvement in quality (Schwoebel & Jones, 1999). For example, feeding readiness and advancement protocols have yielded a decrease in parental nutrition days for a cohort of preterm infants in a multicenter study (Vermont Oxford Network [VON], 2003). Although the primary nurse more efficiently manages the pathway, the case manager serves as a consultant and data collector and reporter. The pathway can be updated and specific outcomes monitored and reported as interdisciplinary teams implement and test, through research, these protocols. Protocols are revised based on input from the research and practice arenas.

## Integrating the Family into the Plan of Care

The core of the care plan must include the parent-infant relationship and the parent-provider relationship. The development of a co-regulatory parent-infant relationship is supported by a continuously expanding component of parent care for the child. For the very preterm infant, this care begins with the parent's simple adoring gaze and gradually advances to holding and complete care as the infant stabilizes and matures. The primary caregiver can use unit resources of literature, videos, and classes to support the parents in their current role and prepare them for future growth.

An individualized process of education will meet the parents' need for information, which in turn will help them manage the stress of having a NICU baby. Research demonstrates that parents have differing needs for information. The parents' cultural background, personalities, and maturity will influence their need for and ability to understand information. Effective communications with the family will enable caregivers to balance technical and infant developmental information in a manner that will foster positive parenting (Loo, Espinosa, Tyler, & Howard, 2003). Caregivers can use unit resources of literature, videos, and classes to support the parents in their current role and prepare them for future growth. Clinical pathways that incorporate developmental care are helpful in balancing the technical information about ventilators and monitors with the parents' need to understand each phase of their infant's neurobehavioral development. Parents can begin focusing on their infant's physiologic and behavioral cues instead of monitor beeps and alarms. The NICU staff has an opportune role in reducing parental stress with open communications and structured education that facilitates positive parenting.

In spite of surfactant, gentle ventilation, and increased attention to nutrition, there are many infants who require significant medical and nursing support for the major part of their hospitalization. It is difficult for parents to envision their child at home while the infant is still attached to monitors, oxygen, and IVs. However, with earlier discharges, the time from "detachment" to home is brief. As we work with infants and families in both designing and implementing developmental care, we advance the scope of our care and teach families the concept of contingent caregiving. Helping families establish a relationship with their child as an integral part of their family provides an excellent foundation for parenting the high-risk infant.

## Monitoring and Evaluating Care

Unit-based clinical pathways can serve the professional need for collecting data and trending outcomes. The data collection tool can be at the bedside or held

*Text continued on p. 459*

The Milton S Hershey Medical Center
Neonatal Intensive Care Unit

Healthcare Provider's Guide to Developmental Care

---

General guidelines for healthcare providers applicable to all infants and families:

- Remember that parents are the single constant in their infant's life and therefore should be a core component of their infant's care.
- During times of stress and distress, parents and infants regress to a less capable level of performance, understanding, or both, and they need time to adapt.
- The NICU environment and lingo are not "natural" for infants and families.
- Anticipate that families will need a great deal of support upon admission; help them connect as parents to their baby; guide them to tap into social and family resources so they can regain a sense of autonomy and control.
- Remember that bonding is essential to caring, and that the bonding process must be sustained over the entire hospitalization.
- Parents need time to grieve the loss of the perfect pregnancy or baby and need opportunities for decision making that allow them to regain a sense of control over their lives.
- Provide a lactation consult for moms who desire to breastfeed.

---

General guidelines for parents applicable to all infants and families:

- Promote sleep and rest; **let a sleeping baby sleep.**
- Spend time at the bedside gazing at and adoring your baby. To get to know your baby, watch activities and expressions.
- Provide containment holding during and after treatments and/or procedures.
- Develop a schedule with your baby's nurse to spend regular time with your baby.
- If you can't be in the nursery daily, set up a telephone schedule to speak with your nurse.
- Consider pumping breast milk, and consider providing directed donor blood.
- Take pictures and videos of your baby and share them with your family and friends.
- Start a journal and write about parenting your special baby.
- Visit the library in the Family Resource Center for additional reading materials.
- Watch the videotape "Getting to Know Your NICU."

---

Figure **22-2** Healthcare provider's guide to developmental care (Excel sheet). (*Courtesy Lois Gates. Copyright 2003 by Pennsylvania State University.*)

*Continued*

## Stage 1: Adjusted Age of 24-28 Weeks

| Infant Characteristics | Caregiver Role | Parent Activities |
|---|---|---|
| *During this time, babies are fragile. They need maximum technologic support. Too much stimulation, such as bright lights, touching, changes in temperature, or loud noises, can stress the baby.* <br>• Babies sleep a lot at this stage and seldom open their eyes. <br>• Babies sleep better in a warm, dim, and quiet environment. <br>• Babies respond to pain and discomfort with increased blood sugar, changes in heart rate, and irregular breathing. <br>• Babies respond to stress by hiccoughs, yawning, and pale color. <br>• Twitches or limpness in the arms and legs represent immature nerves and muscles. <br>• The baby's skin is so fragile that touching and handling must be done carefully. | • Promote sleep and rest by clustering care. <br>• Provide midline orientation, flexion, containment, and boundaries. <br>• Protect the baby from noise and light. <br>• Assess and promote comfort measures and medication to minimize pain and agitation. <br>• Move the baby into the protective environment of the incubator within 24-72 hours. Until then, protect the skin and fluid balance with appropriate extra barriers such as Aquaphor or a humidity tent. <br>• Introduce and encourage the use of Social Services. <br>• Help parents find their role and feel significant in that role. <br>• Encourage parents to write down their observations about and activities with their baby in a journal. | • If your baby is sleeping when you arrive, **let your baby continue to rest.** Sleep will help your baby gain weight and get well. <br>• Accept that each baby is different and that a baby's progress depends on his or her own maturity and illness. <br>• You can calm your baby by gently holding your baby's arms and legs securely against his or her body. Another way to help your baby feel secure is to place one hand on top of your baby's head and use the other hand to cradle the feet. <br>• Select a very special baby blanket or quilt to bring in and use as an incubator cover. This will help your baby by providing a personalized, quiet, and dim environment. <br>• Whisper "sweet nothings" and talk gently with your baby. <br>• Watch the videotapes, "Prematurely Yours" and "NICU Parent Tape I: Parenting the Acutely Ill Infant." |

Figure **22-2**  Cont'd.

Stage 2: Adjusted Age of 27-31 Weeks

| Infant Characteristics | Caregiver Role | Parent Activities |
|---|---|---|
| *During this time, babies acquire autonomic stability. This means the baby's brain is learning to control breathing, heart rate, and blood pressure. Because the baby's brain is still developing, noise and activity can easily overwhelm the baby.*<br>• Babies will have increased periods of being awake, and they will become more alert for short times.<br>• Although the body movements are irregular and squirming, babies are developing increased strength in their legs and arms.<br>• Babies may start to suck on a pacifier, which promotes quiet awakeness and improves digestion.<br>• Babies respond to gentle vocal stimulation, which promotes quiet sleep.<br>• Babies respond to stress with paleness, pauses in breathing (apnea), and limpness. | • Assess babies before, during, and after care; modify care and environment accordingly.<br>• Position babies to support flexion and midline orientation. Add flex prone positioning.<br>• Offer babies a pacifier when they are awake and during tube feedings.<br>• Support autonomic stability by allowing the baby to become acclimated to environmental or physiologic change one step at a time (e.g., speak to the baby before repositioning; allow rest time between vital signs, diaper changing, and feedings).<br>• Encourage parents to appreciate their role and integrate their activities into the plan of care.<br>• Continue the protective environment. | • Spend time at the bedside adoring and appreciating your baby's individuality.<br>• If you are planning to breastfeed, keep pumping every 2 to 3 hours (10 to 12 times per day).<br>• Begin holding your baby as tolerated by the baby. Consider providing "kangaroo care" (holding skin to skin) when your baby becomes eligible. If interested, ask your nurse about this and view the video "Kangaroo Care."<br>• Your baby may begin to tolerate combined activities. For example, talk to your baby while you touch his or her body. Your baby's response will tell you what is good for the baby and what is too much activity.<br>• Review the booklets "Understanding My Signals" and "My Special Start." |

Figure 22-2  Cont'd.

*Continued*

| | Stage 3: Adjusted Age of 29-33 Weeks | |
| --- | --- | --- |
| Infant Characteristics | Caregiver Role | Parent Activities |
| *During this time, babies are in transition from mostly sleeping to a time of sleep and wake cycles. Babies are more alert and awake longer and begin to cry spontaneously.*<br>• Babies gain more control over movements, first in their legs and then in their arms.<br>• Babies may open their eyes for brief periods of time and make eye contact.<br>• Babies respond to stress with paleness, limpness, and pauses in breathing (apnea). | • Encourage sucking on a pacifier during tube feeds.<br>• Evaluate peri-oral sensitivity; introduce positive stimulation as a prefeeding regimen.<br>• Provide positioning and comfort measures when the baby is restless or agitated.<br>• Offer "kangaroo care" to parents when babies reach the criteria; especially encourage breast-feeding moms to provide skin-to-skin holding.<br>• Begin discussing an anticipated timeline for discharge/transfer. Outline developmental expectations and readiness for moving from the NICU.<br>• Schedule parents for infant CPR and car seat classes if indicated.<br>• Consider co-bedding multiples when infants are stable and off IV fluids. Help parents appreciate the multiplicity of the birth as well as each infant's individuality.<br>• Continue to encourage and support parents in their role. Be especially attentive to parents who have experienced loss or whose infants have had setbacks or made poor progress. | • Hold your baby for longer periods. Consider "kangaroo care."<br>• Offer your baby a pacifier during tube feedings.<br>• Add small, colorful pictures to your baby's incubator. These objects will help your baby to focus the eyes. Babies are nearsighted and can only see things up close. They see best when objects are about 8 to 10 inches away.<br>• Learn how to interact with your baby. What are the things your baby likes or doesn't like? What are the best times during the day to interact with your baby? How long does your baby have the energy to respond to you?<br>• Note your baby's sleep and wake cycle. If possible, spend time in the nursery when your baby is likely to be more awake and alert.<br>• Continue to learn your baby's behaviors. You will come to know when your baby is stressed and needs rest and when your baby is relaxed and can be handled.<br>• Select a pediatrician.<br>• Start thinking about bringing your baby home. Talk with your physician about the anticipated transfer or discharge time.<br>• Watch the videotapes, "Feeding your Baby" and "Parent Tape II: Parenting the Growing Premie." |

Figure 22-2  Cont'd.

## Stage 4: Adjusted Age of 32-35 Weeks

| Infant Characteristics | Caregiver Role | Parent Activities |
|---|---|---|
| *During this time, babies begin to communicate the need for food and attention.*<br><br>• Babies begin developing the ability to coordinate sucking and swallowing.<br>• Babies have increased muscle strength and control.<br>• Babies develop visual attention. They can fix and focus on faces and bright objects and follow them with their eyes.<br>• Babies continue to respond to stress with apnea, irregular breathing, paleness, and limpness. | • Evaluate babies for readiness for the transition into an open crib based on temperature support requirements and weight gain.<br>• Assess suck-swallow-breath coordination.<br>• Evaluate the emergence of upper body tone as a prerequisite for oral feeding.<br>• If mom plans to breastfeed, introduce breastfeeding at an adjusted age of 32 to 33 weeks according to baby readiness. Arrange to have the mother meet with the lactation consultant to set up a breastfeeding plan.<br>• Assess bottle-feeding infants at an adjusted age of 33 to 34 weeks to evaluate readiness for oral feedings. Offer feedings based on the infant's level of alertness and ability to sustain tone and attention. Developmentally, babies may make better progress when attempting 2 to 3 short (5 to 10 minute) feeding sessions as opposed to 1 longer session a day. Supplement with tube feeds when an infant demonstrates signs of fatigue (e.g., pallor, change in tone or alertness, decrease in coordination).<br>• Schedule eye exam, hearing screen, and CUS as appropriate.<br>• Consider a baseline PT/OT evaluation. Educate parents about early intervention activities and programs (e.g., play activities, positioning, the importance of "tummy" time).<br>• Support parents in their expanded role of caregiving.<br>• Evaluate for anticipated home needs, such as a monitor, oxygen, tube feedings, medications, and car seat testing.<br>• Solicit parents' reaction to and interpretation of the baby's behavior. | • Encourage your baby to use a pacifier during tube feedings.<br>• Adjust your schedule so you are available to breastfeed or bottle-feed during your baby's more wakeful times.<br>• Learn and perform your baby's routine care, such as diapering, bathing, and taking a temperature.<br>• Discuss the transfer or discharge plan with your baby's physician, such as expected timeline, testing, and care needs after leaving the NICU.<br>• Schedule and take an infant CPR class.<br>• Continue to observe your baby's behavior and learn how your baby communicates with you.<br>• Learn about immunizations.<br>• Take the car seat class before selecting your baby's car seat. |

*Continued*

Figure **22-2** Cont'd.

## Stage 5: Adjusted Age of 34-40 Weeks

| Infant Characteristics | Caregiver Role | Parent Activities |
|---|---|---|
| *During this time, babies mature enough to be capable of social interaction and cry differently when they are tired, hungry, or in pain.*<br>• Babies hold arms and legs flexed.<br>• Vision is maturing, but babies may still take a little longer than older children to focus on an object.<br>• Babies begin to be wakeful before feedings.<br>• Babies are awake for longer periods, can make eye contact, and can follow movement and sounds, or both. | • Consider demand versus scheduled feedings based on calories and ml per day rather than every 3 to 4 hours.<br>• Evaluate nutritional status and transition to discharge formula and/or supplements.<br>• Evaluate for "back to sleep" positioning.<br>• If not being followed by a PT/OT, consider referring parents for education about positioning, early intervention, and early development.<br>• Encourage car seat testing.<br>• Get discharge prescriptions written. Schedule medications for convenient in-home administration. Instruct parents regarding medications.<br>• Help parents anticipate and plan for the stress of the transition from NICU to home.<br>• Evaluate readiness for immunizations. | • Continue to learn the baby's cues for communication and interaction.<br>• Learn the signs and symptoms of illness.<br>• Learn to place your baby correctly in a variety of positions, including your car seat.<br>• Plan to room-in with your baby for a full day or night; do this a day or 2 before discharge to home. Perform all routine care for 2 or 3 consecutive feedings before discharge.<br>• Learn general home and car safety measures for young infants.<br>• Learn about discharge medications and how to administer them.<br>• Contact family and friends for support and help after discharge (e.g., meals, laundry, car pools).<br>• Rest up and prepare for busy days ahead. |

### At Home

• Recognize that it will take a few days for your baby to get used to the different sounds, lighting, and activities in your home. This may result in a bit of fussiness and/or changes in sleeping, waking, or eating activities.
• Schedule yourself as the primary caregiver to help your baby make this transition.
• Keep the family schedule as simple as possible during this time.
• Write out all medications and times and check them off as you give them.
• Write down all follow-up appointments.
• Make notes as questions come to your mind.
• Accept offers of help with other activities (e.g., child care, laundry, shopping).

Figure **22-2** Cont'd.

by the case manager, depending on the type and purpose of information gathered. For instance, the bedside chart might hold a nutrition-monitoring tool that tracks intake, growth, and laboratory profiles for use on daily rounds. However, the case manager might collect outcomes for benchmarking with such organizations as the VON. Along with unit pathway data, institutional outcomes that benchmark family satisfaction, length of stay, acuity indexes, and cost per case can be used to modify the clinical pathway to improve outcomes. Inherently, clinical pathways are never completely done. There should always be room for adjustments based on an ongoing evaluation of the literature and analysis of outcomes.

## OUTCOMES

Clinical pathways are certainly one way to measure outcomes of the implementation of developmental care. Benchmarking against other units that are similar to yours is another way. Both medical and developmental outcomes need to be considered and are outlined in some detail in Chapter 21; these include physiologic stability, growth, achievement of developmental milestones, neurobehavioral development (short- and long-term), parent-infant relationship, parental concerns related to caregiving, length of stay, and complications of the NICU stay (short-and long-term, including infection rates, incidence of retinopathy of prematurity [ROP], intraventricular hemorrhage [IVH], hearing deficits, and learning problems). Programs such as NIDCAP® and Wee Care® (Norwell, MA) are assisting neonatal health professionals to gather data regarding these outcome measures after developmental care has been implemented (Hendricks-Munoz, Prendergast, Caprio, et al., 2002). Until we systematically measure our infant and family outcomes, we will not know for certain how our organizational climate and unit culture is positively or negatively affecting those in our care.

## CONCLUSION

Everyone might not embrace a paradigm shift or change in philosophy from traditional NICU to developmental care overnight. A minimum of 3 to 5 years and even 10 years might be necessary because unit culture and individual attitudes of caregivers can create significant resistance to change. McGrath and Valenzuela (1994) suggest that the best chance for

successfully integrating a developmental philosophy as an organization and implementing IFDC is through patience, endurance, and persistence. Technology, data, task, or disease-focused care, and NICU jargon allow professionals to distance themselves from patients and families. Inherent in the philosophy of IFDC is reaching across the barriers that protect professionals from relationships that might be painful or make them emotionally vulnerable and establishing relationships with patients and their families.

Clearly defined standards and accountabilities, strong leadership, and the use of reflective process for individual and group change coupled with endurance, persistence, and patience might be the combination needed for sustaining the cultural shift to IFDC. The process of becoming a developmental NICU does not just happen all at once. The focus on technology disrupted the relational aspect of caring for patients and their families. It takes a long time to change or go back to what once was a more holistic, humanistic, individual approach, and there are many bumps, bruises, and setbacks along the way. But once you set forward on the road to becoming a family-centered, developmentally supportive unit, you will not be able to go back, because the essence of this model of care is at the heart of why most of us entered a healthcare profession, whatever our disciplinary training may be. It is really caring and behaving toward others as *we* would want them to behave toward our own family members or ourselves. Change is never easy, but the approach to change is just as important as the change itself! The change must be developmentally supported and measured along the way.

## *REFERENCES*

Aiken, L.H., Clarke, S.P., Sloane, D.M., et al. (2002). Hospital nurse staffing and patient mortality, nurse burnout, and job dissatisfaction. *Journal of the American Medical Association (JAMA), 288*(16), 1987-1993.

Aiken, L.H., Clarke, S.P., & Sloane, D.M. (2001). Hospital restructuring: Does it adversely affect care and outcomes? *Journal of Health and Human Services Administration, 23*(4), 416-442.

Aiken, L.H., Smith, J.L., & Lake, E.T. (1994). Lower Medicare mortality among a set of hospitals known for good nursing care. *Medical Care, 32*(8), 771-787.

Als, H. (1982). Toward a synactive theory of development: Promise for the assessment and support of infant individuality. *Infant Mental Health Journal, 3*, 229-243.

Als, H. (1986). A synactive model of neonatal behavioral organization: Framework for the assessment of neurobehavioral development in the premature infant and for support of infants and parents in the neonatal intensive care environment. *Physical, Occupational Therapy and Pediatrics, 6*, 3-55.

Als, H. (1999). Reading the premature infant. In E. Goldson (Ed.). *Nurturing the premature infant: Developmental interventions in the neonatal intensive care nursery* (pp. 18-35). New York: Oxford University Press.

Als, H., & Gilkerson, L. (1997). The role of relationship-based developmentally supportive newborn intensive care in strengthening outcome of preterm infants. *Seminars in Perinatology, 21*, 178-189.

Als, H., Lawhon, G., Brown, E., et al. (1986). Individualized behavioral and environmental care for the very low birth weight preterm infant at high risk for bronchopulmonary dysplasia: Neonatal intensive care unit and developmental outcome. *Pediatrics, 78*, 1123-1132.

Als, H., Lawhon, G., Duffy, F.H., et al. (1994). Individualized developmental care for the very low birth-weight preterm infant: Medical and neurofunctional effects. *Journal of the American Medical Association (JAMA), 272*, 853-858.

American Academy of Pediatrics (AAP)/Canadian Paediatric Society. (2000). Prevention and management of pain and stress in the neonate. *Pediatrics, 105*, 454-461.

Ballweg, D.D. (2001) Implementing developmentally supportive family-centered care in the newborn intensive care unit as quality improvement initiative. *Journal of Perinatal & Neonatal Nursing, 15*(3), 58-73.

Bergman, D. (1999) Evidence-based guidelines and critical pathways for quality improvement. *Pediatrics, 103*(1) 225-232.

Blegen, M.A., & Vaughn, T. (1998). A multisite study of nurse staffing and patient occurrences. *Nursing Economics, 16*(4), 196-203.

Browne, J.V. & Smith-Sharp, S. (1995). The Colorado Consortium of Intensive Care Nurseries: Spinning a web of support for Colorado infants and families. *Zero to Three, 15*, 18-23.

Buehler, D.M., Als, H., Duffy, F.H., et al. (1995). Effectiveness of individualized developmental care for low-risk preterm infants: Behavioral and electrophysiological evidence. *Pediatrics, 96*, 923-932.

Copa, A., Lucinski, L., Olsen, E., et al. (1999). Promoting professional and organizational development: A reflective practice model. *Zero to Three, 20*(1), 3-9.

Corrigan, P.W., Diwan, S., Campion, J., et al. (2002). Transformational leadership and the mental health team. *Administration Policy in Mental Health, 30*(2), 97-108.

Elser, A., McIanahan, M., & Green, T.J. (1996). Advanced practice nurses: Change agents for clinical practice. *Journal of Perinatal & Neonatal Nursing, 10*, 72-78.

Fleisher, B.E., VandenBerg, K., Constantinou, J., et al. (1995). Individualized developmental care for very-low-birth-weight premtuare infants. *Clinical Pediatrics, 34*(10), 523-529.

Flynn, A.M., & Kilgallen, M.E. (1993) Case management: A multidisciplinary approach to the evaluation of cost and quality standards. *Journal of Nursing Care Quality, 8*(1) 58-66.

Folger, J.P., Poole, M.S., & Stutman, R.K. (1997). *Working through conflict: strategies for relationships, groups, and organizations* (3rd ed.). New York, Addison Wesley Longman.

Forsythe, T.J., Maney, L.M., Ramirez, A., et al. (1998). Nursing case management in the NICU: Enhanced coordination for discharge planning. *Neonatal Network, 17*(7), 23-34.

Gaynor, S. (1999). Clinical pathways: A Framework for patient satisfaction. *Journal of Child and Family Nursing, 2*(3): 226-228.

Gilkerson, L., & Als, H. (1995). Role of reflective process in the implementation of developmentally supportive care in the newborn intensive care nursery. *Infants and Young Children, 7*, 20-28.

Gladwell, M. (2000). *The tipping point: How little things can make a big difference.* New York: Little Brown & Company.

Gretebeck, R.J., Shaffer, D., Bishop-Kurylo, D. (1998). Clinical pathways for family-oriented developmental care in the intensive care nursery. *Journal of Perinatal and Neonatal Nursing, 12*(1), 70-80.

Hanson, J.L., Johnson, B.H., Jeppson, E.S., et al. (1994). *Hospitals: Moving forward with family-centered care.* Bethesda, MD: Institute for Family-Centered Care.

Hartz, A.J., Krakauer, H., Kuhn, E.M., et al. (1989). Hospital characteristics and mortality rates. *New England Journal of Medicine, 321*(25), 1720-1725.

Heerman, J.A., & Wilson, M.E. (2000). Nurses' experiences working with families in an NICU during implementation of family-focused developmental care. *Neonatal Network, 19*, 23-29.

Hendricks-Munoz, K.D., Prendergast, C.C., Caprio, M.C., et al. (2002). Developmental care: The impact of Wee Care® developmental care training on short-term infant outcome and hospital costs. *Newborn and Infant Nursing Reviews, 2*(1), 39-45.

Holditch-Davis, D., Blackburn, S.T., & VandenBerg, K. (2003). Newborn and infant neurobehavioral development (pp. 236-284). In C. Kenner & J.W. Lott (Eds.), *Comprehensive neonatal nursing: A physiologic perspective* (3rd ed.). St. Louis: W.B. Saunders.

Horns, K. (1998). Being in tune caregiving. *Journal of Perinatal and Neonatal Nursing, 12*, 38-49.

Ingersoll, G.L., Kirsch, J.C., Merk, S.E., et al. (2000). Relationship or organizational culture and readiness for change to employee commitment to the organization. *Journal of Nursing Administration, 30,* 11-20.

Institute for Family-Centered Care. (1994). *Involving families in advisory roles: Advances in family-centered care.* Bethesda, MD: Institute for Family-Centered Care; pp. 2-6.

Johnson, B.H., Jeppson, E.S., & Redburn, L. (1992). *Caring for children and families: Guidelines for hospitals.* Bethesda, MD: Association for the Care of Children's Health.

Kim, W.C., & Mauborgne, R. (2003). Tipping point leadership. *Harvard Business Reviews, 81*(4), 60-69, 122.

Kimberlin, L., & Bregman, J. (1996) Postconceptional age as the basis for neonatal case management. *Neonatal Network, 15*(2), 5-13.

Kuhle, A. (2000). A necessary discipline: Maximizing case management. *Nursing Watch, 7,* Washington, DC: Nursing Executive Center; pp. 1-15.

Kuokkanen, L., & Katajisto, J. (2003). Promoting or impeding empowerment? Nurses' assessments of their work environment. *Journal of Nursing Administration, 33*(4), 209-215.

Kurz, R.S., & Haddock, C.C. (1989). Leadership: Implications of the literature for health services administration research. *Medical Care Review, 46*(1), 75-94.

Loo, K.K., Espinosa, M., Tyler, R., & Howard, J. (2003) Using knowledge to cope with stress in the NICU: How parents integrate learning to read the physiologic and behavioral cues of the infant. *Neonatal Network; 22*(1), 31-37.

Malloch, K., Neeld, A.P., McMurry, C., et al. (1999). Patient classification systems, Part 2: The third generation. *Journal of Nursing Administration, 29*(9), 33-42.

Malnight, M., & Wahl, J.R.F. (1997). An alternative approach for neonatal clinical pathways. *Neonatal Network, 16*(4), 41-49.

McDaniel, C., & Wolf, G.A. (1992). Transformational leadership in nursing service: A test of theory. *Journal of Nursing Administration, 22*(2), 60-65.

McGrath, J. (2000). Developmentally supportive caregiving and technology in the NICU: Isolation or merger of intervention strategies? *Journal of Perinatal and Neonatal Nursing, 14,* 78-91.

McGrath, J. (2003). Family-centered care (pp. 89-107). In C. Kenner & J.W. Lott (Eds.). *Comprehensive neonatal nursing: A physiologic perspective* (3rd ed.). St. Louis: W.B. Saunders.

McGrath, J., & Valenzuela, G. (1994). Integrating developmentally supportive caregiving into practice through education. *Journal of Perinatal and Neonatal Nursing, 8*(3), 46-57.

Moore, K., Lynn, M.R., McMillen, B.J., et al. (1999). Implementation of the ANA report card. *Journal of Nursing Administration, 29*(6), 48-54.

National Association of Neonatal Nurses (NANN). (1998). *Standards of care for neonatal nursing practice.* Des Plaines, IL: NANN.

National Association of Neonatal Nurses (NANN). (2000). *Guidelines for practice: Infant and family-centered developmental care.* Des Plaines, IL: NANN.

National Center for Family-Centered Care. (1990). *What is family-centered care?.* Washington, DC: Association for the Care of Children's Health (ACCH).

Ohlinger, J., Brown, M.S., Laudert, S., et al. (2003). Development of potentially better practices for the neonatal intensive care unit as a culture of collaboration: Communication, accountability, respect, and empowerment. *Pediatrics, 111*(4)(Pt 2), e471-e481.

Petryshen, P., Stevens, B., Hawkins, J., et al. (1997). Comparing nursing costs for preterm infants receiving conventional vs. developmental care. *Nursing Economics, 15*(3), 138-145, 150.

Robison, L. (2000). *Organizational guide to an effective program of developmentally supportive, family-centered care in the NICU, NIDCAP® Training.* Houston, TX: Texas Children's Hospital.

Robison, L.D. (2003). An organizational guide for an effective developmental program in the NICU. *Journal of Obstetric, Gynecologic, and Neonatal Nursing (JOGNN), 32*(3), 382-383.

Robinson, M.S. (2003). *Transformational leadership defined.* Available online at *www.ethoschannel.com/ personalgrowth/new/1-msr_transformational.html.*

Savage T.A., & Conrad, B. (1992). Vulnerability as a consequence of the neonatal nurse-infant relationship. *Journal of Perinatal and Neonatal Nursing, 6*(3), 64-75.

Schein, E. (1997). *Organizational culture and leadership.* New York: Jossey-Bass.

Schwoebel, A., & Jones, M.L. (1999). A Clinical Pathway System for the Neonatal Intensive Care Nursery. *Journal of Perinatal and Neonatal Nursing, 13*(3), 60-69.

Scott, T., Mannion, R., Davies, H.T., et al. (2003). Implementing culture change in health care: Theory and practice. *International Journal of Quality Health Care, 15*(2), 111-118.

Seago, J.A. (2002). A comparison of two patient classification instruments in an acute care hospital. *Journal of Nursing Administration, 32*(5), 243-249.

Seago, J.A. (2000). Registered nurses, unlicensed assistive personnel, and organizational culture in hospitals. *Journal of Nursing Administration, 30*(5), 278-286.

Seago, J.A. (1999). Evaluation of a hospital work redesign: Patient-Focused care. *Journal of Nursing Administration, 29*(11), 31-38.

Spence, K., Greenwood, J., McDonald, M., et al. (1999). Processing knowledge in practice: Preliminary findings of a study into neonatal intensive care nursing. *Journal of Neonatal Nursing, 5,* 27-30.

Sudia-Robinson, T., & Walden, M. (1999). Problem-based learning in the NICU. *Neonatal Network, 18,* 55-56.

Thomas, M.D., O'Connor, F.W., Albert, M.L., et al. (2001). Case-based teaching and learning experiences. *Issues in Mental Health Nursing, 22,* 517-531.

Tobin, C.R., Sabatte, E., Sandhu, A.S., & Penafiel, E. (1998). A neonatal care map based on gestational age. *Neonatal Network, 17*(2), 41-51.

Tremmel, R. (1993). Zen and the art of reflective practice in teacher education. *Harvard Educational Review, 63,* 434-458.

Vecchi, C.J., Vasquez, L., Radin, T., & Johnson, P. (1996). Neonatal individualized predictive pathway (NIPP): A discharge planning tool for parents. *Neonatal Network, 15*(4), 7-13.

Vermont Oxford Network (VON). (2003). *NICU: Evidence-based quality improvement collaborative for neonatology.* Available online at *www.vtoxford.org/QI/nicq.htm.*

Westrup, B., Kleberg, A., von Eichwald, K., et al. (2000). A randomized, controlled trial to evaluate the effects of the newborn individualized developmental care and assessment program in a Swedish setting. *Pediatrics, 105,* 66-72.

# 23 Implications of Early Intervention Legislation

### Kathleen A. VandenBerg

Understanding the nature and process of early human development in the United States has been a long-term pursuit and fascination of scientists, parents, policymakers, and service providers. This evolution spans the time when the focus was on rigid discipline, viewing children as having "sinful tendencies," to the current sophisticated view, which considers the most recent evidence regarding the science of early childhood and its evolution due to environmental exposures. This evidence now convinces scientists, educators, politicians, and parents that the appreciation of the early years in a human's development matters significantly. The absolute importance of early life experience now has a permanent position in science, in policymaking, and in childrearing practices (Shonkoff & Meisels, 2000). Wolf, Klodewijn, Beelen, et al. (2002) found that in assessing very low birthweight (VLBW) infants at 6 months postconceptional age (PCA), there were many neurobehavioral and developmental deficits that might have been diminished with specific neurobehavioral interventions. These findings, coupled with the scientific view, leads health professionals and families to recognize the need for environmental, individualized, family-centered, developmental care (IFDC) interventions that begin at birth and support positive growth and development.

With this focus on development as influenced by the child's microenvironments and macroenvironments and the importance of a developmental care philosophy, legislation is reviewed that impacts on the early development of a child and its effects on family life.

## EARLY CHILDHOOD EDUCATION

Early childhood education in the United States has developed out of two themes (Lazerson, 1972; Bricker, 1989). The early emphasis on education for the young emerged initially from a focus on social reform for the poor. In the late 1800s to early 1900s, programs for young children living in poverty were initiated by Owen in Scotland, Frobel in Germany, Margaret McMillan in England, and Montessori in Italy (Bricker, 1989; Hanson & Lynch, 1995). All shared similar concerns about the health and abuse of young children living in squalid conditions, who might, it was hoped, thrive physically and intellectually with educational opportunities.

## EARLY DEVELOPMENT: A UNIQUE PERIOD FOR LEARNING

The second theme evident in the literature emphasizes that early development was considered a unique period and an important time in a child's development. This idea states that a child's early years are important, and that the experiences of the first 5 years of life have an impact from that point forward. The power of this idea has grown over the past 200 years, and seems to be finally firmly grounded in our practice, our service delivery, and our childrearing practice in the United States.

The evolving influences that have affected the development of early childhood intervention, have been diverse. Several pathways in early childhood intervention have led us to the place today where political, practical, and theoretic challenges and opportunities are thriving.

Appreciation for the influences of genetics and the environment on the developing brain and the unfolding of human behavior is recently viewed as central to the understanding of this early period in human development. Scientific evidence supports the fact that the first 5 years might be strong and sturdy or replete with risk and vulnerabilities. Whichever pattern is experienced will set the stage for what will follow: a strong foundation with well-developed capabilities or fragility with threats, such as stress or injury or trauma (Shonkoff & Meisels, 2000). A strong, common belief is that early childhood development is susceptible to environmental influences and that the investment in improving and supporting early development increases the odds toward favorable developmental outcomes.

## HISTORICAL ROOTS: THE EVOLUTION OF EARLY CHILDHOOD INTERVENTION

Shonkoff and Meisels (2000) described four sources that have led to a framework for understanding early childhood intervention. These four historical roots have contributed to the existing thinking about early childhood intervention. They are early childhood education, maternal and child health services, special education, and child development research.

### Early Childhood Education

The recognition of the importance of the early years as unique emerged from European philosophic roots of the 17th and 18th centuries. John Locke (1689), in his work *An Essay Concerning Human Understanding: Letter*, suggested that children's minds from birth are like blank slates. This thinking led to a practice of letting the natural unfolding of a child's talents occur. Education in the American colonies reflected the opposite tendencies, and the 17th and 18th centuries saw childrearing practices focusing on rigid discipline and the philosophy that "children should be seen and not heard."

Kindergarten classes originated in Europe, were introduced in the United States in the mid-1800s, and were well established by 1900. The need to assist children growing up in extreme poverty was thought to be addressed through exposing them to middle-class values by educating them early. In addition, it was thought that the family life of slum dwellers through education would be improved. Various curriculum and comprehensive programs focused on services to meet social, physical, emotional, and intellectual needs. Kindergarten classes became a standard component of the United States education system, and brought the concepts of early child development into the education arena.

Nursery school programs also having European roots, developed separately from the kindergarten movement, and gained in popularity in the 1920s and 1930s in the United States. Also developed to serve the poor, these nursery school programs proliferated after the Great Depression and received federal support to create jobs. Nursery schools provided jobs for unemployed teachers and provided daycare facilities for working mothers. Following World War II, child daycare programs increased, with more emphasis on "babysitting" care than meeting educational needs of the young children. From these educational movements came the support of state and federal governments. One of the programs that grew out of the recognition for more structured approaches to development was Head Start.

### HEAD START

The concept of early childhood intervention received a boost in support in the 1960s when concern for the disadvantaged child became an all out "war" effort against poverty. Suddenly, Americans were aware of the effect of poverty on children and developed the concern for the impact of early experience on the early development of young children. A decade of social experimentation was ushered in with experimental preschool programs, including Project Head Start.

Head Start was established through the Economic Opportunity Act of 1964 (PL 88-452). Proponents of Head Start believed that compensatory preschool programs would improve school performance for disadvantaged children born into poverty and, hopefully, would break the cycle of poverty. A later amendment to the Act stipulated that at least 10% of the children enrolled in Head Start have disabilities and that Head Start provide appropriate specialized services to these children. Programs for pregnant mothers, infants and toddlers were also added (Hanson, 2003). Although the Program was hailed as a success with several papers describing its achievements, the Program also had its disappointments. Early childhood intervention professionals learned from Head Start to be explicit and realistic in making promises, goals, and objectives. Head Start did not result in the elimination of school failure, need for welfare, juvenile delinquency, or other social issues related to poverty (Shonkoff & Meisels, 2000). In the 1990s, Early Head Start was developed, with continuous year-round child development services for children of low-income families under 3 years. It was designed to enhance children's physical, social, emotional, and intellectual development and had a strong parental education component.

## MATERNAL AND CHILD HEALTH SERVICES

High mortality rates, poor physical health, and exploitation of children in the work force in the 19th century fueled the concern for the physical health of the young and their mothers. This concern led to legislation. In 1912, the Children's Bureau was established to collect data and provide federal grants to promote the health and development of the nation's children. The Bureau highlighted the linkages between socioeconomic factors and infant and maternal deaths, establishing the focus on public-health nursing services in the 1920s, which stimulated the creation of state child hygiene divisions and permanent maternal and child health centers throughout the country (Shonkoff & Meisels, 2000).

Federal funding followed in 1935 with the Social Security Act (Title V). This legislation formalized federal responsibility for the well-being of children and their mothers. This was explicitly stated in Title V legislation, Part I (Maternal and Child Health Services), which provided funds to the states to provide financial assistance and services designed to promote the general health of mothers and children, including prenatal care, well-baby clinics, school health services, immunization programs, public-health nursing, nutrition services, and health education (Magee & Pratt, 1985). Part II of Title V provided for Services for Crippled Children, which created funds to states to provide services, including case finding, diagnosis, treatment, research, and follow-up care for those with "crippling" diseases, as well as treatment for sensory impairments, seizure disorders, and congenital heart disease. These services reflect the predominant underlying agreement that care and protection of children's

health, especially for the poor or those with disabling conditions, is too important to be left to chance (Shonkoff & Meisels, 2000).

## CHILD DEVELOPMENT RESEARCH

The systematic scholarly study of infant and child development provides another perspective on this era of blossoming legislation and services for young children. Contributions of the academic child development community include launching the debate regarding the influence of the environment on child development versus the genetic makeup of the child (nature-nurture debate), and the impact of the consequences of deprivation in early human relationships (Shonkoff & Phillips, 2000)

Two major influences in human development have been the focus of a professional debate. The inherited abilities (nature) have been pitted against the influence of the environment on development (nurture) in the debate known as *nature-nurture*. The side of the argument one takes in this biologic question determines his/her stand on the fundamental issues regarding the influence of parents and/or the environment on development, how heredity unfolds, and what our genetic makeup means and contributes.

In the 1960s, an unfolding of research in infant and child development demonstrated that the very young were more capable of learning than previously believed. Strong support developed for the idea that infants could learn perceptual and memory tasks. Bloom (1964) produced a well-known publication that stated that much of a child's early cognitive learning took place in the first 4 years of life. Some argued that the brain could demonstrate an amazing capacity, called plasticity. The brain and learning were flexible, and early experience played a major role in a child's development, placing great emphasis on the quality of the early environment (Hunt, 1961). New evidence emerged when the devastation of placing infants in nonstimulating and nonmaternal environments came to light. The publication of research that demonstrated effects of maternal deprivation in the early years strengthened the argument for the influence and importance of the environment in early development (Bowlby, 1973; Spitz, 1946).

One well-known study, conducted by Skeels (1966), had a significant impact on the field of early intervention. Skeels conducted a longitudinal study of two groups of infants who grew up in very different environments. All 26 of the infants studied began their life in an orphanage and were thought to be very low-functioning infants. Thirteen infants were placed in an institution and cared for by a retarded female. After demonstrating significant functional improvement, these 13 infants were placed in adoptive homes. The control group infants remained wards of the state and stayed in the institutional environment. Skeels conducted a 30-year follow-up study, and reported that the 13 infants in the experiment were self supporting and independent. In contrast, of the 12 control infants who remained in the institution, one had died, three were diagnosed as mentally retarded, four were still living in state institutions, one resided in a mental hospital, and the remaining three were in institutions for the mentally retarded. These individuals had a median IQ score of less than third grade. The experiment group completed 12th grade, and were not residents of any institution. This study demonstrated that a young child's growth and development was dependent, in part, on the early context and events in their environment in the formative years. The fact that early human development was susceptible to changing environmental conditions was revolutionary.

## SPECIAL EDUCATION

The earliest services for handicapped individuals as a group were described in the 1800s as residential facilities for the mentally disabled. In the United States, early in the 20th century, residential institutions became purely custodial and eventually housed the handicapped in depressing warehouses. The philosophy was to keep the disabled away from public view, and, thus, institutions became populated with neglected and forgotten individuals. Special Education emerged out of the practice of sending disabled children to distant institutions with limited educational experiences. The post–World War II era began a new interest in vulnerable children. As military personnel were being evaluated for war service, a surprising number of individuals with disabilities

were discovered. As a result, attitudes changed toward the disabled as veterans of the war returned home with varied disabilities. By the 1950s, state and federal legislation began to promote greater access to special education for the needs of this population. By the 1970s, landmark legislation was passed to develop early intervention programs and other federally mandated initiatives to support positive childhood development. This marked the beginning of an era of support and intervention for the handicapped. Unfortunately, at this time the focus of attention was on the handicap and not the individual or the family or the prevention of a handicap. In the 1990s, special education services in the United States shifted again to prevention efforts along with family empowerment for parents of special needs children, and numerous opportunities for these children to live full and active lives in families, classrooms, and in society.

## LEGAL ACCOMPLISHMENTS ON BEHALF OF EARLY INTERVENTIONS

Early childhood intervention during the past 60 years has demonstrated that a major policy commitment in the United States exists to provide early childhood intervention to all children, including handicapped and at-risk infants and toddlers (Hanson, 2003; Bricker, 1989; Turnbull, 1986). However, it was not always so. Before the 1970s, some children with disabilities were denied a public-school education. Services for children with disabilities were segregated, and many children were denied any access to public education. Frustrated parents organized and demanded the right to appropriate services for their children. Infants, toddlers, and preschoolers were not recipients of services at this point; however, a greater investment in the needs of disabled children was witnessed in the 1970s. A new system of services was developed in that decade that served to provide for all children, no matter what the level of disability.

## EDUCATION FOR ALL HANDICAPPED CHILDREN ACT PL 94-142 (1975)

In 1975, the Education for All Handicapped Children Act PL 94-142 guaranteed a public education for all children with disabilities. This legislation mandated individual education plans (IEPs) requiring that they be based on the results of appropriate assessment and the educational plan carried out in the least restrictive environment. The involvement of parents in carrying out the education program was also required. Financial incentives were provided for states to develop educational services for handicapped infants and toddlers, but stopped short of mandating this service (Hanson, 2003; Braddock, Hemp, & Fujiura, 1987; Braddock, Hemp, & Howes, 1987; Turnbull, 1986). Services for infants were not legislated yet, but the National Center for Clinical Infant Programs were founded by a group of concerned scientists and clinicians to focus attention on the needs of children under 3 years of age (Hanson & Lynch, 1995).

## THE INDIVIDUALS WITH DISABILITIES EDUCATION ACT (1986)

In 1986, PL 99-457, the most important legislation that has ever been enacted for the developmentally disabled and high-risk child in the United States, provided a comprehensive, coordinated, multidisciplinary, interagency program that was to be statewide for all handicapped infants and their families. The Individuals with Disabilities Education Act (IDEA) served to significantly construct the service delivery system in the United States and established a national policy of comprehensive early intervention services for all children with disabilities (Turnbull & Turnbull, 1997; Turnbull, 1986).

This law was passed in 1986, but was not fully implemented until 1990; and in 1997 was reauthorized as PL 105-17, and contained three main provisions (Hanson, 2003):

1. Establishment of the Program for Infants and Toddlers (Part C)
2. Provision of Parental Involvement and Advocacy (Part C)
3. Establishment of the Preschool Grant Program (Part B)

### The Program for Infants and Toddlers (Part C of IDEA)

The Program for Infants and Toddlers (Part C of IDEA) is a federal discretionary-grant program that assists states in planning, developing, and implement-

ing a statewide system for all children between the ages of birth and 2 years of age and their families, to provide early intervention services. Children are eligible if they are demonstrating developmental delays or difficulties based on an "appropriate assessment" (Kelly & Barnard, 2000; Meisels & Atkins-Burnett, 2000). All states and territories in the United States participate in this program. To participate, states are required to demonstrate that they can ensure early intervention is available for every eligible child, even children "at risk." To receive Part C funds and implement the program, each state must establish a lead agency to administer the services and appoint an Interagency Coordinating Council (ICC) to assist in the development and implementation of the educational services. The intent of these provisions is to overcome the existing fragmentation in services.

This law states that the family, not the child alone, is the focus of this legislation, and, thus, of this service. Current research reflects the importance of parent involvement and seeks to demonstrate that child outcomes are improved with parental involvement. Moreover, parents of disabled children are invited to advise the program. The varied services that are provided by this legislation might be in the child's home or a community child or infant care setting. Services are multidisciplinary and extensive, including speech-language pathology and audiology services; occupational and physical therapy; psychological services and diagnostic medical services; early identification screening and assessment services; vision services and social work services; assistive technology services, including technology devices, transportation, family counseling and home visits, and special educational instruction (Part C of IDEA Amendment 1997). Professionals providing these services must be qualified and include special educators, speech-language pathologists and audiologists, physical therapists, occupational therapists, social workers, nurses, nutritionists, family therapists, orientation and mobility specialists, and physicians.

### The Preschool Grants Program (Part B of IDEA)

The Preschool Grants Program (Part B of IDEA) provides free and appropriate public education and related services for children with disabilities between the ages of 3 and 5 years. Basically, this extends the services provided by IDEA, including due process, appropriate testing and assessment, individualized service plans, family involvement, and placement in least restrictive environments. The types of services provided under special education for 3- to 5-year-olds is the same as those listed for Part C. The range of conditions that qualifies a child for Part B services includes hearing impairments, speech or language impairments, visual impairments, serious emotional disturbance, orthopedic impairments, mental retardation, autism, traumatic brain injury, and learning disabilities. Eligibility is determined in most states by determining the following criteria: 2.0 standard deviations (SD) below the mean in one developmental area or 1.5 SD below the mean in two or more developmental areas (Hanson, 2003).

## WHAT LEGISLATION MEANS

The Individuals with Disabilities Education Act (IDEA), the landmark legislation for individuals with disabilities, provides the framework and funding for educational services for children with disabilities and their families. These are services that were not provided in the previous decades. Legislation provides these education services at public expense. Additional benefits include appropriate full and individual evaluation with parental consent, by an appropriately trained team in the child's native language, in a nondiscriminatory manner. In addition, an individualized education program states the child's current level of performance and includes measurable goals and objectives with dates, frequency, location, and duration of services. A focus is on child strengths, not deficits. Parental needs and concerns are included, and their right to participate in all aspects of the evaluation must be honored. Parents have full access to their child's educational records and reports. This legislation spells out the appropriate delivery of the educational services, which should include services that take into account the individual's needs in the most appropriate environment—with their peers in their own neighborhood.

## THE COMMITTEE ON INTEGRATING THE SCIENCE OF EARLY CHILDHOOD DEVELOPMENT

The Board on Children and Youth and Families of the National Research Council and the Institute of Medicine (IOM) established a 17-member committee to update scientists and childrearing specialists about the increasing knowledge of the nature of early development and the role of early experience (Shonkoff & Phillips, 2000). During the past several decades, there has been a dramatic growth in policymaking, which has led to the provision of extensive services for the disabled and high-risk children in the United States. Because several policies have now met their objectives, new goals and new approaches are called for. Members of the Committee on Integrating the Science of Early Childhood Development believe that the nation has not capitalized on the knowledge gained from the last 50 years of research regarding the development of children younger than 5 years and the impact of early experience on all aspects of subsequent development. Yet, it is thought that our growing knowledge and research capabilities have only scratched the surface.

Their mission has been to sort out what are erroneous popular beliefs from what is scientific and researched fact to make recommendations for policy, childrearing, and professional development. They have discussed the implications of the new knowledge for early childhood policy, practice, and professional research. This range of review took into account the neural circuitry of the developing brain, the child's social relationships, and cultural values in society and parenting issues. Both normal and disabled children's development was studied. The Committee has derived 10 core concepts of human development from the research that has evolved during the past 50 years (usually called an individualized family service plan [IFSP]) (Box 23-1).

The Committee called for a new national dialogue to rethink the meaning of shared responsibility for children and the strategic investment in their future. They seek to blend the knowledge of a broad range of disciplines and generate an integrated science of early childhood development while avoiding the usual debates of early childhood issues. The focus is to help professionals and parents understand children

BOX **23-1** CORE CONCEPTS IN EARLY CHILDHOOD DEVELOPMENT

1. Human development is shaped by a dynamic and continuous interaction between biology and experience.
2. Culture influences every aspect of human development and is reflected in childrearing beliefs and practices designed to promote healthy adaptation.
3. The growth of self-regulation is a cornerstone of early childhood development that cuts across all domains of behavior.
4. Children are active participants in their own development, reflecting the intrinsic human drive to explore and master one's environment.
5. Human relationships, and the effects of relationships on relationships, are the building blocks of healthy development.
6. The broad range of individual differences among young children often makes it difficult to distinguish normal variations and maturational delays from transient disorders and persistent impairments.
7. The development of children unfolds along individual pathways whose trajectories are characterized by continuities and discontinuities, as well as by a series of significant transitions.
8. Human development is shaped by the ongoing interplay among sources of vulnerability and sources of resilience.
9. The timing of early experiences can matter, but more often than not, the developing child remains vulnerable to risks and open to protective influences throughout the early years of life and into adulthood.
10. The course of development can be altered in early childhood by effective interventions that change the balance between risk and protection, thereby shifting the odds in favor of more adaptive outcomes.

From Shonkoff, J.P., & Phillips, D.A. (2000). *From neurons to neighborhoods: The science of early childhood development.* Washington, DC: National Academies Press.

and deeply appreciate the enormous task for anyone who brings up a child. As Shonkoff and Phillips(2000) states:

The time has come to stop blaming parents, communities, businesses, and government and to shape a shared agenda to ensure both a rewarding childhood and a promising future for all children . . . The charge to society is to blend the skepticism of a scientist, the passion of an advocate, the pragmatism of a policymaker, the creativity of a practitioner, and the devotion of a parent and to use the existing knowledge to ensure both a decent quality of life for all children and a productive future for the nation.

## LEGISLATION AND DEVELOPMENTAL CARE

So what is the linkage between early childhood legislation and developmental care? IDFC is a philosophy that embraces the child and family as part of a larger environment in which they grow and flourish. When

society or the scientific community cannot encourage enough support for educational programs that impact on development, then laws and legal mandates must be shaped. Health policy is derived from healthcare needs. Health policy shapes legislation. But this policy development must be based on scientific evidence to support the right pathway.

We have known for years that the prenatal environment of the fetus can affect the growth of the developing human—for better or worse (Blackburn, 2003). Through this knowledge, programs such as Women, Infants, and Children (WIC) nutrition programs administered through the Department of Agriculture grew. However, often the support for fetal/neonatal growth stopped at the basic facets of feeding/nutrition. Ornoy (2003) reported that even in the face of negative prenatal influences, such as poor maternal nutrition, substance abuse, and lower socioeconomic status, when given an enriched developmental environment, children developed more positively than expected. Although this is only one study, there are growing numbers of similar reports.

If we closely examine the major stages of human brain development, we realize that support for neurobehavioral development is critical. Products such as the Breathing Bear are being developed to support neurobehavioral stability (Novosad, & Thoman, 2003). Other research in this area includes effects of neurobehavioral assessment of feeding and weight gain (Senn & Espy, 2003); cognitive and behavioral outcomes of neonatal intensive care unit graduates (Perlman, 2002); and family-centered care (Griffin, 2003; Moore, Coker, DuBuisson, et al, 2003).

Implications for health professionals then is to take the growing evidence that supports IDFC as a philosophy to promote positive child and family outcomes. To do this, more health professionals must be aware of the current legislation that affects their practice and to become actively involved in pushing for the development and implementation of health policy where gaps are found (Allen, 2003).

## CONCLUSION

In this chapter, we reviewed the early thoughts on child development and the legislative movement in the United States that supports positive child and family outcomes. The ties to developmental care and its partnerships with the family are outlined, and the needs for the future have been explored. We have much yet to learn and much yet to develop when it comes to national policy.

## *REFERENCES*

Allen, L.K. (2003). Nurses need more education in health-care policy making. *Oncology Nursing Forum, 29*(9), 1261-1263.

Blackburn, S.T. (2003). Maternal, fetal and neonatal physiology: A clinical perspective (2nd ed.). St. Louis: W.B. Saunders.

Bloom, B.S. (1964). Stability and change in human characteristics. New York: Wiley and Sons.

Bowlby, J. (1973). *Loss: Sadness and depression (attachment and loss).* New York: Basic Books.

Braddock, D., Hemp, R., & Fujiura, G. (1987). National study of public spending for mental retardation and developmental disabilities. *American Journal of Mental Deficiency, 92*(2), 121-150.

Braddock, D., Hemp, R., & Howes, R. (1987). Financing community services in the United States: Results of a nationwide study. *Mental Retardation, 25*(1), 21-30.

Bricker, D.D. (1989) *Early intervention for at risk and handicapped infants, toddlers, and preschool children* (2nd ed.). Palo Alto, CA: Vort Corp.

Bruder, M.B., & Dunst, C.J. (2000). Expanding learning opportunities for infants and toddlers in natural environments: A chance to reconceptualize early intervention. *Zero to Three, 20*(3), 34-36.

Dunst, C.J., Trivette, C.M., & Deal, A.F. (Eds.). (1994). *Supporting and strengthening families: Methods, strategies and practices.* Cambridge, MA: Brookline Books.

Griffin, T. (2003). Facing challenges to family-centered care. I: Conflicts over visitation. *Pediatric Nursing, 29*(2), 135-137.

Hanson, M.J. (2003) National legislation for early intervention (in press).

Hanson, M.J., & Lynch, E.W. (1995). *Early intervention: Implementing child and family services for infants and toddlers who are at risk or disabled* (2nd ed.). Austin, TX: Pro-Ed.

Head Start, Economic Opportunity and Community Partnership Act of 1964, PL 93-644, 42 U.S.C. #2941 *et seq.*

Hunt, J.McV. (1961). Intelligence and experience. New York: Ronald Press.

Individuals with Disabilities Education Act (IDEA) of 1990. PL 101-476, 20 U.S.C. #1400 *et seq.*

Individuals with Disabilities Education Act Amendments of 1997. (IDEA). PL 105-17, 20 U.S.C. #1400 *et seq.*

Kelly J.F., & Barnard, K.E. (2000) Assessment for parent infant interaction: Implications for early intervention. In J.P. Shonkoff & S.J. Meisels (Eds.), *Handbook of early childhood intervention* (2nd ed.). New York: Cambridge.

Lazerson, J. (1972). The historical antecedents of early childhood education. *Education Digest, 38*, 20-23.

Locke, J. (1689). *An essay concerning human understanding* (letter). Available online at *www.ilt.columbia.edu/publications/Projects/digitexts/locke/understanding/letter.html.*

Magee, E.M. & Pratt, M.W. (1985). *1935-1985: 50 years of US federal support to promote the health of mothers, children, and handicapped children in America.* Vienna, VA: Information, Sciences Research Institute.

Meisels, S.J., & Atkins-Burnett, S. (2000) The elements of early childhood assessment. In J.P. Shonkoff & S.J. Meisels (Eds.), *Handbook of early childhood intervention* (2nd ed.). New York: Cambridge University Press.

Moore, K., Coker, K., DuBuisson, A.B., et al. (2003). Implementing potentially better practices for improving family-centered care in neonatal intensive care units: Successes and challenges. *Pediatrics, 111*(4)(Pt 2), e450-e460.

Novosad, C., & Thoman, E.B. (2003). The breathing bear: An intervention for crying babies and their mothers. *Journal of Development and Behavioral Pediatrics, 24*(2), 89-95.

Ornoy, A. (2003). The impact of intrauterine exposure versus postnatal environment neurodevelopmental toxicity: Long-term neurobehavioral studies in children at risk for developmental disorders. *Toxicology Letters*, *1*, 140-141, 171-181.

Perlman, J.M. (2002). Cognitive and behavioral deficits in premature graduates of intensive care. *Clinical Perinatology*, *29*(4), 779-797.

Senn, T.E., & Espy, K.A. (2003). Effects of neurobehavioral assessment on feeding and weight gain in preterm neonates. *Journal of Developmental and Behavioral Pediatrics*, *24*(2), 85-88.

Shonkoff, J.P., & Meisels, S.J. (2000). *Handbook of early childhood intervention* (2nd ed.). New York: Cambridge University Press.

Shonkoff, J.P., & Phillips, D.A. (Eds.). (2000). *Committee on Integrating the Science of Early Childhood Development, Board on Children, Youth, and Families. Neurons to neighborhoods: The science of early childhood development.* Washington DC: National Academies Press.

Skeels, H.M. (1966). Adult status of children with contrasting early life experiences. *Monographs of Society for Research in Child Development*, *31*(3), Serial No. 105.

Spitz, R. (1946). Hospitalism: A follow-up report: *Psychoanalytic Study of the Child*, *2*, 313-342.

Turnbull, H.R. (1986). *Free appropriate public education: The law and children with disabilities.* Denver: Love Publishing.

Turnbull, A.P., & Turnbull H.R. (1997). *Families, professionals and exceptionality: A special partnership* (3rd ed.). Columbus, Ohio: Charles E. Merrill.

Wolf, M.J., Klodewijn, K., Beelen, A., et al. (2002). Neurobehavioral and developmental profile of very low birthweight preterm infants in early infancy. *Acta Paediatrics*, *91*(8), 930-938.

# 24 Interdisciplinary Competency Validation

## Jana L. Pressler and Lynn B. Rasmussen

Competent caregivers in various healthcare disciplines are essential in providing patients with high-quality care. Competent practice in the healthcare environment is crucial for all aspects of the workforce with the increased acuity of patients and technology being used at the bedside (Lenburg, 1999). As a result, the importance of developing and maintaining competent caregivers, identifying caregivers who are performing less than competently in their caregiving assignments, and re-educating those less competent to help them become competent cannot be overemphasized.

One well-known and more recent competency requirement for neonatal healthcare practice in the intensive care nursery (ICN) and birthing areas is Neonatal Resuscitation Program (NRP) certification. In addition to the NRP, the provision of developmentally supportive care, commonly referred to simply as "developmental care," for high-risk neonates can also be considered a type of competency, although developmental care is not a universal neonatal practice throughout all ICNs at this time (Peters, 1999). In the more than 20 years since Als (1982) first described the concept of developmental care, empiric findings have been published regarding its benefits (Als, 1986; Als, Lawhon, Brown, et al., 1986; Als, Lawhon, Duffy, et al., 1994; Becker, Grunwald, Moorman, et al., 1991, 1993; Buehler, Als, Duffy, et al., 1995; Fleisher, VandenBerg, Constantinou, et al., 1995; Hendricks-Munoz, Prendergast, Caprio, et al., 2002). Nevertheless, there have been a large number of outcomes for which no or conflicting effects were demonstrated in previous studies (Symington & Pinelli, 2001).

Neonatal nurses' consensus is increasing concerning the developmental advantages they observe in infants who have received developmental care.

Empiric evidence supporting its benefits is also increasing. But despite the continuing debate over whether or not randomized, controlled trial (RCT) findings truly support its benefits and warrant it being used to justify evidence-based practice, few will argue that any negative sequelae result from its implementation (Jacobs, Sokol, & Ohllsson, 2002; Symington & Pinelli, 2001). The time might be approaching for developmental care to become a competency requirement or "standard" of practice in the ICN. In this chapter we explore the issue of competency validation as it relates to developmental care. Barriers to implementation of developmental care are discussed; these include a discussion of research and of where methodologic issues, as well as gaps, exist in our knowledge.

## WHAT IS KEEPING DEVELOPMENTALLY SUPPORTIVE CARE FROM BEING FULLY IMPLEMENTED?

Several events must take place before developmental care can serve as a standard of care within most ICNs. One fundamental revision in practice that must occur on a continuing basis is a change in the caregiving expectations of ICN healthcare providers. To set the groundwork, ICN caregivers first must expect that additional education and training concerning developmental care are pre- or co-requisites for employment. Next, concomitant administrative changes must occur, such as revised position descriptions; qualifications for bedside practice; ICN policies and procedures; orientation and continuing education priorities; and skill evaluations essential to optimize health outcomes. Administrators must financially acknowledge that the type and level of developmental care competencies of caregivers have ramifications for the planning of human resources required for the provision of developmental care. Furthermore, once achieved, maintaining the competencies of staff must be ongoing and intermittently reassessed using an appropriate method.

One of the most pivotal changes likely needed, however, is for nurses to assume accountability for leadership roles in conducting their own developmental follow-up studies and documenting the effects of developmental care. Additional follow-up studies (a type of RCT) are needed before the American Academy of Pediatrics (AAP) and individuals involved in compiling the Cochrane Controlled Trials Registry change their positions on its effectiveness (Jacobs, Sokol, & Ohllson, 2002; Symington & Pinelli, 2001) and acknowledge a more profound significance of developmental care in improving infant outcomes. According to Symington and Pinelli (2001):

Before a clear direction for practice can be supported, evidence demonstrating more consistent effects of developmental care interventions on important short- and long-term clinical outcomes is needed. More high-quality, randomized trials, undertaken by different investigators in different settings, are required to assess the effects of developmental care interventions on clinical outcomes (p. 11).

For this to take place, nurses must demonstrate a sophisticated understanding of RCT study designs and findings and more in-depth knowledge of competencies to generate a significant change in the thinking about the scientific merit of developmental care.

## The Resistance of Scientists to New Scientific Discoveries

Convincing physicians and scientists, in general, that a new approach holds significant merit is not a simple or straightforward task. As stated by Barber (1966), in a classic article, an intriguing aspect of the social process of discovery is the resistance on the part of scientists themselves (including physicians) to scientific discovery. This resistance goes against the stereotype of a scientist being "open-minded." Supposedly, the norm of open-mindedness is one of the strongest values of any scientist. However, values or beliefs alone cannot explain human behavior. In addition, no matter how great the value, any value

typically exerts its influence in combination with other cultural and social elements that sometimes promote it, and sometimes restrict it. To look at elements within science that limit open-minded activities, one must construct an accurate portrait of the actual process of scientific discovery and visualize scientists' resistance as a constant phenomenon having specific cultural and social sources.

What does all of this discourse about scientists' resistance and cultural and social stubbornness mean in terms of implementing developmental care? It means that it is imperative that detailed substantiation (RCT evidence) and formal, thorough explanations of developmental care be presented to all involved, in language that all will understand. If explanations are too vague and all-inclusive, proving little by trying to include too much, resistance can erupt and become "contagious." Largely, this is what has happened with some nurses as well as some members of the AAP. When that happens, the reception of new ideas tends to be grudging or hostile. This hostile resistance can be avoided through the inclusion of systematic, objective, and replicable studies. Cultural blinders are a constant source of resistance to innovations of all kinds. Because an established culture (e.g., neonatology) defines a situation for a group of persons, it also can blind those involved to other ways of perceiving situations. Scientists, as well as others, suffer from the irony that "good" scientific ideas currently in place occasionally obstruct the introduction of better ones. Barber (1994) noted that, generally, a new scientific truth does not triumph by convincing its opponents and making them see the light, but unfortunately because its opponents eventually die, and a new generation grows up that is familiar with the new truth. If this is true for developmental care, then it is the responsibility of informed caregivers to educate their co-workers, new employees, and students about the new knowledge concerning developmental care.

## Randomized, Controlled Trial Designs and Subsequent Results

Undoubtedly, research designs are the first concern in developing a stronger argument for use of developmental care. Some of the difficulties with previous

RCT findings reflect basic problems with research design. Symington and Pinelli (2001) reported that of the 31 studies they examined in their meta-analysis, that blindness of randomization, intervention, and adequate outcome measurement were sufficient in only nine studies (29%) and that none of the studies met all of the methodologic quality criteria that they established as warranting valid relevance. What specifically causes a study design to be invalid, and, therefore, not supportive? Campbell and Stanley (1963) articulated 12 common sources of internal and external invalidity in research designs. The sources of internal invalidity included: (1) history, (2) maturation, (3) testing, (4) instrumentation, (5) statistical regression, (6) selection, (7) mortality, (8) interaction of selection and maturation. The sources of external invalidity included: (9) interaction of testing and treatment, (10) interaction of selection and treatment, (11) reactive arrangements, and (12) multiple treatment interference. These sources of invalidity must be examined carefully, because they continue to be very important in research design and evaluation.

The second point that must be considered in RCT studies is power, or the ability of a research design to detect existing relationships if and when they occur. To do that, researchers must conduct a power analysis and determine how much power, or the number of subjects, that they need for their study to be statistically convincing. Each researcher ideally should decide, "In this study, is it worse to commit a type I or a type II error?" For a study involving developmental care as an intervention package, type I and II errors would indicate the following:

Type I Error = Claiming developmental care works, when it does not work

Type II Error = Claiming developmental care does not work, when it does work

According to an experienced biostatistician (Joseph T. Hepworth, personal communication, January 26, 2003), the dilemma reduces to balancing type I and type II errors. It is correct to say that researchers do not want to make a type I error because they do not want to say that developmental care works when it really does not produce the desired effects, because they do not want to waste valuable resources. However, researchers also do not want to make a type II error. Researchers would

not want to say that developmental care does not work, if it really does. That would mean that the intervention package is useful but would not be used because it was falsely believed to be ineffective.

The difficulties with making decisions about power are: (1) deciding whether a type I or II error is worse, and (2) deciding how much an error is worse. If the errors were equally bad, then optimally, researchers would want to set alpha and beta to be equal in the research design. That is, if the researchers set alpha to be 0.05 they would want beta to be 0.05, also. That would mean the researchers would want power to be 0.95 (1-beta). Typically, this design would yield a strong study. However, to obtain a power of 0.95, very large sample sizes are usually required.

It is interesting to examine the usual conventions that are used in research design. Typically researchers set alpha to be 0.05 and power to be 0.80. Given those parameters, a study is designed with an alpha of 0.05 and a beta of 0.20. Researchers are, thus, willing to have four times more type II error than type I error. In essence, researchers are saying that type I error is four times worse than type II error. Effect size also must be considered in the power analysis, but it is difficult to calculate unless one knows what effect (low, medium, or high) they expect an intervention to have on the outcomes of a particular population—thus, complicating the process even more.

Ideally, because the economic impact of developmental care implementation has been singled out as being a critical element before deciding on direction for practice or maintaining a given practice (Symington & Pinelli, 2001), it would be best if researchers could quantify the costs of each error. For example, if they could state that the cost of a type I error would be $1000 and the cost of a type II error would be $250, then they would be correct in setting that 4:1 ratio. This is an important reason for including an analysis of cost of caregiving in RCTs of developmental care.

The third point is that standard components of all analyses help ensure that the reported results are not produced by anomalies in the data—example: outliers, points of high influence, nonrandom missing data, subject selection problems, and attrition problems. These are considerations that must be made when completing the statistical analyses for the study.

Other problems existing with previous RCT of developmental care approaches are varied. The central concern that the AAP has voiced is that most RCTs have not been randomized, double-blind controlled studies. Obviously, those providing the care can rarely, if ever, be blind to developmental care interventions, but they can be blind to the assessors of the outcomes. Some previous problems of developmental care studies include:

1. Lack of random selection of ICN sites
2. Lack of random selection of study participants in some of the studies
3. Lack of random assignment of study participants to groups in some of the studies
4. Clinical trials have been completed in a statistically nonsignificant number of sites ($\sim$7 of more than 200 [Health Forum, 1999] tertiary level ICN sites in the United States) when multisite studies are needed if results from clinical trials are to be generalized
5. If cultural differences or other barriers exist in rural settings, the approach might only work in urbanized sites, because the previous sites used have been urban
6. Too small of a sample size (power too low)

## The Optimal Study Design for Intervention Research

In exploring the effectiveness of an intervention or package of interventions, Hepworth (Personal communication, 2003) states that the best design historically has been an experimental design—a randomized trial with a control group. In that type of design, subjects are randomized to the experimental and control conditions. Through randomization, the groups are deemed equivalent at the beginning of the study, and any differences seen at the end of the study can be attributed to the intervention or interventions. For the most part, establishing the experimental and control groups of the design is simple. The difficult part of the design is deciding exactly what should constitute the experimental and control conditions. Researchers want to keep the experimental and control conditions as

similar as possible except for the "intervention." Any additional differences between the groups could lead to the outcome differences of a group. This is why randomization works as a means to decrease these differences.

Theoretically, randomization keeps the groups equal on all variables in the long run—age, gender, temperament, family's socioeconomic status, and, most importantly, the dependent variable of interest. The only difference will be what happens after the randomization—the intervention. Therefore, what researchers try to do is make the treatment that the groups receive as similar as possible, differing only in those things that they want to report have produced the effect. Exactly what researchers want to control for will depend on the status of the body of knowledge and the questions they are trying to answer.

It is often highly desirable to have studies blinded to rule out effects caused by subjects who know that they are receiving special treatment and/or caregivers who know that they are providing special treatment—hence, the development of the placebo. Although the public typically thinks of sugar pills as placebos, in general they are any "inert" treatments given to the control subjects. Blinding neonatal participants and their families to their group assignment is possible with developmental RCTs. Blinding caregivers to the group assignment of the study subjects is far more difficult, if not impossible. Only if multiple types of intervention approaches were being conducted simultaneously would caregivers have less knowledge of which treatment or treatment package was thought to be the special treatment.

Researchers have to ask themselves where they are with understanding a particular phenomenon. What is known about "developmental care?" Undoubtedly, there are many components and many aspects of developmental care that potentially could produce different outcomes. What researchers like to do in research is to first show that an intervention produces an effect, then conduct incrementally finer-tuned studies to gain understanding concerning exactly what is producing the effect, and the associated when, where, how, and why.

## FOUR KEY CONSTRUCTS PERTINENT TO UNDERSTANDING DEVELOPMENTAL CARE COMPETENCIES

To more fully elucidate and explain what is meant by developmental care competencies, or the substantive piece of an RCT, it is important to define and discuss selected key constructs or complex concepts (Figure 24-1). Knowledge of these constructs will provide the infrastructure needed for a more careful and precise consideration of the content contained within developmental care competencies.

### Competency

What is competency? The most recent edition of the *Webster's New World College Dictionary* (Agnes, 1999) identifies competence and competency as nouns, and defines these terms similarly, as "the condition or quality of being competent; well-qualified; capable; fit; sufficient; adequate; ability; fitness" (p. 298). Two authorities on competence in the workforce refer to competence as those underlying characteristics of individuals that are casually related to criterion-related performance shown to be effective in a job (Spencer & Spencer, 1993). The underlying characteristics are believed to exist as a deep and enduring part of a person's work habits that reflects that person's activities across a variety of job tasks and situations. In the field of nursing as a whole, competencies have become very important considerations, especially in light of the nursing shortage—when job openings are plentiful and applicants are few (Institute of Medicine [IOM],

2003). Among other things, the IOM report states that a core set of competencies must be woven into health-profession education: patient-centered care, interdisciplinary teams, evidence-based practice, continuous quality improvement, and informatics.

Strodtbeck (2003) also recently discussed competencies as they pertain to neonatal nursing. Her conclusions concurred with a premise that Spencer and Spencer (1993) made 10 years earlier—that competency and competence are different. Strodtbeck then built upon Spencer and Spencer's ideas. According to Strodtbeck, competency is an ongoing process that requires that an individual demonstrates the knowledge and corresponding skills that meet the expectations of a specific professional role, whereas competence refers to the skills and abilities of the individual. Strodtbeck's recommendations echo those contained in the report by the IOM, that health professionals must be required to demonstrate competence, not simply pay a license renewal fee, to maintain their authority to practice. Strodtbeck's discussion of competency incorporated the American Nurses Association's (ANA) definitions of continuing competence and professional nursing (ANA, 2000). It is interesting to note that according to the ANA (2000), professional nursing competence behavior is based not solely upon knowledge, but also upon attitudes and beliefs.

Additionally, Benner, Tanner, and Chesla (1996), authorities on levels of expertise in nursing practice, reported that they derived their explanations of knowledge and skills reflective of competence from the Dreyfus Model of Skill Acquisition (Dreyfus,

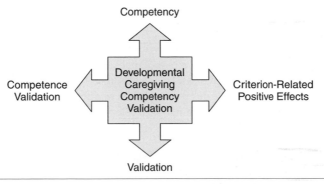

Figure **24-1** Competency validation.

1972; Dreyfus & Dreyfus, 1986). Benner, Tanner, and Chesla (1996) define competence as the increased clinical understanding, technical skills, organizational abilities, and ability to anticipate the likely course of events that typically emerge following 2 years of clinical nursing experience. To clarify what is meant by competency further, it is worthwhile to briefly consider a comment made by a renowned psychometric expert. Known for his development of the Cronbach alpha, and recognized for his expertise on measurement and reliability, Cronbach (1971) stated, "Success on the job depends on nonverbal qualities that are hard to assess" (p. 487).

Cronbach's assertion about job success appears to have been correct. Certain tacit variables that are relatively deeply embedded in a caregiver's personality (e.g., a caregiver's motives, attitudes, values, and self-confidence) can be assumed to significantly affect how caregivers' knowledge and skills are operationalized in clinical settings. However, because they are not outwardly visible, assessing and facilitating the development of those tacit, desirable variables (e.g., high motivation, positive attitudes, self-confidence) can be difficult. Spencer and Spencer (1993) recommended that when a choice exists for how to obtain specific caregiver qualities, it is more cost-effective to select for them initially when hiring, rather than trying to develop them in personnel after the fact.

Unfortunately, ICNs and intermediate care nurseries are not in a position in which they can hire all new personnel or even re-assign a number of staff members, if they do not embody the desired combination of motives, attitudes, values, and self-confidence. Instead, ICN and intermediate care nurseries are faced with working on updating, re-orienting, and re-educating staff. Those involved in continuing education are asked to help staff members achieve and maintain the desired levels of developmental care competencies while simultaneously, promptly, and courteously integrating reinforcement for the desired behaviors and their modifiers (e.g., high motivation, positive attitudes toward life-long learning, self-confidence). It is crucial that these education activities be managed using a gentle and co-regulatory process that is congruent with and sets an example for developmental care (Als & Gilkerson, 1997).

## Criterion-Related Positive Effects

What are criterion-related positive effects? How can nurses be assured that their educative efforts have been successful and are reliable strategies worthy of endorsement? To answer these questions, one must refer to basic psychometric principles. Traditionally psychometricians discuss the terms criterion-referenced or criterion-related when they discuss the reliability of something. "Criterion-related" generally means that something has been measured according to a specific criterion or standard. Therefore, in this case, to have criterion-related reliability, or criterion-related positive effects, developmental care competencies actually should: (1) reflect and/or (2) predict the work completed (hopefully the effects are positive) as measured according to a specific criterion or standard. Furthermore, one can technically distinguish between two types of criterion-related validity (Carmines & Zeller, 1979). If the criterion exists concurrently, then correlating a measure and the criterion at the same point in time assesses *concurrent validity*. If the criterion exists in the future, then correlating the relevant measures with a future criterion assesses *predictive validity*. The logic for both types of criterion-related validity is the same; the only difference concerns the present or future existence of the criterion variable.

It should be acknowledged that criterion-related validity contains an intuitive meaning not shared by other types of validity. Also, because, even under the best of circumstances, performance can be challenging to measure, Cronbach (1971) has recommended that all validation reports include the warning, "insofar as the criterion is truly representative of the outcome we wish to maximize" (p. 488). Here, it is important to emphasize that criterion-validation procedures cannot be applied to all measurement situations in all healthcare settings. As Symington and Pinelli (2001) have pointed out, it is critical that more high-quality RCTs be undertaken by different investigators in different settings to assess the true effects of developmental care on clinical outcomes. A reason criterion-related effects must be examined is that the most relevant criterion variables might not have been identified. For example, it would be difficult to establish an accurate measure of some kinds of personality traits, such as the self-confidence and contentedness sometimes associated with developmental care that could be generalized across populations. Specific types of behavior that people with high or low self-confidence or contentedness demonstrate are not understood to the extent that they could be used to validate measures of those personality traits.

## Validation

What is validation? Understanding the meaning of validation requires one important distinction. This distinction is that "one validates *not a test*, but *one's interpretation of data*" arising from a certain evaluative process (Cronbach, 1971, p. 447). This distinction is central to any validation, because when one validates, s/he is validating the measuring tool in relation to the purpose for which it is being used, not the measuring tool in and of itself. To assess for and validate the existence of competencies, minimum entry-level criteria, or standards for practice effectiveness must be established. Then, the validation of achievement and maintenance of these standards must be completed systematically. Some developmental care competencies have been proposed and are summarized later in this chapter. However, at this time, the actual standards for developmental care practices are hypothetical and nonspecific, in that they have yet to be formally validated using RCTs whereby what constitutes the minimal data set for practice has been tested.

## Competence Validation

What is competence validation? To determine what the previous discussion about competencies, criterion-related positive effects, and validation means with respect to developmental care competencies, competence validation must be a final consideration in establishing the knowledge infrastructure for developmental care. According to Loving (1991, 1993), competence validation within nursing is a special type of validation that refers to a process of identifying some type of competency, or to the overall competency of an individual nurse. Emanating from the ideas of Kuhn (1970) and Polanyi (1962) of "knowing that" and "knowing how", Simpson and Creehan (1998) claim that there are two components essential to any nursing competence

validation: (1) knowledge-based evaluation (knowing "that") and (2) clinical skills verification (knowing "how"). Given that knowledge of "that" and "how" is constantly being revised and updated based on the latest replicated research findings (a.k.a., evidence-based practice), competence validation in nursing exists as a dynamic process that requires thoughtful and intermittent evaluation on an ongoing and planned basis. Therefore, for caregivers to maintain current competencies, they must engage in continuing education programs of one sort or another and partake in regular reading or self-studies to remain abreast of new information and how to better perform particular clinical skills.

Lenburg (1999) advocated using a competency-based model for nursing education as recently as 5 years ago. Lenburg's Competency Outcomes and Performance Assessment (COPA) model might prove helpful in the ongoing creation and validation of competencies related to didactic and clinical aspects of developmental care. According to the COPA model, a competency performance system that is psychometrically sound incorporates the concepts of objectivity, acceptability, consistency, flexibility, and comparability. Using theory and research to develop competencies in a competency performance system is ideal. Burleson's (2001) findings from a study identifying the essential knowledge elements and skills and the competencies for newborn developmental specialists might provide insight into what a developmental care competency system should include.

## DEVELOPMENT OF DEVELOPMENTAL CARE COMPETENCIES

After examining the preceding constructs related to or constituting competency validation, one might deduce that it is premature to begin validating developmental care competencies due to insufficient support by RCTs. However, because preterm infants are continuing to require intensive care, some important benefits have been identified, no negative sequelae to infants who have received developmental care have been shown, and nurses and other caregivers do not want to lose the momentum that has been generated, it seems reasonable to speculate that developmental care is needed and will continue to be needed. Parents and families are beginning to request developmental care, with parents from support groups endorsing it within Internet chats. Therefore, neonatal nurses, as well as others involved in care of infants in ICNs, must forge ahead and become competent developmental caregivers while concomitantly studying its effects.

Where do caregivers begin in their implementation of a developmental care competency system? From a logistical standpoint, it appears that nurses should be first to participate in the implementation of developmental care competencies of the various health professionals involved in caring for newborns and infants. If competency validation for developmental care achieves widespread acceptance, parents, family members, other healthcare providers, and support service workers ought to be the next individuals expected to demonstrate developmental care competencies (Figure 24-2). The fields comprising the particular healthcare or supportive-service workers, in addition to nursing are: medicine, unlicensed nurses' aides, respiratory therapy, physical therapy, infant massage therapists, occupational therapy, clinical psychologists, feeding-team members, speech therapy, special education, radiology technicians, laboratory technicians, social work, unit secretaries, housekeeping, nutrition/dietetics, pharmacy, chaplains, child life specialty, music therapy, maintenance workers, and medical ethics. Students of various disciplines (nurses, medical students, resident physi-

cians, and neonatal fellows) should be included too. All of these groups need relevant information, demonstration of applied knowledge, and competency evaluation or validation as deemed appropriate (Figure 24-3). Each part of the educative process requires effective learning materials, approaches, and evaluative tools. Administrators must also be educated to understand the importance of developmental care and the resources required to implement it.

## Basic Nursing Education

Determining what action should be taken first in the development of developmental care competencies has several possibilities. Ideally, the essential first step in designing a workable system for validating nurse competency in developmental care would be to include it in basic nursing education. In an ideal world, education regarding developmental care for high-risk infants would be included in the core curriculum for nursing students. The National Council of State Boards of Nursing (NCSBN) would be responsible for ensuring the competency of nurses in developmental care, because the National Council Licensure Examination (NCLEX) would test this knowledge. Once licensed, a mechanism for continuing competence could be a mandate for continuing education units in developmental care. However, because a nurse's specialty area is rarely, if ever, included in state boards, an examination for the "generalist" graduate registered nurse, the reality of this approach seems remote.

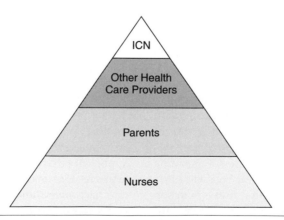

Figure 24-2 Prioritizing competency validation.

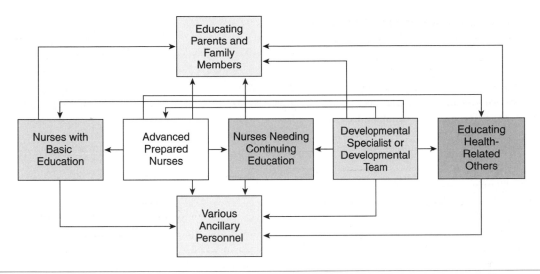

Figure **24-3** Competency in developmental care.

## Continuing Nurse Education Professional Development

Strodtbeck (2003) cautioned that ultimately each nurse must be accountable for his or her own competencies in the practice of neonatal nursing. Aligned with Strodtbeck's thoughts, including the desired competencies in each ICN orientation program could be the most realistic and practical first step in designing a workable system for validating caregiver competency in developmental care. There are several resources available to guide this process. Local competent ICN caregivers can develop program content, or it can be purchased directly through a Newborn Individualized Developmental Care Assessment Program (NIDCAP®) (Boston, MA) trainer or a freelance developmental care expert. Selected resources are listed in Table 24-1. Competencies appropriate to each individual ICN can be adopted from these recommendations into each ICN orientation program as a starting point. Furthermore, many hospitals cross-train nurses to work in more than one clinical area so that orientation to a philosophy of individualized, family-centered, developmental care (IFDC) must be available to these nurses as well. Others employ agency nurses. Therefore, it is critically important that all orientation programs to areas that provide

care to newborns/infant and family care include developmental care competencies.

In a joint venture, the Association of Women's Health, Obstetric, and Neonatal Nursing (AWHONN) and the National Association of Neonatal Nurses (NANN) published recommendations for the orientation and development of neonatal nurses (AWHONN, 1997). In the recommendations' definition of the role of a neonatal nurse, no mention was made of developmental care other than a neonatal nurse "may focus in an area of expertise... such as developmental care" (p. 9). Specific recommendations in that publication concerning developmental care were listed under general considerations for admissions and were very vague: "(1) Provide a suitable environment; (2) Note infant's state and modify exam as needed; (3) Handle infant gently; (4) Warm hands and equipment as needed" (p. 13). In all levels of newborn care units, the verification of clinical skills was recommended and included, "modify the environment to reduce noxious stimuli and pain," and "maximize neurobehavioral development" (AWHONN, 1997, p. 25). Specialty nursing organizations as well as other organizations, such as the Joint Commission on Accreditation of Healthcare Organizations (JCAHO) and the IOM, can play a powerful role in promoting specialized

**Table 24-1**   Sources for Recommended Competencies/Guidelines for Developmental Care

| Title | Authors | Internet Site | Content Summary |
|---|---|---|---|
| Program guide: Newborn Individualized Development Care Assessment Program (NIDCAP®). An education and training program for health professionals (rev. ed.) | Als, H. (2001) Boston, MA: Boston Children's Medical Center Corporation | *www.nidcap.com* (free download) | Developmental education and training program with NIDCAP® competency and reliability testing. Goal: A shift from task-oriented, protocol-based caregiving to individualized, relationship-based care. General topics:<br>• Theoretical framework: Synactive Theory of Development (Als, 1982)<br>• Assessment and documentation of infant's behaviors<br>• Recommendations for modifications of care<br>• Structure of a developmentally supportive environment<br>• Developmentally supportive care interventions and supports<br>• Education and support of parents in the caretaking of their infant<br>• Guidance for facilitation and implementation of developmental care in the ICN |
| Developmental support in the neonatal intensive care unit | Koch (1999) | *www.awhonn.org* | Implement intervention strategies to foster parent-infant interaction. Assess infant behavior according to synactive theory. Assess an infant's unique behavioral style and provide individual intervention programs. Facilitate an infant's neurosocial behavioral organization by organizing care contingent on cues and effecting change within the ICN environment. Didactic content on all the above, along with neuromotor, auditory, and feeding information. |
| Infant developmental care guidelines for practice | NANN (2001) | *www.nann.org* | General principles:<br>• Introduce one intervention at a time.<br>• Cluster caregiving when possible and observe/respond to infant behaviors.<br>• Gently arouse infant before caregiving.<br>• Remain at bedside after caregiving to determine/intervene in infant responses. |

**Table 24-1** Sources for Recommended Competencies/Guidelines for Developmental Care—cont'd

| Title | Authors | Internet Site | Content Summary |
|---|---|---|---|
| | | | • Provide "time-out" when maladaptive signs/symptoms are present<br>• Continually reassess physiologic and behavioral responses to caregiving<br>• Potential interventions that will facilitate adaptation: alter physical surroundings; facilitate handling; facilitate parenting |
| Developmental interventions for preterm and high-risk infants | Staff of The Children's Hospital, Denver, Colorado. Creger (1989) | NA | Six content modules, each with self-tests:<br>• Developmental interventions<br>• Neuromotor development of the premature infant<br>• Development and enhancement of vision in the hospitalized infant<br>• Assessment of the auditory system and follow-up of the Infant at rIsk for hearing loss<br>• Developmentally supportive positioning and therapeutic handling of the hospitalized infant<br>• Neurodevelopmental assessment of feeding abilities and follow-up of the disorganized feeder |
| Basic competencies to begin developmental care in the intensive care nursery | VandenBerg (1993) | NA | Primary knowledge base:<br>• Normal infant development<br>• Atypical infant development<br>• Family dynamics and function<br>Specialized knowledge base:<br>• Fetal and newborn brain development<br>• Medical conditions of premature and full-term infants<br>• Neonatal preterm and full-term infant behaviors and development<br>• Ecology of the ICN<br>• Staffing patterns and the cultural patterns in the ICN<br>• Parenting in the ICN |
| Competencies for developmental care | VandenBerg & Becker (1996) | NA | See Table 1 (pp. 66-67 of article) |

*Continued*

SOURCES FOR RECOMMENDED COMPETENCIES/GUIDELINES FOR DEVELOPMENTAL CARE—CONT'D

|  | Authors | Internet Site | Content Summary |
|---|---|---|---|
| Neuromuscular and sensory systems | Blackburn (2003) | NA | Fetal and neonatal neurodevelopment<br>Referenced recommendations for clinical practice related to the neuromuscular and sensory systems in neonates |
| Newborn and infant neurobehavioral development | Holditch-Davis, Blackburn, & VandenBerg (2003) | NA | Fetal and neonatal central nervous system development<br>Neonatal neurobehavioral development<br>Assessment of neonatal neurobehavioral development<br>ICN environment<br>The developmental intervention approach<br>Guidelines for providing developmental support<br>Effectiveness of individualized developmental care<br>Intervention strategies<br>Application of intervention strategies to specific situations<br>Collaborative care<br>Sleep-wake states<br>State scoring systems<br>Effect of physiologic parameters on state<br>Effect of nursing interventions on state |

*ICN*, Intensive care nursery.

competencies of nurses (Whittaker, Smolenski, & Carson, 2000).

Given that the National Certification Corporation (NCC), Chicago, IL already offers certification examinations in electronic fetal monitoring, breastfeeding, and neonatal nursing, a developmental care competency certification requirement to practice neonatal nursing seems a viable possibility. Developmental care content is covered on the NCC neonatal intensive care nursing examination. However, developmental care is not listed as a content area for either the low-risk neonatal nursing or the maternal newborn nursing examination. Starting in 2003, NCC offers self-learning modules for neonatal continuing education. Perhaps the NCC will consider offering a developmental care self-study module, and/or a developmental care subspecialty examination to meet neonatal nurses' competency validation needs. Even if the NCC offers such an examination, this type of certification most likely would cover only didactic knowledge, not performance of clinical activities, and would be voluntary, rather than a required certification to practice neonatal nursing.

One strategy for providing continuing education concerning developmental care might be to require developmental care competency in specific situations. The environmental and behavioral strategies of developmental care have been recommended as an essential component in the prevention and management of neonatal pain (Franck & Lawhon, 2000).

These nonpharmacologic strategies have been supported by research findings and by significant decreases in demonstrated pain scores (Stevens, Johnston, Franck, et al., 1999; Sizun, Ansquer, Browne, et al., 2002).

Perhaps individual institutions should take responsibility for mounting the first step toward establishing and requiring competency validation of developmental care by neonatal nurses. Nursing leaders at each institution who have developmental care experience, confidence in the existing empiric evidence supporting developmental care practices, and belief in its benefits could oversee the competency validation. As these institutions enact competency requirements, their units could provide developmental care benchmarks for other neonatal care units around the country and internationally. Development of family-centered caregiving benchmarks have already begun to occur within the Vermont Oxford Network (Saunders, Abraham, Crosby, et al., 2003).

## Developmental Nursing Education

Holditch-Davis, Blackburn, and VandenBerg (2003) summarized two formal educational programs presenting a comprehensive approach to the education of healthcare providers about developmental care and its implementation in the ICN. These programs are NIDCAP® and the Wee Care® program (Norwell, MA). In describing the Wee Care Program, Jorgensen (2002) compared its formal educational program for unit implementation of developmental care to the NIDCAP® model. She stated that although most published outcome studies are based on the NIDCAP® model, unpublished outcomes using the Wee Care® model also appear positive. In a recent study of the impact of Wee Care on hospitalized preterm infants, decreased hospital costs and short-term infant outcomes that were evaluated as "beneficial" were demonstrated (Hendricks-Munoz, Prendergast, Caprio, et al., 2002).

## Additional Considerations Regarding Competency Education

Several approaches can be used to educate non-nurse caregivers in developmental care. It is the responsibility of each ICN to establish the level of knowledge and expertise desired by various caregivers and infant contacts, and designate qualified evaluators. For ease in recording evaluations that have been completed, it is advisable to keep a checksheet so that everyone in the particular ICN knows the level of preparation of different individuals (Figure 24-4).

Parents and family members should receive their basic instruction from the infant's bedside nurses, with opportunities given for return demonstrations of caregiving. If the institution employs a developmental care specialist, that individual can work with parents and family members in terms of assessing and validating their caregiving competencies. If the institution does not have a developmental care specialist, then the institution might consider creating a developmental care team involving nurses and other health-related caregivers (e.g., occupational specialist, physical therapist, clinical psychologist) to fulfill these responsibilities. It seems more appropriate for physicians and other non-nurse caregivers to receive their initial instruction and competency validation from a developmental care specialist or developmental care team members who are familiar with the empiric literature on developmental care and can substantiate the scientific basis for different techniques.

All interested professionals are encouraged to attend national presentations on developmental care. There are at least two national conventions at which developmental care interventions are discussed on an annual or biannual basis. These conferences are the University of South Florida's Physical and Developmental Environment of the High-Risk Infant annual meeting in Clearwater Beach, FL, and Contemporary Forum's Developmental Interventions in Neonatal Care Conference (biannual, in different U.S. cities. Should a caregiver desire to become nationally certified in developmental care assessments or to only attend a formal training session, there are nine formal training sites for NIDCAP® certification in the United States (Box 24-1).

Although the focus of this competency discussion has centered on nurses, other disciplines are moving forward on this issue as well. The roles of physical and occupational therapists in the NICU and their discipline-specific competencies are examined in Chapter 26.

| Group | Caregiver Group or Contact Persons | Apprised Only | | Developmental Knowledge Evaluated | | Developmental Care Skills Evaluated | | |
|---|---|---|---|---|---|---|---|---|
| | | Initially | Ongoing & PRN | Initially | Annually & PRN | Initially | Annually & PRN | Nationally Certified |
| 01 | Family Members | | | | | | | |
| 02 | Nurses | | | | | | | NA |
| 03 | Physicians | | | | | | | |
| 04 | Unlicensed Nursing Aides | | | | | | | |
| 05 | Respiratory Therapists | | | | | | | NA |
| 06 | Students | | | | | | | |
| 07 | Physical Therapists | | | | | | | |
| 08 | Infant Massage Therapists | | | | | | | |
| 09 | Occupational Therapists | | | | | | | |
| 10 | Clinical Psychologists | | | | | | | |
| 11 | Feeding Team Members | | | | | | | |
| 12 | Speech Therapists | | | | | | | |
| 13 | Special Educators | | | | | | | |
| 14 | Radiology Technicians | | | | | | | NA |
| 15 | Laboratory Technicians | | | | | | | NA |
| 16 | Social Workers | | | | | | | NA |
| 17 | Unit Secretaries | | | | | | | NA |
| 18 | Housekeepers | | | | | | | NA |
| 19 | Nutritionists/Dieticians | | | | | | | NA |
| 20 | Pharmacists | | | | | | | NA |
| 21 | Chaplains | | | | | | | NA |
| 22 | Child Life Specialists | | | | | | | NA |
| 23 | Music Therapists | | | | | | | NA |
| 24 | Maintenance Workers | | | | | | | NA |
| 25 | Medical Ethicists | | | | | | | NA |

Figure **24-4** Developmental care competency validation checklist for various intensive care nursery personnel.

## ONLINE DEVELOPMENTAL CARE EDUCATION

Two Internet sites were found offering online educational materials concerning family-centered developmental care of neonates. One is the Wee Care® program offered from Children's Medical Ventures Corporation in Norwell, MA. It is located at *www.childmed.com/education/wee_program.asp*. The other is the NIDCAP®, offered by the Boston Children's Hospital, Boston, MA. It is located at *www.nidcap.com/nidcap/*. The techniques discussed by Wee Care® are very practical and generic, and easily applied to all neonates in ICNs and intermediate care nurseries and their families. The techniques discussed in the NIDCAP® are individualized and should be implemented only after an assessment has been made by a certified NIDCAP® tester that includes interventions designed for individual newborns and their families.

### Wee Care Works

The 17-member, interdisciplinary professional team at Wee Care® has devised a program of family-centered developmental care. Using an approach that incorporates interventions involving light, sound, special pacifiers, bumper rolls, blankets,

<u>Box</u> **24-1**   NIDCAP® TRAINING CENTERS*

| Location | Director |
| --- | --- |
| 1. National NIDCAP® Center Boston, MA | Heidelise Als, PhD |
| 2. Sooner NIDCAP® Regional Training Center Oklahoma, OK | Laurie Mouradian, ScD, OTR/L |
| 3. Carolina NIDCAP® Training Center Raleigh, NC | James M. Helm, PhD |
| 4. Colorado NIDCAP® Center Denver, CO | Joy V. Browne, PhD RN |
| 5. West Coast NIDCAP® Training Center Mills Col., Oakland, CA | Kathleen A. VandenBerg, PhD RN |
| 6. St. Luke's NIDCAP® Center Boise, ID | Jerry Hirschfeld, MD |
| 7. Mid-Atlantic NIDCAP® Training Center Camden, NJ | Karen M. Smith, BSN, MEd, RNC; Deana DeMare, PT |
| 8. The NIDCAP® Training Center of Milwaukee, Milwaukee, WI | Laura Robison, MSN RNC |
| 9. Scandinavian NIDCAP® Center Lund & Stockholm, Sweden | Karin Stjernqvist, PhD |
| 10. NIDCAP® Training Center at the University of Connecticut Health Center Farmington, CT | Catherine Daguio, MEd, MPH, OTR/L |

*Listed by order of start date.

and infant seats, they have identified the following results: decreased costs, decreased length of stay, decreased time spent in restraints, fewer numbers of morbidities, increased parent satisfaction, and improved staff morale. At this time, their online education offers specific videotaped programs on: (1) individualized family-focused touch and massage; (2) swaddled bathing; and (3) developmentally supportive positioning. In addition, more comprehensive educational programs with team members on site are available, as well as telephone consultation and follow-up visits.

The premise underlying Wee Care® is that developmentally supportive care should be beneficial for all children in a children's hospital, not solely infants. Consequently, trainees in these education programs are instructed on how to apply the principles across developmental levels. The Wee Care® program asserts that changes made in the hospital environment can enhance patient care, increase patient and family satisfaction, and increase cost-effectiveness institutionwide. They state that although the program was designed to meet the needs of high-risk infants and families of the NICU, it may also be appropriate for extracorporeal membrane oxygenation (ECMO) units, transport teams, surgical populations, and cardiac care.

## NIDCAP®

The NIDCAP® provides education and training in developmental observation and assessment for healthcare professionals responsible for the long- and short-term care of high-risk newborns, preterm infants, and families, and for relevant staff involved in care implementation (Als, 2001). A major focus of the NIDCAP® is its neurodevelopmentally supportive, individualized, and family-centered framework. Better understanding of the developing nervous system can be gleaned through assessment and documentation of infants' competence and behavioral reactions to stress and caregiving. In structuring the physical and social environment to be supportive, it is important to remember that the individual infant's immature nervous system and the family's sense of competence are critical to the care of infants in both the ICN and the home.

The NIDCAP® care approach guides caregivers in shifting from protocol-based to strategic process thinking, and from task-oriented to relationship-based care. This approach sees infants as active participants in their own development, supported by the ongoing co-regulation process of infant and parent development. Developmental care based on the NIDCAP® approach emphasizes the infant's expectation for co-regulatory care and for a close and invested relationship. This approach identifies opportunities for increased effectiveness of ICN care delivery in supporting the newborn and family. Implementation of intensive care in such a framework requires knowledge and understanding of infant, parent, and family development, and of the interaction of the infant's medical issues with her/his development. Because skill and sensitivity are required in supporting and nurturing infants and their family, the NIDCAP® program seeks to provide information, education, and support by provision of reading materials, didactic presentations, observation training, and individual and system guidance and consultation.

In the NIDCAP® behavioral observation methodology, specific estimates of each individual infant's current goal strivings are derived from the direct observation of each infant's behavior in the context of ongoing care delivery. The NIDCAP® and its systematic formal evaluation, called the Assessment of Preterm and Full-Term Infants' Behavior (APIB) (Als, Lester, Tronick, & Brazelton, 1982), are particularly geared to understanding of the preterm and otherwise at-risk newborn's behavior. Both methodologies (the NIDCAP® observation and the APIB) are based in the Synactive Theory of Infant Development (Als, 1979, 1982, 2001) and are designed to specifically document the complexity and sensitivity of the preterm and the at-risk newborn infant by focusing on the infant's autonomic, motoric, state organizational, and attentional functioning as the infant interacts with the caregiver and her/his surroundings.

The online information available at the NIDCAP® website includes a discussion of the NIDCAP®

and provides a download of the *Program Guide on NIDCAP® Nursery Development*. There are no NIDCAP® self-studies or training videos currently available. The goal of all NIDCAP® training and consultation is effective developmental care implementation throughout the nursery. Training is currently available from nine NIDCAP® centers in the United States and one in Sweden (see Box 24-1). Usually, it is thought that moving toward successful delivery of newborn ICN care in a developmental framework requires a minimum of 5 years for full implementation (Als, 2001).

## PRECEPTORS FOR DEVELOPMENTAL CARE

Ideally, developmental care should be part of nurse preceptor programs and something introduced by nurse preceptors in a new nurse's orientation to caregiving in the ICN. In nursing, a preceptor is assigned to serve as a role model of optimal care and to coordinate the orientation of new nurse employees. Most, if not all, ICNs have formal preceptor programs educating experienced nurses about the role and functions of preceptors. Typically, a designated preceptor works alongside one or more new nurses for several weeks, provides instruction concerning selected care practices, and validates competencies at the completion of the orientation program. ICNs that do not use a formal preceptor might rely on several senior staff nurses, a nurse educator, or clinical nurse specialist to perform similar functions to those of a nurse preceptor.

Experienced and inexperienced nurses have different levels of knowledge, skill, confidence, and familiarity with caring for neonates. Therefore, although having a timeframe for acquiring and achieving competent behaviors is helpful for planning for ICN staffing, orientation should be individualized to meet each employee's educational requirements. Before ending an orientation program for an individual nurse, either the designated preceptor or the developmental specialist should be responsible for checking off the new nurse's competency behaviors for developmental care as established specifically by that institution (see Figure 24-4), with definite criteria for what is expected. More discussion about constructing these definitive criteria follows.

## ASSESSING, VALIDATING, AND FURTHERING CAREGIVER DEVELOPMENTAL CARE COMPETENCIES

To assess and validate the fact that caregiver competencies exist, it is of utmost importance to establish minimum entry-level standards of performance. Standards of competency can be described in two ways (Dawes, 1995; Zettle, 1995). They can be discussed in terms of prescriptive competencies for excellence that are "hortatory," or the "thou shalts," and they also can be discussed in terms of the proscriptive competencies that are "minatory," or the "thou shalt nots." The hortatory competencies are positive and consistent with levels of excellence of performance. The minatory competencies are negative, similar to most of the Ten Commandments. *Simply following the minatory rules by not breaking them is not satisfactory*, or regarded adequate to be considered competent. In contrast, the problem with hortatory rules is that there is the hortatory standard itself, and then there is the "not exactly the hortatory standard." The clinical pressures of functioning in an uncertain and imperfect environment lead those who are responsible for enforcing the desired standards to admit that they cannot realistically insist that bedside caregivers understand the competencies completely, perform maximally, and intervene to the highest standards of providing health care. Therefore, those who are responsible for enforcing the standards must make compromises in judging caregivers by hortatory standards.

It is important to recognize that standards of practice must guide caregivers in how they actually practice and what they do—and not how they have been trained, think about practice, or discuss practice. Those who believe in such constraints are accustomed to hearing the common complaint that "science" does not provide sufficient information for practitioners to practice. Although it is true that standards for competency do not yield knowledge of exactly what to do when, caregivers themselves have basic knowledge of providing care and follow basic principles for providing care (e.g., safety, asepsis, ethics).

## THE USE OF RESPECT

Once decisions by an expert collective (e.g., a developmental team) have been made about how competencies are to be assessed and validated, how can competencies be fostered? One of the most powerful ingredients in nurturing relationships and creating fair treatment is the use of respect. *Webster's New World College Dictionary* defines respect for an individual as feeling or showing concern, honor, or esteem for someone and holding that person in high regard (Agnes, 1999). Respect can be operationalized through dialogue, attention, curiosity, healing, empowerment, and by means of self-respect. However, to gain respect, one must give respect (Lawrence-Lightfoot, 2000). Those in charge must be seriously interested in who their staff members are, and in what they have to say. To gain allegiance to developmental care, those staff members in charge must offer their fellow staff their own knowledge and positive reinforcement for what they know, rather than threatening to overpower them. If this does not occur, a quiet but forceful resistance (e.g., a silent informal opposition) to disrespect is likely to coalesce. Although respect is commonly seen as deference to hierarchy driven by duty, and many times based conditionally upon a person's position of authority, respect derived from equality, empathy, and connection in all kinds of relationships might prove to be a more successful use.

## KNOWING WHEN A NURSERY HAS TRUE STANDARDS FOR COMPETENCY

To be realistic about enforcing standards of competency, those in charge can only expect to enforce minatory rules. Therefore, whatever a caregiver does, her/his behavior has to be consistent with what experts in the field believe is known as being true. In any case, for a particular purpose, those in charge might not be able to tell caregivers exactly what to do, such as to follow an exact treatment algorithm that indicates a desirable intervention for each newborn client's condition or behavior of concern. Such exact guidelines do not exist. But those in charge should want caregiving to be consistent with what is believed true. Those in charge of enforcing minatory standards of competency must be willing to take action to halt "out-of-bounds" behavior, to the point of disciplining those who engage in it.

For example, what does saying that a given ICN has high standards for competency in developmental care actually mean?

1. Does this simply mean that an expert collective directs the nursery staff: "to be excellent"?
2. Does this mean that an expert collective ends there with that directive, with expectations that staff will work hard, and as evidence of caregivers' successes, gives out only the highest salary increases and evaluations, no matter what their fellow caregivers do?

Those in charge should not give out the highest salary increases and evaluations to those who only sometimes, rather than always, provide patients with appropriate developmental care when an expert collective states that they have high standards for competency. As difficult as it might be, those in charge of developmental care must be willing to confront less than competent caregivers and tell them that their work does not meet the standards of the nursery for high competency in developmental interventions. Such a statement is a minatory statement, and only when those in charge are willing to endorse these statements does that nursery have true standards for competency.

Training caregivers well in how to perform developmental interventions is not sufficient to ensure good performance. Simply saying, "be good, be excellent, be outstanding," combined with "no matter what you do, I'll reinforce you so that you don't notice that you're making gradual improvements in your performance" is not going to be effective.

Those in charge of ensuring that developmental interventions are performed competently must be willing to say, "This is not acceptable. I could be mistaken, but I'm in a position in which I have to exercise my expert judgment and knowledge, and I have determined that this is not acceptable." If those in charge of a particular ICN are not willing

to inform caregivers when their behavior is unacceptable, there will be no standards for competency, and the ICN of interest will be functioning under only a pretense of developmental competency.

## THE REQUISITE OF CAREFUL PLANNING

A final, but very crucial step in fostering competencies in developmental care is through constructing a plan for action. The word "plan" can be both a noun and a verb, referring to a design that guides action and the acts encompassing the design (Covington, 1987). Planning involves thinking out and documenting acts and purposes beforehand to effectively achieve goals (Scholnick, 1995). Furthermore, the very act of planning has been equated with problem-solving itself because planning plays such a central role in problem-solving (Friedman, Scholnick, & Cocking, 1987). When the costs and risks of making mistakes are high (e.g., the money involved in developmental care training and the money wasted by a lack of endorsement of developmental care by staff), efforts need to be devoted to internal cognitive processing to forego the cost of recovering from making errors and acting inefficiently.

The study of planning is central in trying to explain the interaction of motivation and cognition in intelligent behavior. Planning requires the ability to inhibit actions while thinking through the best way possible to achieve goals. Competency-based workforce planning involves addressing motivation, factual knowledge, intellectual/cognitive level, and interpersonal and psychomotor skills (Simpson & Creehan, 1998). Proven methods for teaching and maintaining competencies exist and have been documented extensively (Griener & Knebel, 2003). Several examples include mastery learning (Block, 1971; Guskey, 1997; MacTurk & Morgan, 1995); discovery learning (Fujishin, 1997); interpersonal skills training (Carcuff, 2000; Wondrak, 1998); cooperative learning (Kagan, 1994); adult education and training (Jarvis, 1995); apprenticeships (Summerfield & Cosgrove, 1994); and internships (Ciofalo, 1992).

## DESIGNING AND MODIFYING DEVELOPMENTAL CARE INTERVENTIONS

In summary, to implement developmental care in an ICN or nursery, those in charge must give their fellow caregivers respect to gain respect for their authority. Second, those in charge of overseeing the implementation must be willing to enforce minatory standards and speak up and take action when care providers are not demonstrating acceptable behavior. Third, a plan must be developed and put into operation for nursery caregivers to both develop and maintain competency in developmental care. Once developmental care competency is established, either a developmental specialist or developmental team needs to assume responsibility for overseeing that competencies are maintained. The overall treatment design must take into consideration the competency levels of those involved in the planning, implementation, evaluation, and revision of care. Refer again to Figure 24-4 for a grid of a plan for developing and maintaining competency levels of various caregivers.

## INCORPORATING DEVELOPMENTAL CARE INTO PHYSICAL EXAMINATIONS

Because they occur at least daily and, usually, more frequently, it seems safe to recommend that all physical examinations of neonates incorporate approaches integral to developmental care without looking further at each and every individual ICN caregiving activity that potentially can be implemented. Direct handling, positioning, lighting, and sound levels at the bed space, bedding, and the inclusion of families should be considered. To do this appropriately, however, neonatal nurse practitioners and physicians must be informed and kept up to date on new RCT evidence concerning the specific developmental care interventions that are most effective.

## PARTIAL RATIONALE FOR COMPETENCY: PREVENTION OF COMPLICATIONS

The word "prevention" grew into its current meaning by the 15th century (Bloom, 1996). The Latin root of prevention "to come before" (Simpson,

1993, p. 111), continues to be the core meaning: to take action before some untoward set of circumstances occurs so as to preclude, delay, or reduce its occurrence in some population or person at risk; and/or to excel. In health care, prevention refers to actions taken by caregivers to minimize and eliminate those social, psychologic, or other conditions known to cause, contribute, or relate to illness and sometimes, to socioeconomic problems. Those actions include establishing conditions in society that enhance the opportunities for individuals, families, and groups to achieve goals. Likewise, these actions include establishing conditions that enhance the evidence of significant negative sorts of circumstances. Caplan (1964) expanded and qualified prevention in psychiatry to include primary, secondary, and tertiary prevention. However, because his distinctions required examples and considerable explanation to achieve clarity, Klein and Goldson (1977) proposed simplifying Caplan's classifications by substituting the terms *treatment* and *rehabilitation* for *secondary* and *tertiary* prevention, respectively.

Complications refer to those sequelae resulting from the incomplete resolution of problems related to a primary diagnosis, or from secondary problems related to one or more secondary diagnoses. As such, prevention of complications might be associated with developmental care by lowering the rate of certain primary complications (e.g., intracranial hemorrhage, chronic respiratory problems) stemming from an initial diagnosis (primary prevention). By preventing primary complications, the rate of disabilities or complications resulting from an initial diagnosis in a nursery (secondary prevention; e.g., reflux and being tube-fed because of uncoordinated oral motor movements) might be reduced, thereby reducing the rate of defective functioning or complications due to an existing disorder (tertiary prevention; e.g., spastic diplegia) and lessening a dying infant's pain and suffering and promoting the personal contentment and social fulfillment to the extent possible of her/his family and friends (palliation). Although the sample sizes were small, developmental care was thought to have shown an impact on some aspects of prevention in six different clinical trials. Als, Duffy, McAnulty, et al. (1996)

demonstrated shorter lengths of hospital stay and decreased healthcare costs in infants who received developmental care, suggesting that complications were fewer in those infants.

## CENTRAL FEATURES AFFECTING SUCCESSFUL IMPLEMENTATION

What factors foster successful implementation of developmental care competency validation within nursing and across health-related fields? More than 20 years ago, Gortner (1980) outlined and discussed five central, generic principles underlying scholarly achievements. Gortner's principles included competency, communality, competition, colleagueship, and continuity. Her principle of *competency* involves knowing "that" and knowing "how." *Communality* entails dialogue and exchange of one's work with others. *Competition* was described as one's developing a capacity to accept critical comments about ideas without intense feelings of personal attack. Competition, according to Gortner, is a part of the reality of scientific activity and means being willing to place ideas on the table for debate and discussion. *Colleagueship* referred to senior scholars mentoring junior scholars and all colleagues exchanging information on a regular and timely basis. Colleagueship included collaborating and cooperating with others in nursing and other disciplines. *Continuity* was defined as the successive and successful improvements in the base of knowledge. The principle of continuity was regarded as fundamental to excellent research programs; to the refinement and ideas over generations of scholars; and to the provision of resources. If neonatal nurses would like to explore whether or not developmental care should be supported as the standard of caregiving, they could begin using Gortner's scholarly principles as their guiding framework. A proposed blueprint for such an endeavor can be found in Table 24-2.

Results of nursing research conducted comparing nurses' knowledge retention of JCAHO required materials through either didactic lecture or written self-learning module suggest that both are essentially equally effective methods for teaching competency-based content (Schlomer, Anderson, Shaw et al., 1997). It appears that for developmental care to turn into multiple scholarly achievements, ICN caregivers must demonstrate a more serious scientific commitment to validating developmental care competency and showing how it affects infant outcomes. Preferably before doing that (or, concurrently), to clarify variables for study, concept analyses are needed on:

1. The concept of the caregiver as an instrument of care
2. The concept of the establishment of infant goals
3. The concept of developmental caregivers working with families
4. The concept of interdisciplinary collaboration

The research conducted must be planned to explore how developmental competency validations of caregivers predict the developmental competencies of the infants receiving developmental interventions.

Exactly how might researchers accurately classify the nature of developmental interventions? Are they technical skills, evidence-based practice, an art, or something a bit different? These classifications require careful scientific study in and of themselves.

If developmental interventions are only technical skills, then once a caregiver learned how to perform them correctly, theoretically, s/he should be capable of implementing them with any individual infant in any setting. If developmental interventions constitute practice that is based on evidence, then once a caregiver was cognizant of and understood the evidence and replication studies supporting the completion of developmental interventions, s/he should be capable of practicing them. If developmental interventions exist as an art, then an understanding of contingencies and contexts are needed for a caregiver to know how, when, and where to implement them. However, an art that cannot be specified in detail cannot be transmitted by prescription, because no prescription for it exists. An art such as this can be passed on only by example, from master to apprentice (Polanyi, 1962). The inclusion of the art of nursing is compatible with the ANA definition of competency as inclusive of beliefs and attitudes as well as knowledge (ANA, 2000). If developmental interventions comprise technical skills, being aware of and understanding evidence supporting their implementation, and a special kind of art that involves connoisseurship, followed by practice doing developmental interventions, then education

TABLE **24-2**  A BEGINNING DRAFT OF A BLUEPRINT FOR SCHOLARSHIP IN STUDYING, IMPLEMENTING, AND EVALUATING DEVELOPMENTAL CARE

| I. Colleagueship | II. Competency Establishment and Validation | Key Scholarship Variables | | | |
| --- | --- | --- | --- | --- | --- |
| | | III. Competitiveness | IV. Continuity | V. Communality | VI. Cost-Effectiveness |
| Study the findings and critique from Canadian Cochrane Report and 2002 meta-analysis published by Jacobs, Sokol, and Ohllsson in the *Journal of Pediatrics*. From the outset, include an economist epidemiologist, developmental expert, and statistician in the development of the project. | A multidisciplinary developmental team should develop minatory standards for developmental care before establishing or validating any corresponding competencies of care providers. Decide which caregivers will be evaluated. Develop a plan for the intervals for evaluation and persons responsible for conducting the evaluations. | Develop a well-thought out, well-designed, competitive RCT research proposal that includes a follow-up phase. Initiate pilot studies (might apply for Dept. of Health's Health Research Formula funds from your state from the Tobacco Settlement Legislation). Submit research grants for funding a larger RCT (might apply for funding from National Institutes's of Health Center for Complementary and Alternative Medicine). | Once funded, initiate studies. Write and submit research reports for publication. Conduct follow-up studies. Make recommendations for revisions in practice as indicated. | The style of communication should be clear, prompt, concise, direct, sensitive, and deliberate among all parties involved. The adequacy of communication should be such that it is effective in meeting the common and specific goals of the respective disciplines involved. | Financial costs of care<br>Morbidities<br>Complications<br>Length of time until taking all feedings enterally<br>Length of time on the ventilator<br>Length of time in restraints<br>Neurobehavioral developmental assessment<br>Quality of sleep/wake states<br>Physiologic parameter status, such as heart rate and oxygen saturation<br>Length of stay<br>Weight gain<br>Parent satisfaction<br>Intensive care nursery morale<br>Mortality |

and being mentored are required to develop competencies in performing these interventions.

## CONCLUSION

In this chapter, we reviewed the issues of competency and the need for competency validation for health professionals committed to individualized, family-centered, developmental care (IFDC). Issues surrounding developmental care as it relates to competency are discussed. We have come a long way to full implementation of developmental care if our many disciplines are acknowledging the need for competencies in this area. Awareness and professional dialogs are the first step toward identifying developmental care competencies and how to measure them. This chapter has raised issues that nurses and multidisciplinary team members can propose in their institutions and in their professional disciplines for further consideration.

## *REFERENCES*

Agnes, M.E. (Ed.). (1999). *Webster's new world college dictionary* (4th ed.). Hoboken, NJ: John Wiley & Sons.

Als, H. (1979). Social interaction: Dynamic matrix for developing behavioral organization. *New Directions for Child Development, 4,* 21-39.

Als, H. (1982). Toward a synactive theory of development: Promise for assessment and support of infant individuality. *Infant Mental Health Journal, 3,* 229-243.

Als, H. (1986). A synactive model of neonatal behavioral organization: Framework for the assessment of neurobehavioral development in the premature infant and for support of infants and parents in the neonatal intensive care environment. *Physical and Occupational Therapy in Pediatrics, 6,* 3-53.

Als, H. (2001). *Program guide: Newborn Individualized Development Care Assessment Program (NIDCAP®), an education and training program for health professionals* (rev. ed.) Boston, MA: Boston Children's Medical Center Corporation.

Als, H., Duffy, F.H., & McAnulty, G.B. (1996). Effectiveness of individualized neurodevelopmental care in the newborn intensive care unit (NICU). *Acta Paediatrica* (Suppl 416), 21-30.

Als, H., & Gilkerson, L. (1997). The role of relationship-based developmentally supportive newborn intensive care in strengthening outcome of preterm infants. *Seminars in Perinatology, 21*(3), 178-189.

Als, H., Lawhon, G., Brown, E., et al. (1986). Individualized behavioral and environmental care for the VLBW preterm infant at high risk for bronchopulmonary dysplasia: NICU and developmental outcome. *Pediatrics 78,* II23-II32.

Als, H., Lawhon, G., Duffy, F.H., et al. (1994). Individualized developmental care for the very low-birthweight preterm infant. Medical and neurofunctional effects. *Journal of the American Medical Association* (*JAMA*), *272*(11), 853-858.

Als, H., Lester, B.M., Tronick, E., & Brazelton, T.B. (1982). Manual for the assessment of preterm infants' behavior (APIB). In H.E. Fitzgerald, B.M. Lester, & M.W. Yogman (Eds.), *Theory and research in behavioral pediatrics, Vol. 1* (pp. 64-133). New York: Plenum.

American Nurses Association (ANA). (2000). *Continued professional competence: Nursing's agenda for the 21st century (a working paper).* Washington, DC: American Nurses Association.

Association of Women's Health, Obstetric, and Neonatal Nurses (AWHONN). (1997). *Neonatal nursing: Orientation and development for registered and advanced practice nurses in basic and intensive care settings.* Washington, DC.: AWHONN.

Barber, B. (1966). Resistance by scientists to scientific discovery. *Science, 134,* 596-602.

Becker, P.T., Grunwald, P.C., Moorman, J., et al. (1991). Outcomes of developmentally supportive nursing care for very low birthweight infants. *Nursing Research, 40,* 150-155.

Becker, P.T., Grunwald, P.C., Moorman, J., et al. (1993). Effects of developmental care on behavioral organization in very-low-birthweight infants. *Nursing Research, 42,* 214-220.

Benner, P.A., Tanner, C.A., & Chesla, C.A. (1996). *Expertise in nursing practice: Caring, clinical judgment, and ethics.* New York: Springer.

Blackburn, S.T. (2003). Neuromuscular and sensory systems. In *Maternal, fetal, and neonatal physiology: A clinical perspective* (2nd ed.; pp. 546-598). St. Louis, MO: W. B. Saunders.

Block, J.H. (Ed.). (1971). *Mastery learning: Theory and practice.* New York: Holt, Rinehart, & Winston.

Bloom, M. (1996). Primary prevention practices. *Issues in children and families' lives, Vol. 5.* Thousand Oaks, CA: Sage Publications.

Buehler, D., Als, H., Duffy, F., et al.. (1995). Effectiveness of individualized developmental care for low-risk preterm infants: behavioral and electrophysiologic evidence. *Pediatrics, 96,* 923-932.

Burleson, R. (2001). *Essential knowledge and skills of the newborn developmental specialist* (unpublished doctoral dissertation). Louisville, KY: The University of Kentucky.

Campbell, D.T., & Stanley, J.C. (1963). Experimental and quasi-experimental designs for research (pp. 1-34). Boston, MA: Houghton Mifflin Co.

Caplan, G. (1964). *Principles of preventive psychiatry.* New York: Basic Books.

Carcuff, R.R. (2000). *The art of helping* (8th ed.). Amherst, MA: Human Resource Development Press.

Carmines, E.G., & Zeller, R.A. (1979). *Reliability and validity assessment* (No. 07-017). Beverly Hills, CA: Sage Publications.

Ciofalo, A. (Ed.). (1992). Internships: Perspectives on experiential learning: A guide to internship management for educators and professionals. Malabar, FL: Krieger.

Covington, M.V. (1987). Instruction in problem solving and planning. In S.L. Friedman, E.K. Scholnick, & R.R. Cocking (Eds.), *Blueprints for thinking* (pp. 469-511). London: Cambridge University Press.

Creger, P. (1989). *Developmental interventions for preterm and high-risk infants: Self-study modules for professionals.* Tuscon, AZ: Therapy Skill Builders.

Cronbach, L.J. (1971). Test validation. In R.L. Thorndike (Ed.), *Educational measurement* (2nd ed.; pp. 443-507). Washington, DC: American Council on Education.

Dawes, R.M. (1995). Standards of practice. In S.C. Hayes, V.M. Follette, R.M. Dawes, & K.E. Grady (Eds.), *Scientific standards of psychological practice: Issues and recommendations* (pp. 31-43). Reno, NV: Context Press.

Dreyfus, H.L. (1972). What computers still can't do (Part II). *Creative Computing, 6*(1), 18-31.

Dreyfus, H.L., & Dreyfus, S.E. (1986). Skill acquisition model. In *Mind over machine: The power of human intuitive expertise in the era of the computer.* New York: Free Press.

Fleisher, B., VandenBerg, K., Constantinou, J., et al. (1995). Individualized developmental care for very-low-birth-weight premature infants. *Clinical Pediatrics, 34,* 523-529.

Franck, L., & Lawhon, G. (2000). Environmental and behavioral strategies to prevent and manage neonatal pain. In K. J. S. Anand, B. J. Stevens, & P. J. McGrath (Eds.), *Pain in neonates* (pp. 203-216). Amsterdam: Elsevier.

Friedman, S.L., Scholnick, E.K., & Cocking, R.R. (1987). Reflections on reflections: What planning is and how it develops. In S.L. Friedman, E.K. Scholnick, & R.R. Cocking (Eds.), *Blueprints for thinking* (pp. 515-534). London, England: Cambridge University Press.

Fujishin, R. (1997). *Discovering the leader within: Running small groups successfully.* San Francisco: Academy Books.

Gortner, S.R. (1980). Nursing science in transition. *Nursing Research, 29,* 180-183.

Greiner, A.C., & Knebel, E. (Eds.). (2003). *Health professions education: A bridge to quality.* Washington, DC: The National Academies Press.

Guskey, T.R. (1997). *Implementing mastery learning* (2nd ed). Belmont, CA: Wadsworth.

Health Forum. (1999). *Hospital statistics, 1999 edition.* Chicago, IL: American Hospital Association Co.

Hendricks-Munoz, K., Prendergast, C., Caprio, M.C., et al. (2002). Developmental care: The impact of Wee Care developmental care training on short-term infant outcome and hospital costs. *Newborn and Infant Nursing Reviews, 2*(1), 39-45.

Hepworth, J.T. (2003). Personal communication. Vanderbilt University, Nashville, TN.

Holditch-Davis, D., Blackburn, S.T., & VandenBerg, K.A. (2003). Newborn and infant neurobehavioral development. In C. Kenner, & J.W. Lott (Eds.), *Comprehensive neonatal nursing: A physiologic perspective* (3rd ed.; pp. 236-284). St. Louis: W.B. Saunders.

Institute of Medicine. (2003). *Health professions education: a bridge to quality.* Available online at *http://books.nap.edu/books/0309087236/html/R1.html.*

Jacobs, S., Sokol, J., & Ohllsson, A. (2002). The newborn individualized developmental care and assessment program is not supported by meta-analyses of the data. *Journal of Pediatrics, 140*(6), 699-706.

Jarvis, P. (1995). *Adult and continuing education: Theory and practice* (2nd ed.). New York: Routledge.

Jorgensen, K. (2002). Moving forward with developmental care: Education and beyond. *Newborn and Infant Nursing Reviews, 2*(1), 5-8.

Kagan, S. (1994). *Cooperative learning* (2nd ed.). San Juan Capistrano, CA: Kagan Cooperative Learning. [1999 printing: Kagan, San Clemente, CA.]

Klein, D.C., & Goldson, S.E. (1977). Primary prevention: An idea whose time has come. *Proceedings of the pilot conference on primary prevention, April 24, 1976* (DHEW Publication No. ADM 77-447). Washington, DC: Government Printing Office.

Koch, S. (1999). Developmental support in the neonatal intensive care unit. In J. Deacon, & P. O'Neill (Eds.) *Core curriculum for neonatal intensive care nursing* (pp. 522-539). Philadelphia: W.B. Saunders.

Kuhn, T.S. (1970). *The structure of scientific revolutions* (2nd ed.). Chicago: The University of Chicago Press.

Lawrence-Lightfoot, S. (2000). *Respect: An exploration.* Reading, MA: Perseus Books.

Lenburg, C. (September 30, 1999). Redesigning expectations for initial and continuing competence for contemporary nursing practice. *Online Journal of Issues in Nursing.* Available online at *www.nursingworld.iorg/ojin/topic10/tpc10_1.htm.*

Loving, G.L. (1991). *Nursing students' perceptions of learning clinical judgment in undergraduate nursing education* (unpublished doctoral dissertation). Austin, TX: The University of Texas at Austin,.

Loving, G.L. (1993). Competence validation and cognitive flexibility: A theoretical model grounded in nursing education. *Journal of Nursing Education, 32,* 415-421.

MacTurk, R.H., & Morgan, G.A. (Eds.). (1995). *Mastery motivation: Origins, conceptualizations and applications.* Stamford, CT: Ablex Publishing Corporation.

National Association of Neonatal Nurses (NANN). (2001). *Infant developmental care guidelines for practice* (2nd ed.). Petaluma, CA: NANN.

Peters, K.L. (1999). Infant handling in the NICU: Does developmental care make a difference? An evaluative review of the literature. *Journal of Perinatal and Neonatal Nursing, 13*(3), 83-109.

Polanyi, M. (1962). *Personal knowledge: Towards a post-critical philosophy.* Chicago: The University of Chicago Press.

Saunders, R.P., Abraham, M.R., Crosby, M.J. et al. (2003). Evaluation and development of potentially better practices for improving family-centered care in neonatal intensive care units. *Pediatrics, 111*(4), e437-e449.

Schlomer, R.S., Anderson, M.A., & Shaw, R. (1997). Teaching strategies and knowledge retention. *Journal of Nursing Staff Development, 13*(5), 249-253.

Scholnick, E.K. (1995). Direction I: Knowing and constructing plans, *SRCD Newsletter, Fall*(1-2), 17.

Simpson, J.A. (Ed.). (1993). *Oxford English dictionary.* New York: Oxford University Press.

Simpson, K.R., & Creehan, P.A. (1998). Introduction to competence validation for providers of perinatal care. In K.R. Simpson, & P.A. Creehan (Eds.), *Competence validation for perinatal care providers: Orientation, continuing education, and evaluation* (pp. xiii-xv). Philadelphia: Lippincott, Williams & Wilkins.

Sizun, J., Ansquer, H., Browne, J., et al. (2002). Developmental care decreases physiologic and behavioral pain expression in preterm neonates. *Journal of Pain, 3*, 446-450.

Spencer, L.M., & Spencer, S.M. (1993*). Competence at work: Models for superior performance.* New York: John Wiley & Sons.

Stevens, B., Johnston, C., Franck, L., et al. (1999). The efficacy of developmentally sensitive behavioral interventions and sucrose for relieving procedural pain in very low birth weight neonate. *Nursing Research, 48*, 35-42.

Strodtbeck, F. (2003). Competency-based education in neonatal nursing. In C. Kenner & J.W. Lott (Eds.), *Comprehensive neonatal nursing: A physiologic perspective* (3rd ed.; pp. 79-88). St. Louis: W.B. Saunders.

Summerfield, C.J., & Cosgrove, H. (Eds.). (1994). Jobs that let you earn while you learn, training programs by experts, combined classroom and on-the-job training. In E.H. Oakes (Ed.), *Ferguson's guide to apprenticeship programs* (2nd ed.). Chicago: Ferguson Publishing.

Symington, A., & Pinelli, J. (2001). Developmental care for promoting development and preventing morbidity in preterm infants (Cochrane Review). In *The Cochrane Library* (Issue 2). Oxford, United Kingdom: Update Software.

VandenBerg, K. (1993). Basic competencies to begin developmental care in the intensive care nursery. *Infants and Young Children, 6*, 52-59.

VandenBerg, K.A., & Becker, A.M. (1996). Developmental care. Developmental competencies for staff in the ICN. *Neonatal Network—Journal of Neonatal Nursing, 15*(5), 65-68.

Whittaker, S., Smolenski, M., & Carson, W. (June 30, 2000). Assuring continued competence—Policy questions and approaches: How should the profession respond? *Online Journal of Issues in Nursing.* Available online at *www.nursingworld.org/ojin/topic10/tpc10_4.htm.*

Wondrak, R.F. (1998). *Interpersonal skills for nurses and health care professionals.* Malden, MA: Blackwell Science.

Zettle, R.D. (1995). Establishing and implementing scientific standards of psychological practice. In S.C. Hayes, V.M. Follette, R.M. Dawes, & K.E. Grady (Eds.), *Scientific standards of psychological practice: Issues and recommendations* (pp. 44-47). Reno, NV: Context Press.

# 25 Developmental Care and Advanced Practice Nursing Education

## Jacqueline M. McGrath

The acceptance of the philosophy of individualized, family-centered developmental care (IFDC) is growing; however, few health professionals have this content as part of their basic or advanced education. But, if developmental care is to be embraced, developmental care education, ideally interdisciplinary education, must be offered at all levels for full integration into practice in the neonatal intensive care unit (NICU). In 2000, with funding from the Department of Health and Human Services (DHHS), Health Resources and Service Administration (HRSA), Bureau of Health Professions (BHP), Arizona State University (ASU) College of Nursing (CON) undertook an innovative master of science in nursing (MS) program that enhanced the nursing of children specialty track within the graduate program with the addition of a neonatal nurse practitioner (NNP) option. The ASU program was designed with developmental and family-centered care as cornerstones of the educational process for advanced practice neonatal and pediatric nurses. Why would such an emphasis be important to future advanced practice nurses (APNs)? How did ASU achieve this goal? In this chapter, the answers to these questions are explored.

## PURPOSE OF THE PROGRAM

As White-Traut (2003) points out in her editorial to a clinical section of the *Journal of Obstetric, Gynecologic, and Neonatal Nursing (JOGNN)*, technology has driven our neonatal practice and education for the past 30 years, but we now realize that machines to support life are not enough. Care is about more than technologic advances and the ability to help a 23-week infant survive, it is about the quality of that survival and what will make the quality of life better for the infant and family. Holistic care that includes technology and traditional medical

and nursing interventions must be coupled with attention to the effects of the environment on the neonate and family. The family is a partner in care. To implement such a philosophic change requires an organizational commitment in the practice arena, and a leadership and organizational commitment in educational institutions as well (Robison, 2003). At ASU, this need for commitment is recognized, as well as a growing need for APNs, especially NNPs.

Despite, the ever-increasing need for NNPs in the state of Arizona, there was no educational program for APNs in this specialty since the closure of a certificate program in the mid-1990s. Although, there were more than 50 openings for NNPs in several different settings, few nurse practitioners wanted to move into the state to take these positions. ASU decided to start a program, but to do so with a different emphasis than the traditional NNP educational options. The desire was to incorporate developmental and family-centered care as two essential aspects of the educational process, thus providing masters degree programs, and prepared APNs who could provide a more comprehensive assessment and plan in the management of the infant and the family. ASU CON already had a firm commitment to families and to promoting positive growth and development of the infants and families as part of their curriculum, and, therefore, the two foci of the new masters option was an extension of this foundation.

The purpose of the program is to prepare APNs to provide comprehensive nursing care to high-risk infants and their families. Upon completion of this program, the graduate NNPs are expected to have competencies that will enable them to:

1. Participate in clinical research.
2. Use research findings in their practice.
3. Communicate scholarly ideas and professional knowledge to colleagues, other disciplines, and the public they served.

4. Critically examine the health of neonatal populations and related health issues.
5. Demonstrate a commitment to lifelong learning.
6. Synthesize advanced knowledge in neonatal nursing, using concepts, principles, and research from nursing, humanities, and sciences to develop advanced nursing practice knowledge that emphasizes the holistic approach.
7. Demonstrate leadership, management, and teaching abilities in advanced practice neonatal nursing.
8. Assume leadership responsibility and accountability for holistic, therapeutic interventions within or across levels of care for diverse neonatal populations, including infants and their families, groups, or communities.
9. Participate in specialty professional nursing organizations and political arenas.

The program has received approval from the Arizona State Board of Nursing (AzSBON) and the National Certifying Corporation (NCC). Graduates of the program are eligible for national certification and employable in states other than Arizona.

## PROGRAM PLAN

The ASU program plan can be undertaken on a full or part-time basis to accommodate as many potential students as possible. The full time plan is outlined in Box 25-1. Emphasis on the integration of family issues focuses on four major areas: developmental care, family-centered care, culturally sensitive care, and integration of Spanish. Because so many families in Arizona speak only Spanish, this content was essential for practice within this community.

The curriculum provides 525 or 570 clock hours of didactic content (dependent on the research option selected by the student) and a minimum of 780 clock hours of clinical content. Out of the total didactic content, 370 clock hours are specifically neonatal-focused. The clock hours are based on 1 clock hour per credit hour of didactic content and 3 clock hours per credit hour of clinical time. The neonatal specific clinical courses are divided as follows:

Advanced Neonatal Assessment—90 hours
Advanced Developmental and Family Centered Nursing Care—90 hours
Neonatal Practicum I—300 hours
Neonatal Practicum II—300 hours.

Thus, graduates have a total of 780 hours of clinical. The Developmental and Family-Centered Care course, which is taught during the first year of full-time study, lays the foundation for providing advanced nursing care and medical management that is developmentally supportive, family-centered, and culturally competent during the clinical courses in the second year of study. One cannot begin to provide comprehensive nursing care for an infant without including the family; therefore, the crux of this course is care of the developing infant within the context of family. Developmental and family theories are used as a foundation for assessment and intervention. These might include Social Exchange and Choice, Feminist Theory, Symbolic Interaction, Family Life Course Development, System Theory, Social Learning Theory, Resilience, and Family Stress Theory-ABCX Model. Normal sensory, cognitive, motor, social/emotional, and language development in children is also addressed. Particular emphasis is given to development from birth until 3 years with additional content related to care of children within their families. The implications of developmental stages, level of developmental skill, and developmental problems for the maintenance of health and management of illness by the APN are emphasized. These are addressed within context of family, as well as social, cultural, ethnic, and religious frameworks. Conversational Spanish is also incorporated for working with families and conveying information about the infant/child. Case management including developmental assessment and intervention with infants/children and families in the nursery as well as after discharge and in the community is also content in the course, along with ethical, societal, and legal issues.

A clinical practicum within the course hours provides the students with essential practice experiences. These experiences include:
- Case management
- Developmental assessments in the NICU with a developmental specialist
- Developmental screening in follow-up clinics
- Play therapy

**Box 25-1   FULL-TIME PROGRAM PLAN**

**Year 01, Fall Semester**

| | |
|---|---|
| Neonatal/Pediatric Embryology and Physiology | 3 credit hours |
| Theoretical Foundations | 3 credit hours |
| Advanced Neonatal Health Assessment | 4 credit hours |
| Research Methods | 3 credit hours |

**Year 01, Spring Semester**

| | |
|---|---|
| Developmental & Family-Centered Neonatal Nursing Care | 4 credit hours |
| Neonatal/Pediatric Pharmacology | 3 credit hours |
| Population Based Health Care | 3 credit hours |
| Current Healthcare Issues | 3 credit hours |

**Year 01, Summer Semester**

| | |
|---|---|
| Advanced Practice Role | 2 credit hours |

**Year 02, Fall Semester**

| | |
|---|---|
| Advanced Neonatal Theory I | 4 credit hours |
| Practicum I | 6 credit hours |
| Research Project or Thesis | 2-3 credit hours |

**Year 02, Spring Semester**

| | |
|---|---|
| Advanced Neonatal Theory II | 4 credit hours |
| Practicum II | 6 credit hours |
| *Research Project or Thesis | 2-3 credit hours |

*Can be taken either semester or divided up across semesters.

- Lactation consultation
- Development of culturally sensitive skills for communication with families in a variety of neonatal units in urban and rural community hospitals
- Specialty clinics such as apnea, bronchopulmonary dysplasia (BPD), spina bifida, cranial facial, and genetics clinics
- Community agencies such as early intervention providers, School for the Blind, School for the Deaf, Project Thrive, home-based schools, pilot parent program, and screening clinics
- Students expected to complete home visits

Additional course requirements include documentation of developmental assessments, literature review on a developmental intervention of choice, exploration of the individualized family service plan/individualized education plan (IFSP/IEP) process and providing education in a grade school or middle school about healthcare professions.

Students in both the neonatal and pediatric APN tracks are required to take the course content together. This allows the students to work together to gain both inpatient and outpatient perspectives that will broaden their foundation for practice. It also provides the students with the opportunity to begin to develop networks within the community that will complement their future practice, whatever the setting.

The decision to provide the developmental and family-centered care content in the first year of the program was integral to the belief that this content would become the foundation for all decision-making and become a pivotal basis for the graduates in their practice. Developmentally supportive caregiving, with a focus on family-centered interventions, was also seen as becoming a standard of care in many NICUs throughout the world. Therefore, as changes in clinical practice occur, these concepts must be integrated into advanced practice neonatal nursing education.

Historically, the early NNP education offered by hospital-based, certificate programs focused primarily on medical management of the high-risk infant. As NNP education moved to graduate nursing education within the university setting, the curriculum has embraced a more holistic approach that encompasses developmentally supportive caregiving and family-centered practices (Beal, Richardson, Dembinski, et al., 1999; Strotbeck, Trotter, & Lott, 1998).

This integration is supported within the graduate competencies suggested by the National Association of Neonatal Nurses (NANN) (1995, 2002a, 2002b) and the National Organization of Nurse Practitioner Faculties (NONPF) (2002). The ASU program actualized this integration by using Als's Synactive Theory of Development (Als & Brazelton, 1981; Als & Gilkerson, 1997) and the developmentally supportive caregiving guidelines recommended by NANN as the foundation of APN education. (D'Apolito, McGrath, & O'Brien, 2000). For example, the curriculum includes holistic assessment, advanced practice procedures with developmental interventions, developmental training, neurobehavioral maturation of the preterm infant, family-centered caregiving, inclusion of cultural diversity within the NICU, the special care infant within the community, and developmental follow-up of NICU graduates.

Graduates of the ASU program come away with the view that developmental and family-centered care is an essential component of care. The competencies expected of program graduates are numerous and comprehensive. A complete listing of these competencies can be found in Box 25-2.

This program embraces a competency-based model that is aligned with the material found in the competency validation chapter, Chapter 24. Competencies are an essential way to move beyond learning objectives and measure application of knowledge in a clinical setting. This program uses competencies required for APNs and especially for neonatal and pediatric practitioners and builds on them to put more emphasis on family and developmental care.

Although this program's emphasis is on nursing education, ideally there will be more opportunities in the future to hold interdisciplinary classes. If we believe that a cornerstone of developmental care is the interdisciplinary coordination, then it makes sense for us to learn together, before we have to work together as a team. Developmental care is a perfect way to bring disciplines together to work on a common goal-positive growth and development of the infant and family. This program is one model for the integration of developmental and family-centered care into the core of neonatal and pediatric APN education. It is hoped that this educational design will serve as a catalyst to get other educational programs at all levels of practice on board.

## CONCLUSION

The ASU program is unique in its emphasis on developmental and family-centered care as foundational knowledge for the neonatal and pediatric APN graduate. It sets the stage for other graduate nursing programs and, hopefully, other disciplines to follow. As we move as a society toward a kinder, gentler form of health care, developmental, individualized, family-centered care makes sense. We need more scientific evidence to support this inclusion in neonatal and pediatric APN curricula, and, therefore, there is a need for formal program evaluations, outcomes, and research protocols to assess the success of this change in education. This program has now graduated two classes, and there is high satisfaction from graduates with this content. Their critical thinking skills appear more holistic, and their inclusion of family is a priority. All graduates have easily found employment, and long-term evaluation of the graduates use of this content is yet to occur.

It is also believed that inclusion of this content will afford the graduates more career opportunities in developmental care and high-risk follow-up. Only time will tell. We also believe that they are armed with knowledge to help us gain the evidence through their research efforts to support the need for and benefits of IFDC. This program marks the entrance of a blending of theory in developmental care/family-centered care with practice and education, the hallmarks of the maturation of our NNP curricular process.

## Box 25-2 ASU NNP Program Terminal Competencies

**A graduate:**

1. Gathers pertinent information systematically and skillfully from all sources: perinatal history, diagnostic tests, and comprehensive physical examination, with behavioral and developmental assessments and provides comprehensive health history and physical assessment.
2. Differentiates normal and abnormal variations for all body systems.
3. Accurately interprets diagnostic tests.
4. Analyzes data from multiple sources in making clinical judgments and in determining the effectiveness of a plan of care.
5. Develops problem lists with associated differential diagnoses.
6. Provides holistic development appropriate to neonatal nursing care to high-risk infants in high-technology tertiary settings.
7. Uses concepts of family-centered care to assess family adaptation, coping skills, and the need for crisis and other interventions.
8. Identifies educational needs of the family and assists with teaching.
9. Ensures routine opportunities for neonate and parent relationships to emerge with development of bonding and attachment.
10. Assists family to restructure daily living activities in ways that meet the needs of the infant and those of other family members.
11. Evaluates infant physiologic and behavioral responses to interventions for revision of management plan.
12. Forms partnerships and communicates with family members regarding the changing healthcare needs of the infant.
13. Initiates and performs measures necessary to resuscitate and stabilize a compromised infant.
14. Accurately and appropriately performs routine diagnostic and therapeutic techniques according to established protocol and current standards for NNP practice.
15. Plans and implements appropriate pharmacologic therapies.
16. Identifies ethical dilemmas involved in the evaluation and management of the high-risk infant.
17. Provides continuing neonatal nursing care to low birthweight infants and vulnerable infants in family settings.
18. Develops therapeutic nurse-client relationship.
19. Demonstrates management of acute and chronic health alterations across the neonatal care continuum.
20. Demonstrates health promotion and health maintenance strategies.
21. Prioritizes and initiates pertinent diagnostic tests.
22. Determines nursing and medical diagnoses, and develops a prioritized comprehensive problem list.
23. Establishes appropriate priorities of care.
24. Collects patient data on an ongoing basis, prioritized according to immediate conditions or needs.
25. Formulates, in collaboration with the family, physician, staff nurse, and other members of the multidisciplinary healthcare team a plan of care that incorporates developmental needs, healthcare maintenance, discharge, and follow-up care as well as needs of the family.
26. Demonstrates management of complex, rapidly changing clinical situations.
27. Evaluates the patient's progress toward attainment of expected outcomes.
28. Systemically evaluates and ensures quality and effectiveness of care.
29. Demonstrates multidisciplinary consultation and collaboration.
30. Initiates referral based on infant/family needs.
31. Seeks appropriate consultation dependent on infant healthcare needs.
32. Facilitates use of organizational resources in caring for the patient.

*Continued*

Box 25-2    ASU NNP Program Terminal Competencies—cont'd

33. Evaluates their clinical practice in relation to professional and ethical standards, relevant laws, statutes, and regulations.
34. Identifies legal components of advanced neonatal nursing practice.
35. Critiques theory and research and participates in research activities for the evaluation, modification, and enhancement of existing practice.
36. Participates in providing in-service education programs and functions as a neonatal clinical resource person within the institution.
37. Assists in developing unit policies and procedures for nursing care of the high-risk infant, and participates in quality assurance measures in the NICU.
38. Develops and implements strategies that have a positive effect on the political and regulatory processes related to healthcare systems and the NNP role.
39. Demonstrates commitment to the NNP role, and identifies mechanisms to determine the future direction of the NNP role.
40. Demonstrates cultural sensitivity and cultural competence.

Adapted from McGrath, J.M. (2002). Integration of developmentally supportive care and family-centered issues into neonatal nurse practitioner education. *Newborn and Infant Nursing Reviews, 2*(1), 35-38.
*NICU,* Neonatal intensive care unit; *NNP,* neonatal nurse practitioner.

## REFERENCES

Als, H., & Brazelton, T. B. (1981). A new model of assessing the behavioral organization in preterm and full-term infants: two case studies. *Journal of the American Academy of Child Psychiatry, 2*(2), 239-263.

Als, H., & Gilkerson, L. (1997). The role of relationship-based developmentally supportive newborn intensive care in strengthening outcome of preterm infants. *Seminars in Perinatology, 21*(3), 178-189.

Beal, J.A., Richardson, D.K., Dembinski, S., et al. (1999). Responsibilities, roles, and staffing patterns of nurse practitioners in the neonatal intensive care unit. *American Journal of Maternal Child Nursing: MCN, 24*(4), 169-175.

D'Apolito, K., McGrath, J.M., & O'Brien, A. (2000). *Guidelines for implementation of developmental care.* Des Plaines, IL: National Association of Neonatal Nurses.

National Association of Neonatal Nurses (NANN). (1995). *Position paper: Graduate education for entry into neonatal nurse practitioner practice.* Petaluma, CA: NANN.

National Association of Neonatal Nurses (NANN). (2002a). *Educational standards for neonatal nurse practitioner programs.* Glenview, IL: NANN. Available online at *www.nann.org.*

National Association of Neonatal Nurses (NANN). (2002b). *Curriculum guidelines for neonatal nurse practitioner education programs.* Glenview, IL: NANN. Available online at *www.nann.org.*

National Organization of Nurse Practitioner Faculty (NONPF) (2002). *Evaluation criteria for nurse practitioner programs: Competencies for advanced practice.* Available online at *www.nonpf.com.*

Robison, L.D. (2003). An organizational guide for an effective developmental program in the NICU. *Journal of Obstetric, Gynecologic, and Neonatal Nursing (JOGNN), 32*(3), 379-386.

Strodtbeck, F., Trotter, C., & Lott, J.W. (1998). Coping with transition: Neonatal nurse practitioner education for the 21st century. *Journal of Pediatric Nursing, 13*(5), 272-278.

White-Traut, R. (2003). The continuing pursuit of optimal developmental care. *Journal of Obstetric, Gynecologic, and Neonatal Nursing (JOGNN), 32*(3), 378.

# 27 Professional Issues and the Future of Developmental Care: Where Will It Be in the 21st Century?

Carole Kenner and Jacqueline M. McGrath

Professional organizations have long been known for their ability to organize, motivate, educate, and advance a profession. The National Association of Neonatal Nurses (NANN) has done this and more for the neonatal nursing specialty. This organization has lead the way in shaping the practice and the environment of neonatal nursing in a way that not only carves out the "niche" for the role of the neonatal nurse within the professional environment but also creates a role that acknowledges infants and families as partners in the environment of the neonatal intensive care unit (NICU). NANN has taken the lead to bring several disciplines together to create a text that reflects the current thinking on individualized, family-centered, developmental care (IFDC). This is an exciting time for neonatal nursing, other health professionals, and parents interested in promoting this philosophy of care. This chapter offers some "predictions" of where developmental care is going in the 21st century and some of the questions still in need of answers, as we forge ahead.

## PROFESSIONAL ASSOCIATIONS AND THEIR ROLE IN DEVELOPMENTAL CARE

Developmental care is a new trend that has gotten a lot of professional and public attention, but as recently as 2002 was listed as a useless therapy in a professional journal. To change this mindset, professional associations that support developmental care need to be vocal and visible on this subject. NANN members have been very vocal about the need to support infants and their families. This support includes a heightened awareness of the macro- and micro-environments of the NICU. The developmental care movement will only work if there is support from all levels of professional education and practice. Nurses, physicians, developmental specialists, occupational and physical therapists, educators, and families who believed in the philosophy of developmental care contributed to the writing of this core curriculum. If the essential content can be identified, then the belief is that more credence will be given to developmental care as a critical part of health professionals' education. It will set a standard for the core knowledge that any professional who has contact with a neonate needs to provide holistic, individualized, infant and family-centered care.

Professional associations such as NANN must take a stand on setting the pace, and having the vision of future care needs of their clients and families. The professional associations lend credibility to the work or standard. However, in the case of the developmental core, the support must be interdisciplinary. It requires a team approach to foster developmental growth of the infant and family.

Professional associations such as NANN, the American Occupational Therapy Association (AOTA), and the Association of Physical and Natural Therapists (APNT), must work together on topics such as the developmental core to broaden the acceptance of this document. Medical associations have been more reluctant to lend a national acceptance to works of this type. But to gain the most impact on practice across disciplines, acceptance is needed to speed up the change process.

Each discipline brings a rich history and perspective that is needed to deliver developmental care. We need a common language, however, to share the vision of the ultimate goal of developmental care. This core represents a bridging across the languages of each of our disciplines with the outcome being a product that will influence practice in an interdisciplinary, coordinated way. Such work requires the putting aside of turf issues and sitting down at the table to work together, not in opposition, for the good of the infant and family. As a consumer of this core, we ask that you do the same. Recognize your discipline's unique contribution to the developmental care team but ultimately see how your discipline's view contributes to healthcare delivery.

## PROFESSIONAL CERTIFICATION IN DEVELOPMENTAL CARE: IS IT NECESSARY?

Professional certification, according to some experts, is just another artificial bureaucratic hoop to jump through. However, the more prevalent view is that certification is an outcome of the educational process. It provides tangible evidence of the degree to which the content has been integrated into one's knowledge. Health professionals are knowledge workers. We use the tools we acquire through practice, experiences, and education. A certification gives further proof that some level of knowledge has been acquired. It provides no assurance that the actual knowledge will be implemented at the bedside. That is where competency levels, checksheets, or similar performance-outcome measures are used. These tools are nice, but do nothing to ensure the actual integration of knowledge into practice. Nevertheless, the certification does demonstrate that there is a minimal level of comprehension of the content that a health professional providing developmental care has achieved.

Certification also lends credence and credibility to the end product, in this case developmental care. If a group or groups have taken the time to create an examination to test the level of knowledge, then this content must be important. In this country, the passage of a certification examination is often a prerequisite of initial or continued employment. Is developmental certification necessary? The answer would seem to be "yes" if health professionals truly believe that developmental care is an essential part of neonatal/family-centered care. This type of

certification will not come quickly or easily, as developmental care has become a turf issue between disciplines. Many opponents to developmental care view it as one more bandwagon for nursing, another passing fad in caregiving strategies, but evidence is mounting to support at least some aspects of this care. It is unlikely that it will go away; continue to change perhaps, but it is here to stay. Consumers/parents are beginning to like what they see when they are exposed to developmental care practices. They are beginning to demand that their infant's care be individualized and support development. The true test of endurance will most likely come when it is "valued" in accreditation standards or as part of the Joint Commission on Accreditation of Healthcare Organizations (JCAHO) review. Another test might be inclusion of content on developmental care on national certification examinations, such as those for neonatal nurses and/or nurse practitioners.

## STRATEGIES FOR ADVANCING DEVELOPMENTAL CARE IN THE 21ST CENTURY

Every aspect of the developmental care curriculum has set forth strategies for advancing the philosophy of IFDC. The essence of the strategies for advancing the practice of developmental care is:

- Acceptance that developmental care is an essential part of individualized, infant/family-centered care
- Commitment that developmental care reflects a change in philosophy of care and is interdisciplinary in nature
- Acceptance that developmental care is a tool that all health professionals partnered with families can and should use with neonates/infants/children
- Acceptance that an "elite group" of trained people will never move the masses forward toward recognition of developmental care as a standard of care
- Change theory must be applied when contemplating the implementation of developmental care
- Commitment to buy-in time: The hook (e.g., education, support, resources) must be provided to gather increasing support for developmental care; marketing the positives about developmental care to the masses before an attempt is made to fully implement this new approach to care delivery is essential

- Provide evidence to support its use; evidence-based practice is essential
- Acknowledge the gaps in evidence to support developmental care
- Conduct well-designed, randomized, controlled clinical trials to demonstrate the effectiveness of developmental care
- Do a cost versus benefits analysis (using an economic model) regarding use of developmental care
- Share the vision with others; if the vision is not shared and the "policy" sits in a manual, developmental care will never be accepted
- See one, do one, teach one; watch experts deliver developmental care, learn how and why to provide such care, practice the techniques, then share the knowledge with others
- Encourage professional associations and parent groups to promote developmental care

## PREDICTIONS FOR DEVELOPMENTAL CARE IN THE 21ST CENTURY

Individualized, family-centered developmental care is growing in importance as an essential part of the health care of infants and families. Where will it go in the future?

The predictions we make are:

1. Developmental care will be embraced as the philosophy of newborn, infant, and family-centered care.
2. Use of a "core curriculum" by health professionals and families will grow and foster its use as a standard of neonatal care.
3. Developmental care will be a model for interdisciplinary education and healthcare management.
4. Developmental care will be a part of standard orientation and continued competency evaluation for health professionals who work with newborns, infants, children, and their families.
5. Developmental care will become the framework from which neonatal care is delivered.
6. Developmental care will be incorporated as an essential part of health professional education—basic and advanced, no matter what the discipline.
7. Families will be partners in care and not visitors in the NICU any longer.
8. Developmental care teams will be an expectation in neonatal care delivery.
9. Evidence will mount to support positive healthy outcomes for newborns, infants, and their families when developmental care is the overarching philosophy of care.
10. Interdisciplinary research studies will increase to examine various aspects of developmental care.

## CONCLUSION

In summary, NANN is grateful for the opportunity to work with such dedicated professionals and parents on this project. But this is only the first step toward integration of developmental care into all NICUs. The core knowledge on development found in these pages must be applied. It must be embraced as a philosophic underpinning of neonatal care. It must be tested through research to determine what works, what does not work, and what needs refinement. Professional associations and parent groups must work together to promote a change in practice that is "owned" by all disciplines and not turfed to one. Now it is your turn to use this knowledge. Go out and spread the word. Developmental care is an essential part of providing good, clinically sound care to every infant and family who must, for some unforeseen reason, enter the healthcare environment, but most especially, those who must traverse the NICU.

# A Sample Protocols and Job Descriptions for Developmental Care

## CO-BEDDING MULTIPLES

### Infant Objectives

- Show improvement in heart/respiratory rate, oxygen requirement, physical growth/development, and motor development in flexor and extensor patterns.
- Show co-regulation and appropriate states consistent and/or interactive with each other, environment, and care providers.

### Benefits

- Enhancement of parent/infant bonding
- Easing of transition to home
- Consistency of care; same RN and same doctor take care of both babies

### Risk

Because this new practice is emerging throughout the country, there is no documented research to support or negate. Risks are unknown at this time. A potential risk might be infection.

### Protocol

- Infants are stable and free from infection/sepsis before being bedded together.
- Infant does not have an endotracheal tube (ETT) and is not under an oxygen hood.
- Infants are in room air or nasal cannula (NC) oxygen.
- If both infants require NC $O_2$, place an emergency $O_2$ tank on wheels at bedside.
- Infants do not have an indwelling catheter (i.e., percutaneous catheter or IV catheter with heplock).

- Infant can be on a cardiorespiratory monitor and/or pulse oximeter.
- Infants might be on gavage feeding.
- Infants can be in cribs or isolettes.
- If one infant requires temperature control via the incubator settings (servo), place the temperature probe on the smaller of the infants or the one with the greatest temperature instability.

### Procedure

- Infection control: provide complete care for each individual infant before beginning care for next infant, with good hand washing between. Keep equipment/supplies separate (i.e., pacifier, monitor).
- Identification: properly labeled ID bands and all equipment color coded (supplies, papers—monitor, pulse oximeter, flow meters—stethoscope, pacifiers, bulb syringe—if necessary, flow sheets, etc.). Ask parents to select color codes for the babies. If infants are dressed, ask parents to select colors and keep them dressed in their respective colored outfits.
- Bed side-by-side, facing each other or one another's back, if able, same position as in utero; ask parents.
- Place boundary and swaddle blanket around both of them, not individually.
- Cluster care, perform vital signs, feeding, etc., on the one that is more alert.
- If necessary to separate, (i.e., one becomes unstable) call parents; separate only as long as necessary.

From Altimier, L., Brown, B., & Tedeschi, L. (2000). *Tri-Health's manual of neonatal nursing policies, procedures, competencies, and clinical pathways.* Glenview, IL: National Association of Neonatal Nurses.

# UNIVERSITY OF ILLINOIS AT CHICAGO MEDICAL CENTER CLINICAL CARE GUIDELINE SUBJECT: KANGAROO CARE (SKIN-TO-SKIN CARE)

## Objective

To establish criteria and procedure for infants/families who wish to participate in kangaroo or skin-to-skin care.

## Position Statements

Skin-to-skin care is a well-established practice that is supportive of both families and the infants. Most infants benefit from the warmth and tactile contact with their parents and frequently demonstrate an improvement in both their behavioral and physiologic responses. This activity is one that the parents can initiate early within the hospitalization period, which thus facilitates the integration of their parental role.

## Standards

The RN will ensure that parents are educated about skin-to-skin care as soon after delivery as possible, even if it will not be feasible to implement it at the time, due to the infant's condition.

The RN will offer skin-to-skin care to parents as soon as the infant meets the criteria, and might request permission from the neonatal fellow or attending if the infant does not meet criteria, but she/he assesses that the infant or family would benefit.

The RN will monitor the family's and infant's response to skin-to-skin care and document findings.

As there are insufficient data to support universal skin-to-skin care for all infants, exclusionary criteria have been established to ensure the safety of the most fragile infants.

Infants who are not eligible for skin-to-skin care are those:

1. Infants who are receiving supplemental humidity.
2. Infants on high-frequency oscillating ventilation.
3. Infants who have indwelling chest tubes.
4. Infants with PPHN (persistent pulmonary hypertension).
5. Infants who are receiving paralytic agents.
6. Infants receiving pressors or sedation at high levels for whom the transfer from the incubator to the parent's body might dangerously counteract the effect of the pressor/sedation.
7. Infant with femoral or radial arterial lines.
8. Infants under respiratory isolation.
9. Infants who are diagnosed with NEC (necrotizing enterocolitis), have open abdominal wounds, or have suspicious abdominal distension.
10. Infants with gastroschisis/omphalocele that has not been fully reduced.

## Procedure

1. The RN/Care Coordinator/Developmentalist will educate parents about skin-to-skin care in the first days of life.
2. When the infant is physiologically able to be placed skin-to-skin, the RN will offer the experience to the parents, explaining the need for their cooperation in: wearing appropriate clothing (shirt that buttons down in front or hospital gown) and staying at least 1 hour with infant.
3. Recliner or rocking chair brought to bedside.
4. Infant is dressed only in a diaper and hat.
5. Infant's temperature is taken before removing from the bed. If below 98° F (36.5° C), measures will be taken to warm the infant before transfer.
6. Infant is moved so that he/she is placed vertically on the parent's chest.
7. After the infant is placed on chest, his/her back is covered with the parent's shirt and one to two blankets.
8. If infant is transferred from the incubator, the temperature control should be set to "air" and the control temperature should be at the current incubator ambient temperature. If the infant has a skin temperature probe on, this should remain on, so that the current skin temperature can be easily monitored.
9. If infant is intubated, solicit the help of another nurse or respiratory therapist.
10. One person will be responsible for the patient, IV lines, and monitoring cables; the other for the ventilator tubing.
11. Infant can be transferred with parent standing or sitting. If standing, one nurse will disconnect

the infant from the ventilator and manage the IV lines and cables while the parent lifts the baby to her chest; the other nurse will move the ventilator tubing out of the incubator and bring to the baby. The parent will then be assisted to sit in the chair. If the parent is sitting, one nurse will disconnect the infant from the ventilator, pick up the baby, IV lines, and cables, and carry to the parent, while the other nurse manages the ventilator tubing.

12. When infant is transferred back, two people again will be needed, one to help the parent out of the chair, and one to guard the ETT and lines. The parent can help contain the infant in the incubator while the others work to secure the lines, tubing, and cables.

13. Infants should be encouraged to suck at the breast while the mother is performing skin-to-skin care. If the mother is expressing milk, she should be encouraged to pump after skin-to-skin care, as this helps stimulate her milk supply.

14. All mothers who are having troubles establishing or maintaining their milk supply should be encouraged to perform skin-to-skin care every time they are with their baby.

15. The infant's temperature should be taken with the thermometer at 1 hour after transfer. If over 99.2° F (37.3° C), remove a blanket. If the temperature has decreased more than 1°, discontinue skin-to-skin care.

16. Documentation in Gemini (computer system) (® United Kingdom) and daily flowsheets: The RN should document the following:

   a. The initial education concerning skin-to-skin care in Gemini (computer system).

   b. Who performed skin-to-skin and for what period of time on the daily flowsheet.

   c. The infant's behavioral responses before, during, and after skin-to-skin care.

   d. Any complications or problems encountered during the skin-to-skin care.

   e. Parental reaction.

From University of Illinois Medical Center at Chicago Women's and Children's Nursing Services. Used with permission by Dhamapuri Vdyasagar, MD; Catherine Theorell, RNC, MSN, NNP, Beena Peters, RN, MS.

The following is an example of the application of a developmental care protocol individualized for a special infant and family.

## CASE STUDY
### Application of Developmental Care: Protocol
#### By Kathleen A. VandenBerg

The following is an example of individualized, family-centered developmental care and how it can be implemented for a high-risk, premature newborn and parents. This program assumes that staff in the neonatal intensive care unit (NICU) and intermediate nursery has received training in the principles, behavioral observation techniques, and intervention strategies of individualized family-centered developmental care. In addition, this example assumes that there is a Developmental Team consisting of infant development specialists and a clinical nurse educator who are certified in the Naturalistic Observation of Newborn Behavior (Als, 1984). The lengthy descriptions for the medical information are written in a language with clear descriptions so that the family can understand every aspect of this son's medical care.

## Developmental History, Including Behavioral Assessments and Developmental Interventions
### The First Week of Life

***Tim's Initial Medical History*** Tim is a 27-week premature newborn born to a 40-year-old, married woman. Tim's mother, Alicia, had spent several weeks on bedrest at home and on the prenatal unit. She received medicine (betamethasone) to help Tim's lungs mature. At birth, Tim weighed 2 lbs, 4 oz (1040 g, 50th%); length measured 13.5 inches (34.5 cm, 20th%); head measured 9.5 inches (24 cm, 10th%) showing that Tim grew appropriately in his mother's womb. The score of Tim's well-being at birth (Apgar) was 3 at 1 minute, and improved to 6 at 5 minutes, and again improved to 7 at 10 minutes with 10 being the best score. Because Tim had difficulty breathing on his own at birth, he had an ETT. This tube was connected to a machine to assist his breathing ventilator and give his body oxygen. The breathing machine (high-frequency oscillatory ventilation) vibrated the air that flowed to Tim's lungs. Tim received a liquid medicine that was slowly dripped down his breathing tube to make it easier for his lungs to expand (Survanta, Ross Laboratories, Columbus, OH). Tim progressed quickly and only needed the support of the ventilator for 1 day. The breathing tube was removed on the second day of his life, and he received air and oxygen through two small, round plastic tubes, one in each side of his nose (continuous positive airway pressure [PAP]). He also received medicine to help prevent infection (ampicillin and cefotaxime).

***Tim's Behavioral Summary at 2 Days of Age*** At 2 days of age Tim was observed for 58 minutes and his behavior described before, during and after routine caregiving. His environment and current medical situation was detailed in a clear write-up describing Tim's medical, environmental, and developmental experience. From this information, a developmental care plan was also written and shared with his parents, who gave input to the plan. The completed care plan was posted at the bedside; a copy was placed in the chart, and a copy was given to the family. The following summary described Tim's behaviors at this time.

Tim was noted to become very upset with being touched and handled, as evidenced by his dramatic arm and leg extension into the air with any handling. He would work up into a pattern of ongoing activity with arms and legs flailing in all directions, his back would arch, and he would squirm and move out of the boundaries that had been placed for him to rest. At these times, his heart rate would increase, and he became dusky in color around his eyes and mouth. His parents, who were tearful and emotional at the bedside, were even more frustrated and felt helpless when they observed his behaviors.

The developmental nurse met with Tim's parents and obtained parental agreement to have Tim participate in the Developmental Program, explaining the goals and activities of the program. She explained that Tim's behavior was very common and that premature infants all had difficulty controlling their arm and leg movements. She suggested ways to help Tim relax and demonstrated positioning techniques, offering a positioning aide to support and maintain his posture in flexion with arms and legs tucked in. She pointed out that Tim was showing his competence during caregiving by being able to maintain his arms and legs in flexion with help from his nurse, and the positioning aide. His parents were shown how they could help Tim maintain flexed positions and especially how much he liked being positioned on his tummy. On his tummy, with his hand near his face, Tim could settle into a restful calmer sleep. Tim appeared to bring his fist near his mouth and try to suck on his hand. His mother also noticed that he liked to grab onto her finger if she placed it in the palm of his hand. The developmental nurse pointed out the stress signals Tim had shown them (squirming, arching, limb extensions, color changes, increased heart rate), and summarized how they could anticipate these signals and help Tim minimize them. Helping him to calm, tuck, and begin to calm himself would lessen the prevalence of his stress signs. After discussing these ideas, a care plan was written and posted at Tim's bedside.

## Tim's Current Behavioral Goals and Developmental Care Plan

Tim appears to be working toward:

1. Achieving some steadiness in heart rate, breathing rate, and color during handling.
2. Maintaining energy and supported flexion during periods of rest and handling.
3. Attempting to achieve calm, restful sleep in between caregiving.
4. Developing self-calming abilities, such as sucking on his hand, bringing his hands to his face, and holding onto mom's or dad's finger.

Recommendations for Tim included:

1. Environmental modifications
   a. Review and discuss the sound environment and sources of sound around Tim. Should separate space be used away from Tim for rounds? Are overhead pagers disrupting his sleep? Would closing the nearby door minimize hallway noise?
   b. Review and discuss effects of nursery lighting for Tim, and consider covering Tim's crib for nighttime and lowering lights to a dimmer level during waking periods during the day. Review sources of light and possibility of indirect light.
   c. Review and discuss environment around bedspace with parents and encourage them to view it as theirs. How could it be arranged to maintain medical care and meet the family's needs? Would a recliner or very comfortable chair be helpful?
   d. Discuss and review the beginning patterns of holding for parents, including hands-on containment on the bed, skin-to-skin holding, and evaluating Tim's and parents readiness for that activity.
2. Bedspace and Bedding
   a. Provide support to softly flex, and maintain comfortable, aligned positioning during all caregiving events and necessary procedures. Blanket rolls, nesting, gentle swaddling, special buntings, and hands-on containment can be used.
   b. Review and discuss self-calming strategies with the family and the provision of a pacifier and available supports in the bedspace, such as bunting and side rolls.
3. Caregiving interaction
   a. Individualized care plan to be reviewed daily on rounds and discussed in team meetings, rounds, and at bedside meetings with the family.
   b. Caregiving events can be clustered and timed to be offered according to Tim's sleeping and waking cycles and medical needs.
   c. All caregiving events will be evaluated regarding their appropriateness (for example, if Tim is too tired/stressed to have his vitals taken and diaper changed all at once, these activities will be reevaluated as to the possibility of taking the vitals off the monitor every other time, and just handling him to change his diaper, to give him more rest.)

4. Preparation for handling and procedures
Complete the following if there is time:
- Check positioning for Tim and stabilize before beginning.
- Check lighting: Is it appropriate for Tim to tolerate?
- Check Tim's state: Is he ready to begin?
- Check Tim's breathing, heart rate, $O_2$ saturations, and color to see if stable before handling.
- Place Tim's hands near his face, if possible, so that he can work to calm himself during handling.

5. During handling and procedures
- Continue to watch Tim for his stress cues.
- If they emerge, stop and contain; take break.
- Move slow enough that he does not build up stress without recovering between parts of care.
- Keep handling gently and maintain supports throughout.

6. Recovery from handling and procedures
- Once activity is completed, reposition carefully, and maintain supports.
- Stay with Tim until he transitions to sleep or calmness and shows he can stay calm, relaxed for several minutes.

## The Fourth Week of Life
### Medical Progress

Tim at this point was 25 days old and weighed 2 lbs. 7 oz. Tim made steady, consistent progress, and after one day of CPAP, he was placed on a nasal cannula, which provided small tubes in his nose for air and oxygen delivery. After 2 weeks on a nasal cannula, Tim was breathing air on his own, no longer requiring any support. He received medicine (caffeine) to help remind him to breath. He had progressed to full feedings and no longer required an IV. He received mother's breastmilk through a feeding tube, which was placed in his nose, to deliver his feedings directly to his stomach every 3 hours.

***Tim's Behavioral Summary*** Tim has developed increasing competence during caregiving by being able to bring his own arms and legs into flexion with the help of his mother or his nurse. He braces his feet on the end of the bedding and is able to keep himself tucked. He continues to make strong efforts to maintain his new, flexed tucked position, and has begun to place his hands on the sides of his face and enjoys keeping his fingers near his mouth. He demonstrates a steady heart rate during caregiving, and shows an increase only during lengthy activities. Tim can rest quietly with relaxed body and hands when held by his parents, who are delighted with his occasional smile.

He shows some moderate sensitivity to being handled as he is dressed, and repositioned after extending his arms and legs, and spreading his fingers and squirming while changing his diaper. He can recover and reposition into a flexed position with the help of his caregiver or parents.

***Tim's Behavioral Goals and Developmental Care Plan*** From his current observation and history, Tim appears to be working toward:

1. Consistent steadiness in heart rate, breathing rate, and color as handled for care
2. Achieving and maintaining consistent, flexed, tucked positions during caregiving/holding
3. Transitioning to sleep or calm quiet awake periods after care is completed
4. Becoming more consistent and effective at using his self-calming strategies and developing his repertoire, including sucking on pacifier, bracing his feet, bringing hands to face and mouth to calm, grasping a finger

### Recommendations for Tim

1. Environment
- Continue to provide a quiet space around the bedside, avoiding overhead pages near his bed, loud voices, and closing the nearby door to the hallway.
- Continue to maintain low levels of lighting, utilizing a darkening crib cover for Tim over his crib during nighttime sleep and dim lighting at bedside (possibly without crib cover, if light is truly dim) during the daytime.
- Continue use of recliner/rocking chair for his parents to consistently hold Tim skin-to-skin.

2. Bedspace and bedding
- Maintain use of appropriate-sized positioning aide or rolled blankets to support his maintaining flexed, tucked positions during resting periods/in between caregiving. Position so that hands are to the face.

- Note movement patterns, encouraging movement within an organized, stable range of smoothness with limbs flexed and avoiding extensions of arms, legs, and fingers. Avoid swaddling, as this inhibits movement.
3. Caregiving interactions
   - Continue to discuss and review his individualized care plan daily on rounds and in interdisciplinary rounds each week and with his family.
   - Note Tim's increasing tolerance for handling and his calm alertness after caregiving events. This does not mean he does not still need support!
   - Introduce self to Tim before caregiving, gently placing hands on his head/body.
   - Slowly remove blanket over Tim and replace with your hands to maintain flexion of limbs as you begin care.
   - If Tim extends his arms, legs, or fingers; fusses; increases his heart rate; or becomes dusky, **STOP**, contain him with limbs tucked in, and wait for him to stabilize. Use gentle support and hand containment.
   - When removing Tim from his bed to weigh him, keep him wrapped in a blanket with limbs tucked, and support him in flexion throughout this activity.
   - Offer pacifier to see if he will suck during caregiving to self-calm.
   - Encourage Tim to grasp and hold on by placing finger in his palm.
   - Continue skin-to-skin holding with parents.
   - Facilitate recovery after care and transition time to relax and sleep or rest after care is completed, staying with him until settled.

## The Tenth Week of Life

*Tim's Medical Summary*  Tim is now 70 days old, or 10 weeks, and is 37 weeks corrected age. He weighs 5 lbs and 1 oz, with a length of 17.2 inches, and his head measures 12.5 inches. He is breastfeeding all of his feedings except two per day, which are bottle-feeding with mother's milk fortified to provide extra protein, vitamins, and calories for Tim. His parents are preparing to take him home in a couple of days.

*Tim's Behavioral Summary*  Tim is a delightful infant who demonstrates increased strength and competence. He makes repeated successful efforts to tuck himself after briefly extending an arm or a leg, and his movements demonstrate consistent smoothness. He can bring his hands to his face to successfully and effectively calm himself. He is able to attain a calm period of spontaneous alertness and make eye contact for a few minutes before looking away. After caregiving, he sucks on his pacifier, and is able to achieve a deep, restful sleep on his own. He is consolable by slowing the activity level. He will become upset if he is rushed, and extends his arms and legs and spreads his fingers. For example, with a recent repositioning, he extended his arm once and then flexed it on his own and began to suck on his own fingers. He appears more robust and energetic, tolerating moderate periods of activity; although he can become fatigued if the activity is prolonged. This shows itself in his irregular breathing and increased paleness in his face. For this reason, the following suggestions were made to his parents upon discharge.

Tim's competencies were celebrated and his sensitivities were noted so that he could continue to receive the support that he would need to continue on his course of development. He still needs sensitive reading of his cues, and a supportive environment that is responsive to his signals, which are becoming clearer and clearer. He is working on learning to be alert and looking and beginning to focus and follow. He is still working on calming himself and will continue to need help in developing his repertoire of successful, effective, self-regulatory maneuvers. He might need help with transitions to sleeping and waking. Too much activity and lengthy outings might disrupt his fragile new ability to get the rest he needs and preserve his energy. His main focus is feeding, gaining weight, growing, and continuing to develop and get to know his wonderful parents.

## Discharge Developmental and Behavioral Recommendations

*Transition to Home Environment*  Tim will still appreciate quiet and restfulness in his environment. It will be helpful to keep lights at a dim level and avoid placing him under bright lighting or taking him near excessively noisy areas. He is not ready for shopping centers and large groups yet. Continue to observe him so that he can tell you how he is experiencing the noise or lights. He can still tell you what is disturbing or tiring him. He might sleep better if a night light is nearby, and if soft music is playing in his room or by his bed, but fade out these additions by the end of the first week.

**1. Bedding and Bedspace** Tim would still love being positioned the same way he was in the hospital. In fact, recreating his "nest" would help him remember to continue to flex and stay tucked when rested. Tim will enjoy sidelying when awake, but remember when he is asleep to be sure he is on his back with no blankets or loose bedding around him. He will need also to have some time on his tummy, so work this in for playtime as you hold him face-to-face lying against your chest, or turn him to his tummy as you dry his back after his bath. You will also notice that Tim will enjoy moving his arms and legs in smaller circles closer to his body. Help him continue to practice grasping and holding on, bracing his feet against the bedding and tucking.

**2. Caregiving and Handling** Tim will do best if you space out some of his caregiving to continue to help him preserve his energy. For example, avoid feeding and bathing all at the same time.

Watch him for his communications about when caregiving or the environment is beginning to overwhelm him. If you see him look tired, pale, or weak, or extend his arms, fingers, or legs, he might be signaling that he needs to take a rest. Giving him breaks will still help him to maintain and build up his strength and energy. Remember he is still trying to gain weight and develop at the same time.

Allowing him to wake on his own for feedings (sleeping no longer than 5 hours) will help him begin to regulate his own sleeping with feeding schedule. Watch for those alert times, and begin to let him gaze at your face. Talk gently and slowly, but do not be surprised if he looks away—he knows he needs a break! He will gradually get used to looking at you, focusing, following your face, and will become more and more interested in engaging in this activity. Looking and following are developing at this stage. You can take your cues from Tim, and trust that he knows what he needs to do to preserve his energy, get to know you, and develop his abilities. Most of all, enjoy him! Know and appreciate all that you are doing to support his growth and development!

The following job description provided by Kathleen VandenBerg serves as samples that can be adapted to different disciplines and institutions.

# SAMPLE JOB DESCRIPTION
## Kathleen A. VandenBerg
## Infant Development Specialist (IDS)
### Qualifications:

Master's level with educational and clinical background in neonatal practice, including primary and specialized knowledge bases in:

1. Neurobiologic, physiologic, and social-emotional development of fetus and newborn and infant development.
2. Family systems and dynamics and parenting issues in the Newborn Intensive Care Unit (NICU).
3. Prenatal, perinatal, and postnatal complications of infant and mother.
4. Fetal, premature, and term behavioral functioning and behavioral organization.
5. Ecology of the NICU, including staffing and cultural pattern.
6. Training and certification to reliability in Newborn Individualized Developmental Care and Assessment Program (NIDCAP®) (Boston, MA), and or Assessment of Preterm Infant Behavior (APIB).
7. Knowledge of implications of medical conditions on developmental processes of premature and newborn infants in the NICU.

### Description of Duties:

The Infant Development Specialist (IDS) will provide comprehensive infant developmental intervention services to newborns, premature, and convalescing babies and their families in the clinical setting of the NICU. Services provided by the IDS are philosophically defined as:

1. Developmentally and behaviorally focused with concentration on the premature and newborn period.
2. Process-oriented and research based.
3. Individualized and family-centered.
4. Theoretic and assessment based.
5. Collaborative with family and interdisciplinary team members.

6. Consistent and in keeping with the medical care needs of infants in NICU.

The developmental plans designed by the IDS will provide assessment-based individualized interventions supportive of the baby's well-modulated and robust behaviors. All developmental assessments and care plans will be initiated after physician order or according to the Developmental Program NICU Protocol (which states that all infants <1500 g will automatically be referred to the Developmental Program). Effective use of self-regulatory competencies and emerging developmental capacities, as well as team building and collaboration with parents and primary nursing staff will be emphasized as an intervention approach. The objective of this focus is to promote optimal consistency in the delivery of contingent intervention strategies and developmentally supportive care and handling to each infant in the program. The IDS might offer direct and/or indirect strategies, methods, and techniques; positional aides; and/or environmental modifications, as appropriate to provide optimal advocacy for the infant and parents, as well as behavioral and developmental protection of the infant's balanced functioning within the NICU. These services will be offered in the context of individualized developmental care model and/or study protocol, and with respect for the medical interventions necessary for the baby's health and well-being, with the focus of providing behavioral organization of infant.

### Specific Duties Include:

**Clinical Program**: Upon referral, the Developmental Program will provide:

a. Introduction of program by lead IDS to family and medical staff and orientation for family to developmental services in NICU and role of infant development specialists.
b. Initial behavioral assessment and implementation of plan to include a discussion of the assessment findings with staff and family.
c. Weekly reassessment and update of developmental care plan to include discussion of progress and developmental issues with parents, staff, and support to create an appropriate environment and pattern of modified caregiving for infant.

d. Establish and maintain contact and ongoing communication with family in spirit of trust-building and collaboration, recognizing the parents are the primary caregivers of their infant.

e. Identify and interpret the infant's behavioral strengths, current developmental functional level and thresholds and sensitivities for handling and activities.

f. Provide and maintain developmental materials supportive of infant's developmental needs. Provide recommendations for positioning, handling, consistency of caregiving, predictability, timing of interventions, support of self-regulation, and support of state regulation and social interaction.

g. Provide and support parents, providing developmental and behavioral information and materials to foster parent-infant relationships and build on their role as members of the healthcare team.

h. Support and encourage parents and caregivers to build confidence in their own observational skills to identify and maintain appropriate levels of infant and parent/caregiver interaction.

i. Interdisciplinary planning with unit staff to provide support for infant and family.

**Mentoring Capacity:** Infant Development Specialist provides for:

a. Developmental and educational opportunities/in-services for families and staff.

b. Understands need to use adult learning theory in education opportunities.

c. Develops appropriate materials and educational materials for staff/families.

d. Mentors staff and other professionals in developmental work.

e. Practices the reflective processing regularly and in collaboration with staff.

f. Provides program evaluation methodology and statistics, as required.

**Provides Leadership and Systems Change:** Provides for:

a. Consistently integrates the developmental perspective into policy-making decisions for NICU.

b. Recognizes opportunities to apply change theory in the NICU and hospital system to effect policy and practice.

c. Collaborates with management and staff to effect systems change and impact on ecology and culture of NICU.

d. Continually evaluates and responds appropriately to parent and staff evaluations.

## CAREGIVING GUIDELINES FOR TOUCH AND INFANT MASSAGE

The following two guidelines for touch and infant massage were developed by the Infant Massage Interest Group (Northern and Yorkshire Region), United Kingdom. Again, although these are included in this section of the book, there is need for more research to determine when infant massage is safely done. The infant's gestational age, severity of illness, and stability must be considered.

### Positive Touch and Containment Holds
#### Aim

To provide a description and rationale for containment holds. These are designed to be used when massage is not appropriate for whatever reason and are applied with no pressure, with the hands resting on the baby. Although, ideally, this touch is done by parents, all members of staff should be encouraged to use it, for settling, calming, or during procedures.

#### Objective

Positive touch is a medium for establishing a working relationship with the family. It is infant led and parent directed—an integral part of a family-centered developmental care program.

### Infant Massage (Preterm and Term)
#### Aim

To introduce massage to parents/caregivers of hospitalized infants. This protocol also acknowledges the existence of appropriate and inappropriate touch.

### POSITIVE TOUCH

| Action | Rationale |
|---|---|
| 1. Assess the needs of the neonate and family. Do not disturb the baby if sleeping. | Touch must be adapted to the individual infant's behavior, physiologic responses, and medical condition, and also the family's needs. |
| 2. Explain to the parents the indications for 'positive touch' and the benefits for baby and parents. | Helps reduce stress by calming the infant, promotes sleep and parental attachment and involvement. |
| 3. Wash hands and remove jewelry before beginning positive touch. | Minimizes the risk of infection, and reduces the risk of abrasions from jewelry. |
| 4. Consider the environment and, when possible, shade the baby's face from the light, and turn down alarm settings (decibels). | Provides a beneficial environment to help eliminate stress. |
| 5. Request baby's permission to be touched. | Enables the baby to prepare and become aware of the beginning of positive, loving touch. |
| 6. Begin with still touch, one hand on head and one on trunk. | Simple introduction of containment holding assists babies in organizing their behavior. |
| 7. When moving from one hold to the next, move one hand at a time; remain in contact with baby throughout. Small, premature, or sensitive babies might need to be kept covered with clothes or a blanket. | Prevents loss of contact, and makes baby feel secure at all times. |
| 8. Continue the hold as long as the baby will allow, observing cues throughout. | Allow baby to communicate with parents through positive behavior and eye contact. Promotes bonding and empowers parents to be involved in baby's development. |
| 9. Evaluate containment/positive touch-in-care plan. | Ensures individualized care has been given, and provides a rationale for the way the baby is positioned at that time. |

## Objective

To reduce stress and the effects of separation.

### Infant Massage

| Action | Rationale |
|---|---|
| 1. Assess the needs of the neonate, and talk to parents about relaxation; practice some simple exercises and visualization. | It is essential that parents understand their role in massage. Infants can sense if someone is feeling tense. Parents are mirrors for their babies, and massage offers parents the opportunity to give themselves some attention. |
| 2. Wash hands, and remove jewelry before beginning massage. | Although you might not be undertaking the massage, this sets a good example for parents. |
| 3. Consider the environment and, when possible, shade the baby's face from the light, and turn down alarm settings (decibels). | Provides a beneficial environment and helps eliminate stress. |
| 4. Request baby's permission to begin. | Lets the baby know that a new experience is about to begin and helps the infant to prepare for it. Also communicates respect. |
| 5. Point out various behavioral states to parents—e.g., waking activity, fussing, and crying. Ask parents to observe their baby and note sleep wake cycles. | Helps parents discover the best massage time for their baby. Best stage for massage is the quiet, alert state, being mindful of the ward environment. |
| 6. Teach the parent massage strokes by demonstration on soft doll. Demonstrate the series of strokes, instructing verbally as progressing. Teach parents to read cues. | Parents can massage with you or watch first, depending on preference. Empowers parent to massage when they feel ready, and makes them feel that they are doing something of value for their baby. |
| 7. Teach touch relaxation, for the parent to condition baby to respond to touch and voice with relaxation. | Positive reinforcement. |
| 8. Encourage parents to continue to offer massage to baby throughout childhood. | Makes parents aware of techniques that are best for each stage of development. |
| 9. Work within the multidisciplinary team to promote infant massage within a safe environment. | Safety should be maintained at all times, and it is important that your colleagues are aware of what is being done. |
| 10. Provide information of how massage can benefit the individual child. | Provides parent with sound knowledge base of why they are providing massage. |
| 11. Evaluate results of massage, and document in care plan. | Provides continuity of care. |

From Wall, A. (2002). Agreeing a standard for infant massage: Not a soft touch. *Journal of Neonatal Nursing, 8*(3), 93–96, as cited in C. Kenner & J.W. Lott (Eds.). (2004). *Neonatal nursing handbook* (pp. 429–435). St. Louis: W.B. Saunders.

# REFERENCES

Als, H. (1984). *Manual for the naturalistic observation of the newborn (preterm and fullterm)* (rev. vol.). Boston: Children's Hospital.

Browne, J.V., VandenBerg, K.A., Ross, E.S., et al. (1999). The newborn developmental specialist: Definition, quali-fications, and preparation for an emerging role in the neonatal intensive care unit. *Infants and Young Children, 11*(4), 53-64.

VandenBerg, K.A. (1993). Basic competencies to begin developmental care in the intensive care nursery. *Infants and Young Children, 6*(2) 52-59.

# B Newborn Individualized Developmental Care Assessment Program (NIDCAP®), Boston, MA—www.nidcap.com/nidcap/

Advances in perinatal and neonatal care have greatly decreased the mortality rates for preterm newborns and newborns otherwise at high risk for developmental compromise. The challenge confronting healthcare professionals caring for these infants and their families is not only to ensure the infants' survival but to optimize their developmental course and outcome. Through assessment and documentation of infant's competence and behavioral thresholds to disorganization, a better understanding of the developing nervous system can be gained. This, in turn, might lead to the provision of developmentally appropriate experiential opportunities for the newborn in the hospital setting and provision of supportive care for the infant's family. Structuring a physical and social environment that is supportive and nurturing of the individual infant's immature or dysmature nervous system and of the family's sense of competence becomes a critical component of care in the newborn intensive care unit (NICU) and of follow-up care in home and community. NIDCAP® has been established to provide education and specific training in developmental observation and assessment for healthcare professionals who have a responsibility for the long- and short-term care of high-risk newborns and preterm infants and their families, and for staff members who are involved in the implementation of their care on a day-to-day basis. An essential focus of the NIDCAP® program is the educational and consultative support and assistance to NICU and special care nursery (SCN) settings toward effective delivery of intensive and special care in a neurodevelopmentally supportive, individualized, and family-centered framework.

## NIDCAP® BACKGROUND

The goal of education and training in the developmental approach to care is to bring about a shift from protocol-based to strategic process thinking, and from task-oriented to relationship-based care. The developmental approach to care sees infants as active structurers of their own developmental trajectories, supported by the ongoing co-regulation process of infant and parent development. The newborn's three evolutionarily adapted and inherited econiches, biologically expected for good-enough development, are the mother's womb, the parents' body and mother's breast, and the family's social group. Preterm newborns unexpectedly have removed themselves from the intrauterine environment and its complex co-regulatory inputs. By virtue of the need for hospital care, they, as well as high-risk, full-term newborns in need of hospitalization, are separated from the expected intimate parent and family environment for prolonged periods. Developmental care takes advantage of the infant's expectation for co-regulatory care and for a close, emotionally attuned and invested relationship. It sees an opportunity for the increased effectiveness of intensive care delivery in supporting the realignment and co-regulation of the newborn and the family. Implementation of intensive care in such a framework requires knowledge and understanding of infant, parent, and family development, and of the interplay of the infant's medical issues with the developmental process. To achieve multidisciplinary collaboration in developmental care implementation, appreciation of each of the professional disciplines coming together in the NICU is necessary, as well as understanding of the organizational structures of the hospital and the nursery. Furthermore, skill and sensitivity are required in supporting and nurturing infant and family. Professionals in such a complex setting must be committed to further their own personal growth, self-knowledge, and emotional maturity. The NIDCAP® program was designed to provide information, education, and support of those aspects by provision of reading materials as well as didactic presentations, observation training, and opportunities for individual and system guidance and consultation. It is the responsibility of each professional participating in training to create additional opportunities as indicated. It is the responsibility of the leadership in a setting to create opportunities for staff development, as well as enhancement of organizational and physical structures as indicated.

In the NIDCAP® model, specific estimation of each individual infant's current goal strivings is derived from the direct observation of each infant's behavior in the context of ongoing care delivery. The infant's behavior provides the guide for the caregiver to estimate the infant's current strengths and active efforts in catalyzing and structuring his or her own development. Direct observation of the infant's behavior with inference of the infant's own goals provides the basis from which to explore opportunities with the family and with professional caregivers to support the infant's goal strivings and differentiating competencies.

A systematic behavioral observation methodology, referred to as NIDCAP® observation, as well as a formal evaluation, the Assessment of Preterm Infant Behavior (APIB), have been developed to assess and increase understanding of the preterm and otherwise at-risk newborn's behavior. Both methodologies, NIDCAP® observation and APIB, are based on the Synactive Theory of Development developed by Dr. Heidelise Als in 1982, and are designed to specifically document the complexity and sensitivity of the preterm and the at-risk newborn infant by focusing on the interplay of the infant's autonomic, motoric, state organizational, and attentional functioning as the infant interacts with the caregiver and world around the infant.

The results of the systematic observations and formal evaluations provide the basis for the estimation of the infant's current goals, which, in turn, leads to the consideration of opportunities in support of the infant's development, such as:

1. The structuring of an appropriate physical environment in the NICU for infant and family
2. The timing and organization of medical and nursing interventions appropriate to the individuality of infant and family
3. The support and nurturance of the parents' cherishing of their infant, and of their confidence in caring for and taking pride in supporting their infant's development
4. The coordination in the developmental framework of the care delivered by special service providers such as respiratory therapists, occupational and physical therapists, social workers, nutritionists, early intervention professionals, public health nurses, and others.

The NIDCAP® approach lends itself to system-based, process-oriented, attuned, and responsive support of individualized developmental care for each infant and family.

Results to date show that medical and developmental outcomes for infants and competence of parents cared for in such a developmental framework are much improved. The APIB provides an additional systematic, formal means for assessment of behavioral functioning of the preterm and otherwise at-risk newborn. In the hands of the professional with advanced background and training in child development and clinical infant psychology, the APIB becomes a diagnostic and prognostic tool, further supporting the caregiver in identifying specific opportunities and issues in complex situations and/or at clinical transition and decision points.

## OVERVIEW OF SPECIFIC NIDCAP® TRAINING COMPONENTS

Effective developmental care implementation on a nursery-wide basis is the goal of all training and consultation provided in the NIDCAP® framework. Training is currently available from 10 NIDCAP® training centers around the country. Based on extensive experience, moving toward successful delivery of newborn intensive care in a developmental framework is typically a 5-year process. It involves:

1. Training of a developmental specialist and a developmental care nurse educator
2. Training of a multidisciplinary leadership support team (approximately 6-7 members)
3. Training of a core group of the nursing staff, and all staff if possible
4. Salaried positions (1.5-2 full-time equivalents [FTEs]) for the developmental specialist and developmental care nurse educator
5. Development of a parent council and/or parent representative working with the team of developmental leadership professionals

Initial training consists of training in infant behavioral observation as well as developmental care planning and implementation based on the behavioral observation (NIDCAP® Level I). This training is embedded in consultation to the NICU regarding environment, developmental team building, and developmental care implementation (NIDCAP® Level II). In addition, training for the developmental specialist and developmental care nurse educator includes training in neurobehavioral assessment (APIB), and consultation with the developmental specialist, the developmental care nurse educator, and the multidisciplinary leadership support team in the facilitation of implementation of developmental care (NIDCAP® Level II). The document *Developmental Care Implementation in a Newborn Intensive Care Unit (NICU): Overview of Training Process, Budget Projections, and Cost Benefit Analysis*, available from the training centers, spells out in more detail the process of implementation. One and one-half to two full-time positions are typically required to effectively support a NICU of between 40 and 50 beds, with between 150 and 180 nursing FTEs, for consistent developmental care implementation.

# C Wee Care® Program, Norwell, MA—www.childmed.com

The Wee Care® program developed by Children's Medical Ventures, Norwell, MA, includes the following components:

- Classroom instruction on developmental theories and cues, sensory system development, environmental issues, family-centered care, and outcomes
- Hands-on workshops focusing on positioning and all aspects of handling and caregiving
- Customized interactive sessions on either Kangaroo care, feeding, or families
- Bedside consultation in the neonatal intensive care unit (NICU) to problem solve daily challenges
- Special presentations for support staff (e.g., respiratory therapy, radiology, clerical, housekeeping) addressing their contribution to developmental care
- Workshops for physical, occupational, and speech therapists focusing on their unique role in the NICU
- Practical ideas for implementation and integration to developmental care throughout the unit and hospital
- Assistance in establishing and mentoring a developmental care committee
- Educational contact hours for nursing staff
- Additional educational sessions, support, and guidance throughout the year

Wee Care® is a clinically relevant, practical program offered by Children's Medical Ventures for the education of the entire NICU staff. The comprehensive program, typically 3 to 5 days in duration, addresses the optimization of the NICU environment and care practices to facilitate the best possible outcomes for premature infants and their families. Wee Care® is taught by a team of clinically active experts in the field and uses classroom-teaching activities, interactive sessions, and hands-on demonstrations of practical skills, in both the classroom and the NICU. The teaching program educates the entire staff, including all support personnel, per their individual needs and roles within the NICU, in the concepts of developmentally supportive, family-centered care. After completion of the basic Wee Care® program, advanced training in developmentally supportive, family-centered care is available from Children's Medical Ventures.

Using this program, research is currently being conducted in these areas:

- Length of stay
- Costs
- Morbidities
- Sound levels
- Ambient lighting
- Restraint hours
- Staff morale
- Parent satisfaction

Source: Children's Medical Ventures. Available online at *www.childmed.com/Education_Programs/invoke.cfm?objectid= CE82CAE0-D7EE-4DD1-973A51AD683E287F&method=display.*

# D Preemie for a Day® Program, Norwell, MA—www.childmed.com

Preemie for a Day® is an interactive, multisensory program that helps caregivers better understand the neonatal intensive care unit (NICU) experience of preterm infants. The unique 4-hour workshop utilizes a variety of teaching modalities that complement the material and address diverse adult learning styles.

The Preemie for a Day® program begins with an overview of developmental care, including a review of up-to-date research and outcomes information. In addition to the overview, participants will have the opportunity to participate in hands-on, small group sessions focused on:

- Admission to the NICU
- Positioning and handling
- Feeding of the preterm infant
- Family involvement and communication

Participants not only learn and discuss ways to improve the care and outcomes of their tiniest patients but also experience the reasons for approaching care in a developmentally supportive manner. Discussion time at the end of the program focuses on shared experiences, obstacles to overcome, and strategies for success.

The program is led by a team of clinically active professionals with a variety of NICU backgrounds, including nursing, medicine, and occupational therapy. Their experiences allow them to present practical and effective ways to change caregiving behaviors in order to integrate developmental care into daily practice.

The Preemie for a Day® program is provided by Children's Medical Ventures, a subsidiary of Respironics, Inc. Since 1991, Children's Medical Ventures has been working to establish developmentally supportive, family-centered care as the standard of care in the newborn intensive care unit with innovative products and education programs. Their interactive programs heighten the awareness of caregivers to the impact that care practices and the environment have on premature infants and their families.

Children's Medical Ventures offers a wide variety of programs including the comprehensive Wee Care® program, the nationally renowned Preemie for a Day® program, and a wide variety of additional offerings. All of the programs are designed to meet the needs of the individual unit, and many of them have a hands-on experiential approach. They also sponsor educational meetings for managers in conjunction with the National Association of Neonatal Nurses and/or other hospital groups.

For more information on any of their education programs, please call Children's Medical Ventures at (866) 866-6750 or e-mail them at *info@childmed.com*.

# Sample Physical Therapy Competencies and Early Intervention Plans

## Neonatal Physical Therapy Competencies, Roles, and Proficiencies (Sweeney et al., 1999)

**COMPETENCY 1: SCREENING, PRIMARY PREVENTION, AND RISK MANAGEMENT**

**Role 1.1 Screen NICU infant population to determine the need for physical therapy services.**

**Clinical Proficiencies**

1.1.1. Identify and interpret infant information by chart review and interview of neonatal caregivers.

1.1.2. Identify and interpret family information related to infant caregiving by interviews of family members.

1.1.3. Observe parent-infant interaction patterns and recognize potential interaction problems during caregiving.

1.1.4. Participate in NICU medical or developmental rounds.

1.1.5. Recognize atypical physiologic or behavioral manifestations in infants.

**Role 1.2 Develop and implement a risk management plan for each infant to prevent physiologic compromise, behavioral stress, and secondary musculoskeletal complications and integumentary disruption.**

**Clinical Proficiencies**

1.2.1. Recognize physiologic stress in an infant by interpreting autonomic responses from the infant and data from monitoring equipment: heart rate, respiratory rate, and breathing pattern, color, oxygen saturation, blood pressure, and temperature.

1.2.2. Identify and interpret infant engagement and disengagement behavioral cues reflected in movement and posture, behavioral state, and attention and interaction.

1.2.3. Conduct prehandling observation of the infant to determine a safe and effective approach to begin examination and intervention.

1.2.4. Formulate a rationale for implementing a risk-management plan for the infant.

1.2.5. Recognize and prevent potential and iatrogenic neuromusculoskeletal, integumentary, and infection complications.

1.2.6. Locate all leads and lines from the infant to the medical equipment and explain the general function of each attached equipment unit.

1.2.7. Handle an infant on physiologic monitors, respiratory equipment, infusion or parenteral feeding lines, and other medical support devices.

1.2.8. Analyze and modify the physical and social environment using environmental support measures (e.g. positioning aids, light and sound control measures) and individualized caregiving procedures.

1.2.9. Educate parents, neonatal caregivers, and community resource representatives on potential injuries from infant products and walkers in home environments.

1.2.10. Modify seating devices and monitor physiologic and behavioral tolerance during predischarge car seat trials.

*Continued*

NEONATAL PHYSICAL THERAPY COMPETENCIES, ROLES, AND PROFICIENCIES (SWEENEY ET AL., 1999)—CONT'D

**Role 1.3 Develop the physical therapy risk management component of the newborn medicine service's risk management program.**

**Clinical Proficiencies**

1.3.1. Establish and document standard operating procedures for managing physiologic risk during observation, infant examinations, and physical therapy interventions.

1.3.2. Establish and document procedures for reporting inadvertent occurrences of adverse events during provision of physical therapy services in the NICU.

## COMPETENCY 2: EXAMINATION AND EVALUATION

**Role 2.1 Examine infants and interpret findings.**

**Clinical Proficiencies**

2.1.1. Conduct clinical examinations and evaluations.

2.1.2. Administer standardized tests and measures.

2.1.3. Evaluate level of functioning and recommend a developmentally appropriate plan of care including strategies for intervention.

## COMPETENCY 3: PLANNING AND IMPLEMENTING NEONATAL INTERVENTION

**Role 3.1 Design, implement, and evaluate intervention plans and strategies in collaboration with the family and neonatal team.**

**Clinical Proficiencies**

3.1.1. Identify measurable long- and-short-range intervention goals and functional outcomes (Msall, 2002).

3.1.2. Determine frequency, intensity, and methods (e.g., direct, consultative) for implementing a developmentally appropriate physical therapy intervention plan.

3.1.3. Implement therapeutic strategies appropriate to gestational age, physiologic tolerance, and state control, including positioning, handling, hydrotherapy, splinting, behavioral organization, oral-motor/feeding, modified infant massage/touch, and adaptive equipment.

3.1.4. Collaborate with neonatal nurses to implement modification of the physical and social environment in the nursery.

3.1.5. Collect data, monitor progress, evaluate effectiveness, and modify therapeutic strategies, plan, and goals accordingly.

3.1.6. Enhance infant-parent interaction and attachment.

3.1.7. Incorporate developmentally appropriate practices and therapeutic strategies into daily caregiving by NICU staff and parents.

3.1.8. Use parent concerns and priorities to guide the design and implementation of intervention.

**Role 3.2 Develop and implement discharge plans in collaboration with caregivers and community resource representatives.**

**Clinical Proficiencies**

3.2.1. Formulate transition plans for discharging infants to their homes and communities.

3.2.2. Create linkages to community resources and NICU follow-up programs.

## COMPETENCY 4: CONSULTATION

**Role 4.1 Consult with health professionals, families, professional and community organizations or agencies, and interested members of the general public.**

**Clinical Proficiencies**

4.1.1. Assess needs and expected outcomes of consultation.

4.1.2. Formulate goals, criteria, timelines, and select consultation models in collaboration with clients.

4.1.3. Identify internal and external procedural and regulatory guidelines.

4.1.4. Collaborate in identifying and analyzing problems and in developing action plans.

4.1.5. Analyze and interpret change process (individual styles and rates of change).

NEONATAL PHYSICAL THERAPY COMPETENCIES, ROLES, AND PROFICIENCIES (SWEENEY ET AL., 1999)—CONT'D

4.1.6. Evaluate outcome and recommend revision of action plans.

4.1.7. Identify expanded resources and potential referrals to other disciplines or services.

## COMPETENCY 5: SCIENTIFIC INQUIRY

**Role 5.1 Incorporate clinical implications from scientific literature into neonatal practice.**
**Clinical Proficiencies**

5.1.1. Review and critically analyze neonatal medicine and pediatric physical therapy literature.

5.1.2. Apply research and practice literature to caregiving plans and interventions.

**Role 5.2 Support or participate in research involving infants, parent, or caregivers in neonatal care units.**
**Clinical Proficiencies**

5.2.1. Create questions or neonatal topics that can be addressed by clinical researchers.

5.2.2. Review the literature to identify related studies, establish a basis for the research question(s) and potential measurement methods, and evaluate designs and statistical methods used in similar studies.

5.2.3. Formulate hypotheses.

5.2.4. Establish and define independent and dependent variables.

5.2.5. Determine research design, including sample size and selection criteria.

5.2.6. Determine research methods, including reliability and validity characteristics of tests and measures.

5.2.7. Analyze and interpret data.

5.2.8. Establish conclusions and clinical implications from the data.

5.2.9. Identify limitations of the study and suggestions for future research.

5.2.10. Disseminate results of the research.

## COMPETENCY 6: CLINICAL EDUCATION AND SELF-LEARNING/PROFESSIONAL DEVELOPMENT

**Role 6.1 Communicate, demonstrate, and evaluate neonatal physical therapy care processes.**
**Clinical Proficiencies**

6.1.1. Identify learner knowledge and skill needs and prepare clinical training that reflects baseline and expected achievement levels.

6.1.2. Establish training objectives and priorities.

6.1.3. Choose teaching methods and format.

6.1.4. Communicate information, demonstrate procedures, arrange practice sessions and repeat demonstrations, and provide feedback with learners on performance.

6.1.5. Evaluate learner performance and teaching effectiveness.

**Role 6.2 Pursue ongoing continuing education in practice topics related to neonatology**
**Clinical Proficiencies**

6.2.1. Self-assess clinical competencies and knowledge limitations in physical therapy for neonates.

6.2.2. Evaluate and select continuing education options to address skill and knowledge deficit areas.

## COMPETENCY 7: ADMINISTRATION

**Role 7.1. Plan and administer a neonatal physical therapy program or service.**
**Clinical Proficiencies**

7.1.1. Develop a mission and philosophy for the neonatal physical therapy program that is consistent with the missions and philosophy of the hospital and newborn medicine service.

7.1.2. Assess the service needs of the target neonatal population.

7.1.3. Select and assign priorities to the physical therapy procedures for neonates that will be offered.

7.1.4. Identify and acquire physical therapy resources for serving neonates, including therapists with precepted training, supplies, and time.

7.1.5. Establish financial support and develop a neonatal physical therapy service budget.

*Continued*

## NEONATAL PHYSICAL THERAPY COMPETENCIES, ROLES, AND PROFICIENCIES (SWEENEY ET AL., 1999)—CONT'D

7.1.6. Develop and implement physical therapy policies and procedures for neonates including referral mechanism, supervision process, protocols for high risk or unusual procedures (e.g., hydrotherapy, extremity taping) and documentation format and timelines.

7.1.7. Establish procedures for managing adverse events, including reporting, following, and clinical teaching.

7.1.8. Identify ethical and legal standards and incorporate them into neonatal physical therapy practice.

**Role 7.2 Evaluate the effectiveness of a neonatal physical therapy program or service.**

**Clinical Proficiencies**

7.2.1. Evaluate and monitor quality of care through review of cases and records with peers.

7.2.2. Evaluate and monitor clinical productivity.

7.2.3. Analyze effectiveness of interventions on infant and family functioning.

7.2.4. Conduct general review of physical therapy program or service with neonatal medical and nursing managers.

## BEGINNINGS INDIVIDUALIZED FAMILY SERVICE PLAN (IFSP)

### (FOR FAMILIES WHOSE BABIES ARE IN THE HOSPITAL NURSERY)

Baby's name:                                                    Birthdate:                    Boy        Girl

Date of referral to:                        Name of hospital:

Part C
Parents'/Guardians' names:

Language(s) spoken at home:                                    Medicaid number/SSN:

Brothers & sisters living in the home:

Others living in the home:

Address:                                                       Home phone:

County:

Phone numbers of other key family members:

**OUR BABY'S HISTORY**
Part C eligible diagnosis:                                     Birth weight:

Actual due date:                                               Date admitted to the hospital:

Anticipated/actual discharge date:

Concerns/problems during pregnancy:

Baby's primary diagnosis at birth:

Our concerns now:

Important tests (hearing screening, vision, etc):

ELIGIBILITY CATEGORIES FOR INFANT AND FAMILY SERVICES IN COLORADO UNDER THE INDIVIDUALS WITH DISABILITIES EDUCATION ACT, PART C (DEVELOPED FOR USE IN NEONATAL INTENSIVE CARE UNITS IN COLORADO)

**CHILDREN WITH CONDITIONS ASSOCIATED WITH SIGNIFICANT DEVELOPMENTAL DELAY:**

A. Chromosomal syndromes: Such as (but not limited to) Down syndrome, Patau syndrome, Edwards syndrome, autosomal deletion syndrome, Turner syndrome, Klinefelter syndrome, fragile X syndrome, 4p syndrome, Apert syndrome, chromosomal deletions, Pierre Robin, trisomy 18, trisomy 13, XYY, DeLange, Peni-Shokeir, Melnich-Fraser, Waardensburg, osteogenesis imperfecta

B. Congenital Syndromes or Conditions:
   1. CNS malformations, such as hydrocephaly, microcephaly, and meningocele, craniosynostosis, agenesis of the corpus callosum, encephalocele
   2. Brain abnormalities, such as evidence of the following in birth records: Seizures, clonic spasms, hypertonia or hypotonia, hyperactivity, lethargy, paralysis/paresis, asymmetric or abnormal reflexes
   3. Fetal alcohol syndrome

C. Sensory Impairments:
   1. Hearing impairment
   2. Deafness
   3. Vision impairment
   4. Blindness

D. Metabolic Disorders: Such as (but not limited to) hypothyroidism (untreated), lipidoses, maple syrup urine disease, galactosemia

E. Prenatal and Perinatal Conditions
   1. TORCH infections (congenital infections including toxoplasmosis, syphilis, rubella, herpes simplex, and cytomegalovirus)
   2. Severe intraventricular hemorrhage (Grades 3 or 4), ventriculomegaly, periventricular leukomalacia
   3. Teratogens
   4. Neonatal seizures, infantile spasms
   5. Cerebral palsy
   6. Intrauterine exposure to illegal drugs
   7. HIV positive
   8. Meningitis

F. Very Low Birthweight (1200 grams or less)

Linda Ikle; revised March 1996.

## The Colorado Consortium of Intensive Care Nurseries Eligibility Categories for Infant and Family Services in Colorado Under the Individuals with Disabilities Education Act, Part C

Please check and/or circle any pertinent diagnoses:

A. Chromosomal syndromes: Such as (but not limited to) Down syndrome, Patau syndrome, Edwards syndrome, Autosomal deletion syndrome, Turner syndrome, Klinefelter syndrome, Fragile X syndrome, 4p syndrome, Apert syndrome, Chromosomal deletions, Pierre Robin, trisomy 18, trisomy 13, XYY, DeLange, Peni-Shokeir, Melnich-Fraser, Waardensburg, osteogenesis imperfecta

B. Congenital Syndromes or Conditions:
   1. CNS malformations, such as hydrocephaly, microcephaly, and meningocele, craniosynostosis, agenesis of the corpus callosum, encephalocele.
   2. Brain abnormalities, such as evidence of the following in birth records: Seizures, clonic spasms, hypertonia, or hypotonia, hyperactivity, lethargy, paralysis/paresis, asymmetrical or abnormal reflexes.

C. Sensory Impairments:
   1. Hearing impairment
   2. Deafness
   3. Vision impairment
   4. Blindness

D. Metabolic disorders: Such as (but not limited to) hypothyroidism (untreated), lipidoses, maple syrup urine disease, galactosemia

E. Prenatal and Perinatal Conditions:
   1. TORCH infections (including toxoplasmosis, syphilis, rubella, herpes simplex, and cytomegalovirus)
   2. Severe intraventricular hemorrhage (Grades 3 or 4), ventriculomegaly, periventricular leukomalacia
   3. Teratogen exposure
   4. Neonatal seizures, infantile spasms
   5. Cerebral palsy
   6. Intrauterine exposure to illegal drugs
   7. HIV positive
   8. Meningitis

F. Very Low Birthweight (1200 grams or less)

G. Other:

Physician's Signature: _____   Date: _____

I understand that by nature of this diagnosis, my baby is *at risk for* developmental disabilities. I have had my baby's eligibility for Early Childhood Connections explained to me and agree to the release of information to the appropriate agency(ies).

Parent Signature: _____   Date: _____

(Infant's Name and Patient
ID Info May Be Stamped Here)

(Hospital Logo and Insignia
May Be Put Here)

These criteria were established by the Colorado NICU Connections Task Force and Dr. Linda Iklé/revised March 1996. This form has been developed by and for the use in The Colorado Consortium of Intensive Care Units. Thanks to the NICU team at Exempla Healthcare, Saint Joseph Hospital for this adaptation.

## The Colorado Consortium of Intensive Care Nurseries/Part C Referral Log

Please fax this form to the Consortium at 303-764-8092 at the end of each month

[Hospital Name]

| Infant's Name or Unique ID | DOB/ Sex/ Race | Primary Part C Diagnosis | Parent's Names & Address (Include County Referred to) | Phone Number | Consent (Y or N) | Date "Beginnings" Initiated | Referred to | Referred by |
|---|---|---|---|---|---|---|---|---|
| | | | | | | | | |
| | | | | | | | | |
| | | | | | | | | |
| | | | | | | | | |

Use the first four letters of the child's last name and the first letter of the first name followed by the birth date in 8 digit format (i.e., 010499). If it is a multiple birth and the children have first names beginning with the same letter, please add a digit at the end of this ID to indicate birth order (1,2,3,4, etc.).

## Early Childhood Connections

### Fact Sheet

### (Sponsored by The Colorado Consortium of Intensive Care Nurseries)

Why refer to Early Childhood Connections? We are located in communities across the state and offer families having a child with or at risk for developmental delays a link to supports and services in their home area. We value education as a way of keeping families in control of the plans for their children and family and in touch with the dreams they have for their child. When a referral is made we:

- Make a connection with the family at home, in the hospital, or at a site of their choosing.
- Bring information about resources, child development, and diagnosis-specific information.
- Connect the family with a person who can coordinate resources the family and baby may need including SSI or Medicaid applications, transportation, child care, and interpreters.
- Assist the family with a plan of action to address specific needs such as early intervention, respite care, daily care and learning activities, making time for yourself and other family members, and including the child in community activities.
- Support the family in building a lifelong circle of support, including parent to parent support.
- Assist in coordinating a comfortable transition from the NICU to home by participating in the discharge planning or the Beginnings IFSP.
- Assist the family to access community resources for paid services by developing an individualized family service plan (Beginnings or other IFSP).

Our focus on development ranges from information about care for the child who is premature to long-term planning for a child with significant needs to assure each an inclusive place in his/her community. Early Childhood Connections refers to Part C of the Individuals with Disabilities Education Act (IDEA) in the state of Colorado.

Call 1-888-777-4041 for more information.

# Neonatal Pain, Agitation, and Sedation Scale (N-PASS)

Pat Hummel, MA, RNC, NNP, PNP & Mary Puchalski, MS, RNC

| Assessment Criteria | Sedation | | Normal | Pain / Agitation | |
|---|---|---|---|---|---|
| | -2 | -1 | 0 | 1 | 2 |
| Crying Irritability | No cry with painful stimuli | Moans or cries minimally with painful stimuli | Appropriate crying<br>Not irritable | Irritable or crying at intervals<br>Consolable | High-pitched or silent-continuous cry<br>Inconsolable |
| Behavior State | No arousal to any stimuli<br>No spontaneous movement | Arouses minimally to stimuli<br>Little spontaneous movement | Appropriate for gestational age | Restless, squirming<br>Awakens frequently | Arching, kicking<br>Constantly awake or<br>Arouses minimally / no movement (not sedated) |
| Facial Expression | Mouth is lax<br>No expression | Minimal expression with stimuli | Relaxed<br>Appropriate | Any pain expression intermittent | Any pain expression continual |
| Extremities Tone | No grasp reflex<br>Flaccid tone | Weak grasp reflex<br>↓ muscle tone | Relaxed hands and feet<br>Normal tone | Intermittent clenched toes, fists or finger splay<br>Body is not tense | Continual clenched toes, fists, or finger splay<br>Body is tense |
| Vital Signs HR, RR, BP, SaO₂ | No variability with stimuli<br>Hypoventilation or apnea | < 10% variability from baseline with stimuli | Within baseline or normal for gestational age | ↑ 10-20% from baseline<br>SaO₂ 76-85% with stimulation - quick ↑ | ↑ > 20% from baseline<br>SaO₂ ≤ 75% with stimulation – slow ↑<br>Out of sync with vent |

© Hummel & Puchalski
Loyola University Health System, Layola University Chicago, 2000

*(Rev. 8/14/01)*

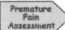

**Premature Pain Assessment**
+ 3 if < 28 weeks gestation / corrected age
+ 2 if 28-31 weeks gestation / corrected age
+ 1 if 32-35 weeks gestation / corrected age

## Assessment of Sedation

- Sedation is scored in addition to pain for each behavioral and physiological criteria to assess the infant's response to stimuli
- Sedation does not need to be assessed/scored with every pain assessment/score
- Sedation is scored from 0 → -2 for each behavioral and physiological criteria, then summed and noted as a negative score (0 → -10)
  - A score of 0 is given if the infant's response to stimuli is normal for their gestational age
- Desired levels of sedation vary according to the situation
  - "Deep sedation" → score of -10 to -5 as goal
  - "Light sedation" → score of -5 to -2 as goal
  - Deep sedation is not recommended unless an infant is receiving ventilatory support, related to the high potential for apnea and hypoventilation
- A negative score without the administration of opioids/ sedatives may indicate:
  - The premature infant's response to prolonged or persistent pain/stress
  - Neurologic depression, sepsis, or other pathology

## Assessment of Pain/Agitation

- Pain assessment is the fifth vital sign – assessment for pain should be included in every vital sign assessment
- Pain is scored from 0 → +2 for each behavioral and physiological criteria, then summed
  - Points are added to the premature infant's pain score based on their gestational age to compensate for their limited ability to behaviorally or physiologically communicate pain
  - Total pain score is documented as a positive number (0 → +10)
- Treatment/interventions are indicated for scores > 3
  - Interventions for known pain/painful stimuli are indicated before the score reaches 3
- The goal of pain treatment/intervention is a score ≤ 3
- More frequent pain assessment indications:
  - Indwelling tubes or lines which may cause pain, especially with movement (e.g. chest tubes) → at least every 2-4 hours
  - Receiving analgesics and/or sedatives → at least every 2-4 hours
  - 30-60 minutes after an analgesic is given for pain behaviors to assess response to medication
  - Post-operative → at least every 2 hours for 24-48 hours, then every 4 hours until off medications

## Pavulon/Paralysis

- It is impossible to behaviorally evaluate a paralyzed infant for pain
- Increases in heart rate and blood pressure may be the only indicator of a need for more analgesia
- Analgesics should be administered continuously by drip or around-the-clock dosing
  - Higher, more frequent doses may be required if the infant is post-op, has a chest tube, or other pathology (such as NEC) that would normally cause pain
  - Opioid doses should be increased by 10% every 3-5 days as tolerance will occur without symptoms of inadequate pain relief

# Scoring Criteria

## Crying / Irritability

−2 → No response to painful stimuli, e.g.:
- No cry with needle sticks
- No reaction to ETT or nares suctioning
- No response to care giving

−1 → Moans, sighs, or cries (audible or silent) minimally to painful stimuli, e.g. needle sticks, ETT or nares suctioning, care giving

0 → Not irritable – appropriate crying
- Cries briefly with normal stimuli
- Easily consoled
- Normal for gestational age

+1 → Infant is irritable/crying at intervals – but can be consoled
- If intubated – intermittent silent cry

+2 → Any of the following:
- Cry is high-pitched
- Infant cries inconsolably
- If intubated – silent continuous cry

## Behavior / State

−2 → Does not arouse or react to any stimuli:
- Eyes continually shut or open
- No spontaneous movement

−1 → Little spontaneous movement, arouses briefly and/or minimally to any stimuli:
- Opens eyes briefly
- Reacts to suctioning
- Withdraws to pain

0 → Behavior and state are gestational age appropriate

+1 → Any of the following:
- Restless, squirming
- Awakens frequently/easily with minimal or no stimuli

+2 → Any of the following:
- Kicking
- Arching
- Constantly awake
- No movement or minimal arousal with stimulation (inappropriate for gestational age or clinical situation, i.e. post-operative)

## Facial Expression

−2 → Any of the following:
- Mouth is lax
- Drooling
- No facial expression at rest or with stimuli

−1 → Minimal facial expression with stimuli

0 → Face is relaxed at rest but not lax – normal expression with stimuli

+1 → Any pain face expression observed intermittently

+2 → Any pain face expression is continual

## Extremities / Tone

−2 → Any of the following:
- No palmar or planter grasp can be elicited
- Flaccid tone

−1 → Any of the following:
- Weak palmar or planter grasp can be elicited
- Decreased tone

0 → Relaxed hands and feet – normal palmar or sole grasp elicited – appropriate tone for gestational age

+1 → Intermittent (<30 seconds duration) observation of toes and/or hands as clenched or fingers splayed
- Body is *not* tense

+2 → Any of the following:
- Frequent (≥30 seconds duration) observation of toes and/or hands as clenched, or fingers splayed
- Body is tense/stiff

## Vital Signs: HR, BP, RR, & $O_2$ Saturations

−2 → Any of the following:
- No variability in vital signs with stimuli
- Hypoventilation
- Apnea
- Ventilated infant – no spontaneous respiratory effort

−1 → Vital signs show little variability with stimuli – less than 10% from baseline

0 → Vital signs and/or oxygen saturations are within normal limits with normal variability – or normal for gestational age

+1 → Any of the following:
- HR, BP, and/or RR are 10-20% above baseline
- With care/stimuli infant desaturates minimally to moderately ($SaO_2$ 76-85%) and recovers quickly (within 2 minutes)

+2 → Any of the following:
- HR, BP, and/or RR are > 20% above baseline
- With care/stimuli infant desaturates severely ($SaO_2$ < 75%) and recovers slowly (> 2 minutes)
- Infant is out of synchrony with the ventilator – fighting the ventilator

Brows:
lowered, drawn together

Forehead:
bulge between brows, vertical furrows

Eyes:
tightly closed

Cheeks:
raised

Nose:
broadened, bulging

Nasolabial fold:
deepened

Mouth:
open, squarish

**Facial expression of physical distress and pain in the infant**

Reproduced with permission from Wong DL, Hess CS: Wong and Whaley's Clincial Manual of Pediatric Nursing, Ed. 5, 2000, Mosby, St. Louis

We value your opinion.
Pat Hummel,
MA, RNC, NNP, PNP
Phone/voice mail: 708-327-9055
Email: phummel@lumc.edu

Mary Puchalski,
MS, RNC
Phone/voice mail: 708-327-9047
Email: mpuchal@lumc.edu

# G Bibliography and Web Resources

This appendix provides a brief synopsis of many print and web resources available to support individualized, family-centered, developmental care (IFDC). This list is not intended to be all inclusive but is a good starting place for resources and information to support your IFDC practices.

## Bibliography: Print Resources

Adams, W.G., Mann, A.M., & Bauchner, H. (2003). Use of an electronic medical record improves the quality of urban pediatric primary care. *Pediatrics, 111*(3), 626-632.
*Includes developmental outcomes in record.*

Aita, M., & Snider, L. (2003). The art of developmental care in the NICU: A concept analysis. *Journal of Advanced Nursing, 41*(3), 223-232.
*Concept analysis was undertaken to increase the knowledge of developmental care and its application to practice and research.*

Alain, C.E., Theunissen, E.L., Chevalier, H., et al. (2003). Developmental changes in distinguishing concurrent auditory objects. *Brain Research and Cognitive Brain Research, 16*(2), 210-218.
*Examines noisy environments related to speech recognition.*

Alexander, G.R., & Slay, M. (2002). Prematurity at birth: Trends, racial disparities, and epidemiology. *Mental Retardation and Developmental Disabilities Research Reviews, 8*(4), 215-220.
*Explores rates of prematurity in relationship to outcomes.*

Ashwal, S., & Rust, R. (2003). Child neurology in the 20th century. *Pediatric Research, 53*(2), 345-361.
*Review of the developing brain.*

Atkinson, J., Anker, S., Nardini, M., et al. (2002). Infant vision screening predicts failures on motor and cognitive tests up to school age. *Strabimus, 10*(3), 187-198.
*Review of vision screening programs.*

Aucott, S., Donohue, P.K., Atkins, E., et al. (2002). Neurodevelopmental care in the NICU. *Mental Retardation and Developmental Disabilities Research Reviews, 8*(4), 298-308.
*Focus of article is on developmental outcomes in relationship to NICU design, interventions, and parent involvement.*

Bhutta, A.T., & Anand, K.J. (2002). Vulnerability of the developing brain. Neuronal mechanisms. *Clinical Perinatology, 29*(3), 357-372.
*Focus is on the developing brain and possible causes of brain dysfunction.*

Byers, J.F. (2003). Components of developmental care and the evidence for their use in the NICU. *MCN: American Journal of Maternal Child Nursing, 28*(3), 174-180.
*This article discusses various aspects of developmental care and the need to use developmentally appropriate interventions that have evidence to support positive outcomes.*

Byers, J.F., Yovaish, W., Lowman, L.B., et al. (2003). Co-bedding versus single-bedding premature multiple-gestation infants in incubators. *Journal of Obstetric, Gynecologic, and Neonatal Nursing (JOGNN), 32*(3), 340-347.
*This article describes use of co-bedding multiples in incubators. It discusses various aspects of co-bedding versus use of single beds for multiple gestation infants.*

Developmental Care/Outcomes. (2003). Patient information: Developmental milestones for infants. *Advance Nurse Practitioner, 11*(2), 35.
*Useful for family teaching.*

Eriksson, M., Bodin, L., Finnstrom, O., et al. (2002). Can severity-of-illness indices for neonatal intensive care predict outcome at 4 years of age? *Acta Paediatrics, 91*(10), 1093-1100.
*Does severity of illness as measured on standardized scales equate to long-term developmental outcomes? This is the underlying question of this article.*

Fallang, B., Saugstad, O.D., Grogaard, J., et al. (2003). Kinematic quality of reaching movements in premature infants. *Pediatric Research, 53*(5), 836-842.
*Motor development and how to assess at an early age is described.*

Feldman, R., Eidelman, A.I., Sirota, L., et al. (2002). Comparison of skin-to-skin (kangaroo) and traditional care: Parenting outcomes and preterm infant development. *Pediatrics, 110*(1) (Pt 1), 16-26.
*Kangaroo care (KC) and parenting are the variables under consideration in this report. The researchers hypothesize that KC positively influences neurodevelopmental organization.*

Foulder-Hughes, L.A., & Cooke, R.W. (2003). Motor, cognitive, and behavioural disorders in children born very preterm. *Developmental Medicine and Child Neurology, 45*(2), 97-103.
*Motor, cognitive, and behavioral outcomes of very immaturely born infants are discussed in relationship to school performance.*

Frank, D.A., Jacobs, R.R., Beeghly, M., et al. (2002). Level of prenatal cocaine exposure and scores on the Bayley Scales of Infant Development: Modifying effects of caregiver, early intervention, and birth weight. *Pediatrics, 110*(6), 1143-1152.

*Using the variable of prenatal cocaine use as the backdrop for developmental scoring, the impact of the role of parents, early intervention, and birthweight is discussed.*

Glascoe, F.P. (2000). Detecting and addressing developmental and behavioral problems in primary care. *Pediatric Nursing, 26*(3), 251-257.

*This article describes the need for increased awareness on the part of primary healthcare providers to detect developmental problems early.*

Glascoe, F.P. (2002). The Brigance Infant and Toddler Screen: Standardization and validation. *Journal of Developmental and Behavioral Pediatrics, 23*(3), 145-150.

*One scale is presented as a screen for developmental growth.*

Grunau, R. (2002). Early pain in preterm infants: A model of long-term effects. *Clinics in Perinatology, 29*(3), 373-394, vii-viii.

*Review article on neonatal pain.*

Halliday, H.L., Ehrenkranz, R.A., & Doyle, L.W. (2003). Early postnatal (<96 hours) corticosteroids for preventing chronic lung disease in preterm infants. *Cochrane Database Systematic Reviews, 1*:CD001146.

*This research-based review includes data on developmental outcomes in this population.*

Hanke, C., Lohaus, A., Gawrilow, C., et al. (2003). Preschool development of very low birth weight children born 1994-1995. *European Journal of Pediatrics, 162*(3), 159-164.

*One of the few articles that examines long-term effects of premature births on developmental outcomes.*

Heermann, J.A., & Wilson, M.E. (2000). Nurses' experiences in working with families in an NICU during implementation of family-focused developmental care. *Neonatal Network, 19*(4), 23-29.

*This article describes one hospital's experience in changing from traditional to developmental care and the nurses' perspectives on this change.*

Jacobs, S.E., Sokol, J., & Ohlsson, A. (2002). The Newborn Individualized Developmental Care and Assessment Program is not supported by meta-analyses of the data. *Journal of Pediatrics, 140*(6), 699-706.

*This article is critical of NIDCAP® versus traditional care in terms of evidence to support better infant developmental outcomes.*

Jones, M.W., & McMurray, J.L. (2001). "Baby steps" neonatal developmental follow-up. *Neonatal Network, 20*(6), 73-78.

*Neonatal follow-up care is discussed, with emphasis on developmental outcomes.*

Katikaneni, L.D., & Wagner, C.L. (2002). Neurodevelopmental outcome of neonatal intensive care graduates: A practical approach to developmental follow-up and intervention strategies for primary care physicians. *Journal of South Carolina Medical Association, 98*(3), 155-160.

*Developmental follow-up care of NICU graduates and their families is discussed from the perspective of primary care physicians.*

Kleberg, A., Westrup, B., Stjernqvist, K., et al. (2002). Indications of improved cognitive development at one year of age among infants born very prematurely who received care based on the Newborn Individualized Developmental Care and Assessment Program (NIDCAP®). *Early Human Development, 68*(2), 83-91.

*A study that examines use of NIDCAP® as a means to improve infant developmental outcomes.*

Korner, A.F. (2003). Evaluating neonatal developmental care. *Journal of Pediatrics, 142*(5), 590.

*An example of how to evaluate use of neonatal developmental care.*

Limperopoulos, C., Majnemer, A., Shevell, M.I., et al. (2002). Predictors of developmental disabilities after open heart surgery in young children with congenital heart defects. *Journal of Pediatrics, 141*(1), 51-58.

*The neurologic outcomes of infants/children who have undergone open heart surgical repair for congenital heart disease are discussed.*

Mainous, R.O. (2002). Infant massage as a component of developmental care: Past, present, and future. *Holistic Nursing Practice, 16*(5), 1-7.

*Infant massage is presented as one facet of developmental care.*

Msall, M.E., & Tremont, M.R. (2002). Measuring functional outcomes after prematurity: Developmental impact of very low birth weight and extremely low birth weight status on childhood disability. *Mental Retardation and Developmental Disabilities Research Reviews, 8*(4), 258-272.

*Using neurobehavioral/functional measurements outcomes of very low birth weight infants were examined. Family interaction was included.*

Ng, E., Taddio, A., & Ohlsson, A. (2003). Intravenous midazolam infusion for sedation of infants in the neonatal intensive care unit. *Cochrane Database Systematic Reviews, 1*:CD002052.

*This systematic, evidence-based review examines use of sedation for infants who are undergoing procedures. This is part of pain management and anticipatory developmental individualized care.*

Nuntnarumit, P., Bada, H.S., Korones, S.B., et al. (2002). Neurobiologic risk score and long-term developmental outcomes of premature infants, birth weight less than 1250 grams. *Journal of Medical Association of Thailand, 85*(Suppl 4), S1135-S1142.

*Although the setting is Thailand, the concept can be globally applied in terms of neurologic risk and developmental outcomes of those infants born prematurely.*

Oberlander, T.F., Grunau, R.E., Fitzgerald, C., et al. (2002). Does parenchymal brain injury affect biobehavioral pain responses in very low birth weight infants at 32 weeks postconceptional age? *Pediatrics, 110*(3), 570-576.

*This article raises the issue of what effect brain injury might have on the very low birthweight infant's ability to respond to or interpret pain.*

Oberlander, T., & Saul, J.P. (2002). Methodological considerations for the use of heart rate variability as a measure

of pain reactivity in vulnerable infants. *Clinical in Perinatology, 29*(3), 427-443.
*A physiologic measure-heart rate variability related to pain is discussed.*

Parker, G., Bhakta, P., Lovett, C.A., et al. (2002). A systematic review of the costs and effectiveness of different models of paediatric home care. *Health Technology and Assessment, 6*(35), 1-118.
*One of the growing number of articles that examines costs in relationship to healthcare delivery. Very low birthweight infants and their outcomes are included in this meta-analysis.*

Pearson, J., & Andersen, K. (2001). Evaluation of a program to promote positive parenting in the neonatal intensive care unit. *Neonatal Network, 20*(4), 43-48.
*This article describes a Parent's Circle Program and its evaluation. Part of this program was describing developmental concepts.*

Perlman, J.M. (2002). Cognitive and behavioral deficits in premature graduates of intensive care. *Clinics in Perinatology, 29*(4), 779-797.
*Issues of age of viability, environmental factors (prenatally and in the NICU), and weight/gestational variation are all discussed. More work is acknowledged as needed in this area of long-term follow-up.*

Pressler, J.L., Hepworth, J.T., Helm, J.M., et al. (2001). Behaviors of very preterm neonates as documented using NIDCAP® observations. *Neonatal Network, 20*(8), 15-24.
*This study explored physiologic/behavioral cues using NIDCAP® scoring to determine changes from week to week postconceptual age (PCA) (from 24 to 30 weeks PCA) of very premature infants.*

Robison, L.D. (2003). An organizational guide for an effective developmental program in the NICU. *Journal of Obstetric Gynecologic, and Neonatal Nursing (JOGNN), 32*(30), 379-386.
*This guide provides recommendations of how to change from traditional to developmental care using a structured approach to the change.*

Ross, E.S., & Browne, J.V. (2002). Developmental progression of feeding skills: An approach to supporting feeding in preterm infants. *Seminars in Neonatology, 7*(6), 469-475.
*Feeding is presented as an aspect of individualized family-centered care.*

Salls, J.S., Silverman, N.L., & Gatty, C.M. (2002). The relationship of infant sleep and play positioning to motor milestone achievement. *American Journal of Occupational Therapists, 56*(5), 577-580.
*Infant sleep and play are described with application to the consideration of impact on sleep-wake cycles on neurodevelopmental outcomes.*

Senn, T.E., & Espy, K.A. (2003). Effects of neurobehavioral assessment on feeding and weight gain in preterm neonates. *Journal of Developmental and Behavioral Pediatrics, 24*(2), 85-88.
*The focus is on feeding of preterm infants in relationship to neurodevelopmental outcomes. This is another aspect of developmental care.*

Standley, J.M. (2002). A meta-analysis of the efficacy of music therapy for premature infants. *Journal of Pediatric Nursing, 17*(2), 107-113.
*Music therapy is part of developmental care. However, we have little evidence to support its inclusion in care. This meta-analysis presents our current knowledge.*

Stanton-Chapman, T.L., Chapman, D.A., Bainbridge, N.L., et al. (2002). Identification of early risk factors for language impairment. *Research and Developmental Disabilities, 23*(6), 390-405.
*Although speech and language delays are not part of the every-day care of many newborn and infant health professionals, this article points to the need for more awareness on long-term consequences of impaired neonatal health.*

Sweet, M.P., Hodgman, J.E., Pena, I., et al. (2003). Two-year outcome of infants weighing 600 grams or less at birth and born 1994 through 1998. *Obstetrics and Gynecology, 101*(1), 18-23.
*Emphasis is on neurodevelopmental outcomes of extremely immature infants. Included is the prenatal history factor that probably resulted in the premature birth.*

Touch, S.M., Epstein, M.L., Pohl, C.A., et al. (2002). The impact of cobedding on sleep patterns in preterm twins. *Clinics in Pediatrics, 41*(6), 425-431.
*Co-bedding is considered by some experts as a part of developmental care; however, it is not without controversy. This article presents one side of the co-bedding story in an examination of prematurely born twins. Physiologic variables are used as a measure of co-bedding success.*

Warren, I. (2002). Facilitating infant adaptation: The nursery environment. *Seminars in Neonatology, 7*(6), 459-467.
*The NICU environment and its impact on physiologic stability is examined.*

Westrup, B., Hellstrom-Westas, L., Stjernqvist, K., et al. (2002). No indications of increased quiet sleep in infants receiving care based on the newborn individualized developmental care and assessment program (NIDCAP®). *Acta Paediatrics, 91*(3), 318-322.
*Sleep-wake patterns are the focus of this report as related to the use of NIDCAP®.*

Westrup, B., Lagercrantz, H., Kleberg, A., et al. (2003). Evaluating neonatal developmental care. *Journal of Pediatrics, 142*(5), 591-592.
*This article outlines how to evaluate use of neonatal developmental care. It is based on an experience in Sweden.*

Westrup, B., Stjernqvist, K., Kleberg, A., et al. (2002). Neonatal individualized care in practice: A Swedish experience. *Seminars in Neonatology, 7*(6), 447-457.
*Application of developmental care using NIDCAP® in Sweden is presented. Discussion includes the lack of evidence to support use of these practices and the need for further research as well as ethical considerations of this type of care.*

White, R.D. (2003). Individual rooms in the NICU—an evolving concept. *Journal of Perinataology, 23*(Suppl 1), S222-S224.

*This article points out the new trend toward single-room NICU designs. The issues of staff and caregiver isolation and communication, financial and space concerns, and benefits for privacy and decreased stimulation for infants are addressed.*

## Family-Centered Care

Allen, R.S., & Shuster, J.L. Jr. (2002). The role of proxies in treatment decisions: Evaluating functional capacity to consent to end-of-life treatments within a family context. *Behavioral Science & Law, 20*(3), 235-252.

Belsk, J., & Fearon, R.M. (2002). Infant-mother attachment security, contextual risk, and early development: A moderational analysis. *Developmental Psychopathology, 14*(2), 293-310.

*This article explores the relationship between attachment and development.*

Besky, J., & Fearon, R.M. (2002). Early attachment security, subsequent maternal sensitivity, and later child development: Does continuity in development depend upon continuity of caregiving? *Attachment and Human Development, 4*(3), 361-387.

*Research findings regarding attachment and development are presented.*

Bortolus, R., Parazzini, F., Trevisanuto, D. (2002). Developmental assessment of preterm and term children at 18 months: Reproducibility and validity of a postal questionnaire to parents. *Acta Paediatrics, 91*(10), 1101-1107.

*A comparison of physician's assessment and parental observations.*

Bracht, M., Kandankery, A., Nodwell, S., et al. (2002). Cultural differences and parental responses to the preterm infant at risk: Strategies for supporting families. *Neonatal Network, 21*(6), 31-38.

*Examines culture as a factor in parenting differences and utilization of available healthcare resources.*

Cowen, P.S., & Reed, D.A. (2002). Effects of respite care for children with developmental disabilities: Evaluation of an intervention for at risk families. *Public Health Nursing, 19*(4), 272-283.

*Discusses respite programs for families with children with developmental disabilities.*

Desai, P.P., Ng, J.B., & Bryant, S.G. (2002). Care of children and families in the CICU: A focus on their developmental, psychosocial, and spiritual needs. *Critical Care Nursing Quarterly, 25*(3), 88-97.

*Holistic approach to care is explored. Includes information on interdisciplinary team members, including child life specialists.*

Dozier, M., Albus, K., Fisher, P.A., et al. (2002). Interventions for foster parents: Implications for developmental theory. *Developmental Psychopathology, 14*(4), 843-860.

*Foster care and parenting under these conditions is the focus of the article. The relationship to these early experiences and growth and development are explored.*

Guttman, H.A. (2002). The epigenesis of the family system as a context for individual development. *Family Process, 41*(3), 533-545.

*This article presents a study that examines the development of an individual within the context of the family. The study population was women with borderline personality disorders, but it holds implications for the consideration of family as it relates to infant development.*

Haight, W.L., Kagle, J.D., & Black, J.E. (2003). Understanding and supporting parent-child relationships during foster care visits: Attachment theory and research. *Social Work, 48*(2), 195-207.

*Emphasis on parent-infant relationships and attachment within the context of a foster care setting.*

Hinojosa, J., Sproat, C.T., Mankhetwit, S., et al. (2002). Shifts in parent-therapist partnerships: Twelve years of change. *American Journal of Occupational Therapy, 56*(5), 556-563.

*A study that explored the attitudes/needs for partnerships with parents from an occupational therapist's perspective is discussed. Each family had a child with a developmental disability.*

Katz, S., & Kessel, L. (2002). Grandparents of children with developmental disabilities: Perceptions, beliefs, and involvement in their care. *Issues in Comprehensive Pediatric Nursing, 25*(2), 113-128.

*This qualitative study describes the experience of having a grandchild with a developmental disability.*

Kumpfer, K.L., Alvarado, R., Smith, P., et al. (2002). Cultural sensitivity and adaptation in family-based prevention interventions. *Preventive Science, 3*(3), 241-246.

*Stresses need for cultural sensitive interventions when working with families to improve infant/child developmental outcomes.*

Lawhon, G. (2002). Facilitation of parenting the premature infant within the newborn intensive care unit. *Journal of Perinatal and Neonatal Nursing, 16*(1), 71-82.

*Discusses parenting in relationship to neurobehavioral infant outcomes.*

Lu, M.C., & Halfon, N. (2003). Racial and ethnic disparities in birth outcomes: A life-course perspective. *Maternal and Child Health, 7*(1), 13-30.

*Health disparities at birth can continue due to differences in development and family attitudes.*

Ohgi, S., Fukuda, M., Moriuchi, H., et al. (2002). Comparison of kangaroo care and standard care: Behavioral organization, development, and temperament in healthy, low-birth-weight infants through 1 year. *Journal of Perinatology, 22*(5), 374-379.

*Kangaroo care (KC) is compared with traditional newborn care, with the emphasis on neurobehavioral outcomes. The researchers suggest that KC promotes positive neurobehavioral organization.*

Pearson, J., & Andersen, K. (2001). Evaluation of a program to promote positive parenting in the neonatal intensive care unit. *Neonatal Network, 20*(4), 43-48.
*In this article, parents' role in neonatal care and a program that is aimed at supporting parents are discussed.*

Ramsey, P.S., & Rouse, D.J. (2002). Therapies administered to mothers at risk for preterm birth and neurodevelopmental outcome in their infants. *Clinics in Perinatology, 29*(4), 725-743.
*This article presents strategies for prevention—from the prenatal side of care to impact on infant neurologic outcomes.*

Thoman, E.B. (2003). Temporal patterns of caregiving for preterm infants indicate individualized developmental care. *Journal of Perinatology, 23*(1), 29-36.
*Comparison of three hospital settings using patterns of caregiving as the variable of interest. The pattern of caregiving appeared to be related to the NICU environment.*

## Web Resources

American Academy of Pediatrics (AAP)
141 Northwest Point Blvd.
Elk Grove Village, IL 60007-1098
Phone: (847) 424-4000
Fax: (847) 434-8000
*www.aap.org*
*Good resource for policies, position statements, and guidelines for perinatal and neonatal care.*

Carpet in Healthcare
*www.carpet-health.org/pdf/CarpetHealthcare.pdf*
*This site offers a combination of industry information and peer-reviewed information such as statements from the Centers for Disease Control on use of carpeting in healthcare delivery areas.*

Children's Medical Ventures
275 Longwater Drive
Norwell, MA 02061
Phone: (888) 766-8443 (parents), (800) 345-6443 (hospitals), or (866) 866-6750 (education)
*www.childmed.com/*
*This company provides onsite training and education as well as sells products to support developmental care.*

Developmental Care Program
Health Sciences Center, University of New Mexico
*http://www.dssw.com/DevCare/*
*Family framework for care. This is just one of many examples of educational/practice programs to be found on the web.*

Developmental Care: Considerations for Touch and Massage in the Neonatal Intensive Care Unit
J. V. Browne, PhD, RN
*www.uchsc.edu/sm/peds/cfii/Joy's%20touch%20 article.html*
*Explores use of touch and massage as part of individualized neonatal care.*

Developmental Care for Promoting Development and Preventing Morbidity in Preterm Infants
*www.nichd.nih.gov/cochrane/symington/symington.htm*
*This is a systematic review by A. Symington and J. Pinelli focusing on developmental care and outcomes.*

Developmental Care Teams in the Neonatal Intensive Care Unit
Ashbaugh, J.B., Leick-Rude, M.K., & Kilbride, H.W. (1999).
*www.nature.com/cgi-taf/DynaPage.taf?file = /jp/journal/v19/n1/abs/7200101a.html*
*Use of developmental care teams within the NICU as a method for promotion of family-centered individualized care.*

Ethics and Parent Collaboration in NICU End of Life Care
T. Sudia-Robinson
*National Institutes of Health (NIH)-funded project on neonatal palliative/end of life care.*
*www.nih.gov/ninr/research/dea/2000grants/pdf/2000 grants_sudia_robinson.pdf*

Infant and Family-Centered Developmental Care
*www.guideline.gov/VIEWS/summary.asp?guideline = 1419&summary_type = brief_summary&view = brief_summary&sSearch_string*
*NANN Guideline that is part of the National Guideline Clearinghouse.*

Institute for Family-Centered Care
7900 Wisconsin Avenue, Suite 405
Bethesda, MD 20814
Phone: (301) 652-0281
Fax: (301) 652-0186
E-mail: *Institute@iffcc.org*
*www.familycenteredcare.org/*
*Good resource for professionals and parents regarding all aspects of parenting.*

National Association of Neonatal Nurses (NANN)
4700 W. Lake Avenue
Glenview, IL 60025-1485
Phone: (847) 375-3660 or (800) 451-3795
Fax: (888) 477-6266
International Fax: (732) 380-3640
E-mail: info@nann.org
www.nann.org
*National Association of Neonatal Nurses is an excellent resource for nurses interested in any aspect of neonatal care.*

NatalU—A University Without Walls—NICU Design
Center Sponsored by Pediatrix and Obstetrix
www.natalu.com
*This site has a threaded discussion group on NICU addressing issues. Dr. Robert White is the moderator. He is chair of the Committee to Establish Recommended Standards for Newborn ICU Design.*

Newborn Individualized Developmental Care and
Assessment Program (NIDCAP®)
www.nidcap.com/nidcap/
*NIDCAP® overview and training centers.*
NICU Design Standards

Recommended Standards for Newborn ICU Design:
Report of the Fifth Consensus Conference on
Newborn ICU Design, January 2002, Clearwater
Beach, FL
www.nd.edu/~kkolberg/DesignStandards.htm
*Recommendations from the Committee to Establish Recommended Standards for Newborn ICU Design for all aspects of NICU design that are aimed at promoting developmentally supportive, family-centered care.*

National Association of Neonatal Nurses (NANN)
Developmental Care/Pain Special Interest Group
www.nann.org/i4a/pages/index.cfm?pageid = 743

*Includes information on NANN policies on pain and developmental care as well as position statements and resources from such sources as American Academy of Pediatrics (AAP).*

The Forgotten Newborn: Family-Focused, Developmental Care in the NICU Neurodevelopment
www.hmcnet.harvard.edu/psych/redbook/95.htm
*This is a report detailing the works of Heidelise Als, PhD and sponsored research in the area of developmental care.*

Children's Hospital, Dayton, Ohio
Realizing the Power of Communication Technology
in the NICU: Judy Smith and Cindy Burger
*http://216.239.53.100/search?q = cache: 4P83HsP2Zu4J:publichealth.usf.edu/conted/pdf/ ie02/smith.pdf + single + room + NICU&hl = en&ie = UTF-8*
*Article describes one hospital's experience with communication technology and redesign, including single-room NICU care.*

NICU Communication Technology Survey: December
2001-January 2002
*http://216.239.57.100/search?q = cache: MIZQu6xPxMsJ:publichealth.usf.edu/conted/pdf/ ie02/smith2.pdf + single + room + NICU&hl = en&ie = UTF-8*
*Issues of communication within NICUs and the number of NICUs considering to a single-room design are discussed.*

Spacelabs Medical
www.spacelabs.com/network/rainbow.html

At Rainbow Babies and Children's Hospital:
Advanced Technology Helps Realize Promise of
High-Tech Healing in a Home-Like Environment
*This article describes single-room design for step down unit within the NICU.*

# Index

Page numbers followed by *b*, *t*, or *f* indicate boxes, tables, or figures, respectively.